KIDNEY TRANSPLANT REJECTION

KIDNEY DISEASE

Editors

J. Stewart Cameron
Professor in Renal Medicine
Clinical Science Laboratories
Guy's Hospital
London, England

Richard J. Glassock
Chairman, Department of Medicine
UCLA School of Medicine and
Harbor-UCLA Medical Center
Torrance, California

Andrew Whelton
Associate Professor of Medicine
The Johns Hopkins University School of Medicine
Baltimore, Maryland

Volume 1 Proteinuria: An Integrated Review, *Amadeo J. Pesce and Martin Roy First*

Volume 2 The Aminoglycosides: Microbiology, Clinical Use, and Toxicology, *edited by Andrew Whelton and Harold C. Neu*

Volume 3 Hepatorenal Disorders, *S. P. Wilkinson*

Volume 4 Acute Renal Failure: Correlations Between Morphology and Function, *edited by Kim Solez and Andrew Whelton*

Volume 5 Renal Tubular Disorders: Pathophysiology, Diagnosis, and Management, *edited by Harvey C. Gonick and Vardaman M. Buckalew, Jr.*

Volume 6 Potassium in Cardiovascular and Renal Medicine: Arrhythmias, Myocardial Infarction, and Hypertension, *edited by Paul K. Whelton, Andrew Whelton, and W. Gordon Walker*

Volume 7 Kidney Transplant Rejection: Diagnosis and Treatment, *edited by G. Melville Williams, James F. Burdick, and Kim Solez*

Other Volumes in Preparation

KIDNEY TRANSPLANT REJECTION

Diagnosis and Treatment

Edited by

G. Melville Williams
James F. Burdick
Kim Solez

The Johns Hopkins University
School of Medicine
Baltimore, Maryland

MARCEL DEKKER, INC. New York and Basel

Library of Congress Cataloging-in-Publication Data

Kidney transplant rejection.

(Kidney disease ; v. 7)
Bibliography: p.
Includes index.
1. Kidneys--Transplantation--Complications and sequelae. 2. Graft rejection--Prevention. 3. Immunosuppressive agents. I. Williams, G. Melville. II. Burdick, James, [date]. III. Solez, Kim, [date]. IV. Series. [DNLM: 1. Graft Rejection. 2. Kidney—transplantation. W1 KI586R v.7 / WJ 368 K455]
RD575.K5 1986 617'.461 86-8810
ISBN 0-8247-7496-5

MARCEL DEKKER, INC.
270 Madison Avenue, New York, New York 10016

Current printing (last digit):
10 9 8 7 6 5 4 3 2 1

PRINTED IN THE UNITED STATES OF AMERICA

ABOUT THE SERIES

This book is the seventh in a series of texts on nephrology intended to cover all aspects of that discipline. Nephrology has grown at a great rate over the past decade, and the available knowledge has outstripped the texts available. The discipline has, however, attained such maturity that a description of any one of its parts becomes more than ephemeral—or worse, outdated before it even appears. We aim to fill some of the many gaps that exist, not only for the specialist in nephrology, but also for the general physician interested in nephrology. In this description, we include the study and management of hypertension, since these two are interwoven at so many points. We welcome comments on the series as it evolves, or suggestions for topics that might be considered for future volumes.

J. Stewart Cameron
London, England

Richard J. Glassock
Torrance, California

Andrew Whelton
Baltimore, Maryland

PREFACE

In the early years of clinical renal transplantation, most surgeons and pathologists thought they could recognize allograft rejection. It was accepted that deterioration of renal function meant rejection and was associated with an intense mononuclear cell interstitial infiltration. Twenty years later, clinical pathological correlations are less clear. Renal failure episodes may be caused by cyclosporine toxicity, cytomegalovirus infection, poor glucose control, and technical complications as well as by rejection. Further, we now realize that significant interstitial lymphocyte infiltrates are present in the majority of grafts and may be intense in some kidneys with normal function and sparse in some destined for complete rejection. Some animal studies have confirmed this view. We have undertaken two clinical studies in the past in which kidney transplants were biopsied at set intervals irrespective of function. Each study has engendered a healthy skepticism regarding the ability of the transplant biopsy to predict rejection, reversibility, and prognosis. Therefore, it seems quite pertinent at this time to take a broad look at the various forms of rejection as we know them clinically and bring together modern studies by distinguished pathologists in the hope of improving our understanding and therapy.

By way of introduction, we would like to present the view that antibody, T lymphocytes mediating "cytotoxicity" or "help" or "delayed type hypersensitivity," and all of the cells with Fc receptors are involved in rejection. At one end of this spectrum, antibody seems clearly to be the predominant effector mechanism in hyperacute rejection. Ironically, 5 to 10 years ago, the worst thing prognostically for the patient was to have a biopsy done at the time of worsening renal function that showed "no evidence of active rejection." The report meant that there were few interstitial lymphoid cells and we had learned that steroid or ALG therapy rarely succeeded in reversing rejection under these histological circumstances. This led to a greater appreciation for the role of antibody in chronic vascular damage. Chronic rejection is probably always a complex mixture of humoral antibody working through both complement-mediated and cell-mediated cytotoxicity, and cellular immunity working through both delayed type hypersensitivity and specific cytotoxic T lymphocytes. At the other end of the spectrum, the acute rejection crises occurring 6 to 20 days following the transplantation are predominantly the result of lymphocyte-mediated cytotoxicity and delayed type hypersensitivity occurring within the kidney.

Perhaps the most controversial of these ideas is the one relating acute rejection to delayed type hypersensitivity. However, this view is supported by considerable evidence. We know from a variety of transfer experiments in experimental animals that the T-helper cell is at least a more consistent mediator of acute rejection than the T-cytotoxic cell. It is now also well established that the cytotoxic factors produced by specific cytotoxic T cells are found in very low concentration, making it likely that cells only in the immediate proximity of the cytotoxic T cell are killed. Thus, it would seem extremely difficult to produce enough cytotoxic T cells to destroy an entire 250-g kidney or its endothelium, and much more attractive to blame the T-helper cells, which are capable of amplifying their presence through the release of lymphokines such as interleukin 2. Finally, it would not be surprising to find a potpourri of cells present in biopsies from patients with acute rejection because of the recruitment phenomena present in delayed type hypersensitivity. Whether T-helper cells are directed toward induction of exquisitely specific cytotoxicity or toward more general delayed type hypersensitivity, the effectiveness of cyclosporine may be explained by its interference with helper cell interleukin 2 production.

For decades it has been the hope of physicians involved in transplantation that a new immunosuppressive agent would be found which would greatly reduce the likelihood of rejection-induced graft loss. In the 1980s this hope has been realized in the form of highly specific monoclonal antibodies and cyclosporine. The advent of cyclosporine has proved to be a giant advance in the field of transplantation. Cyclosporine, however, is a giant with an Achilles' heel, because its nephrotoxicity can sometimes completely negate its beneficial immunosuppressive effect.

From the clinical standpoint, it is important to avoid rejection, but when it occurs a reproducible means of reversing it is a necessity. Clinical trials using the monoclonal antibody OKT-3 have demonstrated unequivocally the central role of the T cell in most acute rejection episodes, since essentially all of these can be reversed with a short course of OKT-3. Given the puzzling patient with recurrent renal failure episodes on cyclosporine therapy, a course of OKT-3 coupled with drastic reductions in other agents "clears the air" and renal function commonly improves greatly. Finally, an even more certain means of producing long-term resignation of the host to its new ingredient will be necessary. Cyclosporine, by virtue of its apparent sparing of suppressor cells, may have provided a serendipitous first step toward this goal. However, the issue of mechanisms of immunoregulation, and possible ways to manipulate them, turns out to be complex.

Should not there be other ways to sort out rejection, nephrotoxicity, and CMV infection? Should not there be a measurable immunological component of rejection that precedes renal functional impairment? Should it not be possible to engineer immunosuppression with far greater precision? We think so, and it is the purpose of this book to see how close we are through the collection of the most recent information available about the biology of the allograft response, the diagnosis of rejection, and new ways to control it. Much is known, and we hope the reader will find in this book the answer to many questions and further will be stimulated to formulate his or her own hypotheses, test them, and increase our knowledge about this rapidly expanding subject.

We are very grateful to the many prominent individuals from around the world who have contributed to this book. We also are most appreciative of the financial support provided by Becton Dickinson, Boehinger-Ingelheim, Ortho Pharmaceutical Corporation, the Upjohn Company, and Sandoz, Inc., to defray costs of the color plates. Finally, we would like to thank our secretaries, Gail Fodel, Pamela Creevey, Donna Wolford, and Nancy Lambert, for keeping us organized during the preparation of this book and for typing and retyping numerous manuscript drafts.

G. Melville Williams
James F. Burdick
Kim Solez

CONTRIBUTORS

J. Thomas August, M.D. Professor and Director, Department of Pharmacology and Experimental Therapeutics, The Johns Hopkins University School of Medicine, Baltimore, Maryland

William E. Beschorner, M.D. Assistant Professor, Departments of Pathology and Oncology, The Johns Hopkins University School of Medicine, Baltimore, Maryland

James F. Burdick, M.D. Associate Professor of Surgery and Director of the Transplant Service, Department of Surgery, The Johns Hopkins University School of Medicine, Baltimore, Maryland

Paul M. Colombani, M.D. Assistant Professor, Department of Surgery and Pediatrics, The Johns Hopkins University School of Medicine, Baltimore, Maryland

Robert Colvin, M.D. Director, Immunopathology Unit, Massachusetts General Hospital, and Associate Professor of Pathology, Department of Pathology, Harvard Medical School, Boston, Massachusetts

A. Benedict Cosimi, M.D. Chief, Clinical Transplant Surgery, Department of Surgery, Massachusetts General Hospital, and Associate Professor of Surgery, Department of Surgery, Harvard Medical School, Boston, Massachusetts

Francis L. Delmonico, M.D. Department of Surgery, Massachusetts General Hospital, and Assistant Professor of Surgery, Department of Surgery, Harvard Medical School, Boston, Massachusetts

Ahmed H. Esa, Ph.D. Postdoctoral Fellow, Department of Oncology, The Johns Hopkins University School of Medicine, Baltimore, Maryland

Stuart M. Flechner, M.D. Associate Professor, Department of Surgery, Divisions of Urology and Organ Transplantation, University of Texas Medical School at Houston, Houston, Texas

Olaf Ganghoff, M.D. Postdoctoral Fellow in Transplant Surgery, Department of Surgery, East Carolina University School of Medicine, Greenville, North Carolina

Uli Gross, M.D. Postdoctoral Fellow in Transplant Surgery, Department of Surgery, East Carolina University School of Medicine, Greenville, North Carolina

Brian W. Haag, M.D.* Fellow in Organ Transplantation, Department of Surgery, University of Chicago, Chicago, Illinois

Douglas W. Hanto, M.D.† Fellow in Transplantation, Department of Surgery, University of Minnesota Health Sciences Center, Minneapolis, Minnesota

Pekka J. Häyry, M.D., Ph.D. Professor of Transplantation, Surgery and Immunology, Transplantation Laboratory, University of Helsinki, Helsinki, Finland

Allan D. Hess, Ph.D. Assistant Professor of Oncology, Immunology and Immunology and Infectious Diseases, The Johns Hopkins University School of Medicine, Baltimore, Maryland

James E. K. Hildreth, D.Phil. (Oxon) Postdoctoral Fellow, Department of Pharmacology and Experimental Therapeutics, The Johns Hopkins University School of Medicine, Baltimore, Maryland

Barry D. Kahan, Ph.D., M.D. Professor of Surgery and Director, Division of Immunology and Organ Transplantation, Department of Surgery, University of Texas Medical School at Houston, Houston, Texas

Paul A. Keown, M.D., Ch.B., M.R.C.P.F.R.C.P. (C) Chief, Division of Nephrology, Department of Medicine, University Hospital, University of Western Ontario, London, Ontario, Canada

Ronald H. Kerman, Ph.D. Associate Professor of Surgery, Department of Surgery and Head, Immune Evaluation Laboratory, Division of Organ Transplantation, University of Texas Medical School at Houston, Houston, Texas

Robin P. Lowry, B.Sc., M.D., F.R.C.P.(C) Assistant Professor, Transplantation Division, Department of Medicine, Royal Victoria Hospital Research Institute, McGill University, Montreal, Quebec, Canada

Daniel J. McGraw, M.D. Intern, Department of Pathology, The Johns Hopkins University School of Medicine, Baltimore, Maryland

Michael J. Mihatsch, M.D. Associate Professor, Department of Pathology, University of Basel, Basel, Switzerland

Patrick A. Murphy, M.D. Associate Professor of Medicine, Department of Medicine, The Johns Hopkins University School of Medicine, Baltimore, Maryland

T. Steen Olsen, M.D. Professor of Pathology, University Institute of Pathology, Municipal Hospital, Aarhus, Denmark

Robert H. Rubin, M.D. Chief of Infectious Disease for Transplantation, Massachusetts General Hospital, and Associate Professor, Department of Medicine, Harvard Medical School, Boston, Massachusetts

Bernhard Ryffel, M.D. Toxicologist, Department of Preclinical Research, Sandoz Ltd., Basel, Switzerland

Helen Siegl, M.D. Professor of Preclinical Research, Sandoz Ltd., Basel, Switzerland

---

Present Affiliations:
*Director of Organ Transplantation, Department of Medical Research, Methodist Hospital Graduate Medical Center, Indianapolis, Indiana
†Assistant Professor of Surgery, Washington University School of Medicine, St. Louis, Missouri

Richard L. Simmons, M.D. Professor of Surgery and Microbiology, Department of Surgery, University of Minnesota Health Sciences Center, Minneapolis, Minnesota

William J. Smith, Ph.D. Assistant Professor, Department of Surgery, Division of Transplantation and Vascular Surgery, The Johns Hopkins University School of Medicine, Baltimore, Maryland

Kim Solez, M.D. Associate Professor of Pathology and Medicine, Department of Pathology, The Johns Hopkins University School of Medicine, Baltimore, Maryland

Calvin R. Stiller, M.D., F.R.C.P. (C) Chief, Multi-organ Transplant Service, University Hospital, University of Western Ontario, London, Ontario, Canada

Frank P. Stuart, M.D. Professor, Department of Surgery, University of Chicago, Chicago, Illinois

Gilbert Thiel, M.D. Professor. Division of Nephrology, Department of Internal Medicine, University of Basel, Basel, Switzerland

Francis T. Thomas, M.D., F.A.C.S. Professor and Chief, Division of Transplantation, Department of Surgery, East Carolina University School of Medicine, Greenville, North Carolina

Judith M. Thomas, Ph.D. Professor, Department of Surgery, East Carolina University School of Medicine, Greenville, North Carolina

Charles T. Van Buren, M.D. Associate Professor, Department of Surgery, Division of Immunology and Organ Transplantation, University of Texas Medical School at Houston, Houston, Texas

Eeva von Willebrand, M.D. Consultant in Clinical Immunology, Transplantation Laboratory, University of Helsinki, Helsinki, Finland

A. Cameron Wallace, M.D. Professor of Pathology and Director of Surgical Pathology, Department of Pathology, University Hospital, University of Western Ontario, London, Ontario, Canada

Carol A. Wideman, R.N. Transplant Coordinator, Department of Surgery, Division of Organ Transplantation, University of Texas Medical School at Houston, Houston, Texas

G. Melville Williams, M.D. Professor of Surgery, Division of Transplantation and Vascular Surgery, The Johns Hopkins University School of Medicine, Baltimore, Maryland

Henry J. Winn, Ph.D. Immunologist, General Surgical Services, Massachusetts General Hospital, Department of Surgery, Harvard Medical School, Boston, Massachusetts

CONTENTS

KIDNEY TRANSPLANT REJECTION

BIOLOGY OF THE ALLOGRAFT RESPONSE

1

PROTEINS AND THE MOLECULAR BASIS OF CELL-MEDIATED IMMUNITY

J. Thomas August and James E. K. Hildreth
The Johns Hopkins University School of Medicine, Baltimore, Maryland

The mechanisms of cell-mediated immunity are extremely complex and involve several cell surface and soluble protein molecules. The identification of these proteins and an understanding of their functions have been augmented greatly by the combined use of in vitro functional assays and the tools of molecular biology. These methods have been especially valuable in identifying and characterizing the proteins involved in T-cell activation and antigen recognition. Several of these structures have been well characterized, and a model has evolved to describe their organization and interactions. Table 1 is a summary of the salient features of protein antigens with known important functions.

MAJOR HISTOCOMPATIBILITY COMPLEX ANTIGENS

Cell surface molecules that play a critical role in self-non-self discrimination are encoded for by the genes of the major histocompatibility complex (MHC) located on chromosome 6. There are three classes of MHC genes: classes I and II, which regulate cell-cell interactions in immune responses and class III, which encodes the C2, C4, and Bf complement components (reviewed in Reference 34).

Class I molecules, the original transplantation antigens, are composed of Mr 40,000-45,000 transmembrane glycoproteins noncovalently associated with the Mr 12,000 β_2-macroglobulin protein. The molecules are expressed on virtually all nucleated cells and normally function as restriction elements for virus-specific cytotoxic T lymphocytes and the target antigens of alloreactive T cells. Cytotoxic T cells tend to recognize antigen in conjunction with the class I molecule. As described below, the recognition of the class I glycoprotein is apparently mediated through the T8 glycoprotein of cytotoxic T lymphocytes and the T-cell receptor complex. The class I protein is highly polymorphic and normally only interacts with T cells of the same allelic specificity [91]. Both the Mr 45,000 and β_2-macroglobulin polypeptides are structurally related to class II MHC and immunoglobulin proteins, and the genes for these proteins are included in the immunoglobulin supergene family (reviewed in References 29 and 75).

Class II antigens consist of two noncovalently associated polypeptides, an α chain of Mr 30,000-35,000 and a β chain of Mr 27,000-30,000. These molecules serve as recognition elements for helper T cells, apparently interacting with the T4 glycoprotein in con-

TABLE 1 Proteins Involved in Immune Response Mechanisms

Protein	MW (reduced)	Distribution	Protein function	Effect of monoclonal antibodies
MHC class I	~45,000	Most nucleated cells	Antigen-specific CTL recognition marker	Block allospecific CTL
MHC class II	~34,000 ~28,000	Antigen presenting cells (e.g. macrophages dendritic cells), β lymphocytes activated T cells	Antigen-specific helper T-cell recognition marker	Inhibit helper T cell induction
T-cell antigen receptor	~40,000 (α) ~40,000 (β)	All mature T lymphocytes	T-cell antigen receptor	Stimulate T-cell proliferation and inhibit antigen-specific T-cell responses
T3	~25,000 (α) ~20,000 (α) ~20,000 (β)	All mature T lymphocytes	Functional association with T-cell antigen	Stimulate T-cell proliferation and inhibit antigen-specific T-cell responses
T4	~62,000	Thymocytes and peripheral T lymphocytes	Antigen-specific adherence between helper T cell and class II MHC	Inhibit T-cell association with cells expressing class II MHC proteins
T8	~34,000 ~46,000	Thymocytes and peripheral T lymphocytes	Antigen-specific adherence between CTL and class I MHC	Inhibit CTL effectors directed at class I MHC-gene products
Interleuken-2 receptor	~52,000	T cells (and B cells)	IL-2 receptor	Inhibit antigen and mitogen-stimulated T-cell proliferation
Interleukin-1	~15,000	Secreted by activated macrophages	Promote secretion of IL-2 and expression of IL-2 receptors	
Interleukin-2	~15,000	Secreted by activated T cells	T-cell growth factor	Inhibit T-cell proliferation
Lymphocyte function associated	175,000 (α) 95,000 (β)	T and B lymphocytes, thymocytes, or granulocytes	Leukocyte adhesion	Inhibit T-cell response to antigens

junction with the T-cell receptor to induce helper function for cell-mediated immunity and for antibody production by B cells. Class II MHC antigens may also serve as target antigens for T4-positive cytotoxic T cells. The class II glycoproteins expressed in large numbers on antigen-presenting cells, such as macrophages and dendritic cells, are also found on B lymphocytes and activated T cells and may be induced in a number of other cells. Class II molecules also contain considerable sequence homology to immunoglobulins and are highly polymorphic, with several distinct families of antigens, including HLA-DR homologous to the murine I-E subregion molecules, and HLA-DS, homologous to murine I-A antigens. Monoclonal antibodies directed at class II glycoproteins have potent invivo and invitro effects, suppressing a variety of processes dependent upon T-lymphocyte interactions with other cell types (reviewed in Reference 32).

GLYCOPROTEINS ON T CELLS

T-Cell Receptor

The surface receptor by which T cells recognize antigen plays a central role in cell-mediated immunity. Antigen recognition initiates a series of events that direct the immediate response of the T cell to this antigen, as well as the response of an array of other cells that act in the immune system, such as B cells, macrophages, and a variety of other accessory cells.

When responding to foreign antigens the individual T cells are specific both for the antigen recognized and the class I or class II products of the MHC complex [91]. Thus, individual T cells appear to recognize simultaneously an epitope of the foreign antigen and a determinant in the polymorphic domain of the MHC products expressed on the surface of the cell presenting the antigen. Major histocompatibility complex-restricted recognition of foreign antigens forms the basis for grouping T cells into two general subsets: (1) cytotoxic T cells that generally recognize antigen in association with class I MHC products, and (2) helper T cells that recognize antigen in association with class II MHC products. However, cytotoxic T cells of the helper phenotype with specificity for class II MHC antigens have been demonstrated [35,49].

Success in identifying the T-cell antigen receptor came with the production of monoclonal antibodies but not other T cells [1,20,30,47,61]. These monoclonal antibodies inhibit a number of functions dependent upon the antigen receptor: binding of T cells to antigen-producing cells, antigen-specific interleukin-2 (IL-2) release, cytotoxic effector function, and antigen-specific proliferation.

The T-cell protein immunoprecipitated by these antibodies is a glycoprotein of about 80,000 daltons (D) composed of sulfhydryl-associated α subunit and β subunit, each about 40,000 D [2,20,48]. Examination of molecules from different T cell clones has revealed subunit heterogeneity. Each polypeptide contains constant regions common to several different T-cell clones and a variable domain, which are clone specific, situated in the amino terminal portion of the molecule. The molecules appear to be noncovalently associated with the T3 glycoprotein. The structures of the receptor molecules are remarkably similar to the immunoglobulin light chains. However, in addition to variable and constant regions there is an additional hydrophobic region anchored in the cell membrane [22,90].

Three classes of T-cell-specific complementary DNA (CDNA) clones have been identified: α, β, and γ [23,56,64,90]. The α and β cDNA clones correspond to the α and β glycopeptides; the protein product of the γ cDNA has not been identified. Sequences of the cloned cDNA revealed the presence of variable, constant, and joining regions remarkably similar in size and sequence to those encoding immunoglobulin proteins. In each case, the genomic DNA encoding these cDNA clones is rearranged in T lymphocytes.

It is not yet clear whether there is a molecular distinction between the T-cell receptors of the different classes of functional T cells. On the basis of the current data, there may be differences between the gene pools controlling the variable regions of these molecules, distinguishing the helper and cytotoxic T cells. Two variable region genes showed approximately 20% similarity between helper and cytotoxic cells. A comparable similarity is present between the constant region of the β subunit and that of the immunoglobulin light chain [20,28,48].

T3

T3 is a cell surface protein complex present on all mature T lymphocytes and a fraction of thymocytes. The proteins appear to be closely associated with the T-cell receptor in a T3-T-cell receptor complex [59]. The T3 molecule consists of three polypeptide chains of Mr 25,000 (T3 γ), Mr 20,000 (T3 δ), and Mr 20,000 (T3 ϵ). The γ and δ chains are glycoproteins, whereas the ϵ chain has no detected oligosaccharides. The three polypeptides are structurally unrelated [85].

cDNA clones that encode the complete amino acid sequence of T3 δ have been isolated. The sequence of this gene corresponds to a 171-amino acid polypeptide with a signal peptide, a 79-amino acid extracellular domain, one transmembrane region, and a 44-amino acid intracellular domain. The predicted Mr of the 13 δ polypeptide is 16,719. The molecule is not homologous to the T-cell receptor or MHC-gene products (immunoglobulin supergene family) [85].

A distinctive feature of this molecule is the effect of anti-T3 monoclonal antibody at a low concentration (10^{-12} M) to induce proliferation of T cells. Antibodies against T3 also inhibit antigen-specific T-cell proliferation and allogenic cytotoxicity [9,58,86]. The insightful hypothesis from these findings was that anti-T3 antibodies react with the T-cell antigen-recognition structure [9]. This suggested association of T3 and the T-cell antigen receptor has been confirmed by a series of experiments involving antibody-induced modulation of T3 from the cell surface; it was found that the specific recognition of antigen by T cells and the effector functions of T4 and T8 cytotoxic clones were linked to cell surface expression of the T3 molecule [59]. A model for these interactions envisions close association of the T-cell antigen receptor molecule and T3 molecules (reviewed in Reference 48). The central role for the T3 glycoprotein in T-cell function and its presence in all mature human T cells has stimulated the trial usage of the OKT3 monoclonal antibody in the treatment of acute renal allograft rejection [10].

T4 and T8

The T4 and T8 cell surface antigens define different T-cell subsets in relation to recognition of the MHC class I and class II glycoproteins. One subset of T cells [Lyt 2^+ in mice and $T8^+$ (Leu 2^+) in human] is correlated with recognition of class I antigens and contains most cells capable of cytotoxic function. Another subset [L3T4 in mice and $T4^+$ (Leu 3^+) in human], recognizes class II MHC antigens and contains the major fraction of helper activity. Murine T cells that respond to class I MHC antigens express high levels of Lyt-2 antigen, and anti-Lyt 2 antibodies block cytotoxic T-cell function [27,54, 68,77]. In contrast, T cells that respond to class II antigens are generally Lyt 2^- and are inhibited by anti-L3T4 antibodies but not be anti-Lyt 2 antibodies [78]. Similar findings were obtained with human cells [7,35,36,39,40,49,58]. Human T lymphocytes with cytotoxic or suppressor function (analogous to the murine Lyt 2 cells) are distinguished by the T8 cell surface glycoprotein, and T8-positive cells interact solely with targets expressing class I MHC molecules. Human T cells with helper/inducer functions specific to class II MHC carry the T4 antigen.

The specificities of the T4 and T8 proteins are substantiated by the effects of monoclonal antibodies inhibit allogenic cytotoxic activity [7,15,58]. Antibodies against the T4 antigens block $T4^+$ T-cell proliferation in vitro and production of IL-2 by T cells in the presence of antigen [15]. Moreover, administration of a monoclonal antibody against the T4 molecule of murine T cells prevented the development of experimental allergic encephalomyelitis and reversed the disease when given to paralyzed animals [87].

The T8 glycoprotein isolated by immunoprecipitation from peripheral blood and lymphocytes was identified by polyacrylamide gel electrophoresis, under reducing conditions, as a Mr 34,000 glycoprotein [69]. Under nonreducing conditions the molecule showed a complex multimeric structure with several components. In thymocytes, a Mr 46,000 polypeptide as well as a Mr 34,000 molecule was present. The Mr 34,000 and Mr 46,000 molecules appeared to differ in both protein and carbohydrate structure. The sequence of cDNA clones reveals that the molecule is a transmembrane glycoprotein with an N-terminal domain homologous to immunoglobulin variable region light chains [44]. Moreover, the gene for T8 is closely linked to the K light chain locus on human chromosome 2 [76].

The T4 molecule consists of a membrane glycoprotein of Mr 62,000 [80]. Genetic polymorphism of this molecule has been detected in the case of individuals with a normal population of inducer/helper T cells but a reduced number of antigenic epitopes reactive with anti-T4 monoclonal antibodies [31,65].

Considerable data suggest that these glycoproteins function as cell adhesion molecules to promote strong adherence between the T cells and target cells. Monoclonal antibodies that bind T4 or T8 appear to inhibit T cell function by diminishing this interaction of the T cell with its target. The ligands that bind to the T4 or T8 molecules have not been identified. Possibly, the specificity of T cell populations and different target cells results from an interaction of T8 or T4 with the class I or class II MHC molecules (reviewed in Reference 46) [7,39,83].

Interleukin-2 Receptor

The immune response to a foreign antigen involves the amplification of thost T lymphocytes with receptors for the antigen. Phenotypic changes in the induced cells include the expression of cell surface receptors for IL-2. Expression of IL-2 receptors is one of the early events after activation by antigen, occurring within the first 4-6 hr [11,55]. The IL-2 receptor is an intrinsic plasma membrane glycoprotein synthesized as a peptide backbone of approximately 33,000 D and then posttranslationally modified by the addition of both N-linked and O-linked oligosaccharides to form the mature molecule of about 50,000-55,000 D [41,50]. The molecule is also sulfated and phosphorylated [42]. Purification of the molecule from a T-cell lymphoma cell line and from activated T lymphocytes has been achieved [84]. The molecules differed slightly in apparent molecular weight but contained the same NH_2-terminal protein sequence. A monoclonal antibody against the IL-2 receptor inhibited both IL-2 binding to cells and multiplication of

IL-2-dependent cell lines. The antibody also blocked antigen- and mitogen-induced T-cell proliferation, the generation of cytolytic T lymphocytes in allogeneic cell coculture, and T-cell-dependent activation of B-cell immunoglobulin production [13]. Purified IL-2 reversed the inhibitory effects of the antibody.

SOLUBLE FACTORS

Interleukin-1

A critical event in the initiation of the immune response is the activation of helper T cells by interleukin-1 (IL-1) produced by macrophages and monocytes (reviewed in Reference 14). These cells can be stimulated to produce IL-1 by a variety of agents, including microbes, microbial products, inflammatory agents, plant lectins, and antigens. The protein, initially called the lymphocyte activation factor [16], appears to function by acting on T cells to promote the secretion of optimum amounts of IL-2 and to induce the expression of IL-2 receptors on the T-cell surface [33]. Interleukin-1 also has been associated with a number of other activities: endogenous pyrogen [53], collagenase synthesis by fibroblasts [57] and rheumatoid synovial cells [51], release of acute phase reactants by the liver [73], and fibroblast proliferation [67].

Interleukin-1 has recently been purified as a Mr 15,000 molecule [66]. Concentrations of the purified material of 10^{-10} M gave half-maximal stimulation in a thymocyte proliferation assay. A human IL-1 cDNA of 1580 bases that encodes a polypeptide of 269 amino acids, Mr 35,000, has been obtained from endotoxin-stimulated monocytes [5]. A similar cDNA has also been obtained from mouse cells [43]. The natural glycoprotein of about Mr 15,000, with high biologic activity, is the carboxy terminus of the Mr 35,000 precursor. The receptor for IL-1 has not been identified.

Interleukin-2

Interleukin-2, originally called T-cell growth factor [52], is released into tissue culture media by human T cells when activated by antigens or mitogens. Media containing IL-2 has made it possible to clone and propagate T cells in vitro. The molecule purified from human T leukemia cells or peripheral mononuclear cells [74] is highly homologous to the polypeptide of Mr 14,800 predicted from the nucleotide sequence of cDNA clones [79]. The structure of the molecule has also been confirmed by peptide mapping and protein sequencing [60]. Purified IL-2 has been found to enhance thymocyte mitogenesis, stimulate the proliferation in vitro of antigen-specific helper or killer T-cell lines, augment the lytic activity of natural killer cells, and induce the development of plaque-forming B cells (reviewed in Reference 17). Antibodies to purified mouse IL-2 inhibit a variety of immune responses: antigen- and lectin-stimulated T-cell mitogenesis, cytotoxic lymphocyte generation in vitro, and T-cell helper function for antibody production in culture [13,18]. In addition, anti-IL-2 antibodies injected into mice reduce the in vivo development of alloreactive cytotoxic lymphocytes in response to allogeneic cells [18].

OTHER IMPORTANT MOLECULES IN IMMUNE RESPONSES: LYMPHOCYTE FUNCTION-ASSOCIATED ANTIGEN

T cells respond to foreign antigens only when those antigens are presented on the surface of other cells that bear the appropriate MHC antigens [91]. In addition to the T-cell specific proteins already described, other cell membrane proteins are important in the generation of immune responses.

One of the best characterized of these other proteins is the lymphocyte function-associated antigen (LFA-1) [12,25,36,37,62,63,88]. This molecule is one of a family of leukocyte cell surface antigens that contain two noncovalently associated subunits: a common β subunit of Mr 95,000 and a cell-specific α subunit. The LFA-1 molecule is expressed on T and B lymphocytes, thymocytes, macrophages, granulocytes, and subpopulation of bone marrow cells and contains an α subunit of Mr 175,000. The macrophage-specific Mac-1 antigen contains an α subunit of Mr 165,000 [24,38,70,71]. An α subunit of Mr 150,000 of unknown function has also been identified on macrophages and monocytes [24,63]. The murine LFA-1 molecule is polymorphic and has been found to correspond to the Ly15 cell membrane alloantigen [26].

A monoclonal antibody against murine Mac-1 cross-reacts with human monocytes [4] and has been shown to inhibit binding of C3bi-coated erythrocytes to murine and human macrophages [6, 70, 71]. These and similar results of [24, 89] indicate that the Mac-1 antigen is closely associated with or represents the type 3 compliment receptor (CR_3). Human Mac-1 antigen (HMac-1) appears to be identical in tissue distribution and structure to the OKM-1 and Mo 1 human monocyte antigens [8, 24, 81, 82].

Monoclonal antibodies against LFA-1 block a wide variety of T-cell functions, including the mixed lymphocyte reaction, response to mitogens, and lysis of target cells by cytotoxic T lymphocytes [12,19,24,25,88]. In general, the HLFA α-specific antibody inhibits only T-cell-associated functions and the HMac-1 α-specific antibody inhibits only a monocyte/macrophage-associated function, but anti-β antibodies inhibit all functions tested [24]. It is possible that the functional specificity of the HMac-1 and HLFA antigens is determined by the α subunits whereas the primary functional molecule is the shared β subunit. Antibodies directed against the LFA molecules have also been reported to prolong allograft survival in a mouse model system [21].

There is strong evidence that the anti-HLFA antibodies inhibit T-cell functions by preventing the conjugation of T cells with other cells [35,45]. It thus appears that the HLFA and HMac-1 antigens may serve as leukocyte adhesion molecules. It is of interest that both adhesion of CTL to target cells (blocked by anti-LFA-1 antibodies) and adhesion through CR_3 (blocked by anti-Mac-1 antibodies) occur through a Mg^{2+}-dependent step [63].

Recently, a clinical syndrome characterized by recurrent bacterial infections, delayed wound healing, and granulocytoses has been described (reviewed in Reference 3). This deficiency has been associated with a defect in the β subunit of the LFA-1 and Mac-1 molecules, corresponding to a deficiency in the adherence and other functions of granulocytes and mononuclear leukocytes [72].

ACKNOWLEDGMENTS

This research is supported in part by grants from the National Institutes of Health (P01 A1 19373-02), the Office of Naval Research (N00014-82-K-0221), and the Johnson and Johnson Focused Giving Program. Hildreth is a Gustavus and Louise Pfeiffer Scholar in Pharmacology and Experimental Therapeutics

REFERENCES

1. Acuto, O., Hussey, R. E., Fitzgerald, K. A., Protentis, J. P., Meuer, S. C., Schlossman, S. F., and Reinherz, E. L. The human T cell receptor; Appearance in ontogeny and biochemical relationship of α and β subunits on IL-2 dependent clones and T cell tumors. *Cell* 34:717-726, 1983.
2. Allison, J. P., McIntyre, B. W., and Bloch, D. Tumor-specific antigen of murine T lymphoma cells defined with monoclonal antibody. *J. Immunol.* 129:2293-2300, 1982.
3. Anderson, D. C., Schmalstieg, F. C., Kohl, S., Arnaout, M. A. Hughes, B. J., Tosi, M. F., Buffone, G. J., Brinkley, B. R., Dickey, W. D., Abramson, J. S., Springer, T. A., Boser, L. A., Hollers, J. M., and Smith, C. W. Abnormalities of polymorphonuclear leukocyte function associated with a heritable deficiency of a high molecular weight surface glycoprotein (GP138): Common relationship to diminished cell adherence. *J. Clin. Invest.* 74:536-551, 1984.
4. Ault, K. A., and Springer, T. A. Cross-reaction of a rat-anti-mouse phagocyte-specific monoclonal antibody (anti-Mac-1) with human monocytes and natural killer cells. *J. Immunol.* 126:359-364, 1981.
5. Auron, P. E., Webb, A. C., Rosenwasser, L. J., Mucci, S. F., Rich, A., Wolff, S. M., and Dinarello, C. A. Nucleotide sequence of human monocyte interleukin 1 precursor cDNA. *Proc. Natl. Acad. Sci. USA* 81:7907-7911 (]984.
6. Beller, D. I., Springer, T. A., and Schreiber, R. D. Anti-Mac-1 selectively inhibits the mouse and human type three complement receptor. *J. Exp. Med.* 156:1000-1009.
7. Biddison, W. E., Rao, P. E., Talle, M. A., Goldstein, G., and Shaw, S. Possible involvement of the OKT4 molecule in T cell recognition of class II HLA antigens. Evidence from studies of cytotoxic T lymphocytes specific for SB antigens. *J. Exp. Med.* 156: 1065-1076 (1982).
8. Breard, J., Reinherz, E. L., King, P. C., Goldstein, G., and Schlossman, S. F. A monoclonal antibody reactive with human peripheral blood monocytes. *J. Immunol.* 124: 1943-1948, 1980.
9. Chang, T. W., Kung, P. C., Gingras, S. P., and Goldstein, G. Does OKT3 monoclonal antibody react with an antigen-recognition structure on human T cells. *Proc. Natl. Acad. Sci. USA* 78:1805-1808, 1981.
10. Cosimi, A. B., Burton, R. C., Colvin, R. B., Goldstein, G., Delmonico, F. L., LaQuaglia, M. P., Tolkoff-Rubin, N., Rubin, R. H., Herrin, J. T., and Russell, P. S. Treatment of acute renal allograft rejection with OKT3 monoclonal antibody. *Transplantation* 32: 535-539, 1981.
11. Cotner, T., Williams, J. M., Christenson, L., Shapiro, H. M., Strom, T. B., and Strominger, J. Simultaneous flow cytometric analysis of human T-cell activation antigen expression and DNA content. *J. Exp. Med.* 157:461-472, 1983.
12. Davignon, D., Martz, E., Reynolds, T., Kurtzinger, K., and Springer, T. A. Monoclonal antibody to a novel lymphocyte function-associated antigen (LFA-1): Mechanism of blocking of T lymphocyte-mediated killing and effects on other T and B lymphocyte functions. *J. Immunol.* 127:590-595, 1981.
13. Depper, J. M., Leonard, W. J., Robb, R. J., Waldmann, T. A., and Greene, W. C. Blockade of the interleukin-2 receptor by anti-tac antibody: Inhibition of human lymphocyte activation. *J. Immunol.* 131:690-696, 1983.
14. Dinarello, C. A. Interleukin-1. *Rev. Infect. Dis.* 6:51-95, 1984.
15. Engleman, E. C., Benike, C. J., Glickman, E., and Evans, R. L. Antibodies to membrane structures that distinguish suppressor/cytotoxic and helper T lymphocyte subpopulations block the mixed leukocyte reaction in man. *J. Exp. Med.* 153:193, 1981.
16. Gery, I., Gershon, R. K., and Waksman, B. Potentiation of the T lymphocyte response to mitogens. I. The responding cell. *J. Exp. Med.* 136:128-142, 1972.

17. Gillis, S., Mochizuki, D. Y., Conlon, P. J., Hefeneider, S. H., Ramthun, C. A., Gillis, A. E., Frank, M. B., Henney, C. S., and Watson, J. D. Molecular characterization of interleukin 2, *Immunol. Rev.* 63:167-209, 1982.
18. Granelli-Piperno, A., Andrus, L., and Reich, E. Antibodies to interleukin 2. Effects of immune responses in vitro and in vivo. *J. Exp. Med.* 160:738-750, 1984.
19. Gromkowski, S. H., Heagy, W., and Martz, E. Blocking of CTL-mediated killing by monoclonal antibodies to LFA-1 and Lyt-2,3. II. Evidence that trypsin pretreatment of target cells removes a non-H-2 molecule important in killing. *J. Immunol.* 134:70-77, 1985.
20. Haskins, K., Kappler, J., and Marrack, P. The major histocompatibility complex-restricted antigen receptor on T cells. *Annu. Rev. Immunol.* 2:51-66, 1984.
21. Heagy, W., Waltenbaugh, C., and Martz, E. Potent ability of anti-LFA-1 monoclonal antibody to prolong allograft survival. *Transplantation* 37:520-523, 1984.
22. Hedrick, S. M., Cohen, D. I., Nielsen, E. A., and Davis, M. M. Isolation of cDNA clones encoding T cell-specific membrane-associated proteins. *Nature* 308:149-153, 1984.
23. Hedrick, S. M., Nielsen, E. A., Kavaler, J., Cohen, D. I., and Davis, M. M. Sequence relationships between putative T cell receptor polypeptides and immunoblobulins. *Nature* 308:153-158, 1984.
24. Hildreth, J. E. K., and August, J. T. The human lymphocyte function-associated (HLFA) antigen and a related macrophage differentiation antigen (HMac-1): Functional effects of subunit specific monoclonal antibodies. *J. Immunol.* in press.
25. Hildreth, J. E. K., Gotch, F. M., Hildreth, P. D. K., and McMichael, A. J. A human lymphocyte-associated antigen involved in cell-mediated lympholysis. *Eur. J. Immunol.* 13:202-208, 1983.
26. Hogarth, P. M., Walker, I. D., McKenzie, I. F. C., and Springer, T. A. The Ly-15 alloantigenic system: A genetically determined polymorphism of the murine lymphocyte function-associated antigen-1 molecule. *Proc. Natl. Acad. Sci. USA* 82:526-530, 1985.
27. Hollander, N. E., Pillemer, and Weissman, I. L. Blocking effect of Lyt-2 antibodies on T cell functions. *J. Exp. Med.* 152:674-687, 1980.
28. Hood, L., Kronenberg, M., and Hunkapiller, T. T-cell antigen receptors and the immunoglobulin supergene family. *Cell* 40:225-229, 1985.
29. Hood, L., Steinmetz, M., and Malissen, B. Genes of the major histocompatability complex of the mouse. *Annu. Rev. Immunol.* 1:529-568, 1983.
30. Kappler, J., Kubo, R., Haskins, K., White, J., and Marrack, P. The mouse T cell receptor: Comparison of MHC-restricted receptors on two T cell receptor: Comparison of MHC-restricted receptors on two T cell hybridomas. *Cell* 34:727-737, 1983.
31. Karol, R. A., Eng, J., Dennison, D. K., Faris, E., and Marcus, D. M. Hereditary abnormalities of the OKT4 human lymphocyte epitope in two families. *J. Clin. Immunol.* 4:71-74, 19xx.
32. Kaufman, J. F., Auffray, C., Korman, A. J., Shackelford, D. A., and Strominger, J. The class II molecules of the human and murine major histocompatability complex. *Cell* 36:1-13, 1984.
33. Kaye, J., Gillis, S., Mizel, S. B., Shevach, E. M., Malek, T. R., Dinarello, C. A., Lachman, L. B., and Janeway, C. A. Growth of a cloned helper T cell line induced by a monoclonal antibody specific for the antigen receptor: Interleukin 1 is required for the expression of receptors for interleukin 2, *J. Immunol.* 133:1339-1345, 1984.
34. Klein, J., Juretic, A., Baxevanis, C. N., and Nagy, Z. A. The traditional and a new version of the mouse H-2 complex. *Nature* 291:455-460, 1981.

35. Krensky, A. M., Clayberger, C., Reiss, C. S., Strominger, J. L., and Burakoff, S. J. Specificity of OKT4+ cytotoxic T lymphocyte clones. *J. Immunol.* 129:2001-2003, 1982.
36. Kung, P. C., Goldstein, G., Reinherz, E. L., and Schlossman, S. F. Monoclonal antibodies defining distinctive human T cell surface antigens. *Science* 206:347-349, 1979.
37. Kurzinger, K., Reynolds, T., Germain, R. N., Davignon, D., Martz, E., and Springer, T. A. A novel lymphocyte function-associated antigen (LFA-1): Cellular distribution, quantitative expression, and structure. *J. Immunol.* 127:596-602, 1981.
38. Kurzinger, K., and Springer, T. A. Purification and structural characterization of LFA-1, a lymphocyte function-associated antigen, and Mac-1, a related macrophage differentiation antigen associated with the type three complement receptor. *J. Biol. Chem.* 257:12412-12418, 1982.
39. Landegren, U., Ranstedt, V., Axberg, I., Ullberg, M., Jondal, M., and Wigzell, H. Selective inhibition of human T cell cytotoxicity at levels of target recognition or inhibition of lysis by monoclonal OKT3 and Leu-2a antibodies. *J. Exp. Med.* 155:1579-1584, 1982.
40. Ledbetter, J. A., Evans, R. L., Lipinski, M., Cunningham-Rundles, C., Good, R. A., and Herzenberg, L. A. Evolutionary conservation of surface molecules that distinguish T lymphocyte helper/inducer and suppressor/cytotoxic subpopulations in mouse and man. *J. Exp. Med.* 153:310-323, 1981.
41. Leonard, W. J., Depper, J. M., Crabtree, G. R., Rudikoff, S., Pumphrey, J., Robb. R. J., Kronke, M., Svetlik, P. B., Peffer, N. J., Waldman, T. A., and Greene, W. C. Molecular cloning and expression of cDNAs for the human interleukin-2 receptor. *Nature* 311: 626-631, 1984.
42. Leonard, W. J., Depper, J. M., Kronke, M., Robb, R. J., Waldmann, T. A., and Greene, W. C. The human receptor for T-cell growth factor. Evidence for variable post-translational processing, phosphorylation, sulfation, and the ability of precursor forms of the receptor to bind T-cell growth factor. *J. Biol. Chem.* 260:1872-1880, 1985.
43. Littman, D. R., Thomas, Y., Maddon, P. J., Chess, L., and Axel, R. The isolation and sequence of the gene encoding T8: A molecule defining functional classes of T lymphocytes. *Cell* 40:237-246, 1985.
44. Lomedico, P. T., Gubler, U., Hellmann, C. P., Dukovich, M., Giri, J. G., Pan, Y. E., Collier, K., Semionow, R., Chua, A. O., and Mizel, S. B. Cloning and expression of murine interleukin-1 cDNA in *Escherichia coli. Nature* 312:458-462, 1984.
45. Martz, E., and Gromkowski, S. H. Lymphocyte function-associated antigens: Regulation of lymphocyte adhesions in vitro and immunity in vivo. In *Mechanisms of Cell-Mediated Cytotoxicity,* Vol. II, P. Henkart and E. Martz, eds. Plenum Press, New York, 1984, pp. 1-17.
46. Martz, E., Heagy, W., and Gromkowski, S. H. The mechanism of CTL-mediated killing: Monoclonal antibody analysis of the roles of killer and target cell membrane proteins. *Immunol. Rev.* 72:73, 1983.
47. McIntyre, B. W., and Allison, J. P. The mouse T cell receptor: Structural heterogeneity of molecules of normal T cells defined by xenoantiserum. *Cell* 34:739-746, 1983.
48. Meuer, S. C., Acuto, O., Hercend, T., Schlossman, S. F., and Reinherz, E. L. The human T-cell receptor. *Annu. Rev. Immunol.* 2:23-50, 1984.
49. Meuer, S. C., Schlossman, S. F., and Reinhertz, E. L. Clonal analysis of human cytotoxic T lymphocytes: T4+ and T8+ effector T-cells recognize products of different major histocompatibility complex region. *Proc. Natl. Acad. Sci. USA* 79:4395-4399, 1982.
50. Miyawaki, T., Yachie, A., Uwadana, N., Ohzeki, S., Nagaoki, T., and Taniguchi, N. Functional significance of Tac antigen expressed on activated human T lymphocytes:

Tac antigen interacts with T-cell growth factor in cellular proliferation. *J. Immunol.* 129:2474-2478, 1982.

51. Mizel, S. B., Dayer, J. M. Krane, S. M., and Mergenhagen, S. E. Stimulation of rheumatoid synovial cell collagenase and prostaglandin production by partially purified LAF (IL-1). *Proc. Natl. Acad. Sci. USA* 78:2474-2477, 1981.
52. Morgan, D. S., Ruscetti, F. W., and Gallo, R. C. Selective in vitro growth of T lymphocytes from normal human bone marrows. *Science* 193:1007-1008, 1976.
53. Murphy, P. A., Simon, P. L., and Willoughby, W. F. Endogenous pyrogens made by rabbit peritoneal exudate cells are identical with lymphocyte activating factors made by rabbit alveolar macrophages. *J. Immunol.* 124:2498-2501, 1980.
54. Nakayama, E., Shiku, H., Stockert, E., Oettgen, H. F., and Old, L. J. Cytotoxic T cells: Lyt phenotype and blocking of killing activity by Lyt antisera. *Proc. Natl. Acad. Sci. USA* 76:1977-1981, 1979.
55. Neckers, L. M., and Cossman, J. Transferrin receptor induction in mitogen-stimulated human T lymphocytes is required for DNA synthesis and cell division and is regulated by interleukin 2. *Proc. Natl. Acad. Sci. USA* 80:3494-3498, 1983.
56. Patten, P., Yokota, T., Rothbard, J., Chien, Y., Arai, K., and Davis, M. Structure, expression and divergence of T-cell receptor β-chain variable regions. *Nature* 312: 40-46, 1984.
57. Postlethwaite, A. E., Lachman, L. B., Mainardi, C. L., and Kang, A. H. Interleukin 1 stimulation of collagenase production by cultured fibroblasts. *J. Exp. Med.* 157: 801-806, 1983.
58. Reinherz, E. L., Hussey, R. E., Fitzgerald, K., Snow, P., Terhorst, C., and Schlossman, S. F. Antibody directed at a surface structure inhibits cytolytic but not suppressor function of human T lymphocytes. *Nature* 294:168-170, 1981.
59. Reinherz, E. L., Meuer, S., Fitzgerald, K. A., Hussey, R. E., Levine, H., and Schlossman, S. F. Antigen recognition by human T lymphocytes is linked to surface expression of the T3 molecular complex. *Cell* 30:735-743, 1982.
60. Robb, R. J., Kutny, R. M., Panico, M., Morris, H. R., and Chowdhry, V. Amino acid sequence and post-translational modification of human interleukin 2. *Proc. Natl. Acad. Sci. USA* 81:6486-6490, 1984.
61. Samelson, L. E., Germain, R. N., and Schwartz, R. H. Monoclonal antibodies against the antigen receptor on a cloned T-cell hybrid. *Proc. Natl. Acad. Sci. USA* 80:6972-6976, 1983.
62. Sanchez-Madrid, F., Krensky, A. M., Ware, C. F., Robbins, E., Strominger, J. L., Burakoff, S. J., and Springer, T. A. Three distinct antigens associated with human T-lymphocyte-mediated cytolysis: LFA-1, LFA-2, and LFA-3. *Proc. Natl. Acad. Sci. USA* 79:7489-7493, 1982.
63. Sanchez-Madrid, F., Nagy, J. A., Robbins, E., Simon, P., and Springer, T. A. A human leukocyte differentiation antigen family with distinct α-subunits and a common β-unit: The lymphocyte function-associated antigen (LFA-1), the C3bi complement receptor (OKM1/Mac-1), and the p150,95 molecule. *J. Exp. Med.* 158: 1785-1803, 1983.
64. Saito, H., Kranz, D. M., Takagaki, Y., Hayday, A. C., Eisen, H. N., and Tonegawa, S. Complete primary structure of a heterodimeric T cell receptor deduced from cDNA sequences. *Nature* 309:757-762, 1984.
65. Sato, M., Hayashi, Y., Yoshida, H., Yanagawa, T., and Yura, Y. A family with hereditary lack of $T4^4$ inducer/helper T-cell subsets in peripheral blood lymphocytes. *J. Immunol.* 132:1071-1073, 1984.
66. Schmidt, J. A. Purification and partial biochemical characterization of normal human interleukin 1. *J. Exp. Med.* 160:772-787, 1984.
67. Schmidt, J. A., Mizel, S. B., Cohen, D., and Green, I. Interleukin 1, a potential regulator of fibroblast proliferation. *J. Immunol.* 128:2177-2182, 1982.

68. Shinohara, N., and Sachs, D. H. Mouse alloantibodies capable of blocking cytotoxic T cell function. I. Relationship between the antigen reactive with blocking antibodies and the Lyt-2 locus. *J. Exp. Med.* 150:432-444, 1979.
69. Snow, P. M., and Terhorst, C. The T8 antigen is a multimeric complex of two distinct subunits on human thymocytes but consists of homomultimeric forms on peripheral blood T lymphocytes. *J. Biol. Chem.* 258:14675-14681, 1983.
70. Springer, T. A., Davignon, D., Ho, M. K., Kurzinger, K., Martz, E., and Sanchez-Madrid, F. LFA-1 and Lyt-2,3, molecules associated with T lymphocyte-mediated killing; and Mac-1, an LFA-1 homologue associated with complement receptor function. *Immunol. Rev.* 68:111-135, 1982.
71. Springer, T., Galfre, G., Secher, D. S., and Milstein, C. Mac-1: A macrophage differentiation antigen identified by monoclonal antibody. *Eur. J. Immunol.* 9:301-306, 1979.
72. Springer, T. A., Thompson, W. S., Miller, L. J., Schmalstieg, F. C., and Anderson, D. C. Inherited deficiency of the Mac-1, LFA-1, p150,95 glycoprotein family and its molecular basis. *J. Exp. Med.* 160:1901-1918, 1984.
73. Stein, M. B., Vogel, S. N., Sipe, J. D., Murphy, P. A., Mizel, S. B., Oppenheim, J. J., and Rosenstreich, D. L. The role of macrophages in the acute phase response: SAA induction is closely related to lymphocyte activating factor and endogenous pyrogen. *Cell. Immunol.* 63:164-176, 1981.
74. Stern, A. S., Pan, Y-C. E., Urdal, D. L., Mochizuki, D. Y., DeChiara, S., Blacher, R., Wideman, J., and Gillis, S. Purification to homogeneity and partial characterization of interleukin 2 from a human T-cell leukemia. *Proc. Natl. Acad. Sci. USA* 81:871-875, 1984.
75. Strominger, J. L., Engelhard, V. H., Fuks, A., Guild, B. C., Hyafil, F., Kaufman, J. F., Korman, A. J., Kostyk, T. G., Krangel, M. S., Lancet, D., Lopez de Castro, J. A., Mann, D. L., Orr, H. T., Parham, P. R., Parker, K. C., Ploegh, H. L., Pober, J. S., Robb, R. J., and Shackelford, D. A. Biochemical analysis of products of the MHC. In *The Role of the Major Histocompatability Complex in Immunobiology,* M. E. Dorf, ed., Garland Press, New York, 1981, pp. 115-172.
76. Sukhatme, V. P., Vollmer, A. C., Erikson, J., Isobe, M., Croce, C., and Parnes, J. R. Gene for the human T-cell differentiation antigen Leu-2/T8 is closely linked to the k light chain locus on chromosome 2. *J. Exp. Med.* 161:429-434, 1985.
77. Swain, S. L. Significance of Lyt phenotypes: Lyt-2 antibodies block activities of T cells that recognize class I major histocompatibility complex antigens regardless of their function. *Proc. Natl. Acad. Sci. USA* 78:7101-7105, 1981.
78. Swain, S. L., Dialynas, D. P., Fitch, F. W., and English, M. Monoclonal antibody to L3T4 blocks the function of T-cells specific for class 2 major histocompatibility complex antigens. *J. Immunol.* 132:1118-1123, 1984.
79. Taniguchi, T., Matsui, H., Fujita, T. Takaoka, C., Kashima, N., Yoshimoto, R., and Hamuro, J. Structure and expression of a cloned cDNA for human interleukin-2. *Nature* 302:305-309, 1983.
80. Terhorst, C., van Agthoven, A., Reinhertz, E. L., and Schlossman, S. F. Biochemical analysis of human T lymphocyte differentiation antigens T4 and T5. *Science* 209: 520-521, 1980.
81. Todd, R. F., III, Nadler, L. M., and Schlossman, S. F. Antigens on human monocytes identified by monoclonal antibodies. *J. Immunol.* 126:1435, 1981.
82. Todd, R. F., III, Van Agthoven, A., Schlossman, S. F., and Terhorst, C. Structural analysis of differentiation antigens Mo1 and Mo2 on human monocytes. *Hybridoma* 1:329-337, 1982.
83. Tsoukas, C. D., Carson, D. A., Fong, S., and Vaughan, J. H. Molecular interactions in human T cell-mediated cytotoxicity to EBV. II. Monoclonal antibody OKT3 in-

hibits a post-killer-target recognition/adhesion step. *J. Immunol.* 129:1421-1425, 1982.

84. Urdal, D. L., March, C. J., Gillis, S., Larsen, A., and Dower, S. K. Purification and chemical characterization of the receptor for interleukin 2 from activated human T lymphocytes and from a human T-cell lymphoma cell line. *Proc. Natl. Acad. Sci. USA* 81:6481-6485, 1984.
85. van den Elsen, P., Shepley, B. A., Borst, J., Coligan, J. E., Markham, A. F., Orkin, S., and Terhorst, C. Isolation of cNDA clones encoding the 20K T3 glycoprotein of human T-cell receptor complex. *Nature* 312:413-418, 1984.
86. van Wauwe, F. P., DeMay, J. R., and Goosener, J. G. OKT3: A monoclonal anti-human T lymphocyte antibody with potent mitogenic properties. *J. Immunol.* 124: 2708-2713, 1980.
87. Waldor, M. K., Sriram, S., Hardy, R., Herzenberg, L. A., Lanier, L., Lim, M., and Steinman, L. Reversal of experimental allergic encephalomyelitis with monoclonal antibody to a T-cell subset marker. *Science* 227:415-417, 1985.
88. Ware, C. F., Sanchez-Madrid, F., Krensky, A. M., Burakoff, S. J., Strominger, J. L., and Springer, T. A. Human lymphocyte function associated antigen-1 (LFA-1): Identification of multiple antigenic epitopes and their relationship to CTL-mediated cytotoxicity. *J. Immunol.* 131:1182-1188, 1983.
89. Wright, S. D., Rao, P. E., Van Voorhis, W. C., Craigmyle, L. S., Iida, K., Talle, M. A., Westberg, E. F., Goldstein, G., and Silverstein, S. C. Identification of the C3bi receptor of human monocytes and macrophages by using monoclonal antibodies. *Proc. Natl. Acad. Sci. USA* 80:5699-5703, 1983.
90. Yanagi, Y., Yoshikai, Y., Leggett, K., Clark, S. P., Aleksander, I., and Mak. T. W. A human T cell-specific cDNA clone encodes a protein having extensive homology to immunoglobulin chains. *Nature* 308:145-148, 1984.
91. Zinkernagel, R. M., and Doherty, P. C. H-2 compatibility requirement for T cell mediated lysis of target infected with lymphocytic choriomeningitis virus. Different cytotoxic T cell specificities are associated with structures coded in H-2K of H-2D. *J. Exp. Med.* 141:1427-1436, 1975.

2

ANTIBODY-MEDIATED REJECTION

Henry J. Winn
Massachusetts General Hospital and Harvard Medical School, Boston, Massachusetts

It has not been possible to clearly define the role of humoral antibodies in the rejection of allografted tissues, in part because our knowledge of the effector functions of these molecules is incomplete, but in greater measure because their effects are widely variable, depending upon the type of tissue that has been transplanted and the genetic relationship between the donor and recipient. It has been found, for example, that xenografts of primarily vascularized organs can be routinely destroyed in acute fashion by preformed, "naturally occurring" antibodies or by antibody formed in response to the foreign tissue itself, whereas skin grafts that possess no major histocompatibility complex (MHC) antigens that are foreign to their new hosts fail to provoke detectable humoral responses, and their rejection appears to be mediated largely, if not exclusively, by immunologically specific mononuclear cells. These represent the extremes of a broad spectrum of combinations of donors and recipients, in which the outcome of transplantation is affected by humoral antibody in variable and often unpredictable ways. There are even instances in which antibodies specifically reactive with graft antigens have been shown to be responsible for prolongation rather than curtailment of the survival of allografts [5,14,16]. The expression of this phenomenon, termed immunologic enhancement, is also variable and strongly influenced by the nature of the graft and the immunogenetic relationship between its donor and recipient.

Systematic studies of the participation of humoral antibodies in the rejection of allografts in humans have not, of course, been carried out, and most of our knowledge of the role of these agents in transplantation biology has come from animal experimentation. Here we present a brief review of these studies, which is intended to emphasize those features that are likely to be of relevance to transplantation in humans. This is followed by a discussion of our current views on the importance in renal transplantation of antibodies reactive with HLA or major blood antigens.

ANIMAL STUDIES

The first systematic studies of the host response to allografts were carried out at a time when humoral antibody was widely considered to be the only specifically acting component of immune responses. It was a matter of great surprise, therefore, to find that transplantation immunity could not be routinely transferred to new recipients by infusions of sera obtained from animals that had previously rejected the test grafts. Indeed, failure to transfer immunity was observed in almost all cases except those involving the use of lymphoid cell tumors as allografts. The principal finding that emerged from these studies, with respect to graft rejection, was that susceptibility to destruction by humoral antibody was determined, to a large extent, by the density of the relevant antigens on the surface of the target cells. Thus lymphoid cells, both normal and malignant, have high concentrations of MHC antigens on their plasma membranes, and they are highly susceptible to anti-MHC sera in vivo as well as in vitro [12,14,15]. Because of the difficulty of obtaining viable singly suspended cells from tissues other than those of the lymphoreticular system, the sensitivity of such cells to humoral antibodies has not been widely studied. It has, however, been a simple matter to study the sensitivities of some malignant cells derived from nonlymphoid tissues. It is generally found that cells prepared from transplanted sarcomas or carcinomas are significantly more resistant than lymphoid cells to alloantibodies both in vivo and in vitro, and these differences in sensitivity are correlated with the density of cell surface antigens [14].

Subsequent studies have shown that the susceptibility of nucleated cells to humoral antibody can be significantly influenced by factors other than cell surface antigen density, as, for example, the ability of cells to shed or internalize molecules that have reacted with antibodies, the fluidity of the plasma membrane, the internalization of incompletely assembled effector complexes, or the ability to synthesize new membranes, perhaps as a repair mechanism. However, these factors may operate, as discussed below, to emphasize the importance of antibody concentration as well as antigen density. Thus, the modulation of antigens, the internalization of effector molecules, or the repair of damage may be less effective in protecting cells when antibody is introduced in vivo or in vitro rapidly, continuously, and in high concentration. Clearly, increasing antigen density will also work in favor of more rapid mobilization of effector substances and decreased effectiveness of protective mechanisms. Perhaps the importance of antigen density on the cell surface is best illustrated by the observation that with respect to individual alloantigenic systems homozygous cells of defined type are invariably more sensitive to humoral antibody specifically reactive with the products of one allele of the system than are heterozygous cells, a point that certainly is related to the differences in antigen concentration on the surfaces of the cells of homozygotes and heterozygotes [12,14]. Whatever the precise mechanisms involved may be, it is clear that in experimental animals there are many tissues that when grafted to allogeneic recipients are remarkably resistant to destruction by humoral antibody, and early on in the development of the modern era of transplantation biology, this observation lead to a dominant interest in cellular mechanisms of rejection.

Recently, there have been systematic efforts to define the role of humoral antibodies in the destruction of grafts of normal tissues and organs. These studies have involved free grafts of skin as well as primarily vascularized grafts of hearts and kidneys. The general plan has been to place the grafts on animals whose immune responses have been suppressed by thymectomy and a brief course of antilymphocytic serum (ALS), to exclude any significant contribution of specific immune substances from the host. Anti-graft sera are subsequently injected into these recipients, and their effects on the grafts are determined by gross inspection as well as by microscopic examination of fixed or frozen sections of the grafts. The major findings of these studies are summarized here.

Initial studies dealt with the fate of xenografts because it was believed that they would be more vulnerable than allografts to attack by humoral antibodies. This view was based on the notion that xenografts present more foreign epitopes on their cell surface molecules than do allografts and would, therefore, interact more intensely with host immune substances. This, indeed, turned out to be the case, as will become evident below.

Rat skin that had been transplanted to immunosuppressed mice was tested for its vulnerability to humoral antibody 12-16 days postgrafting. This interval was chosen, in part, to allow the grafts to become completely healed into place, with essentially normal vascular and lymphatic connection to their hosts, and in part to avoid completely any confounding effects of the slowly recovering responsiveness of the recipient mice. The intravenous administration of as little as 0.1 ml of mouse anti-rat serum resulted in the induction of an intense inflammatory response in the graft within 30-45 min. These responses, which consisted initially of hyperemia and edema, rapidly increased in intensity, leading within hours to hemorrhage and necrosis of graft tissue. Almost all of the grafts were completely destroyed or very badly and irreversibly damaged 24 hr after administration of antiserum [1,17]. In subsequent studies it was shown that rat skin grafts could be damaged by rat alloantisera, though, as anticipated, the reactions were less intense, and in some instances the inflammatory responses subsided before the grafted tissue was irreversibly damaged. Of particular interest here is the observation that skin from donors that were heterozygous for the histocompatibility determinants under study was less susceptible to antibody-mediated damage than was skin from homozygous donors. Thus, the importance of antigen density is reaffirmed in these studies carried out in vivo with skin.

In these same studies it was found that the concentration of antibody, rather than the total amount of antibody injected, was of crucial importance in the induction of graft damage. Thus the rapid injection of 0.5 ml of antigraft serum, in a single dose, was much more effective in causing acute damage than were five injections of 0.1 ml of serum injected at intervals of 1-2 hr. This is probably attributable to shedding or internalization of antibody-antigen complexes, repair of early damage, or development of refractoriness to phlogistic agents. It seems to reflect the need for the induction of an explosive response for extensive damage to occur.

These observations on the effects of humoral antibodies, and especially those of alloantibodies, seemed initially to run counter to earlier reports on the resistance of established skin grafts to these immune agents. However, it soon became apparent that the vulnerability of skin to antibodies had been obscured in earlier studies by the fact that the sensitivity of skin to antibody-mediated damage is decisively influenced by the interval of time between placement of the grafts and the administration of antiserum. Contrary to widely held views on the special vulnerability of grafts that are healing into place, it was found that antiserum injected at the time of grafting, or within 5-6 days thereafter, had little detectable influence on the course or time of survival of the transplanted skin. This period of insusceptibility was rapidly succeeded by a state of sensitivity to humoral antibody that, in immunosuppressed hosts, reaches a peak of intensity at about 14-16 days after grafting and persists at decreasing levels for an additional 3 weeks. Grafts that survive beyond that period of time regain their resistance to antiserum, and this state is maintained for the duration of survival of the grafts [10,11].

Early attempts to influence the course of skin grafts by means of antisera had focused on the period immediately surrounding the time of transplantation, and in a few cases the effects of antisera on long-standing grafts carried on tolerant animals had been studied. It is not surprising, therefore, that the grafts were usually found to be insensitive, or that in the few cases in which destructive effects of sera were encountered, the observations were difficult to reproduce.

In an extensive analysis of the variations in the sensitivity of skin grafts to humoral antibodies, it was concluded that the phenomenon could be fully accounted for on the basis of the finding that the vascular bed serves as the primary target in the destruction of grafts by antiserum [10,11]. This was especially evident in the case of long-surviving grafts, in which it was found that the loss of sensitivity to antiserum was highly correlated with the gradual replacement of a donor-type endothelium in the microvasculature of the graft by cells derived from the recipient. Thus in grafts examined at peak sensitivity, it was shown by immunohistochemical techniques that endothelial cells were of donor type only, whereas in grafts that survived for 100 days or longer virtually all the endothelial cells were of host origin. Grafts examined at intermediate points contained varying proportions of donor-type and host-type endothelium.

The resistance of freshly placed grafts to antiserum was attributed to the fact that vascularization of the skin was not evident until 4-5 days after transplantation. After the grafts had become vascularized, sensitivity to antiserum developed only gradually. This persistent resistance has not been fully explained but is thought to be due to the poor responsiveness of newly formed vessels to vasoactive substances [10].

In support of these views on the crucial role of vascular endothelium in the response of grafts to antiserum are the observations made on primarily vascularized grafts of hearts and kidneys [3]. In grafts of this kind there is little neovascularization. Such grafts are highly sensitive to antiserum immediately following transplantation, and they remain sensitive for a long, indefinite, period of time thereafter. This persistent sensitivity seems likely to be related to the fact that the endothelium of the microvasculature of the grafted hearts remains of donor origin. It is not difficult to see how the small segments of donor vessels that are retained in skin grafts, and that are joined at both ends to recipient vessels, could undergo replacement of their endothelial lining by host cells, whereas the microvascular bed of the primarily vascularized hearts, which is continuous at both ends with extensive networks of donor-derived vessels, would be expected to retain donor-type endothelial cells.

The importance of the microvascular bed in the interaction of grafts with humoral antibody is further illustrated by the following observations. If antisera specifically reactive with donor antigens are injected intravenously into recipients whose grafts are sensitive to antibody, and the grafts are removed and examined microscopically for the deposition of immune globulin, by immunofluorescent techniques, staining is found only on the luminal surfaces of small vessels. However, if grafts are removed from recipients that have not been challenged with antiserum and examined microscopically by immunofluorescent techniques in which a thin section is flooded with antigraft serum and then treated with FITC anti-immunoglobulin, many cells in addition to endothelial cells are stained.

Furthermore, when mice-bearing grafts that have become resistant to antibodies are injected with antigraft serum and the grafts removed and examined as above, no fluorescent staining is observed; when sections of these grafts are treated with antigraft serum followed by FITC anti-immunoglobulin, endothelial cells remain unstained but other cells of donor origin become fluorescent. Thus, many cellular elements in the graft are capable of reacting with the antigraft serum, but the crucial reactivity in vivo is restricted largely, or solely, to endothelial cells of small blood vessels.

It is important to note that grafts in which donor endothelium has been replaced by host cells and that are, accordingly, resistant to antisera are susceptible to rejection by cellular mechanisms either on their primary hosts or when transplanted to recipients syngeneic with these primary hosts. Moreover, freshly placed grafts that have not yet acquired sensitivity to antisera are readily destroyed by immune cells. These observations underscore the prime importance of cells in the usual circumstances in which grafts are rejected.

The mechanisms involved in the destruction of grafted tissues by humoral antibody have not been fully elucidated, but it is clear that they involve a wide variety of effector agents—complement, granulocytes, mononuclear cells, platelets, and vasoactive substances. The importance of any particular effector varies according to the kinds and amounts of antibody molecules present in the host, the specificity of the antibody molecules, the density of the cell surface antigens with which they react, the nature of the graft, and the species of the recipient of the graft. In most, perhaps all, cases multiple mechanisms are brought into play, and it is extremely difficult to dissect out the process into defined pathways or to determine the relative importance of the various effectors that are activated. This is not of major concern from a clinical point of view for, as indicated below, much of the difficulty posed by the action of humoral antibody can be avoided through the use of screening procedures that identify those individuals whose sera contain antibodies that would be expected to cause graft damage. Such sensitized patients should be given kidneys only from those donors whose cells show no reactivity with the patients' sera.

In spite of the complexity of antibody-mediated destruction of grafts and the wide differences in the detailed courses of such processes in different species and even within the same species in different circumstances, the immediate and principal effects on organ grafts are invariably found to be alterations in the structure and function of small vessels within the graft. All subsequent damage to the graft can be traced to this vascular damage, as already discussed. Both interspecies and intraspecies differences in the course of antibody-mediated destruction are reflections of the remarkable versatility of immune responses, which clearly evolved under selective forces not directly related to transplantation. A large number of classes and subclasses of immunoglobulin molecules has evolved, and each of these selectively activates a different array of effector processes designed to afford protection against a variety of pathogeneic agents. It is not surprising, therefore, to find great variability in the ways in which humoral responses affect grafted tissues, and it is to be expected that such responses may at times seem ill suited for the destruction of grafts. Indeed, as pointed out earlier, humoral antibodies may in some circumstances lead to extended rather than shortened survival times of allografts. This phenomenon, known as immunologic enhancement, is discussed below.

Enhancement due to antiserum alone is most readily and consistently observed with allografts of certain transplanted tumors in mice. The immediate effects of antiserum in these experimental systems is a striking and specific inhibition of host responsiveness to graft antigens. Not surprisingly, this state of nonresponsiveness is observed only if the recipients are grafted within a few days of the administration of antiserum. Why a state of unresponsiveness or low responsiveness should persist for long periods of time after treatment with antiserum only at the time of grafting is not understood. It may be due to selective loss of donor dendritic cells, which constitute a very potent source of immunogens in allotransplantation, or to some alteration in the active responses of the host. In any case, it is clear that enhancement is observed only if the graft is not destroyed by the antiserum. Hence, tumors that are highly resistant to antiserum have generally been employed in studies on enhancement.

ENHANCEMENT

The term "enhancement" was originally applied to a phenomenon in which treatment of intended recipients of allografts of certain tumors with homogenates of the tumor, which had been frozen and thawed, led to prolonged survival of subsequent implants of living tumor cells. In effect, a procedure that had been designed to immunize had produced the opposite effect, tendering the treated animal less resistant to tumor growth than were normal untreated animals. Later it was found that a similar effect could be produced if the intended recipients were treated instead with small amounts of host antidonor serum. Because treatment with the homogenate of tumor induced low levels of humoral antibody, it was concluded that both phenomena had similar mechanisms. In one case, antibody was acquired actively, and, in the other case, passively. In fact, this has never been firmly established, and it seems likely that treatment with homogenate may have effects beyond the induction of humoral antibody. Accordingly, we shall not consider that phenomenon here, but rather confine this brief discussion to so-called passive enhancement.

Prolongation of graft survival times by alloantisera is not restricted to transplanted tumors. Enhancement has been observed for skin [9], kidneys, and several other normal tissues [5]. Generally, this has required the use of special donor-recipient combinations, and in some cases carefully adjusted doses of antiserum that caused inhibition of host responses with little or no damage to the grafts. It is conceivable that further manipulation of the kinds (classes and subclasses) and amounts of antibodies may facilitate prolonged survival of other types of grafts, including those that have been found to be expecially sensitive to relatively large amounts of unfractionated antisera. The phenomenon is not discussed in further detail here because its occurrence in humans has not been documented. The beneficial effects of blood transfusions on the outcome of renal transplantation in humans have at times been loosely attributed to enhancement, but evidence to support this suggestion has not been forthcoming. The possibility of modifying patients' responses through administration of humoral antibodies is by no means excluded, but problems of specificity, dose, and immunoglobulin class are formidable.

HUMORAL ANTIBODY IN CLINICAL TRANSPLANTATION

Our knowledge of the role of humoral antibody in transplantation in the human has not, of course, come from experiments designed to obtain such information, but, rather, it has accrued largely as a by-product of the early years of renal transplantation, when our understanding of transplantation immunology was relatively crude and could not serve to anticipate the effect of humoral agents on grafted tissues. As indicated below, two major immunogenetic systems (ABH and HLA) have been responsible for the antibodies that have thus far been found to have important effects on renal allografts in humans.

MAJOR BLOOD GROUP ANTIBODIES

Shortly after the introduction of renal allotransplantation as a form of therapy for end-stage renal disease, it was noted, in retrospective analyses, that major blood group (ABO) incompatibilities between donors and recipients were associated with poor function and early rejection of grafted kidneys. Thus, in those cases in which kidneys from type A, B, or AB donors were placed in recipients whose tissues lacked such antigens, there was a high incidence of early acute rejection of the grafts. Close observations in several instances suggested that such grafts were destroyed within a few hours of completion of vascular anastomoses, and this rapid time course in conjunction with the finding of infiltration of neutrophilic leukocytes and widespread edema has been taken as strong evidence for the involvement of anti-A and anti-B antibodies. This view is entirely consistent with the fact that A and B antigens are present on vascular endothelium of many organs, including kidneys, and are, accordingly, readily accessible for reactivity with circulating antibodies leading to the activation of effector substances that would produce the intense, destructive inflammatory responses observed in the grafts. Curiously, in some instances ABO incompatibilities between donor and recipient seem to have had little effect on the outcome of transplantation. Close analysis of these cases reveals a high preponderance of A_2 donors [2]. In view of the absence of naturally occuring anti-A_2, these findings are not surprising, and there have been suggestions that, from an immunogenetic point of view, type A_2 kidneys be regarded as essentially the same as those from type O donors.

There are also a few reported examples of the survival of renal allografts in the face of A_1 or B incompatibilities. The explanation for these occurrences is not clear, but it should be noted that, although the presence of anti-A_1 and anti-B in the sera of individuals whose tissues do not contain such antigens is very common, there are cases in which the expected antibodies are found in very low concentrations or not at all. Perhaps this accounts for these surprising observations. In any event, there are no carefully documented instances of the survival of an ABO-incompatible kidney in a recipient with readily detectable antibodies of the appropriate specificity, and it seems reasonable to suggest that such incompatibility be avoided. Kidneys from type O individuals can, of course, be used for recipients of all major blood types and, as already suggested, this may be true for A_2 kidneys as well. There has been no well-documented report of the involvement in renal transplantation of antibodies specifically reactive with other red blood cell antigens.

ANTI-HLA ANTIBODIES

Anti-HLA antibodies are found in the sera of a significant number of individuals who are candidates for renal transplantation. The presence of such antibodies can be accounted for on the basis of the receipt of transfusions of whole blood, the rejection of previously placed allografts, or stimulation during pregnancy by paternally derived antigens present on embryonic or fetal tissues. Whatever their origin, anti-HLA antibodies pose a problem in organ transplantation. Because of the widespread distribution of HLA antigens on various cells and tissues throughout the body, these antibodies can react with a variety of cells, including endothelial cells of allografts. As in the case of the major blood group antibodies already discussed, the presence in intended recipients of anti-HLA antibodies reactive with donor cells is associated with early, acute destruction of renal grafts. The observations leading to this conclusion were made at a time when the human MHC was only poorly defined and the dire effects of anti-HLA antibodies could not have been anticipated. It is now a relatively simple matter to screen the sera of candidates for transplantation for antibodies reactive with the cells of potential donors to avoid these catastrophic events. It is important in such undertakings to employ sensitive test systems [6] and to apply them to samples of serum prepared from blood taken at various intervals prior to transplantation. Obviously, such samples should include some that have been prepared from blood drawn at a point close to the time of testing. Indeed, in three recent studies it has been suggested that close analysis of such samples may be essential to the process of recipient selection [4,7,13]. These studies included a number of patients in whom there were alterations in serologic reactivity such that reactivity found in early samples of serum was not detectable in later samples. Careful analysis of these sera made it clear that the titer for some HLA specificities had gradually diminished with time to a point where they were not detectable even when the most sensitive tests were employed. These patients received renal allografts from donors who would have been judged unacceptable on the basis of cross-matches carried out with early samples of serum, but not on the basis of tests carried out with serum prepared from blood drawn within 4-6 months prior to testing. There was no evidence of early acute damage to the grafts, and although rejection responses were observed in some of these patients during the first 3 weeks after transplantation, there was no indication that these were due to humoral antibody. Moreover, reactivity with donor cells was not detected after placement of the grafts, and nothing in the clinical courses of these patients indicated that they were sensitized to graft antigens.

The gradual loss of sensitization with respect to some HLA specificities that has been observed in these patients provides hope for at least a partial resolution of the problems posed by the large numbers of highly sensitized individuals who are candidates for renal transplantation. It may be possible to devise procedures for accelerating the decline in sensitivity to extend the benefits of transplantation to greater numbers of this special group. Perhaps, for example, selected immunosuppressive agents may be useful in such efforts.

Individuals who have become sensitized to HLA antigens, and especially those individuals who have become sensitized as a result of transplantation, may bear cellular as well as humoral immune substances, and these cells may play a role in some forms of early acute rejection. This seems not to be the case for the very early form, so-called hyperacute rejection, but there are other instances of early accelerated rejection in which immune cells may play an important role, as discussed elsewhere in this volume.

From time to time it has been suggested that the presence in candidates for transplantation of antibodies reactive with the lymphoid cells of potential donors is not always a contraindication to the use of such donor organs for transplantation. There is growing acceptance of this view, which, in spite of appearances, is not at variance with the point of view just expressed. Not all antigens expressed on the surfaces of lymphoid cells are expressed on all other cells throughout the body. Indeed, many of these, including some HLA antigens, have a very restricted tissue distribution. The HLA-DQ antigens, for example, are readily detected on some mononuclear blood cells and on extravascular dendritic cells, but not on the endothelial cells found in kidneys. It is not surprising, therefore, that some antibodies reactive with donor leukocytes have little or no effect on organ grafts from these same donors. Clearly, this is a matter of specificity rather than one of resistance to the effects of humoral antibody.

CHRONIC REJECTION

A major role for humoral antibody in the early acute rejection of renal allografts has been relatively easy to establish on the basis of a striking correlation between this form of rejection, frequently referred to as hyperacute, and the presence in the graft recipients of preformed antibodies specifically reactive with donor antigens. The presence of such antibodies prior to transplantation, the very early onset and intensity of the destructive process, and the absence of any significant lymphocytic infiltration of the graft argue strongly for a prime role of humoral antibody. Chronic rejection, on the other hand, occurs months or years after transplantation in recipients whose immune responses have been continuously suppressed. It is not clear in these patients whether the low-grade responses that lead to this chronic attack are primarily cellular or humoral in nature, and it seems likely that they are mixed responses of variable composition. Nevertheless, the appearance of humoral antibodies specifically reactive with donor antigens has been documented in a number of patients, and in at least one study a striking correlation was found between the presence of these antibodies and the occurrence of the obliterative arteritis that is characteristic of chronic rejection [8]. It may be that some recipients have preformed antibody that escapes detection prior to transplantation and increases in concentration in response to graft antigens. Secondary responses are known to be more difficult to suppress than are primary responses. Here, again, the importance of a very sensitive test for preformed humoral antibody is underscored.

It seems unlikely that humoral antibody could have such devastating effects if present at the time of transplantation and be without significant effect if formed in response to the graft. It is, however, not possible at this time to separate the effects of low-grade humoral and cellular responses in this patients, and it must be kept in mind that the allograft serves as a trap for immune substances, thereby making the interpretation of measurements of them in the circulation ambiguous. The issue is not whether humoral or cellular immune substances are responsible for chronic rejection but the extent to which each of these major classes contributes to rejection in individual cases.

SUMMARY AND CONCLUDING COMMENT

In the usual circumstances in which renal transplantation is carried out in humans the problem of rejection is thought to be created largely, in many cases perhaps exclusively, by cellular responses of the graft recipient, and therapy is properly directed to suppression of the induction and expression of such cellular responses. However, it should be noted that suppression of T-cell function is invariably accompanied by the suppression of humoral antibody formation as well, either because of direct effects on B cells or because helper activity is greatly diminished. Thus B cells may, through their immunoglobulin products, pose a potential threat to transplanted organs, but the threat is masked by more vigorous and less tractable T-cell responses.

Problems with humoral antibody relate principally to states of presensitization found in a significant number of candidates for renal transplantation. These problems are dealt with largely through the employment of screening procedures that are designed to guard against the placement of organs into individuals whose sera contain antibodies reactive with donor cells. The antibodies of concern are those that react with major blood group (ABH) antigens or with antigens of the major histocompatibility complex (HLA). Occasionally, antibodies that react with some subpopulations of donor lymphoid cells have been found not to have adverse effects on organs transplanted from such donors. In such cases it turns out that the antibodies in question cannot be shown to be reactive with antigens in the graft itself. There is no documented instance in which a renal allograft has been observed to go undamaged in a recipient whose sera contains antibodies reactive with endothelial cell surface antigens of the graft, and there has been no report of a beneficial effect of humoral antibodies on the course of renal allografts in humans.

Humoral antibody seems to play a role in some cases of chronic rejection. This may at times be traceable to low-grade presensitization that is gradually elevated to threshold levels by graft antigens, or it may arise de novo because the graft presents a particularly strong stimulus to the recipient. It is, in any case, difficult if not impossible to demonstrate a role for humoral antibody in individual cases. The insidious and unmanageable courses of some cases of chronic rejection are consistent with a role for humoral responses, which are usually very difficult to reverse.

Recent observations on the gradual and spontaneous decrease in the spectrum, as well as the intensity of sensitization in some individuals awaiting renal allografts, hold some promise for the resolution of the problem of the highly sensitized patient. Perhaps in the future the decline in sensitization may be initiated or hastened by active intervention. Certainly, the ability to terminate a state of humoral sensitization, together with the widespread use of sensitive techniques for the detection of sensitization, would be expected to reduce humoral responsiveness to a relatively minor problem in renal transplantation in humans.

REFERENCES

1. Baldamus, C. A., McKenzie, I. F. C., Winn, H. J., and Russell, P. S. Acute destruction by humoral antibody of rat skin grafted to mice. *J. Immunol.* 110:1532-1541, 1973.
2. Brynger, H., Rydberg, B., Samuelsson, B., and Sandberg, L. Experience with 14 renal transplants with kidneys from blood group A (subgroup A2) to O recipients. *Transplant Proc.* 16:1175-1176, 1984.
3. Burdick, J. F., Russell, P. S., and Winn, H. J. Sensitivity of long-standing xenografts of rat hearts to humoral antibodies. *J. Immunol.* 123:1732-1735, 1979.
4. Cardella, C. J., Falk, J. A., Nicholson, M. J., Harding, M., and Cook, G. T. Successful renal transplantation in patients with T-cell reactivity to donor. *Lancet* 2:1240, 1982.
5. Carpenter, C. B., d'Apice, A. J. F., and Abbas, A. K. The role of antibodies in the rejection and enhancement of organ allografts. *Adv. Immunol.* 22:1-55, 1976.
6. Fuller, T. C., Phelan, D., Gebel, H. M., and Rodey, G. E. Antigenic specificity of antibody reactive in the antiglobulin-augmented lymphocytotoxicity test. *Transplantation* 34:24, 1982.
7. Fuller, T. C., Forbes, J. B., and Delmonico, F. L. Renal transplantation with a positive historical donor crossmatch. *Transplant Proc.* 17:113, 1985.
8. Jeannet, M., Pinn, V. W., Flax, M. H., Winn, H. J., and Russell, P. S. Humoral antibodies in renal allotransplantation in man. *N. Engl. J. Med.* 282:111-117, 1970.
9. Jeekel, J., McKenzie, I. F. C., and Winn, H. J. Immunological enhancement of skin grafts in the mouse. *J. Immunol.* 108:1017-1024, 1972.
10. Jooste, S. V., Colvin, R. B., Soper, W. D., and Winn, H. J. The vascular bed as the primary target in the destruction of skin grafts by antiserum I. Resistance of freshly-placed skin graft to antiserum. *J. Exp. Med.* 154:1319-1331, 1981.
11. Jooste, S. V., Colvin, R. B., and Winn, H. J. The vascular bed as the primary target in

the destruction of skin grafts by antiserum II. Loss of sensitivity to antiserum in long term skin grafts. *J. Exp. Med.* 154:1332-1341, 1981.

12. Jooste, S. V., and Winn, H. J. Acute destruction of rat skin grafts by alloantisera. *J. Immunol.* 114:933-938, 1975.
13. Norman, D. J., Barry, J. M., and Wetzsteon, P. J. Successful cadaver kidney transplantation in patients highly sensitized to blood transfusions. Unimportance of the most reactive serum in the pretransplant crossmatch. *Transplantation* 39:253, 1985.
14. Winn, H. J. The participation of complement in isoimmune reaction. *Ann. N.Y. Acad. Sci.* 101:23-44, 1962.
15. Winn, H. J. Humoral antibody in allograft reactions. *Transplant. Proc.* 2:83-91, 1970.
16. Winn, H. J. Mechanisms of immunological enhancement. In *Progress in Immunology II,* Vol. 3, L. Brent and J. Holborow, eds. North-Holland Publishing, Amsterdam, 1974, pp. 207-216.
17. Winn, H. J., Baldamus, C. A., Jooste, S. V., and Russell, P. S. Acute destruction by humoral antibody of rat skin grafted to mice: The role of complement and polymorphonuclear leukocytes. *J. Exp. Med.* 137:893-910, 1973.

3

MECHANISMS OF CELL-MEDIATED REJECTION

Francis T. Thomas, Judith M. Thomas, Olaf Ganghoff, and Uli Gross
East Carolina University School of Medicine, Greenville, North Carolina

Since Medawar's early studies [97] demonstrating the immunologic basis of allograft rejection, a variety of experimental in vivo and in vitro models have been developed to study the various immunologic mechanisms responsible for allograft rejection. It appears that allografts are susceptible to destruction by both immunologically specific cellular and humoral mechanisms and also by various nonspecific inflammatory mechanisms [3,51,88]. With increasing study, the alloimmune response has proven to be extremely complex, and the precise nature of the various effector mechanisms remains controversial [41,88,96, 147]. Although the functions of T-lymphocyte populations appear to dominate the alloimmune response, other mononuclear cell populations, including cells of the macrophage/ monocyte lineage, dendritic cells, B lymphocytes, and null lymphocytes of the natural killer/killer cell type, have each been implicated at some level of the rejection process. In addition to the cells mediating allograft destruction, there may be present within the graft and lymphoid tissues suppressor cells that regulate the effector responses. Under such heterogeneous conditions, it is not easy to identify the relevant effector cell mechanism. The problem of pinpointing the critical effector population is a primary research focus and is important for the development of more accurate diagnosis and management of clinical rejection.

GENERAL CONSIDERATIONS FOR MODELS OF ALLOGRAFT REJECTION

In any overview of effector mechanisms involved in allograft rejection, it is useful to bear in mind that the *type of tissue transplanted* influences the nature of the effector mechanisms generated to destroy it. There are apparent differences in the rejection of skin grafts, primary vascularized organ allografts (kidneys, hearts, and others), and dissociated cell grafts, such as bone marrow transplants. Skin grafts, for example, are unusually susceptible to rapid rejection. Factors that may explain differences in the sensitivity of various types of solid allografts to rejection include lymphatic drainage, access of the host circulation to the graft by ingrowing host capillaries or direct anastomoses between recipient and donor blood vessels, and the extent to which recipient alloreactive cells come into contact with donor alloantigen presenting cell populations that express major histocompatibility complex (MHC) class II antigens, including tissue macrophages, dendritic cells

(Langerhans cells in skin), endothelial cells, and passenger leukocytes in the graft. As discussed in other chapters in this volume, there is convincing evidence to suggest that dendritic cells within the allograft are a major immunologic stimulus for elicitation of the rejection process [47,79,81].

For studies of cellular immune effector mechanisms within in vivo transplant models, the *immunosuppressive status of the recipient* can be a major variable. It is important to consider whether an immunosuppressed state exists or has been induced iatrogenically in the recipient and if so what type and treatment schedule of immunosuppressive agent is used (i.e., irradiation, antilymphocyte antibodies, cyclosporin, and steroids, among others). Apparent differences in the specificity and immunoregulatory action of such immunosuppressive treatment modalities are only beginning to be understood. It is not surprising, therefore, that a variable spectrum of histopathologic and immunohistopathologic features is encountered in rejecting allografts of immunosuppressed recipients. This is particularly true in human transplant recipients in whom the heterogeneity of pathologic parameters associated with rejection often limits diagnostic accuracy as well as varying the immunobiologic and clinical features of the rejection process. In contrast, the rejection of solid allografts in most normal, unmodified transplant recipients exhibits notably consistent histopathologic features. The conventional pattern is cellular rejection involving a patchy migration of heterogenous populations of infiltrating leukocytes through blood vessel walls associated with increased vascular permeability, accumulation of infiltrating cells within the interstitium, and endothelial changes. The infiltrating cells exhibit a preponderance of mixed lymphocyte and monocyte/macrophage subpopulations associated with varying degrees of tissue destruction and loss of graft function. It is also apparent that different immunosuppressive regimens can influence both the intensity of rejection activity and the nature of intragraft inflammatory responses [51].

Another consideration in studies of rejection effector mechanisms is the *species of origin* of the recipient-donor combination. There are dissimilarities in the susceptibility of different species to some alloimmune effector mechanisms. For example, complement-fixing antibodies against donor MHC alloantigens will often induce hyperacute rejection in the human, whereas seemingly analagous antibodies in certain rat strains can enhance or prolong the survival of a rat allograft indefinitely. The biologic basis for such discrepancies is not fully understood, but immunogenetic differences, particularly in the expression of class II MHC antigens on endothelial cells, have been suggested as a possible explanation [36,46]. A variety of procedures, including injection of limited amounts of specific antibodies, tissue antigens, or antigen-antibody complexes, may abrogate the rejection response resulting in prolonged graft tolerance in rats but apparently have limited effects in higher mammals. Despite some difficulties in extrapolation of rodent data to higher mammals, inbred rodent models have unique advantages for basic studies of allograft rejection, including availability of syngeneic, congenic, and allogeneic strains that permit control of histocompatibility factors in experimental design, economy, ease of handling, resilience to infection, and lower priority in animal welfare groups' concerns than the higher mammals.

RECENT APPROACHES TO DEFINE THE CELLULAR EFFECTOR MECHANISMS OF REJECTION

With the current impact of technological advances in the field of immunology, research efforts to elucidate the cellular and molecular basis of allograft rejection have intensified. Particularly relevant has been the development of monoclonal antibody reagents to identify and fractionate lymphocyte subpopulations [59,116] and macrophage/monocyte subpopulations [150] on the basis of surface phenotypic characteristics. Equally important has been the development of sensitive methods for analysis, such as fluorescent-activated cell sorters [58], enzyme-linked immunoassays [103], immunochemical staining techniques, such as the immunoperoxidase-biotin-avidin system [63], and T-cell cloning techniques [76]. Recent investigations on the effector mechanisms of graft rejection have mainly included (1) use of lymphocyte subset-specific monoclonal antibodies for direct analysis of infiltrating cells in tissue sections and in fine needle aspirates of rejecting allografts and for monitoring of lymphocyte subsets in the circulation and peripheral lymphoid tissues of recipients during rejection; (2) studies of functional properties of cultured and cloned lymphocytes obtained from the circulation, peripheral lymphoid tissues, and from the rejecting allograft; and (3) adoptive transfer studies using isolated lymphocyte subsets to transfer alloimmune reactivity from one animal to another.

TYPES OF REJECTION

Hyperacute Rejection

Hyperacute rejection occurs rapidly, often within minutes of establishing blood flow. The donor organ becomes mottled, cyanotic, and swollen, and transplant function ceases. Histologically, the reaction is characterized by heavy platelet deposition, endothelial damage in both large and small vessels, prominent polymorphonuclear (PMN) leukocyte infiltration, and relatively scant lymphocyte infiltration [35,161]. Antibodies have been shown to be deposited within the rejected kidneys, and this type of rejection is generally thought to be due to preformed humoral antibody directed against donor alloantigens. Theoretically, this reaction ought to be entirely preventable by proper cross-matching. In practice, improved techniques of cross-matching markedly reduced the incidence of hyperacute rejection, although this reaction still occurs in perhaps 0.1-1% of kidney transplants. The cross-match techniques require nonphysiologic conditions, such as addition of rabbit rather than human complement to demonstrate cytotoxic alloantibody. Thus, the exact etiology of hyperacute rejection has perhaps not been fully elucidated. Some investigators have suggested heightened cell-mediated immunity may be involved in hyperacute rejection [31], but if so, the nature of the effector mechanisms remain speculative.

Acute Rejection

Acute allograft rejection continues to be the most common cause of allograft loss in transplantation. Acute rejection episodes occur frequently in perhaps 75% or more of human related donor allografts and over 95% of cadaver allografts. Although the majority of acute rejection crises are initially reversed with steroids and/or ALG, there is evidence to indicate that acute allograft rejection continues to be seen with all types of immunosuppression, including recently improved regimens of cyclosporin and ALG. Thus, acute allograft rejection continues to be the main problem in posttransplant management of patients at the present time and can even occur in HLA identical donor-recipient pairs.

Woodruff first noted that acute rejection occurred far more commonly in the initial 6 weeks after allografting and decreased in both incidence and severity after this time [164]. Early clinical investigations noted that acute rejection seemed to occur in what could be described as a "crisis," literally an acute reaction occurring over a period of only hours to days [64]. Biopsy studies demonstrated that the inflammatory process was usually of much longer duration than the clinical reaction and that the inflammatory process seemed to build up to a crescendo, culminating in the clinical picture of acute rejection. It was noted that these "crises" could be reversed by the short-term (3-5 days) administration of high doses of steroids. Unfortunately, although the first rejection was usually reversed, the host often experienced a second or subsequent rejection crisis that was refractory to the steroid therapy, and the graft was lost to rejection.

The histopathologic features of acute rejection were described early in the history of transplant immunobiology, and there is considerable information on the pathology of allograft rejections from studies using light microscopy and electron microscopy [13,33,113, 119]. The reaction is characterized by an acute mononuclear cell infiltrate often associated with arteritis and perivascular cuffing of mononuclear cells. In virtually all organ allografts, rejection is associated with heavy patches of mononuclear cell infiltration in the interstitium of the allograft. In general, the infiltrating mononuclear cells are heterogeneous and consist of T cells, macrophages, B cells, and large granular lymphocytes (LGL), with occasional PMN, eosinophils, and basophils.

The pattern of cellular infiltration vary between organs and even within the same organ. In some instances, immunohistochemical studies have shown evidence of selected migration of mononuclear subsets to the interstitium or portions of it [40,88]. It is often difficult to interpret the results of histopathologic studies on biopsies of rejecting allografts, partly because of the uneven distribution of infiltrating cells in different areas of the rejecting allograft. There are also difficulties in establishing accurate correlations between morphologic and functional properties of mononuclear subpopulations. Furthermore, there are convincing data to indicate immunocompetent cells rapidly traffic in and out of allografts, presenting at any one time a transient glimpse rather than a complete picture of a dynamic process [3]. Many of the lymphoid cells found in the allograft may be bystanders, since a significant amount of lymphocyte traffic is known to be nonspecific [62,77,130]. Polymorphonuclear leukocytes, basophils, and eosinophils in rejecting allografts probably represent incidentally recruited cells that are not centrally related to the rejection process.

A common feature of human allograft rejection is endothelial damage. Since the primary interface between host and allograft is represented by the endothelial cells, which in humans express both class I and class II MHC antigens, it is not surprising that endothelial cells are poised targets for immunologic attack [5,48,111]. In contrast, class II MHC antigens are absent on rat endothelium [46,47], which may explain why endothelial damage is often less conspicuous in acutely rejecting rat allografts [19,145] and why alloantibodies reactive with donor class II MHC antigen specificities are benign or even beneficial to rat organ allografts but apparently deleterious to human organ allografts [46].

Recent studies of Hanto and colleagues have described how vascular permeability changes in the microvasculature may increase the traffic of immunocompetent cells into the allograft interstitium [61]. It is not known, however, if vascular permeability is a critical part of the alloactivation sequence since migration of cells in and out of the organ allografts can occur regularly, often with little evidence of immunologic injury. It has been suggested that the degree of vascular injury and presence of antibody-producing cells in the graft has the poorest prognosis for survival of the allograft [13,117,147]. Cellular infiltration within the interstitium of a graft can often be rapidly and completely reversed by immunosuppressive agents, especially the steroids, whereas vascular damage is more resistant to reversal by immunosuppressive drugs. Endothelial damage is usually associated with endothelial repair, including infiltration by macrophages and foamy cells with fat products, smooth muscle proliferation, and processes that resemble the pathologic picture of ordinary atherosclerosis.

Immunobiologists have long recognized that the acute rejection process can take two forms: (1) unmodified acute rejection, which normally occurs 5-7 days posttransplant in an immunocompetent host not treated to reduce rejection activity, and (2) modified acute rejection, which occurs in hosts treated with an immunosuppressive agent to dampen the alloimmune response. Modified acute rejection takes a milder form than unmodified acute rejection and often does not demonstrate many of the dramatic effects of unmodified rejection, such as rapid and complete loss of graft function, severe swelling of the allograft, and a systemic picture of marked inflammation with fever and tenderness at the graft site. This difference has been especially prominent with improved immunosuppressive agents and treatment protocols. A logical corollary of these findings, of course, would be that the cell-mediated immune process of allograft reactivity must also be modified by many of these treatments. In the human, in whom the immune system has been modified in virtually every transplant performed, the pattern of cell-mediated immunity is highly variable. However, immunosuppressive agents can serve as immunobiologic probes by which one may gain understanding of immunologic parameters relevant to allograft rejection by studying the modified host. In fact, it was largely from associative immune monitoring studies in recipients who were rendered severely T-cell depleted by drug therapy that the importance of T cells in acute human allograft rejection began to be appreciated [21,133]. Similarly, the importance of humoral immunity in blood vessel damage in graft rejection has become apparent following observations in transplant recipients treated with immunosuppressive agents that abrogate the cellular infiltration patterns but do not effectively block humoral rejection.

Chronic Rejection

Studies of long-term transplant patients have revealed the great majority of acute rejection episodes occur within the first 90 days posttransplant (except in the case of the heart, in which some late acute rejections may be seen). In contrast, chronic rejection can continue in an inexorable course. Patterns of chronic rejection take many different forms in different organs. In the kidney, a triad of pathologic findings include arteriosclerosis and nephrosclerosis related to endothelial damage, interstitial fibrosis related to damage and repair of elements in the interstitium, and glomerulonephritis resulting from damage in the glomeruli [114]. In human kidney transplants, the glomeruli appear to be a prime site of immunologic attack in chronic rejection. The role of cell-mediated immunity in glomerular damage in allografts is not well understood, partly because glomerular epithelial and mesangial cells may be damaged by recurrent disease, immune complexes, and many other pathologic processes unrelated to rejections. In the heart, the target of the chronic rejection process is mainly the large epicardial coronary vessels, although the smaller vessels are also altered to some degree. In the liver, where chronic rejection is perhaps least understood, the pathologic process resembles atherosclerosis and seems to take the form of cholestasis for the most part. Clearly, the most prominent target organ for most types of chronic rejection is the arterial endothelium. Although the mechanism of the chronic rejection pathologic process is not understood, earlier studies have indicated this type of rejection is mediated by antibody [66,112,114]. Studies from our laboratory suggested that antibody-dependent cell-mediated cytotoxicity (ADCC) may be important in chronic rejection [141,142]. Patients with demonstrable anti-donor ADCC have shown a high incidence of chronic rejection, and conversely, kidney transplant patients without detectable ADCC have exhibited a lower incidence of chronic rejection [75]. Since chronic rejection is the largest cause of graft loss over a prolonged period of time, it constitutes an important immunobiologic process that needs to be better understood if the survival of incompatible allografts is to be prolonged for great periods of time.

THE CENTRAL ROLE OF T CELLS IN REJECTION

It is generally recognized that thymus-derived (T) lymphocytes have an essential role in acute allograft rejection. Hosts naturally or experimentally deprived of T cells, including the nude mouse or thymectomized, irradiated, bone marrow reconstituted recipients, are unable to reject allografts in a first set fashion [98,118,165], a deficiency that is readily overcome in experimental transplant models by repopulating the host with viable syngeneic T cells [23,24,41,42,85,99,147]. In human transplant recipients effectively depleted of circulating T cells by prophylactic treatment with rabbit anti-thymocyte globulin, acute rejection rarely occurs during the period of T-cell lymphopenia, but often occurs during or after recovery of T-cell levels [135].

Current evidence implicates T-cell involvement at many levels of the alloimmune response including antigen recognition, immunoregulation, and cytolytic effector function. However, the actual cellular and molecular mechanism by which T lymphocytes orchestrate the rejection scenario and the donor-specific versus nonspecific nature of the response remains to be firmly established. The problem is complex since alloaggressive donor-directed T-cell activity may consist, on one hand, of direct cytotoxicity mediated by antigen-specific cytolytic T cells and, on the other hand, of inflammatory T-cell activity primarily related to the elaboration of a variety of lymphokines by noncytotoxic T cells. The soluble lymphokines can regulate (amplify or suppress) a specific or nonspecific antidonor response as well as recruit and activate other cells, such as macrophages, to execute antidonor cytotoxicity.

DIVERSIFICATION OF THE T-CELL SYSTEM INTO DISTINCT SUBSETS

The mature postthymic T-cell population has proven to be heterogeneous both in the expression of cell membrane differentiation antigens and in functional properties [14,59,116]. Based upon functional parameters, T cells can be grouped into major populations that mediate either delayed-type hypersensitivity (DTH)-associated mediator release (Tdth), helper (Th), inducer (Ti), cytotoxic (Tc), or suppressor (Ts) activities. Based on the expression of cell membrane differentiation markers, the T-cell system appears to contain two dominant subpopulations. In humans and several nonhuman primate species, the T-cell population is subdivided into the T4 and T8 subsets, respectively [116]. In mice the analogous T-cell subsets are the Ly 1^+ and Ly 2^+ populations [59], and in rats they are the W3/25^+ and $OX8^+$ populations, respectively [92].

The human $T4^+$, murine Ly 1^+, and rat W3/25^+ subsets principally contain T cells that express helper and inducer activities and constitute the main population of responding cells in allogeneic one-way mixed lymphocyte culture responses (MLR). In allogeneic responses, this T-cell subset tends to respond to I region encoded (class II) MHC gene products [123]. Furthermore, the antigen-specific function of the Th/i subset is usually restricted by I region encoded alloantigens. Cells of the T-helper subset are usually activated by antigen present in conjunction with class II antigens on antigen-presenting cells. Sensitized T cells expressing the Th/i subset phenotype produce lymphokines upon contact with antigen and mediate delayed-type hypersensitivity reactions. Release of lymphokines, such as macrophage activation factor [70], γ interferon [109], and interleukin-2 (IL-2) [32], can elicit a local accumulation of nonspecific accessory cells. Although most lymphokines are not directly destructive to tissue, the local influx of activated accessory mononuclear cells can indirectly induce pathologic changes characteristic of delayed hypersensitivity reaction.

The human $T8^+$, murine Ly 2^+, and rat $OX8^+$ subsets comprise cells that express antigen-specific, MHC-restricted, cytotoxic effector activity, cytotoxic precursor cells that can be elicited by in vitro allogeneic stimulation, and suppressor cells that negatively regulate cellular and humoral immune responses. The response of this T-cell subset is usually dependent upon the activity of the helper or inducer T-cell subset and/or the soluble products released by activated Th/i cells, such as interleukin 2 [32]. Class I MHC alloantigens have a major role in the immunologic specificity and restriction properties of the Ts/c subset. In alloimmune responses cytotoxic T lymphocytes (CTL) respond mainly to class I MHC alloantigens, and cytotoxic responses to viral and soluble antigen or hapten-conjugated cells are restricted by class I MHC antigens [123].

Although there is strong evidence supporting the concept of T-cell diversification on the basis of monoclonal antibody-defined subsets, the subdivisions may be artificial. Multiple functions are attributed to each of these subsets, and some functional overlap has been observed. For example, cloned CTL lines have been shown to express helper activity [160] and to produce lymphokines capable of activating macrophages [70,109]. Furthermore, cloned T-cell lines with the helper/inducer phenotype have been shown to be cytotoxic against MHC class II antigen targets [78,125] and also to class I antigen targets [128]. These overlapping functions of T-cell subsets make it difficult to draw valid inferences about the in vivo biologic properties of T-cell subsets defined only by surface markers.

There are recent data indicating T-cell subsets may be further subdivided on the basis of monoclonal antibody-defined surface markers. Additional differentiation antigens expressed on the human $T4^+$ subset (e.g., TQ1, 2H4, Leu 8) appear to distinguish suppressor-inducer T cells and mixed leukocyte culture-reactive T cells from the T cells that provide helper function for B cells [37,38,80,101,102]. It is yet unclear how the DTH function of human $T4^+$ cells fits into these phenotypic subdivisions.

The cytotoxic and suppressive properties of human $T8^+$ cells and the analogous Tc/s subsets of other species have been difficult to distinguish on the basis of surface membrane markers. The Ly 1-Ly 2/3 phenotype of the cytotoxic/suppressor T-cell subset in mice appears to be variable and depends on the nature of the antigens used for immunization [59]. However, the expression of Qa-1 and I-J antigens can distinguish the Ly $2/3^+$ cells with suppressor activity [95]. In humans, the cells involved in immunoregulatory circuits are less well defined. Recent evidence indicates human suppressor $T8^+$ cells may be distinguished from $T8^+$ cytotoxic cells by the presence of Leu 15/D12 marker [20] and by the expression of HLA-DR (Ia) antigens [38]. The use of simultaneous multiparameter fluorescence to define relevant subdivisions of T4 and T8 subsets infiltrating rejecting allografts is likely to provide new insights into the cellular immune mechanism of graft rejection. For example, recent studies of fine needle aspirates of human kidneys in our laboratory suggest that rejecting kidneys contain elevated numbers of Leu 2^+, Leu 15^- T cells (putatively cytotoxic cells) compared to nonrejecting human kidneys that have higher levels of Leu $2a^+$, Leu 15^+ cells (putatively suppressor cells; U. Gross, P. Cunningham, et al., unpublished observations).

THE CONTROVERSY OVER WHICH T-CELL SUBSET IS THE EFFECTOR OF REJECTION

Two dominant hypotheses have been elaborated to explain the cell-mediated effector mechanism of allograft rejection. Early studies based largely upon histologic and ultrastructural analysis of rejection allografts suggested T cells cause rejection by a delayed-type hypersensitivity mechanism [11]. According to the DTH concept of graft rejection, small numbers of antigen-specific sensitized T cells entering the graft would locally release a variety of lymphokines. Among the most well studied lymphokines is IL-2, which is required for the differentiation of cytotoxic T-cell precursors into functionally active cytotoxic T cells [32] and also for optimal cytotoxic function of natural killer cells and K cells mediating antibody-dependent cellular cytotoxicity [69]. Other T-cell lymphokines, such as macrophage activating factor [70] and γ interferon [34,109], activate macrophages to become cytotoxic. These lymphokines also enhance the expression of Ia antigens on macrophages, which in turn can augment macrophage antigen-presenting capability for reactive T cells [7]. Such lymphokines could presumably bring about intragraft localization and activation of mixed populations of nonspecific cells, particularly macrophages, resulting in damage to the surrounding tissue. This DTH mechanism is theoretically very economical in that the function of very few specifically sensitized T-helper cells could be efficiently amplified to cause large areas of tissue destruction via nonspecific effector cell activity.

On the other hand, the putative nonspecificity of the inflammatory effector cells involved in DTH is difficult to reconcile with early studies in allophenic mice showing specific destruction of individual allogeneic cells within a mixed population [100]. The allophenic mouse is obtained experimentally by fusing early embryo blastomeres of different MHC genotypes and is a genetic mosaic with phenotypically distinguishable MHC subpopulations of cells in any tissue. Mintz and Silvers studied allograft rejection in an allophenic mouse model containing a mosaic of C3H ($H2^k$, $H2^k$) and C57BL ($H2^b$, $H2^b$) genotypes. After transplanting an allophenic skin graft to either an H2k/H2k recipient or an $H2^b$/$H2^b$ recipient, the incompatible melanocytes were focally destroyed while closely adjacent, histocompatible melanocytes remained viable. The extraordinary specificity of the rejection process in these experiments, that is, identification and destruction of single cells in mosaic skin grafts, suggests a highly specific, discriminating effector mechanism, such as T-cell-mediated cytotoxicity, is operative.

In vitro studies demonstrated that stimulation of responding lymphocytes with allogenic cells differing at the major histocompatibility complex elicits both proliferative and cytotoxic responses to the stimulated cells [49]. As more became understood about the characteristics and fine immunologic specificity of cytotoxic T lymphocytes, the CTL hypothesis of graft rejection emerged as an alternative to the earlier DTH hypothesis [4,18, 149]. The expansion and elicitation of alloantigen-specific cytotoxic effector cells has proven to be a multifaceted process, involving the interaction of mononuclear phagocytes, multiple T-cell subsets, and soluble factors, including interleukins 1 and 2. Furthermore, the prediction of functional activity of T-lymphocyte populations on the basis of surface differentiation antigens seems to be more complicated than previously considered. For example, T cells derived from a single clone have been found to express multiple functions, including both DTH and CTL activity [25]. At present, much of the evidence supporting exclusive DTH or CTL hypotheses of rejection remains circumstantial, and no single mechanism has been unequivocally proven to mediate the rejection process.

STUDIES FROM ADOPTIVE TRANSFER MODELS IN RODENTS

In the past few years, the CTL concept of graft rejection has been called into question as a result of adoptive transfer studies in rodents [23,84,85]. In the adoptive transfer type of experimental model, immunoincompetent hosts can be reconstituted with defined lymphoid cell populations, which theoretically permits analysis of a particular cell population or cellular immune mechanism. Using thymectomized, irradiated, adult mice repopulated with syngeneic bone marrow (ATXBM mice), Loveland and McKenzie [85] attempted to reconstitute the ability to reject allografts by infusing fractionated syngeneic T-cell subpopulations. They fractionated sensitized T cells into Ly 1^+ (T helper/inducer) and Ly 1^- (T cytotoxic/suppressor) subsets, and they showed that transfer of Ly 1^+ T lymphocytes from spleen and lymph nodes could lead to rejection of skin allografts. Furthermore, the Ly 1^+-reconstituted recipients exhibited positive DTH responses following rejection. In contrast, when Ly 1^+ cells were depleted from the reconstituting inoculum, challenge skin grafts failed to undergo rejection. Similar patterns were obtained for allograft responses generated to H2 alloantigens using either skin, melanoma, or lymphoma transplants and lead to the conclusion that Ly 1^+ cells are necessary and sufficient to mediate rejection in immunodeficient ATXBM mice [86]. In keeping with this view, other studies have shown cloned T-helper cells can mediate in vivo allograft rejection in mice when inoculated into syngeneic recipients [74]. Furthermore, the known immunostimulatory activity of vitamin A in promoting allograft rejection has been shown by adoptive transfer studies to be mediated by T cells with an Ly 1^+ phenotype [90].

Studies in ATXBM rats reconstituted with syngeneic bone marrow from T-cell-deficient donors have also indicated that infusion of sensitized syngeneic splenic T-helper cells ($OX8^-$, $W3/25^+$) can induce a rapid rejection of cardiac and renal allografts in the rat [41, 54]. Infusion of sensitized $OX8^+$ cytotoxic cells along with exogenous interleukin 2-rich culture supernatants failed to promote allograft rejection. Thus, the T-cell subset containing strong in vitro cytotoxic activity did not induce rejection in the ATXBM rat, despite the administration of lymphokines. However, in two studies the $OX8^+$ cells did exhibit a striking synergy with $OX8^-$, $W3/25^+$ cells in accelerating the tempo of rejection, and $OX8^+$ T cells were shown to infiltrate the cardiac allografts more extensively than the $W3/25^+$, $OX8^-$ population [43,54]. Collectively, the results of these adoptive transfer studies implicate a pivotal role for the Th/i subset in the rejection of allografts in the ATXBM model, but they do not exclude a major role of CTL. There are many lingering questions from these studies. How complete is the depletion of T cells in the recipients? Is the function of transferred CTL altered or inhibited in an abnormal immunologic environment favoring unresponsiveness? Could the failure of the Tc/s subset to induce rejection in ATXBM recipients be related to suppressor cell activity transferred within the reconstituting subset, which might be intensified in the ATXBM host environment? These studies do strongly suggest, however, that if cytotoxic T cells have a role in the rejection process, they probably do not mediate allograft rejection in ATXBM rodent recipients without the support of cells that express phenotypic properties of the Th/i subset.

An implicit assumption in the ATXBM/T-cell subset repopulation studies mentioned above is that the host alloimmune system is inert, since ATXBM hosts do not acutely reject allografts. Actually, it is quite difficult to develop a truly T-cell-free adult host, and it is known that nude mice [39] and ATXBM recipients [30] have alloreactive cytotoxic T-cell precursors. The adoptive transfer experiments do not exclude the possibility that inactive precursor CTL in the recipients might become activated by products of the reconstituting T-helper/inducer cell subset and go on to actually mediate the allogeneic tissue destruction process. There are other data from adoptive transfer studies in ATXBM recipients and rats that can be interpreted to support the hypothesis that CTL do mediate allograft rejection. Dallman and Mason [23] showed that, although they could induce skin allograft rejection in ATXBM rats by infusing the W3/25$^+$ subset of syngeneic thoracic duct T cells, the rejected allografts became predominantly infiltrated with cells with the OX8$^+$ phenotype. In contrast, adoptively transferred OX8$^+$ thoracic duct T cells failed either to restore a rejection response or to result in heavy infiltration of the graft with OX8$^+$ cells. This experiment suggested that the T-cell-deprived ATXBM rat reconstituted with OX8$^-$ T cells contains a population of OX8$^+$ precursor cells that can be triggered to respond to allogeneic tissue in the presence of the transferred T-helper/inducer cells. Rat Th/i are known to be the main producers of IL-2, which is required for amplification and differentiation of CTL precursors [16]. The CTL precursors in ATXBM animals could be derived from radioresistant host cells or from donor cells that escaped the depletion procedure.

In support of this view are the findings of LeFrancois and Bevan [82], who performed adoptive transfer studies in a stringent ATXBM mouse model in which the syngeneic bone marrow was T-cell depleted by a combination of two methods. The bone marrow donors received an in vivo treatment with antithymocyte serum before harvesting the marrow, which was further depleted of residual T cells by in vitro incubation with a mixture of T-cell-specific monoclonal antibodies. These investigators showed that Thy 1.2 ATXBM mice that receive either adoptively transferred Ly 1$^+$ or Ly 2$^+$ spleen T cells from a congenic Thy 1.1 donor can reject skin allografts expressing minor histocompatibility antigens. Moreover, the results indicated that the recipients adoptively transferred with Ly 2-depleted Thy 1.1 T cells develop graft-specific CTL of host (i.e., Thy 1.2) origin. Thus, on the basis of these elegant studies, the notion that CTL mediate allograft destruction certainly cannot be laid to rest and remains a viable hypothesis.

T-CELL SUBSETS IN HUMAN KIDNEY ALLOGRAFTS

In the human, fine needle aspiration studies have indicated that acute graft rejection is associated with a major infiltration of the OKT8$^+$ cytotoxic-suppressor T-cell subset and less infiltration by the OKT4 helper/inducer T-cell subset [44,155]. In addition, infiltrating cells extracted from acutely rejecting human allografts have been shown to exhibit donor-directed T-cell cytotoxic activity [145,146,156]. Phenotypic analyses of infiltrating cells in situ in frozen or fixed specimens of acutely rejecting allografts have also shown that the cytotoxic/suppressor T-cell subset is usually represented in larger numbers than the helper T-cell subset [45,53]. Conversely, in quiescent or nonrejecting human allografts, as in nonrejecting allografts in irradiated, enhanced, or cyclosporin-treated rats [10], the number of infiltrating cells expressing the phenotype of the T-helper/inducer subset tends to be higher than the number of cells expressing the cytotoxic/suppressor phenotype. Thus, this pattern seems to prevail in both experimental animal and human allografts undergoing acute rejection. There is some disagreement on this point, and several investigators have demonstrated an opposite pattern with a preponderance of the T-helper subset in rejecting grafts [12,40,153]. In general the phenotypic ratios of Th/i and Tc/s subsets in rejecting human allografts do not have clear prognostic indications for the reversibility of the rejection episode with immunosuppressive agents. However, one group has suggested that, although the Tc/s subset predominates in acute rejection episodes, the irreversibility of rejection is associated with high levels of Th/i cells in the graft [53,155]. Perhaps finer analyses of these major T-cell subsets with activation markers and also additional markers to distinguish components with helper versus suppressor inducer or cytotoxic versus suppressor effector activity will improve our understanding of cellular mechanisms that mediate graft rejection in humans.

OTHER ASSOCIATIONS BETWEEN CTL ACTIVITY AND ALLOGRAFT REJECTION

The hypothesis implicating alloantigen-directed CTL as principal mediators of allograft rejection is supported by several additional lines of evidence. In most mammalian species, cytotoxic lymphocytes are regularly induced during allograft rejection [1,2,17,18,52,126, 136,149]. In contrast, allospecific anti-donor CTL are infrequently detected in tolerant recipients [9,73,89,94,131,136]. Furthermore, the results of some studies indicate the allospecific reactivity of cytotoxic precursors to donor cells may become deficient or suppressed in operationally tolerant allograft recipients [15,60,68,120], including successful human transplant recipients [28,139,140,143,144,163]. During allograft rejection, effector cells exhibiting specific antidonor cytotoxicity have been recovered from peripheral lymphoid tissue, the circulation, the rejecting allograft [51,147], and artificial sponge matrix allografts [1,2]. Furthermore, recent evidence indicates that cloned CTL lines can result in alloantigen-specific, MHC-restricted, dose-dependent tissue destruction of allogeneic skin [110,152] and ascites tumors [110] when injected into nonimmunosuppressed recipients.

On the other hand, comparative studies of T-cell responses to minor histocompatibility antigens in skin allograft recipients have shown the appearance of a DTH response to alloantigens gave a better correlation than the CTL response, which was frequently observed after, not before, rejection [124]. Furthermore, the high number of sensitized effector cells required to kill relevant allogeneic target cells in vitro (commonly a 100:1 ratio) and the prolonged incubation period required to detect significant cytotoxicity in vitro (usually 4-8 hr) has caused investigators to doubt the in vivo efficiency of the CTL effector pathway compared to the DTH effector pathway, in which small amounts of lymphokine released by antigen-specific T cells can bring about major tissue destruction via the recruitment and activation of accessory cells. In studies of lymphocyte trafficking in a mouse sponge matrix allograft model, however, Ascher and colleagues demonstrated that precursor CTL are recruited to the allograft and undergo maturation directly within the allograft [1]. Recent studies show cloned CTL upon contact with specific antigen can release lymphokines, such as interleukin-2 which is required for expansion of CTL [87,115], and γ interferon [70] which is capable of activating macrophages. Thus, in addition to being sufficient, discriminative killers of allogeneic target cells, CTL may be able to locally regulate their own activity and that of accessory macrophages.

Another approach to the study of effector mechanisms in rejection has been to abrogate the rejection process in adult recipients with a tolerance-inducing immunosuppressive treatment protocol and correlate the presence or absence of in vitro defined effector mechanisms with survival or rejection of the allograft. Using this type of approach, Bradley et al. [10] treated DA strain rat renal allograft recipients with either cyclosporin A (CsA) or enhancing alloantibody to prevent rejection and compared specific antidonor CTL activity and nonspecific natural killer (NK) cell-like activity in the two treated recipient groups and in unmodified recipients with rejecting allografts. They found CsA-treated and enhanced recipients exhibited a specific deficiency of antidonor CTL activity while largely retaining nonspecific cytotoxicity. Thus, the immunosuppressive effectiveness of CsA and enhancing antibody in promoting allograft acceptance was associated with the absence of specific donor-directed CTL activity. Our studies in primate allograft recipients have led us to a similar conclusion. We have utilized a primate model of renal allograft tolerance in which long-term survival of MHC-incompatible rhesus monkey allografts can be obtained following treatment with ATG and donor bone marrow in the absence of chronic immunosuppression [134,137]. In this model of transplant tolerance, in vivo generated antidonor CTL activity is specifically deficient compared with nontolerant controls, but the CTL responses of tolerant recipients to third party and the nonspecific NK activity to K562 are similar to that of normal controls [136]. The specific absence of antidonor CTL responses in nonrejecting rodent and primate organ allograft recipients suggests by inference that this effector mechanism is important in organ allograft rejection.

NK Cells

Studies of human kidney [53,91,159], human heart [91], and rat kidney allografts [104] indicate that large granular lymphocytes (LGL) are among the first cells to appear during rejection. The LGL population has been shown in most species to contain natural killer cells, which destroy certain tumor and virally infected target cells in the absence of known prior immunization [56,57]. The precise lineage of these cells is not clearly established. However, the NK cell population is known to be derived from bone marrow and expresses unique phenotypic characteristics as well as other phenotypic characteristics associated partially with T lymphocytes and also with monocyte and myeloid cells [72,151].

Natural killer cells are believed to have a role in the control of malignancies and viral infections [56,57] and in rejection of bone marrow transplants [71]. Their possible role in the rejection of organ allografts is still unknown. Recent findings indicate human NK cells may recognize transferrin receptors that are expressed on malignant cell lines [154]. Since transferrin receptors are also expressed on activated lymphocytes, it has been postulated that NK cell activity may represent a homeostatic control mechanism for regulating blast cell transformation in malignant, hematopoietic, and immunostimulated lymphoid cell populations.

Serial studies of LGL and NK activity in rat renal allografts revealed striking differences in the timing and location of NK and CTL activity in the spleen and graft [104]. Nemlander and Hayry observed sequential phases of high NK activity, first in the spleen, then in the graft, and again in the spleen, suggesting an NK traffic circuit between spleen and allograft. Peak intragraft NK activity occurred very early and was not synchronized with peak CTL activity, which occurred at the time of rejection. Beschorner's findings in human renal allografts also indicate that NK-like cells (phenotypically Leu 7^{+}) accumulate in allografts very early in the course of rejection episodes before clinical manifestations of rejection are evident [8]. On the basis of these reports, it is questionable that NK cells act as final effectors of kidney allograft rejection, since NK activity seems to both peak and decline well before rejection is discernible. Furthermore, the presence of active NK-like cells in allografted organs does not clarify if and how NK activity might be linked to the rejection process. Active NK cells have also been recovered from nonrejecting rat kidney allografts in enhanced or cyclosporin-treated hosts [10]. Furthermore, no target for NK cells has been found in renal allografts [105]. Thus, the role of NK mechanisms in allograft rejection remains poorly understood.

It is possible that NK cells have a role in the maturation or regulation of CTL and/or other immunocompetent cells [22]. Natural killer cells have documented immunoregulatory activity, the best known of which is their ability to produce interferon in response to stimulation with adjuvants, viruses, mitogens, and other agents [55]. By producing interferon, NK cells could provide an accessory function to activate local macrophages [112] and/or suppress lymphoproliferative responses and antibody production [67].

Antibody-Dependent Cellular Cytotoxicity

The population of killer (K) cells mediating antibody-dependent cellular cytotoxicity (ADCC) is phenotypically indistinguishable from the NK population [55]. In addition to sharing common membrane antigen phenotypes, both NK and K cells have IgG Fc receptors capable of affixing cytophilic antibody. In normal individuals, there is usually a high correlation between ADCC and NK activity, although there are documented dissociations of NK and K activity in immunosuppressed [27,83] and in tumor-bearing hosts [107]. Unlike NK cells, which are directly cytotoxic to certain sensitive targets in vitro, K cells are indiscriminantly cytotoxic to most nucleated target cells provided the latter are sensitized with IgG antibody. There are also instances in which K cells appear to exert direct cytotoxic activity when they are armed with cytophilic antibodies via Fc receptors [56].

The apparent phenotypic similarities between K and NK cells suggest the same cell might mediate both cytotoxic activities. Since NK cells have been found in rejecting allografts, the question is raised whether K cell activity (i.e., ADCC) could be involved in graft rejection. The available data are controversial on this point but overall suggest ADCC may be an ancillary allograft effector mechanism.

Tilney and colleagues demonstrated high levels of antidonor ADCC activity within the infiltrating cell population of rejecting rat heart allografts in unmodified recipients [129,146,149]. Furthermore, at least half the cells recovered from rejecting grafts were found to exhibit Fc receptors. Recent studies of Nemlander et al. have shown strong donor-directed ADCC in the spleens of unmodified rats rejecting renal allografts, although lower levels were found in the graft [105]. Our group has monitored donor-directed ADCC in the peripheral blood of rhesus monkey kidney allograft recipients that received either no immunosuppression or ATG immunosuppression [136]. In unmodified rejection, CTL activity was regularly demonstrable, but ADCC was not demonstrable. In contrast, delayed rejection occurring in ATG-treated primates was consistently associated with both donor-directed CTL and ADCC activity. Thus, depending on the duration of transplant function, as well as the presence and possibly the type of immunosuppression used, the relative importance of ADCC in rejection may vary considerably.

In human transplant recipients, specific donor-directed ADCC has been associated with acute rejection in some studies [29,79,126,127,132], but in other studies ADCC has been infrequently detected during rejection [162]. Several reports have demonstrated the presence of antidonor ADCC in recipients with functioning transplants and consequently suggested it does not represent a relevant effector mechanism of rejection. We monitored antidonor ADCC in a series of long-term recipients (2-10 years posttransplant) and found a highly significant association with clinical and histopathologic indications of chronic rejection [141]. The ADCC-positive individuals all had functioning allografts, but the graft function was progressively deteriorating. Thus, on the basis of available information, ADCC would appear to represent a highly sensitive, ancillary effector mechanism that may have an important role in delayed or chronic rejection in immunosuppressed hosts and/or perhaps in genetic recipient/donor combinations that tend to preferentially elicit alloantibody responses.

MACROPHAGES IN REJECTION

Virtually all experimental and clinical studies of infiltrating cells from acutely rejecting allografts show a high proportion of macrophages, with the most frequent range 20-60% [19,45,158]. The role of mononuclear phagocytes, possibly macrophage subpopulations, in the process of allograft rejection is not well understood. Several lines of evidence indicate that increased vascular permeability, fibronectin, and T-cell-derived lymphokines—MAF, γ interferon, and others—are responsible for localization of macrophages in areas of inflammatory injury, including allograft sites. It is difficult to establish the extent to which macrophages are active effectors of allograft destruction or are involved in an accessory role, such as amplification of the alloimmune T-cell response, or in repair, or merely represent inactive bystanders. For example, macrophages appear to infiltrate both rejecting allografts as well as nonrejecting grafts in syngeneic recipients and in ATXBM allogeneic recipients [93]. On the other hand, infiltrating macrophages in rejecting allografts have been shown to exert antidonor cytotoxicity [157,158]. Perhaps a heterogenicity of cytotoxic effector populations is required by the variable sensitivity of target cell types to different cellular cytotoxicity mechanisms. The observation of Christmas and MacPherson showing the differential distribution of macrophages in the interstitium of rejecting cardiac allografts and lymphocytes in the perivascular areas [19] is particularly intriguing in the light of their finding that only the adherent infiltrating cell population exhibited cytotoxicity to the myocardial cells [88].

It has been suggested that the presence of large numbers of macrophages in the rejecting allograft is associated with a poor prognosis [50]. However, it is not established whether the prevalence of cells of the monocyte/macrophage series is a cause or consequence of irreversible tissue injury, a question of considerable importance for purposes of therapeutic intervention. Attempts to study the role of macrophages in rejection are confounded by a number of variables and by the inability to establish in vivo models of macrophage depletion. As discussed by MacPherson, all models of macrophage depletion, including antimacrophage serum and poisoning of reticuloendothelial cells, fail to achieve effective ablation of either macrophage numbers or activity. Perhaps the best we are left with is a strong suggestion that macrophages may well be an important effector cell in allograft rejection and a strong belief in the great need for better studies of these poorly understood cells in the future.

Macrophage Production of IL-1

It has long been recognized that the macrophage has an important function in antigen processing for optimal elicitation of in vitro alloimmune responses. More recently, it has been shown that cells of the monocyte/macrophage lineage produce the lymphokine interleukin-1 (IL-1). The role of the macrophage in inducing acute inflammation and in amplifying allograft reactivity could well be related to IL-1 production. This lymphokine has systemic effects, producing fever and negative nitrogen balance, and can also trigger a cascade of local inflammatory activities [26,108]. Interleukin-1 stimulates T-helper cells to produce IL-2, which in turn leads to expansion and amplification of activated cytotoxic

T-cell clones and other T-cell-dependent immune responses. In addition, this lymphokine acts to stimulate B-cell proliferation and augments suppressor T-cell activity as well as natural killer activity, probably primarily through its action in stimulating the production of IL-2. Interleukin-1 is also known to stimulate fibroblast proliferation [121], which might contribute to the chronic inflammatory processes seen in chronic allograft rejection.

The effects of pharmacologic agents on IL-1 production are important considerations for the clinical management of transplant recipients. For example, nonsteroidal anti-inflammatory agents do not decrease IL-1 production and can actually enhance IL-2 release [108]. Cyclosporin, a potent inhibitor of IL-2 production, apparently has no direct effect on IL-1 production. In contrast, both in vitro and in vivo pharmacologic doses of steroids act to strongly inhibit or suppress completely the production of IL-1 [26]. This would seem to provide a rationale to support the use of high doses of steroids in the early posttransplant period when inflammatory reactions involving IL-1 may be occurring in the recently transplanted allograft.

Our understanding is still rudimentary regarding the biochemical mechanisms that regulate IL-1 production by macrophages as well as the in vivo relevance to cellular immune effector mechanisms of graft rejection. Much work will be necessary in this area before it is known what pharmacologic agents might be useful in the modulation of production and/or activity of this potent stimulator of inflammation.

IMMUNOCOMPETENT CELL MIGRATION PATTERNS DURING REJECTION

Hematopoietic cells are known to have characteristic migration patterns. For example, the vast majority of polymorphonuclear leukocytes appear to be marginated in the small capillaries of the body, and only a small portion circulate freely within the peripheral bloodstream. Lymphocytes migrate in massive numbers between the bloodstream and the lymphatic vessel space, finally converging via the lymphatics to the thoracic duct, where they are returned to the bloodstream. Early studies showed modification of the lymphatic drainage of a skin allograft can change the patterns of rejection of [6]. On the other hand, the isolation of a primarily vascularized kidney allograft from its lymphatic connections was shown not to prevent or modify the rejection response [65].

During the course of allograft rejection, immunocompetent cells appear to migrate among various lymphoid depots in the body, the peripheral circulation, the lymphatic circulatory channels, and the allograft [3,51]. The allograft is often distant from lymphoid compartments, and presumably, the migration patterns of lymphoid cells are related to immunologic mechanisms designed to recruit and concentrate immunocompetent cells in the allograft. Nemlander et al. [106] studied the flow of white cell traffic to and from rat renal allografts in unmodified hosts and found the traffic was bidirectional and increased exponentially until day 4. Thereafter, proliferative activity occurred within the specific compartment with little intercompartmental exchange.

Most of the infiltrating cells found in allografts do not exhibit donor-specific reactivity [2,3,51,62,130]. The reason that large numbers of nonspecific immunocompetent cells accumulate early after transplantation is not clear. Certainly, the ischemic injury and the trauma of reimplantation could elicit inflammatory stimuli associated with wound healing. In fine needle aspirates of monkey kidney allografts taken hours after transplantation, data from our laboratory indicate infiltrating cells contain about 40% $OKM1^+$ cells with cytologic characteristics of monocytes and macrophages (U. Gross, unpublished observations). In rat allograft models the early inflammatory cell influx during the first 4-5 days has been found to be largely nonspecific, containing high levels of macrophages and NK cells [23,94,104]. Even with syngeneic grafts and allografts in immunoincompetent ATXBM rats, infiltrating macrophages are prominent early after transplantation [23].

In addition to the nonspecific inflammatory cells infiltrating allografts, studies of unmodified sponge matrix allografts [3] and vascularized organ allografts [51] have shown there is an accumulation of specific donor-reactive cytotoxic cells and helper cells in the peripheral lymphoid compartments and in the allograft. In the experience of Hayry's group, the profile of CTL activity follows the T-cell blastogenesis profile with generation of immunoblasts in situ. In the rat renal allograft, donor-specific CTL are usually found in the spleen within 4-5 days posttransplant and simultaneously or shortly thereafter within the allograft [105]. Circulating T cells also exhibit direct cytotoxicity against donor target cells, but CTL activity is demonstrable in the blood of rats only after rejection. This pattern may be variable, however, as our studies in rhesus monkeys have regularly detected antidonor CTL in the circulation before kidney allograft rejection [136]. In unmodified rejection, there seems to be a much higher level of CTL activity in the allograft than in any of the systemic lymphoid depots [105]. Whether this represents the local differentiation and expansion of donor-reactive CTL or selective migration of these cells into the graft is not certain. However, the elegant study of Ascher et al. [1] supports the former notion. These investigators placed sponge matrix allografts on recipient mice and then irradiated the recipients on day 5 with one of the grafts selectively shielded from irradiation. Anti-donor cytotoxic cells developed to a much higher level in the unshielded sponge matrix allograft, leading to the conclusion that CTL recruitment to the graft is independent of the host lymphoid system after day 5. This result supports the findings of Nemlander's group indicating there is little cellular exchange between rat lymphoid compartments and the allograft after day 4 [106]. Presumably, cytolytic precursors present in the allograft matured in situ into cytolytic cells sometime after day 5. If this presumption is correct, then the migration of lymphocytes and inflammatory cells and antidonor cells into the allograft is probably most important in the early stages of rejection and less important during the latter stages when specific alloaggressive mechanisms within the allograft may become independent of lymphoreticular traffic.

SUMMARY

In summary, recent studies of alloaggressive events involved in graft rejection indicate that the rejection reaction consists of a constellation of effector mechanisms. These destructive processes, which include both immunologically specific and nonspecific inflammatory components, are heterogeneous in nature and may vary greatly with the immunosuppressive status and species of the transplant recipient. Although a large volume of information has been accrued about intragraft rejection mechanisms, a comprehensive concept of the process of allograft destruction has yet to be formulated. Much of the evidence reviewed in this chapter implicates cytotoxic T cells as primary effectors of most acute allograft rejection reactions. However, noncytotoxic T cells and non-T-cell mechanisms also play a role in rejection. As more is learned about this complex biologic response, development of more effective and specific immunosuppression for transplantation is likely to follow.

ACKNOWLEDGMENTS

We are grateful to Maureen Fox and Angie Cox for their excellent assistance and patience in helping prepare this manuscript.

REFERENCES

1. Ascher, N. L., Chen, S., Hoffman, R., and Simmons, R. L. Maturation of cytotoxic effector cells at the site of allograft rejection. *Transplant. Proc.* 13:1105-1107, 1981.
2. Ascher, N. L., Ferguson, R. M., Hoffman, R., and Simmons, R. L. Partial characterization of cytotoxic cells infiltrating sponge matrix allografts. *Transplant* 27:254-259, 1979.
3. Ascher, N. L., Hoffman, R., Hanto, D., and Simmons, R. Cellular basis of allograft rejection. *Immunol. Rev.* 77:217-232, 1984.
4. Bach, F., Bach, M., and Sondel, P. Differential function of major histocompatibility complex antigens in T-lymphocyte activation. *Nature* 259:273-278, 1976.
5. Baldwin, W. M., Class, P., van Es, A., and van Rood, J. HLA A, B, Dr and endothelial-specific antigens in kidney graft rejection. *Immunol. Today* 1:110-111, 1980.
6. Barker, C., and Billingham, R. The role of regional lymphatics in the skin homograft response. *Transplantation* 5:962-967, 1967.
7. Beller, D. I., and Unanue, E. R. Regulation of macrophage populations. I. Preferential induction of Ia^- rich peritoneal exudates by immunologic stimuli. *J. Immunol.* 124:1426-1432, 1981.
8. Beshorner, W., Burdick, J., Williams, G., and Solez, K. The presence of Leu 7 reactive lymphocytes in renal allografts undergoing acute rejection. *Transplant. Proc.* 17: 618-622, 1985.
9. Biesecker, J., Fitch, F., Rowley, D., Scollard, D., and Stuart, F. Cellular and humoral immunity after allogeneic transplantation in the rat. II. Comparison of a ^{51}Cr release assay and modified microcytotoxicity assay for detection of cellular immunity and blocking serum factors. *Transplantation* 16:421-431, 1973.
10. Bradley, J. A., Mason, D. W., and Morris, P. J. Evidence that rat renal allografts are rejecting cytotoxic T cells and not by nonspecific effectors. *Transplantation* 39:169-175, 1985.
11. Brent, L., Brown, I., and Medawar, P. Quantitative studies on tissue transplantation immunity. IV. Hypersensitivity reactions associated with the rejection of homografts. *Proc. R. Soc. Lond.* [*Biol.*] 156:187-209, 1962.
12. Burdick, J., Beschorner, W., Smith, W., McGraw, D., Bender, W., Williams, G., and Solez, K. Lymphocytes in early renal allograft biopsies. *Transplant. Proc.* 17:562-563, 1985.
13. Busch, G. J., Garovoy, M. R., and Tilney, N. L. Variant forms of arteritis in human renal allografts. *Transplant. Proc.* 11:100-103, 1979.
14. Cantor, H. T lymphocytes. In *Fundamental Immunology,* W. E. Paul, ed. Raven Press, New York, 1984, pp. 51-74.
15. Cantor, H., and Simpson, E. Regulation of the immune response by subclasses of T lymphocytes. I. Interactions between pre-killer T cells and regulatory T cells obtained from peripheral lymphoid tissues of mice. *Eur. J. Immunol.* 5:330-336, 1975.
16. Cantrell, O., Robins, R., and Baldwin, R. W. Rat lymphocyte subsets: Cellular requirements for the generation of T cell growth factor. *Cell. Immunol.* 70:367-372, 1982.
17. Canty, T. G., and Wunderlick, J. P. Quantitative assessment of cellular and humoral responses to skin and tumor allografts. *Transplantation* 11:111-116, 1971.

18. Cerottini, J. C., and Brunner, K. T. Cell-mediated cytotoxicity, allograft rejection and tumor immunity. *Adv. Immunol.* 18:67-132, 1974.
19. Christmas, S. E., and MacPherson, G. G. The role of mononuclear phagocytes in cardiac allograft rejection in the rat. I. Ultrastructural and cytochemical features. *Cell. Immunol.* 69:248-270, 1982.
20. Clement, L., Dagg, M., and Landay, A. Characterization of human lymphocyte subpopulations: Alloreactive cytotoxic T-lymphocyte precursor and effector cells are phenotypically distinct from Leu 2^+ suppressor cells. *J. Clin. Immunol.* 4:395-402, 1984.
21. Cosimi, A. B., Wortis, H., Delmonico, F., and Russell, P. Randomized clinical trial of antithymocyte globulin in cadaver renal allograft recipients: Importance of T cell monitoring. *Surgery* 80:155-161, 1976.
22. Cudkowicz, G., and Hochman, P. S. Do natural killer cells engage in regulated reaction against self to ensure homeostasis? *Immunol. Rev.* 44:13-44, 1979.
23. Dallman, M. J., and Mason, D. W. Role of thymus-derived and thymus independent cells in murine skin graft rejection. *Transplantation* 33:221-223, 1982.
24. Dallman, M. J., Mason, D. W., and Webb, M. The roles of host and donor cells in the rejection of skin allografts by T cell-deprived rats injected with syngeneic T cells. *Eur. J. Immunol.* 12:511-518, 1982.
25. Dennert, G., Weiss, S., and Warner, J. T cells may express multiple activities: Specific allohelp, cytolysis and delayed-type hypersensitivity are expressed by a cloned T cell line *Proc. Natl. Acad. Sci. USA* 78:4540-4543, 1981.
26. Dinarello, C. A. Interleukin-1 and the pathogenesis of the acute-phase response. *N. Engl. J. Med.* 311:1413-1418, 1984.
27. Dokhelar, M. C., Wiels, J., Lipinski, M., Tetand, C., Devergie, A., Gluckman, E., and Tursz, T. Natural killer cell activity in human bone marrow recipients. *Transplantation* 31:61-65, 1981.
28. Dosseter, J., Liburd, E., and Kovithavongs, T. Suppressor cells and loss of in vitro killer cell inductiveness to donor cells in the peripheral blood lymphocytes of allograft recipients. *Transplant. Proc.* 11:1260-1262, 1979.
29. Dumble, L., Clunie, G., MacDonald, I., Bowes, L., and Kincaid-Smith, P. Prediction of renal allograft rejection responses to steroids from ADCC responses to in vitro steroids. *Transplant. Proc.* 15:1145-1147, 1983.
30. Duprez, J., Hamilton, B., and Burakoff, S. Generation of cytolytic T lymphocytes in thymectomized, irradiated, and bone marrow reconstituted mice. *J. Exp. Med.* 156:844-859, 1982.
31. Eichwald, E. J., Bernhard, E. J., and Jorgensen, C. Cell mediated hyperacute rejection. VIII. The recipient's role in adoptive transfer. *Transplantation* 39:219-220, 1985.
32. Farrar, J., Benjamin, W., Hilfiker, M., Howard, M., Farrar, W., and Fuller-Farrar, J. The biochemistry, biology and role of interleukin 2 in the induction of cytotoxic T cell and antibody forming B cell responses. *Immunol. Rev.* 63:129-166, 1982.
33. Feldman, J., and Lee, S. Renal homotransplantation in rats. I. Allogeneic recipients. *J. Exp. Med.* 126:783-794, 1967.
34. Fischer, D., Golightly, G., and Koren, H. Potentiation of the cytolytic activity of peripheral blood monocytes by lymphokines and interferon. *J. Immunol.* 130:1220-1225, 1983.
35. Forbes, R., and Guttmann, R. Mechanisms of humoral-mediated cardiac allograft rejection in vivo controlled comparative morphologic studies utilizing inbred rat models. *Heart Transplant* 1:196-202, 1982.
36. Forbes, R., and Guttmann, R. Pathogenetic studies of cardiac allograft rejection using inbred rat models. *Immunol. Rev.* 77:5-30, 1984.

37. Gatenby, P., Kansas, G., Xian, C., Evans, R., and Engelman, E. Dissection of immunoregulatory subpopulations of T lymphocytes within the helper and suppressor sublineages in man. *J. Immunol.* 129:1997-2000, 1982.
38. Gatenby, P., Kotzin, B., Kansas, G., and Engleman, E. Immunoglobulin secretion in the human autologous mixed leukocyte reaction. *J. Exp. Med.* 156:55-67, 1982.
39. Gillis, S., Union, N., Baker, P., and Smith, K. The in vitro generation and sustained culture of nude mouse cytotoxic T lymphocytes. *J. Exp. Med.* 149:1460-1476, 1979.
40. Hall, B., Bishop, G., Farnsworth, A., Duggin, G. G., Horvath, J. S., Sheil, A. G. R., and Tiller, D. J. Identification of the cellular subpopulations infiltrating rejecting cadaver renal allografts: Preponderance of the T4 subset of T cells. *Transplantation* 37:564-570, 1984.
41. Hall, B., and Dorsch, S. Cells mediating allograft rejection. *Immunol. Rev.* 77:31-59, 1984.
42. Hall, B., and Dorsch, S. The cellular basis of allograft rejection in vivo. I. The cellular requirements for first set rejection of heart grafts. *J. Exp. Med.* 148:878-889, 1978.
43. Hall, B., Gurley, K., and Dorsch, S. Do T helper-inducer cells mediate rejection without T cytotoxic-suppressor cells? *Transplant. Proc.* 17:233-234, 1984.
44. Hammer, C., Land, W., Stadler, J., Killer, C., and Brendel, W. Lymphocyte subclasses in rejecting kidney grafts detected by monoclonal antibodies. *Transplant. Proc.* 15: 356-360, 1983.
45. Hancock, W. Analysis of intragraft effector mechanisms associated with human renal allograft rejection: Immunohistological studies with monoclonal antibodies. *Immunol. Rev.* 77:61-84, 1984.
46. Hart, D. N. The effects of antibodies on organ allograft survival. *Heart Transplant.* 2: 143-150, 1983.
47. Hart, D., and Fabre, J. Demonstration and characterization of Ia positive dendritic cells in the interstitial connective tissues of rat heart and other tissues except brain. *J. Exp. Med.* 154:347-361, 1981.
48. Hart, D. N., Fuggle, W. V., Williams, K. A., Fabre, J. W., Ting, A., and Morris, P. J. Localization of HLA, ABC and DR antigens in human kidney. *Transplantation* 31: 428-433, 1981.
49. Hayry, P., and Defendi, V. Mixed lymphocyte cultures produce effector cells: Model in vitro for allograft rejection. *Science* 168:133-135, 1970.
50. Hayry, P., and von Willebrand, E. Transplant aspiration cytology in diagnostic evaluation of renal allografts. *Transplant. Proc.* 13:1575-1578, 1981.
51. Hayry, P., von Willebrand, E., Parthenais, E., Nemlander, A., Soots, A., Lautenschlager, I., Alfoldy, P., and Renkonen, R. The inflammatory mechanisms of allograft rejection. *Immunol. Rev.* 77:85-142, 1984.
52. Hayry, P., von Willebrand, E., and Soots, A. In situ effector mechanisms of allograft rejection. III. Kinetics of the inflammatory response and generation of donor directed killer cells. *Scand. J. Immunol.* 10:95-108, 1979.
53. Hayry, P. Intragraft events in allograft destruction. *Transplantation* 38:1-6, 1984.
54. Heidecke, C., Kupiec-Weglinski, J., Lear, P., Abud-Filho, M., Araujo, J., Araneda, D., Strom, T., and Tilney, N. Interactions between T lymphocyte subsets supported by interleukin 2-rich lymphokines produce acute rejection of vasculatized cardiac allografts in T cell deprived rats. *J. Immunol.* 133:582-588, 1984.
55. Herberman, R. Immunoregulation and natural killer cells. *Mol. Immunol.* 19:1313-1321, 1982.
56. Herberman, R., Kjeu, J., and Kay, H. Natural killer cells: Characteristics and regulation of activity. *Immunol. Rev.* 44:43-70, 1979.

57. Herberman, R., and Ortaldo, J. Natural killer cells: Their role in defenses against disease. *Science* 214:24-27, 1981.
58. Herzenberg, L. A., and Herzenberg, L. A. Analysis and separation using the fluorescence actuated cell sorter (FACS). In *Handbook of Experimental Immunology*, Vol. 2, D. M. Weir, ed. J. B. Lippincott, Philadelphia, 1978, pp. 22.1-22.21.
59. Hogarth, P. M., and McKenzie, I. F. C. Lymphocyte antigens. In *Fundamental Immunology*, W. E. Paul, ed. Raven Press, New York, 1984, pp. 457-477.
60. Holan, J., Chunta, J., and Hasek, M. Specific suppression of antigen reactive cells in neonatal transplant tolerance. *Nature* 274:895-897, 1978.
61. Hanto, D., Hopt, U., Hoffman, R., and Simmons, R. Lymphocyte recruitment, regional blood flow, and vascular permeability at sites of allogeneic cellular interactions. *J. Immunol.* 129:2437-2443, 1982.
62. Hopt, U. T., Sullivan, W., Hoffman, R., and Simmons, R. L. Migration and cell recruiting activity of specifically sensitized lymphocyte in sponge matrix allografts. *Transplantation* 30:411-416, 1980.
63. Hsu, S., Raine, L., and Fanger, H. Use of avidin-biotin-peroxidase complex (ABC) in immunoperoxidase techniques: A comparison between ABC and unlabelled antibody (PAP) procedures. *J. Histochem. Cytochem.* 29:577-580, 1981.
64. Hume, D. The immunological consequences of organ homotransplantation in man. *Harvey Lect.* 64:261-388, 1970.
65. Hume, D., and Egdahl, R. Progressive destruction of renal homografts isolated from the regional lymphatics of the host. *Surgery* 38:194-201, 1958.
66. Jeannet, M., Pinn, V., Flax, M., Winn, H., and Russell, P. Humoral antibodies in renal allotransplantation in man. *N. Engl. J. Med.* 282:111-117, 1970.
67. Johnson, H. M., and Baron, S. Evaluation of interferon and interferon inducers on the immune response. *Pharmacol. Ther. A* 1:349-375, 1977.
68. Kamada, N., Davies, H., and Roser, B. J. Fully allogeneic liver grafting and the induction of donor-specific unreactivity. *Transplant. Proc.* 13:837-841, 1981.
69. Kewase, I., Brooks, C., Kuribayashi, K., Glabuenaga, S., Newman, W., Gillis, S., and Henney, C. S. Interleukin 2 induces interferon production: Participation of macrophages and NK-like cells. *J. Immunol.* 131:228-292, 1983.
70. Kelso, A., Glasebrook, A., Kanagwa, O., and Brunner, K. Production of macrophage-activating factor by T-lymphocyte clones and correlation with other lymphokine activities. *J. Immunol.* 129:550-556, 1982.
71. Kiessling, R., Hochman, P. S., Haller, O., Shearer, G. M., Wigzell, H., and Cudkowicz, G. Evidence for a similar or common mechanism for natural killer cell activity and resistance to hematopoietic grafts. *Eur. J. Immunol.* 7:655-663, 1977.
72. Kiessling, R., and Wigzell, H. An analysis of the murine NK cell as to structure, function and biological relevance. *Immunol. Rev.* 44:165-208, 1979.
73. Kilshaw, P. J., Brent, L., Brooks, C. G., New, R. C., and Pinto, M. Studies on the mechanism of specific unresponsiveness to skin allografts in mice. *Transplant. Proc.* 7: 385-387, 1975.
74. Kim, B., Rosenstein, M., Weiland, D., Eberlein, T. J., and Rosenberg, S. A. Clonal analysis of the lymphoid cells mediating skin allograft rejection. *Transplantation* 36: 525-532, 1983.
75. Kirchoff, C., Thomas, F., Edwards, E., and Thomas, J. Value of pre and posttransplant studies of antidonor antibody-dependent cellular cytotoxicity (ADCC). *Transplant. Proc.* 13:1565-1568, 1981.
76. Kontainen, S., Simpson, E., Bohrer, E., Beverly, P., Hezenberg, L., Fitzpatrick, W., Vogt, P., Torano, A., McKenzie, I. F., and Feldman, M. T-cell lines producing antigen specific suppressor factors. *Nature* 274:477-479, 1978.
77. Koster, F., and McGregor, D. The mediators of cellular immunity. II. Migration of

immunologically committed lymphocytes into inflammatory exudates. *J. Exp. Med.* 133:400-409, 1971.

78. Krensky, A., Reiss, C., Mier, J., Strominger, J., and Burkaroff, S. Long term human cytolytic T cell lines allospecific for HLA DR6 antigen are OKT4$^+$. *Proc. Natl. Acad. Sci. USA* 79:2365-2369 (1982).
79. Lafferty, K., Prowse, S., Simeonovic, C., and Warren, H. S. Immunobiology of tissue transplantation: A return to the passenger leucocyte concept. In *Annual Review of Immunology,* W. E. Paul, C. G. Fathman, and H. Metzgar, eds. Annual Reviews, Inc., Palo Alto, California, 1983, pp. 143-173.
80. Lanier, L. L., Engelman, E. G., Gatenby, P., Babcock, G. F., Warner, N. L., and Herzenberg, L. A. Correlation of functional properties of human lymphoid cell subsets and surface markers using multiparameter analysis and flow cytometry. *Immunol. Rev.* 74:143-160, 1983.
81. Lechler, R., and Batchelor, J. Restoration of immunogeneity to passenger cell depleted kidney allografts by the addition of donor strain dendritic cells. *J. Exp. Med.* 155:31-41, 1982.
82. LeFrancois, L., and Bevan, M. A reexamination of the role of Ly T-2-positive T cells in murine skin graft rejection. *J. Exp. Med.* 159:57-67, 1984.
83. Lipinski, M., Tursz, T., Kreis, H., Finale, Y., and Amiel, J. L. Dissociation of natural killer cell activity and antibody-dependent cell-mediated cytotoxicity in kidney allograft recipients receiving high-dose immunosuppressive therapy. *Transplantation* 29: 214-218, 1980.
84. Loveland, B. E., Hogarth, P., Ceredig, R., and McKenzie, I. F. C. Cells mediating allograft rejection in the mouse. I. Ly-1 cells mediate skin graft rejection. *J. Exp. Med.* 153:1044-1057, 1981.
85. Loveland, B. E., and McKenzie, I. F. C. Which T cells cause graft rejection? *Transplantation* 33:217-221, 1982.
86. Loveland, B. E., and McKenzie, I. F. C. Cells mediating graft rejection in the mouse. II. The Ly phenotypes of cells producing tumor allograft rejection. *Transplantation* 33:174-180, 1982.
87. MacDonald, H. R., Sekaly, R., Kanagawa, O., Thiernesse, N., Taswell, C., Cerottini, J., Weiss, A., Glasebrook, A., Ewgers, H., Kelso, A., Brunner, K., and Bron, C. Cytolytic T. lymphocyte clones. *Immunobiology* 161:84-106, 1082.
88. MacPherson, G., and Christmas, S. E. The role of the macrophage in cardiac allograft rejection in the rat. *Immunol. Rev.* 77:143-166, 1984.
89. Maki, T., Gottschalk, R., Homsy, F. N., Okazaki, H., Wood, M. L., and Monaco, A. P. In vitro analysis of immune reactivity in ALS-treated, bone marrow injected mice bearing enhanced skin allografts. *Transplant. Proc.* 13:596:598, 1981.
90. Malkovsky, M., Edwards, A., Hunt, R., Palmer, L., and Medawar, P. T cell mediated enhancement of host versus graft reactivity in mice fed a diet enriched in vitamin A acetate. *Nature* 302:338-340, 1983.
91. Marboe, C. C., Knowles, D. M., Chess, L., Reemtsma, K., and Fenoglio, J. J. The immunologic and ultrastructural characterization of the cellular infiltrate in acute cardiac allograft rejection: Prevalence of cells with the natural killer (NK) phenotype. *Clin. Immunol. Immunopathol.* 27:141-151, 1983.
92. Mason, D., Brideau, R., McMaster, W. R., Webb, M., White, R., and Williams, A. Monoclonal antibodies that define T-lymphocyte subsets in the rat. In *Monoclonal Antibodies. Hydridomas: A New Dimension in Biological Analyses,* R. Kennett, T. McKearn, and K. Bechtol, eds. Plenum Press, New York, 1980, pp. 251-274.
93. Mason, D. W., Dallman, M. J., Arthur, R. P., and Morris, P. J. Mechanisms of allograft rejection: The roles of cytotoxic T cells and delayed-type hypersensitivity. *Immunol. Rev.* 77:167-184, 1984.

94. Mason, D. W., and Morris, P. J. Inhibition of the accumulation, in rat kideny allografts, of specific—but not nonspecific—cytotoxic cells by cyclosporine. *Transplantation* 37:46-51, 1984.
95. McDougal, J., Shen, F., Cort, S., and Barot, J. Feedback suppression: Phenotypes of T cell subsets involved in the Ly-1 cell-induced immunoregulatory circuit. *J. Immunol.* 125:1157-1160, 1980.
96. McKenzie, I. F. C. Alloaggression. *Transplant. Proc.* 15:269-273, 1983.
97. Medawar, P. B. The behavior and fate of skin autografts and skin homografts in rabbits. *J. Anat.* 78:176-199, 1944.
98. Miller, J. F. A. P. Role of the thymus in transplantation tolerance and immunity. In *Transplantation, Ciba Foundation Symposium,* A. Wolstenholme and A. Cameron, eds. Churchill-Livingstone, London, 1962, pp. 397-408.
99. Miller, J. F. A. P., and Osboa, D. Current concepts of immunological functions of the thymus. *Physiol. Rev.* 47:437-519, 1967.
100. Mintz, B., and Silvers, W. Histocompatibility antigens on melanoblasts and hair follicle cells: Cell-localized homograft rejection in allophenic skin grafts. *Transplantation* 9:497-505, 1970.
101. Morimoto, C., Distaso, J., Cheney, J., Reinherz, E., and Schlassman, S. Cellular interaction between subsets of T8 population for maximal suppression of antigen-specific antibody response. *Cell. Immunol.* 88:75-84, 1984.
102. Morimoto, C., Letvin, N., Distaso, J., Aldrich, W., and Schlossman, S. The isolation and characterization of the human suppressor inducer T cell subset. *J. Immunol.* 134: 1508-1515, 1985.
103. Nakane, P., and Pierce, G. Enzyme labelled antibodies: Preparation and applications for the localization of antigens. *J. Histochem. Cytochem.* 14:929-931, 1966.
104. Nemlander, A., Saskela, E., and Hayry, P. Are natural killer cells involved in allograft rejection? *Eur. J. Immunol.* 13:348-350, 1983.
105. Nemlander, A., Soots, A., and Hayry, P. In situ effector pathways of allograft destruction. 1. Generation of the cellular effector response in the graft and graft recipient. *Cell. Immunol.* 89:409-419, 1984.
106. Nemlander, A., Soots, A., von Willebrand, E., and Hayry, P. Redistribution of renal allograft responding leucocytes during rejection. *J. Exp. Med.* 156:1087-1100, 1982.
107. Ono, M., Tanaka, N., and Orita, K. Dissociation of natural killer activity and antibody-dependent cellular cytotoxicity in spleen cells of tumor bearing mice. *Acta Med. Okayama* 37:367-376, 1983.
108. Oppenheim, J. J., and Gery, I. Interleukin 1 is more than an interleukin. *Immunol. Today* 3:113-119, 1982.
109. Pace, J., Russell, S., Schreiber, R., Altman, W., and Katz, D. Macrophage activation: Priming activity of a T-cell hybridoma is attributable to interferon-gamma. *Proc. Natl. Acad. Sci. USA* 80:3782-3786, 1983.
110. Palladino, M. A., Welte, K., Carroll, A., and Oettgen, H. Characterization of interleukin 2 (IL-2) dependent cytotoxic T cell clones. V. Transfer of resistance to allografts and tumor grafts requires exogenosis IL-2. *Cell. Immunol.* 86:299-307, 1984.
111. Paul, L., van Es, L., and Baldwin, W. M. Antigens in human renal allografts. *Clin. Immunol. Immunopathol.* 19:206-223, 1981.
112. Pierce, J., Kay, S., and Lee, H. M. Donor-specific IgG antibody and the chronic rejection of human renal allografts. *Surgery* 78:14-21, 1975.
113. Porter, K. Renal transplantation. In *Pathology of the Kidney,* R. H. Heptinstall, ed. Little, Brown, Boston, 1966, pp. 601-643.
114. Porter, K. The effect of antibodies on human renal allografts. *Transplant. Proc.* 8: 189-197, 1976.
115. Prystowski, M., Ely, J., Beller, D., Ersenberg, L., Goldman, S., Goldman, M., Gold-

wasser, E., Ihle, J., Quintans, J., Remold, H., Vogel, S., and Fich, F. Alloreactive cloned T cells. *J. Immunol.* 129:2337-2344, 1982.

116. Reinherz, E. L., and Schlossman, S. F. The differentiation and function of human T lymphocytes. *Cell* 19:821-827, 1980.
117. Renkonen, R., Soots, A., von Willebrand, E., and Hayry, P. Lymphoid cell subclasses in rejecting renal allografts in the rat. *Cell. Immunol.* 77:187-195, 1983.
118. Rolstad, B., and Ford, W. Immune response of rats deficient in thymus derived lymphocytes to strong transplantation antigens (Ag-B), graft versus host activity, allograft rejection and the factor of immunization. *Transplantation* 17:405-415, 1974.
119. Rowlands, D., Hill, G., and Zmijewski, G. The pathology of renal homograft rejection. *Am. J. Pathol.* 85:774-804, 1977.
120. Russell, P., Chase, C., Colvin, R., and Plate, J. Kidney transplantation in mice: An analysis of the immune status of mice bearing long-term H-2 incompatible transplants. *J. Exp. Med.* 147:1449-1468, 1979.
121. Schmidt, J., Mizel, S., Cohen, D., and Green, I. Interleukin 1, a potential regulator of fibroblast proliferation. *J. Immunol.* 128:2177-2182, 1982.
122. Schulz, R. M., Papamatheakis, J. D., and Chirigos, M. A. Interferon: An inducer of macrophage activation by polyanious. *Science* 197:674-676, 1977.
123. Schwartz, R. The role of gene products of the major histocompatibility complex in T cell activation and cellular interactions. In *Fundamental Immunology,* W. E. Paul, ed. Raven Press, New York, 1984, pp. 379-437.
124. Simpson, E. The role of H-4 as a minor histocompatibility antigen. *Immunol. Today* 3:97-98, 1982.
125. Spitz, H., Borst, J., Terhorst, C., and deVries, J. The role of T cell differentiation markers in antigen specific and lectin-dependent cellular cytotoxicity mediated by $T8^+$ and $T4^+$ human cytotoxic T cell clones directed at class I and calss II MHC antigens. *J. Immunol.* 129:1563-1569, 1982.
126. Stiller, C., Dossetor, J., Carpernter, C. B., and Myburgh, J. Immunologic monitoring of the transplant recipient. *Transplant. Proc.* 4:1245-1254, 1977.
127. Stiller, C., Sinclair, N., McGirr, D., Jernikar, A., and Ullan, R. Diagnostic and prognostic value of donor specific posttransplant immune responses: Clinical correlates and in vitro variables. *Transplant. Proc.* 10:525-530, 1978.
128. Strassman, G., and Bach, F. $OKT4^+$ cytotoxic T cells can lyse targets via class I molecules and can be blocked by monoclonal antibody against T4 molecules. *J. Immunol.* 133:1705-1709, 1984.
129. Strom, T., Tilney, N., Carpenter, C., and Busch, G. Identity and cytotoxic capacity of cells infiltrating renal allografts. *N. Engl. J. Med.* 292:1257-1263, 1975.
130. Strom, T. B., Tilney, N. L., Paradyez, J., Bancewicz, J., and Carpenter, C. B. Cellular components of allograft rejection: Identity, specificity and cytotoxic function of cells infiltrating acutely rejecting allografts. *J. Immunol.* 118:2020-2026, 1977.
131. Stuart, F. P., Scollard, D. M., McKearn, T. J., and Fitch, F. W. Cellular and humoral immunity after allogeneic renal transplantation in the rat. *Transplantation* 22:455-466, 1976.
132. Suthanthrian, M., and Garovoy, D. M. Immunologic monitoring of the renal transplant patient. *Urol. Clin. North Am.* 10:315-325, 1983.
133. Thomas, F. Differential effects of immunosuppressive agents on T and B lymphocytes. *Proc. Natl. Dialy. Transplant Forum* 4:124, 1974.
134. Thomas, F. T., Carver, F. M., Foil, M. B., Pryor, W. H., Larkin, E. W., Hall, W. R., Haisch, C. E., and Thomas, J. M. Long-term incompatible kidney survival in outbred higher primates without chronic immunosuppression. *Ann. Surg.* 198:370-378, 1983.

135. Thomas, F. T., Lee, H. M., Lower, R. R., and Thomas, J. J. Immunological monitoring as a guide to the management of transplant recipients. *Surg. Clin. North. Am.* 59:253-281, 1979.
136. Thomas, J., et al., 1986, in press.
137. Thomas, J. M., Carver, F. M., Foil, M. B., Hall, W. R., Adams, C., Fahrenbruch, G. B., and Thomas, F. T. Renal allograft tolerance in outbred rhesus monkeys induced with ATG and donor bone marrow. *Transplantation* 36:104-106, 1983.
138. Thomas, J., Carver, M., Scott, J., Williams, E., and Thomas, F. Effect of rabbit anti-human thymocyte globulin on lymphocyte subpopulations and functions following allotransplantation in the rhesus monkey. *Transplantation* 27:163-170, 1979.
139. Thomas, J., Thomas, F., Edwards, E., Hoffmann, S., and Lee, H. M. Regulation of T cell mediated cytotoxic allograft response in human transplant recipients. *Transplant. Proc.* 13:1594-1598, 1981.
140. Thomas, J., Thomas, F., Hoffman, S., Johns, C., and Lee, H. M. Macrophage related suppressor cells in human renal transplant recipients. *Surgery* 86:266-272, 1979.
141. Thomas, J., Thomas, F., Kaplan, A. M., and Lee, H. M. Antibody-dependent cellular cytotoxicity and chronic renal allograft rejection. *Transplantation* 22:94-100, 1976.
142. Thomas, J., Thomas, F., and Lee, H. M. Studies of lymphocyte-dependent antibody in human chronic renal allograft rejection. *Transplant. Proc.* 9:65-68, 1977.
143. Thomas, J., Thomas, F., and Lee, H. M. Why do HLA non-identical renal allografts survive 10 years or more? *Transplant. Proc.* 8:85-89, 1977.
144. Thomas, J., Thomas, F., Mendez-Picon, G., and Lee, H. M. Immunologic monitoring of long surviving renal transplant recipients. *Surgery* 81:125-131, 1977.
145. Tilney, N. L. The extent of immunological injury to the vasculature of cardiac allografts in the rat. *Transplantation* 17:561-567, 1974.
146. Tilney, N. L., Garovoy, M. R., Busch, G. J., Strom, T. B., Graves, M. J., and Carpenter, C. B. Rejected human renal allografts. *Transplantation* 28:421-426, 1979.
147. Tilney, N. L., Kupiec-Weglinski, J., Heidecke, C., Lear, P., and Strom, T. Mechanisms of rejection and prolongation of vascularized organ allografts. *Immunol. Rev.* 77:185-216, 1984.
148. Tilney, N. L., MacLennon, I., Strom, T. B., and Baldwin, W. Effect of thymectomy, thoracic duct drainage, and radiation on T & B lymphocyte distribution and cardiac allograft survival in rats. *Transplantation* 31:26-30, 1981.
149. Tilney, N. L., Strom, T. B., MacPherson, S. G., and Carpenter, C. B. Surface properties and functional characteristics of infiltrating cells harvested from acutely rejecting cardiac allografts in inbred rats. *Transplantation* 20:323-330, 1975.
150. Todd, R., and Schlossman, S. Differentiation antigens on human monocytes and macrophages defined by monoclonal antibodies. In *Mononuclear Phagocyte Biology*, A. Volkman, ed. Marcel Dekker, New York, 1984, pp. 129-150.
151. Trinchieri, G., and Perussia, B. Human natural killer cells: Biologic and pathologic aspects. *Lab. Invest.* 50:489-513, 1984.
152. Tyler, J. D., Galli, S., Snider, M., Dvorak, A., and Steinmuller, D. Cloned LyT-2^{+} cytolytic T lymphocytes destroy allogeneic tissue in vivo. *J. Exp. Med.* 159:234-243, 1984.
153. van Es, A., Meyer, C., Oljans, P. J., Tanke, H. J., and van Es, L. A. Mononuclear cells in renal allografts. Correlation with peripheral blood T lymphocyte subpopulations and graft prognosis. *Transplantation* 37:134-139, 1984.
154. Vodinelich, L., Sutherland, R., Schneider, C., Newman, R., and Greaves, M. Receptor for transferrin may be a target structure for natural killer cells. *Proc. Natl. Acad. Sci. USA* 80:835-839, 1983.
155. von Willebrand, E. OKT4/T8 ratio in the blood and in the graft during episodes of human renal allograft rejection. *Cell. Immunol.* 77:196-201, 1983.

156. von Willebrand, E., and Hayry, P. Composition and in vitro cytotoxicity of cellular infiltrates in rejecting human kidney allografts. *Cell. Immunol.* 41:358-372, 1978.
157. von Willebrand, E., Soots, A., and Hayry, P. In situ effector mechanisms in rat kidney allograft rejection. *Cell. Immunol.* 46:309-326, 1979.
158. von Willebrand, E., Soots, A., and Hayry, P. In situ effector mechanisms in rat kidney allograft rejection. II. Heterogeneity of the effector cells in the inflammatory infiltrate vs. that in the spleen of the recipient rat. *Cell. Immunol.* 46:327-336, 1979.
159. Weber, B., Welte, M., Hammer, C., Stadler, J., Koller, C., Caspo, C., Land, W., Hillebrand, G., and Castro, M. Increase of natural killer cells in rejecting grafts. *Transplant. Proc.* 16:1177-1178, 1984.
160. Widmer, M. B., Roopenian, D. C., and Bach, F. H. Cytolytic T lymphocyte clones with helper cell characteristics. *Transplant. Proc.* 15:393:395, 1983.
161. Williams, G. M., Hume, D., Hudson, R., Morris, P., Kano, K., and Milgrom, F. Hyperacute renal homograft rejection in man. *N. Engl. J. Med.* 279:611-618, 1968.
162. Williams, K., and Morris, P. Retrospective screening for lymphocyte-dependent antibody in recipient of renal transplants. *Clin. Exp. Immunol.* 27:191-197, 1977.
163. Wonigeit, K., and Pilchmayr, R. *Dialys. Transplant.* 6:58, 1977.
164. Woodruff, M. F. A. The transplantation of homologous tissue and its surgical applications. *Ann. R. Coll. Surg. Engl.* 11:173-195, 1952.
165. Wortis, H. Immunological responses of nude mice. *Clin. Exp. Immunol.* 8:305-317, 1971.

4

THE INTERLEUKINS

Patrick A. Murphy
The Johns Hopkins University School of Medicine, Baltimore, Maryland

Essentially all immune responses involve the formation of associations between cells of different types, followed by interactions between them. These associations are visible microscopically, are stable enough to allow clumps to be semipurified from uninvolved cells, and are immunologically specific in that B and T cells in such clusters have receptors for the same antigen. Associations are established after 14-20 hr incubations in vitro of spleen cells plus specific antigen, and they precede lymphocyte multiplication [36]. As a rule, immunologic responses are complex: antibodies of several different classes are made; T-cell populations may be cytotoxic (Tc), helper (Th), or suppressor (Ts); important parts of the response may be mediated by antigen nonspecific cells responding to bound antibody or fixed complement. Even when a response can be attributed entirely to one cell type, as antibody responses to B cells, the stimulation and clonal expansion of these B cells take place under the guidance of other cells. Typically, IgM secretion by B cells requires both T cells and macrophages in the early stages of the response, although once B-cell proliferation and differentiation have occurred, antibody secretion can continue for a time in the absence of other cells.

The cellular requirements for some immunologic responses can be replaced by soluble factors. In general, these are proteins that are secreted into culture media by antigen-stimulated cells of the same type as those replaced by the factor. Thus, single B cells can be induced to differentiate, proliferate, and synthesize immunoglobulin by anti-IgM antibody (which substitutes for an antigen stimulus) [52]. However, the process requires at least three and probably four protein growth factors: B-cell growth factor, two other factors derived from T cells, and probably a trace of the macrophage-derived interleukin 1.

In many cases, factors that allow particular immunologic responses to proceed can also be obtained as culture supernates of cloned cell lines. Sometimes the cell must be stimulated to secrete the factor, and sometimes factor secretion is spontaneous. Most of the factors secreted by cell lines are indistinguishable from the natural products. Many of them have been purified to homogeneity, and for some the genes have been cloned.

In early work, scientists described a biologic activity that was essential to whatever immunologic response they were interested in. However, it was soon realized that many apparently disparate biologic activities were being mediated by the same substances. For example, at an international meeting at Ermatingen in 1979, a number of investigators decided that they were all working on the same factor. Since it was a messenger molecule that transmitted instructions from one cell of the immune system (the macrophage) to another (a specialized T cell), and since it was hoped that it would be the first of many, it was christened interleukin-1. At the same meeting, T-cell growth factor was designated interleukin-2, effecting another great simplification. The letter to the editor of the *Journal of Immunology* was signed by no fewer than 34 people [1].

There has not been much more progress in interleukin nomenclature in the last 5 years. Interleukin-3 was discovered in the supernates of activated T cells and has been purified to homogeneity, and the gene has been cloned [84]. However, it has not been possible as yet to assign it an unambiguous role in any immune response [83]. And perhaps because of this premature naming of a factor as an interleukin before its function was well established, there is no interleukin-4. Rather, there has been a retreat to the naming of factors in terms of what they do. Thus, even though γ interferon is clearly a polyfunctional molecule essential to several important immunologic responses, it is still known by its original name.

Another reason for caution in the naming of new factors is the discovery that particular factors may appear to be essential under some circumstances, but not under others. Also, there is a general realization that the in vitro systems that we study are not necessarily related to happenings in vivo. Thus, Nossal has recently shown that cloned single B cells can be induced to proliferate by the addition of large amounts of purified interleukin-2, in the apparent absence of any other factor [59]. However, the medium contained fetal calf serum (whose composition is poorly known and probably contains at least platelet-derived growth factor), and huge amounts of mercaptoethanol (100 mM). Furthermore, the proliferation observed was much less than that seen with the "natural" stimulus for B cells, B-cell growth factor. What relation these experiments, in which cloned B cells respond to a T-cell growth factor, have to real life is problematic. In real life, no B cell responds in isolation from T cells and macrophages.

Since the present state of knowledge about interleukins is in flux, what will be done here is to describe those interleukins and lymphokines about which most is known. There is no definitive evidence that any of them are essential either to allograft rejection or to allograft tolerance. However, there are some very suggestive observations, and these will be referred to in their place.

INTERLEUKIN-1

Interleukin-1 (IL-1) is a protein whose molecular weight is usually given as about 15,000 daltons (D) [18]. Its main cellular source is monocytes and macrophages, although there is evidence that under some circumstances it may be secreted by other cells. These include keratinocytes from skin [70], renal mesangial cells [44], and neuroglia [19]. Also, some malignant cells of macrophage type [6] and certain transformed epithelial cell lines can be sources of IL-1 [70].

In most species, including the human, IL-1 exists in two main forms: one has an isoelectric point (pI) of about 7, and the other has a pI of about 5. The pI 5 form shows microheterogeneity. There is considerable evidence that the pI 7 and pI 5 forms of IL-1 are coded for by different genes. Both forms appear to be synthesized inside the macrophage as precursors of about 33,000 D [3,43]. During or shortly after secretion, these are cleaved to the common 15,000 D forms. Further cleavages do not necessarily destroy biologic activity, and a form of molecular weight 4000 D is found circulating in the serum of infected human patients [12]. As yet, there is no evidence that the pI 7 and pI 5 forms of IL-1 differ in biologic activity, but obviously that remains possible.

Interleukin-1 is not present in resting monocytes or macrophages; it is synthesized when the cells are exposed to suitable stimuli [8,50]. Some effective stimuli are immunologically nonspecific. Thus, Gram-positive and Gram-negative bacteria, such bacterial products as peptidoglycan, endotoxin, and some exotoxins, fungal cell walls, and certain viruses, are all able to induce IL-1 synthesis and secretion by macrophages from animals that have not been previously exposed to the organisms. Parenthetically, it is probably no accident that many of the substances on this list are commonly used as immunologic adjuvants. Other stimuli are definitely immunologic: antigen-antibody complexes are effective, as are lymphokines of unknown nature secreted by T cells that have been exposed to antigen. (All stimuli are reviewed in Reference 18.)

Very few immunologic reactions can proceed in the absence of antigen-presenting cells. In addition to antigen, such cells must present Ia determinants that are recognized as self by T cells. Until quite recently it was thought that the macrophage was the normal antigen-presenting cell. Now there is controversy over whether a nonphagocytic cell, the dendritic cell of Steinman, may account for much or all of the antigen-presenting capacities usually ascribed to macrophages [35]. Dendritic cells are present at an incidence of about 1 per 100 macrophages, so it is difficult to exclude their presence from macrophage populations.

The orthodox account of how IL-1 may promote immunologic reactions is that macrophages are present in essentially all body tissues, respond to chemotactic substances, and seek out and phagocytose foreign materials. Frequently these foreign materials are organisms that stimulate macrophages to secrete IL-1 directly. If the substances themselves are bland, the macrophage processes and displays antigen for inspection by neighboring T cells. T cells recognizing antigen would stimulate macrophage IL-1 synthesis and secretion by means of the aforementioned lymphokine. Interleukin-1 would then participate in the generation of antigen-specific B- and T-cell clones by the mechanisms discussed below. If the dendritic cell hypothesis proves correct, the above would be modified by saying that dendritic cells are responsible for displaying antigen. At this point it has apparently been difficult to show that purified dendritic cells do secrete IL-1, and indeed they may secrete other immunostimulant substances [11].

A further modification of the general hypothesis is that under some circumstances other cells may replace the macrophage. Ia-positive IL-1-secreting cells are found in skin (keratinocytes), blood vessels (endothelium) [7], glomeruli (mesangial cells), and the brain (neuroglia). It is easy to imagine circumstances under which macrophages would not be strictly necessary for an immune response in those areas. For example, vascular endothelial cells might be quite important sources of antigen presentation for graft rejection, especially once the rejection has started. Steinman has impressive evidence that dendritic cells are by far the most efficient cells at stimulating resting T cells. However, before T cells proliferate they need to be restimulated by an antigen-presenting, Ia-positive (and probably IL-1-producing) cell. Restimulation can be done by a wide variety of cells, including macrophages and B cells [36].

Interleukin-1 acts on a subset of T cells and induces them to secrete interleukin-2 (IL-2). In the mouse, the IL-1 target cell is found among the large mature cortical thymocytes, which are Ly-1^+, 23^+, and which do not display receptors for peanut agglutinin. A cell line with these characteristics has been developed (LBRM 33-1A5). In the thymus, IL-1 target cells are in phase G_0 of the cell cycle, and the effect of IL-1 is to move them into a state in which they become sensitive to antigen or lectin. Antigen causes IL-1-primed cells to secrete IL-2, but of course the response is restricted to those T cells with the correct antigen receptor. Lectins, such as phytohemagglutinin (PHA), cause IL-2 secretion by all IL-1-primed cells. Similar observations have been made with the IA5 cell line. In the absence of IL-1 and lectin, these cells secrete a small amount of IL-2, which they consume themselves to facilitate growth. If IL-1 and lectin are presented together, the cell line secretes excess IL-2, which accumulates in the medium [13,22].

One of the safety mechanisms of the immune system is that cells require a double stimulus before a response occurs. In the case of IL-1-responsive T cells, timing is crucial. The optimum response occurs when IL-1 and antigen or lectin are presented together. Adding the IL-1 before or after the lectin causes a progressive decline in response, and if the asynchrony reaches 24 hr, the response is essentially zero [13].

In summary, the main immunologic purpose of IL-1, as far as we know, is to induce the secretion of IL-2. Once that has been accomplished, IL-1 is irrelevant and it plays no direct part in the clonal expansion of T cells that characterizes almost all immune responses. However, it is essential to start the process, and it has been shown that IL-1 can replace the antigen-presenting cell requirement in a whole variety of in vitro immune responses, such as the IgM response to sheep red cells, the mixed lymphocyte reaction, the development of cytotoxic T cells, and the development of suppressor T cells in response to histamine.

Because of the central position of IL-1 in the initiation of essentially all immune responses, there is much current interest in the generation of IL-1 agonists and antagonists that might prove useful in therapy. The human [3] and mouse IL-1 [43] genes have recently been cloned, and protein sequences have been predicted. The human gene is a pI 7 type, the mouse a pI 5. At the protein level there is only about 20% homology between the two forms of IL-1. This is enough to suggest that they are related, but sufficiently different to suggest that, even in the same species, pI 5 and 7 IL-1 will prove to be specified by different genes. Both IL-1 genes predict protein sequences devoid of the hydrophobic leader peptides that normally allow proteins to be secreted from cells. And data from many species indicate that most IL-1 is intracellular. Extracellular release of IL-1 is potentiated by cell-damaging agents, such as silica. It may be that the IL-1 important in immune responses is passed directly to T cells clustered about the antigen-presenting cell. In that case, soluble IL-1 in the medium would be an artefact, of more significance in pathology than in physiology. And soluble extracellular IL-1 agonists and inhibitors might prove to be of little therapeutic value.

Interleukin-1 has many actions other than initiating immune responses. It seems to be identical with the endogenous pyrogens, which are the mediators of all clinical and experimental fevers other than those due to disease of the nervous system [51]. Interleukin-1 acts on neutrophils, causing them to degranulate their specific granules to the exterior of the cell [39]. The apolactoferrin released in this way probably mediates the fall in serum iron characteristic of severe infections [78]. There is much evidence that IL-1 acts on the liver to cause alterations in plasma protein synthesis. Albumin synthesis is markedly slowed, and synthesis of some proteins not present in normal serum is initiated. The most prominent of these are C-reactive protein and the serum amyloid A-associated protein [58]. Overall, liver protein synthesis is increased during infection, and the amino acids required for this process are supplied by muscle and bone matrix, whose proteins are broken down at a greatly increased rate. It has recently been shown that IL-1 acts directly on muscle cells to cause increased protein breakdown and release of amino acids to the medium [4].

Thus, the present picture of IL-1 is complex. It is synthesized by macrophages in the earliest stages of response to almost any foreign material. If the inflammatory response is weak and few cells die, then all the IL-1 produced will be expended locally, and its main function is to initiate T-cell proliferation and potentiate immune responses of all types. With the onset of tissue damage or cell death, IL-1 gets into the draining lymphatics and into the bloodstream. Circulating IL-1 induces most of the acute phase changes characteristic of infection, including fever.

The case of fever is of some interest. It has been shown that fever strongly potentiates the action of IL-1 on T cells [27]. Since fever is characteristic of rejection crises, and since IL-1 is presumably involved both in the rejection and the fever, it might make sense to suppress fever in this specific situation.

INTERLEUKIN-2

Interleukin-2 is much less pleiotrophic than IL-1; as far as we know it acts only on immunocytes, and its main target is T cells. It was originally described as T-cell growth factor, which is essential to the growth of all normal T cells, helper (Th), suppressor (Ts), and cytotoxic (Tc) [72]. Because of this, IL-2 is essential to any immune response that involves the clonal expansion of T cells. In the real world, that means almost all immune responses. Interleukin-2 has been specifically shown to be necessary in the development of Th cells for the anti-sheep red blood cell (RBC) response, for the mixed lymphocyte reaction, for the development of both virus-specific and tumor-specific Tc cells, and for the development of Ts cells [23]. Certain T-cell lines and hydridomas are IL-2 independent. Frequently this is because they produce sufficient IL-2 to satisfy their own growth requirements. However, some transformed T-cell lines appear to be genuinely IL-2 independent: they do not secrete IL-2 and do not even have receptors for it.

Interleukin-2 is a glycoprotein. Human IL-2 has a molecular weight of about 15,000, and isoelectric focusing, as expected for a glycoprotein, shows microheterogeneity. Most of the activity focuses around pH 6.5. Interleukin-2 produced by human T-cell lines, or in other species, may vary considerably from these specifications. Molecular weights up to 50,000 D and isoelectric points as low as 4.5 have been reported. More recent studies, reviewed below, have essentially resolved these discrepancies.

Taniguchi and coworkers cloned the human IL-2 gene from the T-cell lymphoma line JURKAT [75]. This line constitutively produces very large quantities of IL-2 and has been used by many investigators because it is a homogeneous population. The gene predicted a polypeptide of 153 amino acids with a molecular weight of 17,632 D. However, there was a hydrophobic "signal peptide" of 20 amino acids, with a Ser_{20}-Ala_{21} sequence that was a likely point for proteolytic attack. Removal of the signal peptide predicted a protein of 15,420 D. There were no likely N-glycosylation sites (Asn $\times$ Ser or Asn $\times$ Thr). This is interesting, because JURKAT IL-2 is mostly not glycosylated, unlike IL-2 from normal cells. The gene was expressed both in *Escherichia coli* and in frog oocytes, and the JURKAT cells were found to have one copy of the gene per cell.

Shortly afterward, the IL-2 gene was cloned from spleen cells [17] and from peripheral blood lymphocytes [67]. The genes were substantially identical with that from the JURKAT cell line. Recombinant human IL-2 has been made in large quantity from *E. coli* and is identical in all respects with highly purified IL-2 from normal T cells or from T-cell lines [67].

Evidence that the putative IL-2 genes really did code for IL-2 was provided by Robb et al., who purified to homogeneity and sequenced four different molecular forms of

JURKAT IL-2: one was the unmodified protein predicted by DNA sequence; two were glycosylated at position 3, one with *N*-acetylgalactosamine and one with sialic acid; and fourth lacked the first two amino acids, which had presumably been removed by a protease. All variations were confined to the first tryptic peptide. An –SS– bond was identified between Cys_{58} and Cys_{105} [66].

It was already known that reduction and alkylation destroyed the biologic activity of IL-2. And although IL-2 activity could be expressed in *E. coli,* the activity was low and much immunoreactive IL-2 was insoluble. By analogy with other proteins expressed in *E. coli,* it was thought likely that the IL-2 molecule was folding in the wrong way, perhaps by –SS– bond formation involving the third Cys residue of the molecule, at position 125. Serine differs from cysteine only in that the sulfur atom of cysteine is replaced by oxygen, and –SS– bond formation is impossible. Site-specific mutations were therefore induced at codons 58, 105, and 125, which replaced the natural codon with one specifying Ser. Interleukin-2 so mutated at position 58 had 0.5% of the usual activity, and IL-2 with serine at position 105 had only 2% of the usual activity. Interleukin-2 with a $Cys_{125} \rightarrow Ser_{125}$ mutation had 130% of the activity of the natural molecule, and furthermore was freely soluble. Thus, genetic engineering confirmed the essential Cys_{58}-Cys_{105} –SS– bond, and the mutation at position 125 actually gave a superior product, because incorrect molecular folding was rendered impossible [82].

Much of the variation in molecular properties between natural specimens of IL-2 is explained by glycosylation differences. It is clear that glycosylation makes <5% difference to the biologic activity of IL-2, at least as regards those variants secreted by the JURKAT line [66]. However, IL-2 from human tonsil seems to be quite heavily glycosylated; whether the gene is altered in tonsil cells is not known. Heavy glycosylation could explain some of the variations in apparent molecular weight. However, it is likely that dimers and perhaps polymers of IL-2 account for molecular weights above 20,000 D. Nothing is known about how the monomers bind together; one obvious possibility is by –SS– bonding between the Cys_{125} residues.

Interleukin-2 receptors were originally demonstrated using biosynthetically labeled natural IL-2. This was allowed to bind to T cells for a variable period of time, then the mixtures were centrifuged over an oil that floated the medium but allowed the cells to sediment through. Bound and free IL-2 could thus be measured separately [64]. It was found that receptors were few on resting cells but increased greatly in cells activated by antigen or lectin. Under some circumstances, small quantities of IL-2 appear to be able to induce expression of the IL-2 receptor [63]. Obviously, this would constitute a positive feedback loop for the immune response.

More recently, two types of IL-2 receptor have been demonstrated on human cells, one of low affinity and the other of high affinity. This resolved certain discrepancies in older data. Both types of receptor bound IL-2, and both reacted with the anti-receptor antibody, anti-Tac. It was thought that the receptors had the same polypeptide chain, but that one form was modified after translation in a way that lowered affinity for IL-2 [65].

Urdal and coworkers have developed three monoclonal antibodies to the IL-2 receptor, all of which compete with each other as well as with IL-2, so presumably they are recognizing one structure. All three antibodies precipitated the same antigen from detergent lysates of T cells. Normal cells gave a glycoprotein of 55,000-60,000 molecular weight, whereas receptor from a T lymphoma was definitely smaller at 50,000-55,000. The receptor was purified by affinity chromatography on monoclonal antibody columns followed by reverse phase high-performance liquid chromatography (HPLC). It gave one band on sodium dodecyl sulfate (SDS) PAGE gels, and on sequencing a unique NH_2 terminal was found. DNA probes were made specifying the NH_2 terminal sequence and were used to pull out and clone the receptor gene. The cloned gene confirmed the partial sequence and gave the rest of the sequence.

The IL-2 receptor gene was not homologous to any other known gene; in particular it was not homologous to any of the known viral oncogenes. The specific activity of purified receptor was 1.26 fmol/μg, and there seemed to be about 95,000 receptors per cell [77]. Of these, most would be of low affinity, but only a few thousand molecules of IL-2 are needed to drive the cell.

Interleukin-2 is the only lymphokine known that allows antigen-primed T cells to grow exponentially. In fact, by growing T cells in the presence of antigen and IL-2 and repeatedly cloning at limiting dilutions, it has been possible to develop normal T-cell lines that are antigen specific and whose effector type may be Tc, Th, or Ts. All such lines remain dependent on IL-2 for growth [68]. The defect in the nude mouse appears to be an inability to secrete IL-2, and only IL-2 allows the development of antigen-specific cytotoxic T cells from the spleens of such mice [81].

The process of IL-2 secretion by T cells responding to antigen or mitogen was found to be absolutely dependent on the presence of a small number of macrophages. Interleukin-1 could replace this macrophage requirement. The hypothesis already referred to was developed, in which IL-1 is an essential signal for the release of IL-2. This was confirmed by the discovery of the IL-1-sensitive, IL-2-secreting T-cell line, LBRM 1A5.

Interleukin-1-responsive, IL-2-secreting T cells are a small minority of the T-cell population, less than 5% of cells in the thymus and correspondingly few elsewhere. They are the large, mature, cortisone-resistant thymocytes, and it is thought that they do not themselves differentiate into Tc, Th, or Ts cells. Rather, the IL-2 they secrete is taken up by the small immature cells that make up about 90% of the total T-cell population. Normally, these cells are resting, and they do not express IL-2 receptors. Therefore, they respond sluggishly or not at all to IL-2 alone. Antigen stimulates these cells to move from G_0 into G_1 and to synthesize and display IL-2 receptors. If IL-2 is supplied, exponential growth follows. Thus, although both IL-1 and IL-2 are entirely without antigenic specificity, nevertheless most of the immune response is specific for the antigen presented. Both the IL-1 target cell and the IL-2 target cell require antigen as a second signal, and T-cells with the wrong specificity are unlikely to multiply to any extent. On the other hand, it is not surprising that small but significant rises may be observed in the levels of antibodies and T cells specific for irrelevant antigens. This is one reason antibody rises have never been very reliable for the diagnosis of infectious diseases.

If a T-cell population is stimulated with lectin rather than antigen, the response is polyclonal, because all T cells receive a double signal. Under these circumstances it is possible to study DNA and RNA synthesis in the whole population, and observe G_0-G_1 transitions by cytofluorimetry using acridine orange. With this dye, red fluorescence measures RNA content and green fluorescence measures DNA. Normal human peripheral blood leukocytes contain one genome equivalent of DNA and very little RNA (G_0 cells). In the presence of PHA, some RNA is synthesized, but the process stops after 12-14 hr with about twice the basal level of RNA (G_{1a} cells). If IL-2 is available as well, the cells synthesize about six times the resting level of RNA (G_{1b}), and they proceed on to S phase, [^{3}H] TdR incorporation, and eventual cell division [40].

One of the problems with the organization of the lymphokine system as described so far is that it is difficult to understand how any immune response gets expressed. Since Ts cells develop along with Th and Tc cells, why are responses not simply shut off? The answer appears to be that a normal immune response has an asynchrony between Tc and Th, and Ts development, with Tc and Th cells developing first, and Ts cells later. Recent studies are beginning to suggest a molecular mechanism for this arrangement. All human T cells have an antigen on their surface recognized by the mouse monoclonal antibody OKT3. This is related to the T-cell antigen receptor, which is composed of two noncovalently associated chains. In Tc or Th cells, triggering of the receptor by OKT3 antibody, antigen, or anti-idiotype antibody leads to expression of IL-2 receptors and to proliferation if IL-2 is provided. Indeed, if the stimulus is presented as an array on Sepharose beads, rather than in soluble form, Tc and Th precursor cells will secrete their own IL-2 and direct their own proliferation. However, when Ts cell receptors are triggered, the initial response is not merely not to proliferate, but to become refractory to exogenous IL-2. The IL-2 refractoriness is not due to lack of IL-2 receptors, and it is temporary, returning to normal after 4 days. This provides a very neat explanation of the observed behavior, in which suppressor cell development occurs late in the immune response, when antigen is waning, and Ts development can occur under the influence of IL-2 secreted by other cells [5].

Both polyclonal and monoclonal antibodies have been raised that neutralize the activity of IL-2. These antibodies do not block the actions of IL-1, IL-3, γ interferon (IFNγ), B cell growth factor (BSF-1p or BCGF), or antigen-specific Tc differentiation factors. However, as expected, they blocked the mixed lymphocyte reaction, the generation of Tc cells, and the primary and secondary PFC responses to sheep red cells. Also, when given to whole animals, the yield of Tc cells was sharply reduced [23].

Some clinically important immunosuppressives produce interesting effects on IL-2. Dexamethasone and other steroids have multiple effects, and it is not clear which of them are most important clinically. However, one well-authenticated steroid effect is to block IL-2 production by activated T cells [40]. Cyclosporin A (CsA) has been examined in detail. Cyclosporin acts primarily on T cells: B cells and macrophages function normally in its presence. It has been known for some time that CsA blocks IL-2 release by activated T cells, but two recent papers have thrown light on the mechanism. Kronke et al. studied a subclone of the JURKAT cell line, which had to be induced to secrete IL-2 by phytohemagglutinin and phorbolmyristic acetate (PMA). Interleukin-2-specific mRNA was measured in whole-cell lysates, in polyadenylated RNA sized on sucrose gradients, and as freshly synthesized mRNA in isolated nuclei incubated with [^{32}P] UTP and other cold nucleotides. The probe was a 1.1 kb human IL-2 gene cloned in *E. coli.* The IL-2 message was at very low levels in uninduced cells, was strongly expressed in all three situations within an hour of stimulation, peaked at 6 hr, and then declined. Cyclosporin essentially abolished IL-2-specific mRNA synthesis in a concentration of 0.3 μg/ml or more, and inhibition was clearly visible at 0.01 μg/ml.

The cells remained viable, and there was no significant depression of DNA, RNA, or protein synthesis in general. The failure to find IL-2-specific mRNA was not due to an increased rate of breakdown, or to failure to transport it from nucleus to cytoplasm, because nascent mRNA synthesis in isolated nuclei was severely depressed. Interleukin-2 receptor expression was not suppressed as measured by anti-Tac binding. Also, HLA antigen expression (constitutive) and HT3 antigen expression (inducible) also remained normal. In short, CsA seemed to produce a block in the transcription of IL-2 DNA into mRNA. This fits very well with the observed effects of CsA, which can prevent T-cell activation by antigen or lectin but cannot prevent IL-2-driven proliferation in activated T cells [41].

T cells contain a protein, cytophilin, which binds CsA with fairly high affinity (K = 2×10^{-7} M). This has been purified to homogeneity and binds almost exactly one molecule of CsA per molecule of protein. It was partially sequenced and proved to be unrelated to any other known protein. It was also found in mouse and human thymus and in human peripheral blood mature T cells [26]. At present it is not known whether the CsA protein complex has anything to do with the inhibition of IL-2-specific mRNA, but obviously one possibility is that the complex functions as a repressor.

Taken together, these data suggest very strongly that CsA is immunosuppressive because it prevents the synthesis of IL-2.

So far, IL-2 has been discussed in terms of its proliferative action on T cells, but some of its actions do not require that the target cells proliferate. As already discussed, IL-2 can induce the formation of IL-2 receptors on T cells [63]. It also causes the expression of receptors for transferrin on T cells, although the immunologic significance of that is not clear. Interleukin-2 stimulates T cells to synthesize and secrete two important lymphokines, IFNγ and B-cell growth factor (BSF-lp). These are discussed below. Cell division is not usually necessary for lymphokine release, although in practice they often go together. Incidentally, another immunosuppressive effect of dexamethasone is to block IL-2-mediated IFNγ secretion [63].

Interleukin-2 also has effects on at least two immunocytes that are not T cells. There are reports from several laboratories that IL-2 causes B cells to proliferate and to synthesize antibody. The quantities of IL-2 required were rather large, and it is not certain that they were physiologic. In one report, IL-2 was effective as the only lymphokine known to be present [59]. In the other, it synergized with several other lymphokines and could not stimulate B-cell proliferation by itself [52]. B cells do have some IL-2 receptors (<1000 per cell as measured by anti-Tac binding), so it is possible that IL-2 has some direct B-cell effects [52]. However, it does not seem likely that a B cell with <1000 IL-2 receptors could compete effectively in vivo with a T cell with $>90{,}000$ receptors.

Interleukin-2 also has major effects on natural killer (NK) cells. These are a population of large granular lymphocytes that constitute about 5% of peripheral blood lymphocytes and have the capacity to kill cells of many spontaneous or induced tumors. The granules have been isolated by disrupting the cells and are themselves cytolytic [28]. The granules of "cytotoxic T cells," which may or may not be the same as the granules of NK cells, have been shown to contain six different proteins. Of these, two are capable of assembling in arrays that act as transmembrane channels and lyse the target cell [60].

Interleukin-2 can induce a short-term increase in NK activity of human peripheral blood leukocytes. The increase is present before there is any demonstrable secretion of IFNγ. However, NK cells do secrete IFNγ in response to IL-2, and IFNγ is itself known to activate NK cells. It may be, therefore, that the IL-2 effect occurs because of autostimulation of NK cells by the IFNγ they secrete. The increased activity is due both to an increase in numbers of NK cells (possibly due to maturation from a precursor cell) and an increased cytolytic activity of each individual cell [76].

Interleukin-2 also allows the establishment of long-term cultures of NK cells. After 3 or 4 days in such cultures, NK activity is raised to a point at which tumor cells not sensitive to ordinary NK cells are killed. Natural killer cells from patients with cancer generally cannot kill dissociated cells of the autologous tumor. After 3-4 days in culture with IL-2, patients' NK cells do kill the autologous tumor [25]. Hence, the intense commercial interest in IL-2 as a possible anti-tumor agent.

INTERLEUKIN-3

Interleukin-3 is a glycoprotein of molecular weight about 26,000 D found in the supernates of T cells stimulated with antigen or mitogens. The first biologic activity ascribed to it was the ability to induce the enzyme 20 α-hydroxysteroid dehydrogenase (20α-SDH) in spleen cells from nude mice. This enzyme is associated with mature T cells, and it was thought that IL-3 must be involved in the regulation of T-cell differentiation [33]. However, when IL-3 was used to promote the growth of bone marrow cells, instead of the expected T cells, most of the lines differentiated into mast cells. Interleukin-3 appeared also to promote the growth of erythroid, megakaryocytic, eosinophil, granulocyte, and macrophage colonies from bone marrow. In other words, it behaved as a classic colony-stimulating factor (CSF) [21,83].

Interleukin-3 is produced constituitively and in high yield by the mouse tumor line WEHI-3. Significantly, most people think that the cell type of this line is myelomonocytic leukemia. In any event, cell supernates were concentrated and purified by chromatography on DEAE cellulose, hydroxylapatite, Sephadex G75, and a reverse phase HPLC system. The purified IL-3 was homogeneous on SDS-PAGE. It was successfully iodinated and shown to bind to IL-3-dependent cell lines. Also, an antibody was raised that precipitated the purified protein and simultaneously abolished IL-3 activity.

Interleukin-3 had some unusual properties. It was unaffected by boiling. It was heavily glycosylated, and some variation in the molecular weight and charge of purified IL-3 was found. However, the N-terminal amino acid sequence was the same for all variants. A total of nine amino acids were identified, and the IL-3 sequence seemed to be unique. It was confirmed that homogeneous IL-3 had all the CSF activities already referred to, as well as the ability to induce 20α-SDH in *nu/nu* cells [34].

Recently, the IL-3 gene from a mouse T-cell line has been cloned. The gene contained a single open reading frame of 166 codons, but it was not clear which of three available methionine residues represented the usual start point. The sequence of nine amino acids obtained from the protein was found just after a stretch of 20 hydrophobic amino acids, which probably served as a signal peptide and was removed during secretion of IL-3. If that is accepted, the secreted molecule contains 134 amino acids with four available N-glycosylation sites [47,84].

The availability of cloned genes for IL-3 will presumably allow the synthesis of large amounts of recombinant IL-3. It will then be possible, it is hoped, to decide whether IL-3 is actively involved in the developing immune response or whether it is merely a cell differentiation factor that ensures adequate numbers of B cells, T cells, and macrophages from which immune responses can be developed. Palacios has recently shown that a myeloid cell line dependent on IL-3 for growth did not have receptors for IL-3 and that the IL-3 dependence could be partially replaced by exogenous ATP. An IL-3-dependent lymphoid cell line did have IL-3 receptors, and the IL-3 dependence was absolute. However, to add to the confusion about just what IL-3 does, it was a pre-B-cell line [57].

γ INTERFERON

The IFN are induced proteins, secreted into the medium by animal cells, which protect other cells from viral infections by modifying intracellular functions. There is an enormous literature on IFN which was reviewed in a recent monograph [73]. Much of this literature is rapidly becoming irrelevant because it concerns mixtures of unknown IFN heavily contaminated with other proteins. But that period did bequeath us the present IFN nomenclature.

Initially, IFNα referred to the type obtained from blood leukocytes, IFNβ was obtained from fibroblasts, and IFNγ was obtained from lymphocytes stimulated with antigen, lectin, or histoincompatible cells. It has now been discovered that leukocytes can secrete some IFNβ and that fibroblasts can secrete IFNα. A recent committee recommended that they be lumped together as type I IFN, and that IFNγ be known as type II [74]. This nomenclature has not yet become general and will not be used here.

Genes for IFNα have been cloned, and recombinant IFNα is available. There are at least 14 genes for IFNα, each specifying a slightly different protein. The gene for IFNβ appears to be single, and there is only 15% homology with IFNα. Neither of these forms of IFN has much immunologic significance, and they will not be discussed further. However, it is conceivable that IFNα and β cause the suppression in delayed hypersensitivity and cell-mediated immunity characteristic of generalized viral infections, such as measles.

γ Interferon is a glycoprotein that is immunologically unrelated to other IFN and is chemically different in that it is inactivated at pH 2. The usual molecular weight of human IFNγ is 35,000-70,000 D. The usual inducers of IFNα and β are viruses and double-stranded RNA, but other substances, such as bacteria, fungi, microbial products, and various chemicals, are also effective. T cells acted on by these stimuli make IFNα, just as do other cells. However, when T cells participate in immunologic reactions, they secrete mainly IFNγ, and IFNγ is not secreted by other cell types. γ Interferon is thus a lymphokine, a soluble product of activated T cells. There is clear evidence that the major stimulus for IFNγ release by T cells is IL-2 [37].

γ Interferon is a perfectly genuine IFN and protects many different kinds of cells from viral infections with efficiencies comparable to those of IFNα and β. It also has the mild depressive effect on the replication of normal cells characteristic of other IFN. Depending on when it is given, IFNγ (and other IFN) can either suppress or enhance immune responses of all types. Suppression is generally seen when IFN and antigen are given about the same time, because B- and T-cell replication is impeded. Enhancement is seen when IFN is delayed for 3-4 days after antigen, when Ts cells are normally beginning to multiply (reviewed in Reference 20). γ Interferon, like other IFN, also inhibits replication of many tumors to a greater extent than it inhibits replication of normal cells. For this reason, there is intense interest in the use of large quantities of IFNγ as an anti-tumor agent, particularly because its antiproliferative effect is about 100 times as strong as that of IFNα and β.

Despite all the above, it seems likely that the main actions of IFNγ take place locally in lymph nodes and other tissues of the immune system and that its principal importance is in the maturation of phagocytic and cytolytic killer cells of many different kinds. Evidence to support this idea is beginning to accumulate since recombinant IFNγ has become available in the last couple of years and it was at last possible to study IFNγ in isolation from other interferons and lymphokines.

The human IFNγ gene has recently been cloned using mRNA from peripheral blood leukocytes treated with staphylococcal enterotoxin B plus desacetylthymosine α. The mRNA was sized by electrophoresis on agarose, and it was found that the 18S mRNA fraction caused IFNγ secretion when injected into frog oocytes. This mRNA was reverse transcribed to DNA and cloned by the usual methods. The putative gene contained 166 codons, and there was a 20-residue hydrophobic probable signal peptide with a Gly-Cys probable cleavage site. The probable structure of the secreted IFNγ was a protein of molecular weight 17,110 D, much smaller than most reported weights for IFNγ. There were only two Cys residues, at positions 1 and 3, so it did not seem probable that –SS– bonds could contribute much to secondary structure. This agreed with evidence that IFNγ is not destroyed by reduction and alkylation. The high pI of 8.6 was explained by a 27:19 predominance of basic residues over acidic ones. Two glycosylation sites were present: Asn-Gly-Thr at positions 28-30, and Asn-Tyr-Ser at 100-102. The cloned gene was transfected into *E. coli* and into monkey cells, and biologically active IFNγ was secreted in both cases. Human peripheral leukocytes seemed to contain one IFNγ gene per cell [24].

The unexpectedly low molecular weight was confirmed by Prat et al. [62]. They obtained a monoclonal antibody against murine IFNγ by the usual methods of cell fusion and hybrid selection. This monoclone was used to screen cell extracts from the murine T-cell lymphoma line L12-R4 after stimulation with PMA. If the cells were stimulated in the presence of labeled methionine, it was possible to precipitate two ^{35}S-labeled peptides from such cells, with apparent molecular weights of 16,800 and 17,800 D. If the cells were stimulated in the presence of [^{3}H] glucosamine, the same two peptides were labeled with ^{3}H, confirming that they were glycosylated. Obviously, the authors intend to clone the murine IFNγ gene, because they added that there was about 40% homology between human and murine IFNγ.

The discrepancy in molecular weight between the gene products and the IFNγ found in cell supernates has now been resolved [10]. Two monoclonal anti IFNγ antibodies were made, which were to serve as the basis of a solid phase immunoassay. Since immunodeterminants occur only once per protein molecule, one monoclonal was needed to fix IFNγ to the solid support and the other to detect it once there. Unexpectedly, it was found that the assay was just as effective if a single antibody was used for both purposes. That can only mean that secreted IFNγ is polymeric, hence the molecular weights of 35,000 D (dimer) to 70,000 D (tetramer).

Nathan et al. have clearly shown that IFNγ is the only important lymphokine that can activate macrophages to kill intracellular parasites, such as *Listeria, Toxoplasma,* and *Leishmania.* Macrophages treated with IFNγ secreted large quantities of superoxide, singlet oxygen, and other reactive oxygen compounds after triggering with PMA. Such macrophages were able to kill the above-mentioned intracellular parasites, as well as others. The activity was shown with highly purified natural IFNγ, as well as recombinant IFNγ, and was abolished with a monoclonal antibody against IFNγ. A series of other lymphokines and biologic factors was also tested for the ability to activate macrophages to the killer state. They were IFNα, IFNβ, three forms of CSF, MIF, TNF, IL-1, and IL-2. All were negative [53]. It has also been shown that macrophages have an IFNγ receptor and that IFNγ can activate macrophages to kill tumors [9].

There is a great deal of older evidence suggesting that IFNγ enhances the function of phagocytic and cytolytic cells. Macrophages exposed to IFNγ grow larger, spread further on solid surfaces, express more Fc receptors, and phagocytose more particles [80]. The effect of IFNγ on the activity of NK cells was discussed. There is a good deal of evidence suggesting that NK cells are not a homogeneous population and that IFNγ may enhance the killing activity of some types, whereas IL-2 enhances that of others [29,46]. γ Interferon also probably enhances the development and/or activity of Tc cells and of the null, or K, cells that mediate antibody-dependent cytotoxicity. Cytotoxic T-cell development is totally dependent on IL-2, but it is also blocked by antisera against IFNγ [56]. There is much disagreement about what, if anything, is required for the development of Tc and K cells besides IL-2 and IFNγ. None of these systems has yet been examined with recombinant IFNγ, monoclonal antibodies against IFNγ, or in clearly defined cell populations. However, all these areas are under intense investigation at present, and answers will be forthcoming. Obviously, if IFNγ antagonists can be developed, they may be of use in controlling some types of graft rejection.

Another type of activity mediated by IFNγ is its ability to cause many different kinds of cells to modify their surface antigens. Increased Fc receptor display by macrophages was referred to, but increased Fc receptor display is also seen on both B cells and T cells [2]. Other cell surface markers, such as HLA or H2 antigens, β_2-microglobulin, Ia antigens, Ly antigens, and specific antigen receptors on T cells, have all been observed to increase in various cell populations treated with IFN (reviewed in Reference 80). When it was tested, IFNγ was much more effective in inducing these changes than were IFNα and β. Just how altered display of surface proteins of B and T cells affects immune function is not yet clear.

Glucocorticoids suppress the secretion of IFNγ and other lymphokines by T cells. Since they also suppress secretion of IL-2, it had been assumed that this latter reaction was primary. However, there are alloreactive T-cell clones that liberate IFNγ and CSF as well as IL-2 when stimulated with concanavalin A (ConA). The secretion of all three factors is suppressed by dexamethasone at concentrations between 10^{-8} and 10^{-6} M, and the secretion of IFNγ and CSF cannot be restored by supplying the cells with exogenous IL-2. Furthermore, the corticosteroid effect on IFNγ secretion was demonstrable in T-cell clones that were IL-2 independent and did not secrete IL-2. The dexamethasone effect was not due to cell death; the cells continued to proliferate at a normal rate but did not secrete lymphokines. Cytotoxic T-cell clones were less susceptible to dexamethasone-mediated suppression of lymphokine secretion than non-Tc clones [38].

B-CELL GROWTH FACTOR AND OTHER LYMPHOKINES DIRECTING THE DEVELOPMENT OF IMMUNOGLOBULIN: SECRETING CELLS

B cells undergo an orderly pattern of differentiation in which surface markers, genetic reorganizations, and syntheses of portions of immunoglobulins occur in a definite sequence. The earliest pre-B cells have neither cytoplasmic nor surface Ig, and both heavy and light chain immunoglobulin genes are in the germ line arrangement. During the next stage, in the mouse, the markers Lyb-2 and Ly-5 become demonstrable, the IgM heavy chain genes are rearranged, and the Mac-1 antigen is lost. This is a large pre-B cell. In the small pre-B cell, the Th B marker is added and light chain gene rearrangements occur. These cells often have cytoplasmic μ or δ chains. In the next stage, the cell expresses surface IgM and IgD and is a B cell. Upon stimulation, these cells differentiate further, add a complement receptor, and finally secrete a little IgM. They may continue to secrete IgM, or may change the class of antibody produced to IgG (all varieties), IgA, or IgE. These Ig-secreting cells are immunoblasts, most of which follow the suicidal final differentiation path to plasma cells, which secrete large quantities of immunoglobulin but have a life span of only a few days [16].

The whole of this differentiation is almost certainly under very tight control. However, although a multitude of soluble factors has been described that affect B-cell differentiation in some way, there is at the moment no agreement about which of them are necessary, the sequence in which they act, and whether any of the phenomena observed in vitro are relevant to immune responses in vivo. For example, it is possible to trigger B cells, not only in the absence of antigen, but through a membrane protein that is not immunoglobulin [15]. Whether, as the authors claim, this is the only physiologic method of activating B cells to secrete antibody to T-dependent antigens remains to be seen.

There does appear to be agreement that B cells that have developed as far as expressing immunoglobulin on their surfaces (sIg-positive B cells) are in a resting state and will not spontaneously differentiate unless stimulated. A total of four types of signal are thought to exist.

1. An inductive signal, which is most usually thought of as antigen. Antigen can be mimicked by stimulating the cells with anti-μ antibody, which cross-links the cell sIg in approximately the same way that antigen would [52]. Inductive signals are thought to allow the B cell to express receptors for growth factors. However, by themselves they do not stimulate B-cell replication. The effects of antigen on resting B cells have recently been studied in more detail. Cells stimulated with anti-μ, or antigen, enter the G_1 phase of cell cycle without DNA synthesis but with increased amounts of RNA, an increase in cell size, and increased expression of Ia antigens [49]. The earliest observable events are a decrease in membrane potential and an influx of calcium; whether these events are causal of the entry into G_1 is not known [48,61]. The expression of Ia determinants is maximal in G_1 and declines during S to a point where it is even less than that of resting B cells. Thus, it looks as if the effect of antigen is to cause the expression of Ia determinants, which in turn makes the B cell very susceptible to T-cell help. Both Th cells and soluble factors derived from them require Ia antigen display before they can be effective. There is evidence that under some circumstances both T cells [15] and T-cell helper factors [42,45] may be able to induce B cells and then sustain their growth once induced, in the absence of antigen. This can occur because resting B cells do display a little Ia antigen, and induction promotes increased Ia display, which in turn makes T-cell help more effective. But it seems likely that in vivo, B cells are induced by antigen, and T-cell help makes the induced cells proliferate.
2. Growth factors, which stimulate mitosis in induced B cells. The most well defined of these is B-cell growth factor (BSF-lp). Growth factors in and of themselves do not usually stimulate IgG secretion.
3. Differentiation factors, which stimulate the secretion of Ig. Polyclonal B-cell activators, such as lipopolysaccharide (LPS), usually lead to the secretion of mostly IgM, with some IgG_3 and IgG_{2b}. These antibody classes are thought to be T independent. Secretion of other antibody classes requires the next class of factor.
4. Class switching factors, which cause or promote the genetic rearrangements that allow secretion of IgG_1, IgG_{2a}, IgA, or IgE. All such class switches appear to be mediated by T cells or products derived from them.

An international committee of lymphokine experts met in Kyoto and agreed on a nomenclature and a method of approach to the various soluble factors that influence the growth of B cells once they have been induced. It was agreed that factors well characterized biochemically and functionally in more than one laboratory would be given the designation BSF, for B-cell stimulation factor. A numerical suffix is to describe the order of discovery, and a *P* (provisional) is attached to the designation of any factor that has not been purified to homogeneity or cloned. Under these rules, the only thoroughly established B-cell lymphokine was B-cell growth factor, referred to as BCGF in older literature. This is now BSF-lp. All other lymphokines affecting B-cell development have a complicated three-part temporary nomenclature that gives the cell of origin, the factor activity, and the name of the principal author.

B-cell growth factor is capable of stimulating DNA synthesis in B cells that have bound antigen or have been stimulated with polyclonal activators, such as LPS. It is secreted by normal T cells stimulated with antigen and by a variety of T-cell lines, hybridomas, and tumors [30,31]. It is a glycoprotein of molecular weight 12,000-15,000 D by SDS-PAGE. Because of the glycosylation, it shows microheterogeneity of isoelectric point. It has not been purified to homogeneity, nor has the gene been cloned, but it is clearly separable from IL-2 and other known lymphokines.

The BSF-lp exists in the cytoplasm of T lymphocytes as a precursor of molecular weight 60,000-80,000 D. When T cells are stimulated with antigen or lectin, the intracellular pool diminishes and the extracellular small-molecular-weight form appears. Partial digestion of the intracellular form with trypsin yielded active BSF-lp of lower molecular weight. Messenger RNA was isolated from stimulated T cells, either by digesting polysomes or by isolating the polyadenylated fraction on oligo-DT columns. Both forms sedimented at 16-20S on sucrose gradients, and both could cause *Xenopus* oocytes to secrete biologically active BSF-lp. This size of mRNA corresponds to a protein of about 70,000 D [69]. Obviously, the gene is going to be cloned in the next few months.

The BSF-lp has no action on T cells and cannot substitute for either IL-1 or IL-2 in assays requiring those factors. It does not by itself stimulate small resting B cells to enter the cell cycle, but it does increase the expression of several surface markers, especially the Ia markers [54]. Once B cells have been induced by antigen, anti-μ, or LPS, BSF-lp promotes their entry into S phase and cell division. Such B cells can be maintained in cycle for long periods of time, but not yet indefinitely. In the absence of other factors, the B cells do not secrete immunoglobulin [69]. The action of BSF-lp is without antigenic specificity; it acts on any induced B cell. Under normal circumstances, the specificity of the immune response is maintained because only B cells induced by antigen are sensitive to BSF-lp.

There are receptors for BSF-lp on activated B cells, as judged by the ability of such cells to remove it from solution, even at low temperature. Most workers have thought that there were no receptors on resting B cells, but in view of the fact that BSF-lp induces Ia antigen expression in resting B cells [54], receptors must be present at some low level. The receptor has not yet been identified with any particular membrane protein, nor is there a good assay for it, so these questions must be left in abeyance at present.

Probably all B-cell proliferative responses require at least a trace of IL-1. Fetal calf serum is well known to have "good" batches that support immunologic responses and "bad" batches that do not. It seems probable that good batches are so because they contain traces of IL-1 secreted by fetal calf monocytes. Melchers, who is probably the only person in the world who can grow B cells in a serum-free medium, finds an absolute dependence on macrophages or their soluble products even for responses to polyclonal activators, such as LPS [14]. Only about 1 macrophage per 1000 B cells is required, and it is difficult or impossible to reduce macrophage contamination of B cells to below this level. Even Melchers can only do it about half the time. This explains many apparently conflicting results in the literature, in which IL-1 is apparently not required for responses to LPS. There is overwhelming evidence from many sources that macrophages or IL-1 are required for B-cell responses to T-dependent antigens. And Paul and his colleagues have found that IL-1 is necessary for B-cell proliferation in response to anti-μ antibody [32].

B-cell differentiation factors act on dividing B cells and promote the secretion of immunoglobulin. In the system of Paul, B cells are induced by anti-μ and stimulated to grow by BSF-lp, and two T-cell-derived factors are required to make them secrete IgM. Both come under the general category of T-cell-replacing factors (TRF): one is derived from the cell line B_{151} K_{12} and is required soon after BSF-lp; the other is found in the supernate of the EL-4 line, and is required later in the response. This latter activity can be replaced by IL-2, but IL-2 does not account for all the activity in an EL-4 supernate [52]. Other workers have similar multiple TRF, which one way or another are involved in stimulating IgM synthesis by B cells. None has been purified, nor is there agreement between laboratories on how many there are and how they act. Nossal even believes that the single lymphokine IL-2 can in large doses replace BSF-lp and all TRF [59].

Lymphokines that cause B cells to switch heavy chains while retaining the same combining site probably exist. It is not quite clear that they act on B cells secreting IgM and cause them to rearrange their genomes to secrete IgG_1, Ig_{2a}, IgA, or IgE. They could in theory work by encouraging the growth of B cells already committed to secreting IgG_1. In any event, they are class specific; a given factor promotes the secretion of a particular class of immunoglobulin. They have thus been given such names as BCDF (B-cell differentiation factor) γ_1, BCDFα, and so forth. The present knowledge of these factors is reviewed in Reference 79.

SUMMARY

Immune responses occur when cells have joined themselves into clumps in which macrophages or dendritic cells embrace with their processes T cells and B cells with common antigenic specificity. The different cells in these clumps communicate at very close range, and it may be that mechanisms of which we know nothing are involved. Nonetheless, soluble hormones secreted by immunocytes have been purified that can partially or completely replace the cell requirements for some immune responses. Those involved early in immune responses are quite well defined, both functionally and biochemically. They are probably involved in allograft rejection and in allograft tolerance. Immunosuppressives, such as corticosteroids and cyclosporin A, can be shown to interfere with the secretion of lymphokines, which are probably important in promoting allograft rejection. Soluble hormones affecting the late stages of the immune response have been described in profusion, but their place in mediating immune responses is not yet settled.

REFERENCES

1. Aarden, L. A., Brunner, T. K., Cerrotini, J. C., et al. Revised nomenclature for antigen nonspecific T cell proliferation and helper factors. *J. Immunol.* 123:2928-2829, 1979.
2. Agnet, M. High affinity binding of ^{125}I labelled mouse interferon to a specific cell surface receptor. *Nature* 284:459-461, 1980.
3. Auron, P. C., Webb, A. C., Rosenwasser, L. J., Mucci, S. F., Rich, A., Wolff, S. M., Dinarello, C. Nucleotide sequence of human monocyte interleukin 1 precursor cDNA. *Proc. Natl. Acad. Sci. USA* 81:7907-7911, 1984.
4. Baracos, V., Rodeman, H. P., Dinarello, C. A., and Goldberg, A. L. Stimulation of muscle protein degradation and prostaglandin E_2 release by interleukin-1. *N. Engl. J. Med.* 308:553-558, 1983.
5. Bensussan, A., Acuto, O., Hussey, R. C., Milanese, C., and Reinherz, E. L. T3-Ti receptor triggering of $T8^+$ suppressor T cells leads to unresponsiveness to interleukin 2. *Nature* 311:565-567, 1984.
6. Bodel, P. Spontaneous pyrogen production by mouse histiocytic and myelomonocytic tumor cell lines in vitro. *J. Exp. Med.* 147:1503-1516, 1978.

7. Burger, D. R., and Vetto, R. M. Vascular endothelium as a major participant in T lymphocyte immunity. *Cell. Immunol.* 70:357-361, 1982.
8. Cebula, T. A., Hanson, D. F., Moore, D. M., and Murphy, P. A. Synthesis of four endogenous pyrogens by rabbit macrophages. *J. Lab. Clin. Med.* 94:95-105, 1979.
9. Celada, A, Gray, P. W., Rinderknecht, E., and Schreiber, R. D. Evidence for a γ interferon receptor that regulates macrophage tumoricidal activity. *J. Exp. Med.* 160:55-74, 1984.
10. Chang, T. W., McKinney, S., Liu, V., Kung, P. C., Vilcek, J., and Le, J. Use of monoclonal antibodies as sensitive and specific probes for biologically active human γ interferon. *Proc. Natl. Acad. Sci. USA* 81:5219-5222, 1984.
11. Clayberger, C., DeKruyff, R. H., Fay, R., and Cantor, H. Identification of a unique B cell stimulating factor produced by a cloned dendritic cell. *Proc. Natl. Acad. Sci. USA* 82:183-187, 1985.
12. Clowes, G. H. A., George, B. C., Villee, C. A., and Saravis, C. A. Muscle proteolysis induced by a circulating peptide in patients with sepsis or trauma. *N. Engl. J. Med.* 308:545-552, 1983.
13. Conlon, P. A rapid biological assay for the detection of interleukin 1. *J. Immunol.* 131:1280-1282, 1983.
14. Corbel, C., and Melchers, F. Synergism of accessory cells and of soluble α factors derived from them in the activation of B cells to proliferation. *Immunol. Rev.* 78:51-74, 1984.
15. Coutinho, A., Pobor, G., Petterson, S., Leandersson, T., Forsgren, S., Periera, P., Bandeira, A., and Martinez-A., C. T cell dependent B cell activation. *Immunol. Rev.* 78:211-224, 1984.
16. Davidson, W. F., Frederickson, T. N., Rudikoff, E. K., Coffman, R. L., Hartley, J. W., and Morse, H. C., III. A unique series of lymphomas related to the Ly-1$^+$ lineage of B lymphocyte differentiation. *J. Immunol.* 133:744-753, 1984.
17. Devos, R., Plaetinck, G., Cheroutre, H., Simons, G., Degrave, W., Tavernier, J., Remaut, E., and Fiers, W. Molecular cloning of human interleukin 2 cDNA, and its expression in *E. coli. Nucleic Acids Res.* II:4307-4323, 1984.
18. Dinarello, C. A. Interleukin I. *Rev. Infect. Dis.* 6:51-95, 1984.
19. Fontana, A., Kristensen, F., Dubs, R., Gemsa, D., and Weber, E. Production of prostaglandin E and an interleukin-1 like factor from cultured astrocytes and C6 glioma cells. *J. Immunol.* 129:2413-2419, 1982.
20. Friedman, R. M., and Vogel, S. N. Interferons with special emphasis on the immune system. *Immunol. Rev.* 34:97-140, 1983.
21. Garland, J. M., and Dexter, T. M. Relationship of haemopoietic growth factor to lymphocytes and interleukin 3: A short review. *Lymphokine Res.* 2:13-22, 1983.
22. Gillis, S., and Mizel, S. B. T cell lymphoma model for the analysis of interleukin 1 mediated T cell activation. *Proc. Natl. Acad. Sci. USA* 78:1133-1137, 1981.
23. Granelli-Pipierno, A., Andrus, L., and Reich, E. Antibodies to interleukin 2, effects on immune responses in vitro and in vivo. *J. Exp. Med.* 160:738-750, 1984.
24. Gray, P. W., Leung, D. W., Rennica, D., Yelverton, E., Najarian, R., Simonsen, C. C., Derynck, R., Sherwood, P. J., Wallace, D. M., Berger, S. L., Levinson, A. D., and Goeddel, D. V. Expression of human immune interferon cDNA in *E. coli* and monkey cells. *Nature* 295:503-508, 1982.
25. Grimm, E. A., Gorelik, E., Rosenstein, M. M., and Rosenberg, S. A. The lymphokine activated killer cell phenomenon: In vitro and in vivo studies. In *Interleukins, Lymphokines and Cytokines,* J. J. Oppenheim and S. Cohen, eds. Academic Press, New York, 1983, pp. 739-748.
26. Handshumaker, R. E., Harding, M. W., Rice, J., Drugge, R. J., and Speicher, D. W. Cytophilin: A specific cytosolic binding protein for cyclosporin A. *Science* 226:544-547, 1984.

27. Hanson, D. F., Murphy, P. A., Silicano, R., and Shin, H. S. The effect of temperature on the activation of thymocytes by interleukins I and II. *J. Immunol.* 130:216-221, 1983.
28. Henkart, R. A., Millard, P. J., Reynolds, C. W., and Henkart, M. P. Cytolytic activity of purified cytoplasmic granules from rat cytotoxic large granular lymphocyte tumors. *J. Exp. Med.* 160:75-83, 1984.
29. Henney, C. S., Kuribayashi, K., Kern, D. E., and Gillis, S. Interleukin 2 augments natural killer cell activity. *Nature* 291:335-338, 1981.
30. Howard, M., Farrar, J., Hilfiker, M., Johnson, B., Takatsu, K., Hamaoka, T., and Paul, W. E. Identification of a T cell derived B cell growth factor distinct from interleukin 2. *J. Exp. Med.* 155:914-923, 1982.
31. Howard, M., Matis, L., Malek, T., Shevach, E., Kell, W., Cohen, D., Nakanishi, K., and Paul, W. E. Interleukin 2 induces antigen reactive T cell lines to secrete BCGF-1. *J. Exp. Med.* 158:2024-2039, 1983.
32. Howard, M., Mizel, S. B., Lachmann, L., Ansel, J., Johnson, B., and Paul, W. E. Role of interleukin 1 in anti immunoglobulin induced B cell proliferation. *J. Exp. Med.* 157:1529-1543, 1983.
33. Ihle, J. N., Pepersack, L., and Rebar, L. Regulation of T cell differentiation: In vitro induction of 20-alpha hydroxysteroid dehydrogenase in splenic lymphocytes is mediated by a unique lymphokine. *J. Immunol.* 126:2184-2189, 1981.
34. Ihle, J. N., Keller, J., Henderson, L., Klein, F., and Palaszynski, E. Procedures for the purification of IL-3 to homogeneity. *J. Immunol.* 129:2431-2436, 1982.
35. Inaba, K., Steinman, R. M., Van Voorhis, W. C., and Muramatsu, S. Dendritic cells are critical accessory cells for thymus dependent antibody responses in mouse and in man. *Proc. Natl. Acad. Sci. USA* 80:6041-6047, 1983.
36. Inaba, K., and Steinman, R. M. Resting and sensitized T lymphocytes exhibit distinct stimulatory requirements for growth and lymphokine release. *J. Exp. Med.* 160:1717-1735, 1984.
37. Kasahara, T., Hooks, J. J., Daugherty, S. F., and Oppenheim, J. J. Interleukin 2 mediated immune interferon (IFN-γ) production by human T cells and T cell subsets. *J. Immunol.* 130:1784-1789, 1983.
38. Kelso, A., and Munck, A. Glucocorticoid inhibition of lymphokine secretion by alloreactive T lymphocyte clones. *J. Immunol.* 133:784-791, 1984.
39. Klempner, M. S., Dinarello, C. A., and Gallin, J. I. Human leukocytic pyrogen induces release of specific granule contents from human neutrophils. *J. Clin. Invest.* 61:1330-1336, 1978.
40. Kristensen, F., Bettens, F., Walker, C., Joncourt, F., and de Weck, A. Human lymphocyte proliferation: Relationship between cell cycle events and interleukin 2 production. In *Interleukins, Lymphokines and Cytokines,* J. J. Oppenheim and S. Cohen, eds. Academic Press, New York, 1982, pp. 43-49.
41. Kronke, M., Leonard, W. J., Depper, J. M., Arya, S. K., Wong-Stahl, F., Gallo, R. C., Waldmann, T. A., and Greene, W. C. Cyclosporin A inhibits T cell growth factor gene expression at the level of mRNA transcription. *Proc. Natl. Acad. Sci. USA* 81:5214-5218, 1984.
42. LeClerq, L., Bismuth, G., and Theze, J. Antigen specific T cell clone supernatant is sufficient to induce both polyclonal proliferation and differentiation of small resting B lymphocytes. *Proc. Natl. Acad. Sci. USA* 81:6491-6495, 1984.
43. Lomedico, P. T., Gubler, U., Hellman, C. P., Dukovich, M., Giri, J. G., Pan, Y. E., Collier, K., Semionow, R., Chua, A. O., and Mizel, S. B. Cloning and expression of murine interleukin 1 cDNA in *Escherichia coli. Nature* 312:458-462, 1984.
44. Lovett, D. H., Sterzek, R. B., Ryan, J. L., and Atkins, E. Production of an endogenous pyrogen by glomerular mesangial cells. *J. Immunol.* 134:670-672, 1985.

45. Melchers, F., Andersson, J., Leonhardt, W., and Schreier, M. H. H2 unrestricted polyclonal maturation without replication of small B cells induced by antigen-activated T cell factors. *Eur. J. Immunol.* 10:679-685, 1980.
46. Mineto, N., Reid, L., and Bloom, B. R. On the heterogeneity of murine natural killer cells. *J. Exp. Med.* 154:750-762, 1980.
47. Miyataka, S., Yokota, T., Lee, F., and Arai, K.-I. Structure of the chromosomal gene for murine interleukin 3. *Proc. Natl. Acad. Sci. USA* 82:316-320, 1985.
48. Monroe, J. G., and Cambier, J. C. B cell plasma membrane depolarization and hyper Ia antigen expression induced by receptor immunoglobulin cross-linking are coupled. *J. Exp. Med.* 1589-1599, 1982.
49. Monroe, J. E., and Cambier, J. C. Level of mIa expression on mitogen stimulated murine B lymphocytes is dependent on position in cell cycle. *J. Immunol.* 130:626-631, 1983.
50. Moore, D. M., Murphy, P. A., Chesney, P. J., and Wood, W. B., Jr. Synthesis of endogenous pyrogen by rabbit leukocytes. *J. Exp. Med.* 137:1263-1274, 1973.
51. Murphy, P. A., Simon, P. L., and Willoughby, W. F. Endogenous pyrogens made by peritoneal exudate cells are identical with lymphocyte activating factors made by rabbit alveolar macrophages. *J. Immunol.* 124:2498-2501, 1980.
52. Nakamishi, K., Malek, T. R., Smith, K. A., Hamaoka, T., Shevach, E. M., and Paul, W. E. Both IL-2 and a second T cell derived factor in EL-4 supernates have activity as differentiation factors in IgM synthesis. *J. Exp. Med.* 160:1605-1621, 1984.
53. Nathan, C. F., Prendergast, T. J., Weibe, W. E., Stanley, E. R., Platzer, E., Remold, H. G., Welte, K., Rubin, B. Y., and Murray, H. W. Activation of human macrophages: Comparison of other cytokines with interferon γ. *J. Exp. Med.* 160:600-605, 1984.
54. Noelle, R., Krammer, P. H., Ohara, J., Uhr, J. W., and Vitetta, E. S. Increased expression of Ia antigens on resting B cells: An additional role for B cell growth factor. *Proc. Natl. Acad. Sci. USA* 81:6149-6153, 1984.
55. Ortaldo, J. R., Mason, R. T., Gerard, J. P., Henderson, L. E., Farrar, W., Hopkins, R. F., Herberman, R. B., and Rabin, H. Effects of natural and recombinant IL-2 on regulation of IFNγ production and natural killer activity. *J. Immunol.* 133:779-783, 1984.
56. Osbourne, L. C., Georgiades, J. A., and Johnson, H. M. Classification of interferons with antibody to immune interferon. *Cell. Immunol.* 53:65-70, 1980.
57. Palacios, R., and Garland, J. Distinct mechanisms may account for the growth promoting activity of interleukin 3 on cells of lymphoid and myeloid origin. *Proc. Natl. Acad. Sci. USA* 81:1208-1211, 1984.
58. Pepys, M. B., and Baltz, M. L. Acute phase proteins with special reference to C reactive protein and serum amyloid A protein. *Adv. Immunol.* 34:141-212, 1983.
59. Pike, B. L., Raubitschek, A., and Nossal, G. J. B. Human interleukin 2 can promote the growth and differentiation of single hapten specific B cells in the presence of specific antigen. *Proc. Natl. Acad. Sci. USA* 81:7917-7920, 1984.
60. Podeck, E. R., and Konigsberg, P. J. Cytolytic T cell granules: Isolation, structure, biochemical and functional characteristics. *J. Exp. Med.* 160:695-710, 1984.
61. Pozzan, T., Arslan, P., Tsien, R. Y., and Rink, T. J. Anti immunoglobulin, cytoplasmic free calcium, and capping in B lymphocytes. *J. Cell Biol.* 94:335-340, 1982.
62. Prat, M., Gribaudo, G., Comoglio, P. M., Cavallo, G., and Landolfo, S. Monoclonal antibodies against murine gamma interferon. *Proc. Natl. Acad. Sci. USA* 81:4515-4519, 1984.
63. Reem, G. H., and Yeh, N. H. Interleukin 2 regulates expression of its own receptor and synthesis of gamma interferon by human T lymphocytes. *Science* 225:429-430, 1984.
64. Robb, R. J., Munck, A., and Smith, K. T cell growth factor receptors: Quantitation, specificity and biological relevance. *J. Exp. Med.* 154:1455-1475, 1981.
65. Robb, R. J., Greene, W. C., and Rusk, C. M. Low and high affinity receptors for interleukin 2. *J. Exp. Med.* 160:1126-1146, 1984.

66. Robb, R. J., Kutney, R. M., Panico, M., Morris, H. R., and Chowdhry, V. Amino acid sequence and post-translational modification of human interleukin 2. *Proc. Natl. Acad. Sci. USA* 81:6486-6490, 1984.
67. Rosenberg, S. A., Grimm, E. A., McGrogan, M., Doyle, M., Kawasaki, E., Koths, K., and Mark, D. F. Biological activity of recombinant human interleukin 2 produced in *Escherichia coli. Science* 223:1413-1415, 1984.
68. Ruscetti, F. W., Morgan, D., and Gallo, R. C. Functional and morphologic characterization of human T cells continuously grown in vitro. *J. Immunol.* 119:131-138, 1977.
69. Sahasrabuddhe, C. G., Morgan, J., Sharma, S., Mehta, S., Martin, B., Wright, D., and Maizel, A. Evidence for an intracellular precursor for human B cell growth factor. *Proc. Natl. Acad. Sci. USA* 81:7902-7906, 1984.
70. Sauder, D. N., Carter, C. S., Katz, S. I., and Oppenheim, J. J. Epidermal cell production of thymocyte activating factor (ETAF). *J. Invest. Dermarol.* 79:34-39, 1982.
71. Schmidt, J. A. Purification and partial biochemical characterization of normal human interleukin 1. *J. Exp. Med.* 160:772-787, 1984.
72. Smith, K. A., and Ruschetti, F. W. T cell growth factor and the culture of cloned functional T cells. *Adv. Immunol.* 31:137-176, 1981.
73. Stewart, W. E., II. *The Interferon System.* Springer-Verlag, New York, 1979.
74. Stewart, W. E., II. Interferon nomenclature. *Nature* 286:110, 1980.
75. Taniguchi, T., Matsui, H., Fujita, T., Takaoka, C., Kashima, N., Yoshimoto, R., and Hamuro, J. Structure and expression of a cloned cDNA for human interleukin 2. *Nature* 302:305-310, 1983.
76. Trinchieri, G., Matsumoto-Kobayashi, M., Clark, S. C., Seehra, J., London, L., and Perussia, B. Response of resting human peripheral blood natural killer cells to interleukin 2. *J. Exp. Med.* 160:1147-1169, 1984.
77. Urdal, D. L., March, C. J., Gillis, S., Larsen, A., and Dower, S. K. Purification and chemical characterization of the receptor for interleukin 2 from activated human T lymphocytes and from a human T cell lymphoma line. *Proc. Natl. Acad. Sci. USA* 51:6481-6485, 1984.
78. Van Snick, J. L., Masson, P. L., and Heremans, J. F. The involvement of lactoferrin in the hyposideremia of acute inflammation. *J. Exp. Med.* 140:1068-1084, 1974.
79. Vitetta, E. S., Brooks, K., Chen, Y. W., Isakson, P., Jones, S., Layton, J., Mishra, G. C., Pure, E., Weiss, E., Word, C., Yuan, D., Tucker, P., Uhr, J. W., and Krammer, P. H. T cell derived lymphokines that induce IgM and IgG secretion in activated murine B cells. *Immunol. Rev.* 78:137-157, 1984.
80. Vogel, S. N., Weeden, L. L., Moore, R. N., and Rosenstreich, D. L. Correction of defective macrophage differentiation in C3H/HeJ mice by an interferon like molecule. *J. Immunol.* 128:380-387, 1982.
81. Wagner, H., Hardt, C., Heig, K., Rollinghoff, M., and Pfizenmaier, K. T cell derived helper factor allows in vivo induction of cytotoxic T cells in nu/nu mice. *Nature* 284: 278-280, 1980.
82. Wang, A., Lu, S. D., and Mark, D. F. Site specific mutagenesis of the human interleukin 2 gene. *Science* 224:1431-1432, 1984.
83. Watson, J. D., and Prestidge, R. L. Interleukin 3 and colony stimulating factors. *Immunol. Today* 4:278-280, 1983.
84. Yokota, T., Lee, F., Rennick, D., Hall, C., Arai, N., Mosmann, T., Nabel, G., Cantor, H., and Arai, I.-I. Isolation and characterization of a mouse c DNA clone that expresses mast cell growth factor activity in monkey cells. *Proc. Natl. Acad. Sci. USA* 81:1070-1074, 1984.

5

IMMUNOLOGIC ENHANCEMENT AND ITS RELATIONSHIP TO CLINICAL TRANSPLANTATION

Robin P. Lowry
Royal Victoria Hospital Research Institute, McGill University, Montreal, Quebec, Canada

Immunologic enhancement has been defined [98] as

> . . . the successful establishment or prolonged survival (conversely, delayed rejection) of an allogeneic graft as a consequence of interaction between the graft and specific antiserum in the host. The demonstrated requirement for contact of the graft with antigraft antibody as the initiating factor in immunologic enhancement distinguishes this phenomenon from the various manifestations of induced unresponsiveness, designated by such terms as acquired tolerance, immunologic unresponsiveness, immune paralysis and others.

It is the belief of the author that the phenomenon of immunologic enhancement underlies the now well accepted observation that pretransplant transfusion augments survival of renal allografts in humans [156]. Some of the experimental and clinical data supporting this thesis will be presented in this chapter.

The phenomenon of enhancement has been extensively reviewed on a number of occasions [11,26,57,87,138,186,204], and accordingly we will provide only a brief outline of some of the important observations leading to our current understanding of antibody-induced immunosuppression. The mechanism whereby immunologic enhancement promotes allograft survival will be discussed in terms of the known or presumed effects of enhancing antibody on the (allo)immune response and recent thoughts about the mechanism of graft rejection. Finally, we will briefly review available evidence that would link the apparently nonspecific beneficial effect of random transfusion in clinical transplantation with the phenomenon of specific immunologic enhancement.

IMMUNOLOGIC ENHANCEMENT: HISTORICAL PERSPECTIVE

Studies in Tumor Systems: The Initial Observation of Enhancement Phenomena

In 1907, Flexner and Jobling reported that the injection of a heat-treated (56°C for 30 min) tumor emulsion would promote the growth of a transplantable sarcoma in rats [60]. These authors noted that if the emulsion was injected 10-30 days prior to inoculation with viable tumor, the tumor would grow to a larger size and was less likely to undergo spontaneous regression than would untreated controls. Further, they noted that if the injection of tumor emulsion was repeated at 10-day intervals once or twice, the conditions favoring tumor growth were maintained or even increased. The observations that paradoxical promotion of tumor growth may be obtained in preimmunized hosts was soon confirmed by other investigators and subsequently documented in other species [28,32, 74,109].

Progress in the study of tumor promotion phenomena paralleled conceptual advances in the developing science of immunology. In the early 1930s, Casey used the term "enhancement" and suggested that enhancement was mediated by immunologic factors, having observed that enhancement phenomena demonstrated remarkable specificity [29,30], in keeping with the known specificity of immune reactions in general. Briefly, he noted that the inoculation of rabbits with rabbit tumor would promote the growth of tumor in that species but would do nothing to promote the growth of a mouse tumor in mice, and vice versa. Subsequently, Snell, working with inbred mice, recognized that the immunologic specificity of the enhancement phenomena documented by Casey was related to histocompatibility antigens borne by transplantable tumors and not to tumor antigens per se [95,178]. Kaliss [96] is credited with the important observation that the passive transfer of serum, from animals previously inoculated, to promote survival of a specific allogeneic tumor, would promote the survival of that tumor in naive recipients (i.e., *passive enhancement*). In subsequent studies (reviewed in Reference 97), he demonstrated that the mediators of enhancement were globulins, most likely gamma globulin, and so established the immunologically specific character of this phenomena. Kaliss further suggested that *active enhancement,* achieved by inoculating the prospective host with allogeneic tissues of the donor strain, was related to the presence of antibody and was therefore much akin to the passive creation of an enhanced state by transfer of serum containing antibodies to the alloantigens borne by the graft. He suggested [98] that passive enhancement was more uniformly successful than active enhancement because active immunization of the prospective recipient could give rise to transplantation immunity (capable of leading to accelerated rejection of the graft), as well as to an enhanced state (capable of leading to increased survival of the graft).

These and numerous other studies by a large number of investigators working in tumor systems permitted some conclusions to be drawn about the phenomena of enhancement with more general applicability. Specifically, with relevance to the thesis being presented in this chapter, it was noted that the mode of antigen presentation, the quantity of antigen administered, the route of administration, and the immunization schedule appeared to be important determinants of whether the inoculation of the prospective recipient would result in graft rejection or promotion.

Mode of antigen presentation. Presensitization using a solid organ graft or by inoculation with dissociated cells tended to favor immunization and rejection of the subsequent graft, whereas inoculation with cell extracts, killed cells, or cell emulsions would have favored enhancement.

Antigen dose. Small doses of antigen tended to favor immunization for rejection; larger doses would have favored enhancement.

Route of immunization. Intradermal injection of antigen would have sensitized for rejection; intravenous administration of antigen favored enhancement.

Timing of sensitization. A short time span between inoculation and challenge favored rejection; a greater delay prior to grafting would have favored enhancement.

As will be discussed later, it is of considerable interest that factors in the field of transplant immunology that would direct the immune reaction toward rejection or enhancement-facilitation are reminiscent of similar factors in early immunology that direct the reaction toward cell-mediated or delayed hypersensitivity, due to the function of specifically sensitized cells, or to antibody formation and humorally mediated (anaphylactic or arthus) types of sensitivity. Specifically, the factors recognized that would favor delayed hypersensitivity versus antibody formation were the following: intradermal versus intravenous inoculation, incorporation of antigen into complete Freund's Adjuvant (CFA) versus aqueous suspensions of antigen, small doses of antigen versus high, single immunization versus hyperimmunization, and sensitivity testing shortly after immunization versus a longer delay. These characteristics suggest that a large intravenous infusion of antigen (i.e., a blood transfusion) would tend to lead to the formation of antibody, not delayed-type hypersensitivity, to the alloantigen(s) contained therein.

Enhancement of Nontumor Allografts

Immunologic enhancement phenomena, initially described in tumor models, were subsequently reproduced in other experimental systems. Specific antisera were shown to inhibit graft-versus-host (GVH) disease in newborn mice receiving allogeneic spleen cells [203]. Immunologic enhancement was said to be responsible for increased survival times of skin grafts in rabbits pretreated with intravenous injections of living dissociated epidermal cells or whole blood from the specific donor [15]. Though in general skin grafts proved very difficult to enhance, slight prolongation of skin allografts was obtained in rats and guinea pigs [83,142].

In the majority of the early studies of active enhancement of nontumor allografts, it was, however, hard to attribute the prolongation of graft survival to an enhancing effect of antibodies since in general such studies did not specifically determine whether antigraft antibody was present in the serum at the time of transplantation. Nelson, in 1961, was the first to show that the passive transfer of serum from animals prepared as for active enhancement, to new recipients, would promote skin allograft survival in guinea pigs [141]. This was an important observation since it suggested that, despite whatever other suppressive mechanisms were induced by prior inoculation of the prospective recipient with antigen, the presence of antibody as an agent capable of promoting enhancement had been demonstrated. In the late 1960s, it was noted that kidney allografts were particularly sensitive to enhancement. Stuart et al. (1968) reported that enhancement of renal (LEW × BN)F_1 allografts was obtained in LEW rats by the following immunologic manipulations: active immunization with donor strain (BN) spleen cells, inoculation of recipients with specific hyperimmune alloantiserum (LEW anti-BN hyperimmune serum), or combined treatment with alloantiserum and antigen [187].

Needless to say, both active and passive enhancement phenomena were subsequently further explored in numerous experimental organ transplantation models. The following are some of the observations made. Cardiac allografts were less easy to enhance than kidney allografts [195]. Some donor-recipient combinations were easier to enhance than others [51,52]. Semiallogeneic grafts from F1 hybrid donors were easier to enhance than fully allogeneic grafts [51,52,132]. Though enhancement of vascularized organ allografts could be obtained in rats with relative ease, much more difficulty was encountered in attempting to reporduce these results in higher mammals [93,130,132,182]. Additional studies provided information on the passively enhancing activities of alloantisera with diverse target specificities (antibody to both class I and class II alloantigens, as well as antibody to other target specificities, was capable of causing enhancement [40,68,94, 180], the nature of the antigen preparations effective in inducing active enhancement (mononuclear leukocytes, bone marrow cells [145], and occasionally red blood cells [213] and platelets [12] have been shown to produce active enhancement), the dosage of cells required to induce active enhancement and the pretreatment interval [145], the effect of enhancement on the alloimmune response (reviewed in References 26, 138, and 186), and the nature of the immunoglobulins responsible for enhancement (reviewed in Reference 205). Many of these topics will be discussed, to a greater or lesser extent, in the sections that follow.

UNDERSTANDING ENHANCEMENT: LESSONS FROM EARLY IMMUNOLOGY

It has been repeatedly observed since the early 1900s that passively administered antibody is able to suppress various aspects of the immune response to a wide number of antigens. These early studies have provided considerable insight into the phenomenon of enhancement.

Effect of Antibody on the Humoral Immune Response (Feedback Regulation by Antibody)

The regulatory effects of antibody on the immune response were extensively reviewed by Uhr and Möller in the early 1960s [199]. Smith, in 1909, first emphasized the role of excess antibody in decreasing the immune response after antigen injection [177]. Briefly, he noted that, although injection of toxin-antitoxin mixtures into guinea pigs led to active immunity, the provision of excess antitoxin significantly reduced such immunity and might extinguish it altogether. A humoral immune response to erythrocyte Rh antigens and other weak immunogens was shown to be effectively suppressed by passive antibody transfer even after primary immunization had taken place [36]. Suppression of secondary responses was seen to be markedly less effective than suppression of primary antibody responses [198]. This was true for diphtheria toxin in guinea pigs as well as sheep red blood cells in rats or mice. IgG antibodies generated after hyperimmunization were found to be more suppressive than IgM antibodies, obtained shortly after immunization, in suppressing humoral immune responses [59].

Effects of Antibody on Cellular Immunity

Antibody has also been shown to inhibit delayed-type hypersensitivity (DTH). In early studies (reviewed in Reference 199), DTH to protein antigens appeared to be quite insensitive to suppression by antibody, but this was probably due to the experimental techniques employed. For example, complexes of toxoid and antitoxin were injected together, in CFA, into guinea pigs and induced DTH indistinguishable from that induced by free toxoid in adjuvant. All attempts to demonstrate suppression of DTH in such systems failed despite the use of large amounts of highly avid antitoxins. These findings appeared paradoxical at the time since antibody-mediated suppression of induction and expression of transplant immunity (presumed to be at least partly a manifestation of cell-mediated immunity) had been clearly demonstrated. Subsequently, however, Crowle and Hu [37], Axelrad [7], and others reported that either prior inoculation with antigen or passive transfer of specific antibody could suppress DTH. Axelrad noted, in addition, that combined pretreatment with both antigen and specific antibody was more efficacious in suppressing DTH than providing either antigen or antibody alone.

Particularly enlightening articles on the effect of antibody on delayed-type hypersensitivity were published by MacKaness, Lagrange, Miller, and coworkers [106,107,124, 125]. These investigators examined the mechanisms that regulate T-cell activity in animals that have been immunized without adjuvants or selective immunosuppressants (i.e., cyclophosphamide) commonly used to induce a state of DTH. Their important observations are reviewed in some detail below.

Inverse Correlation Between Antibody Formation and Delayed-Type Hypersensitivity

Mice inoculated with small doses of sheep red blood cells (SRBC) intravenously (10^3-10^5 SRBC) manifest (Figure 1) increasing DTH to SRBC, (assessed by footpad challenge with an optimal number of SRBC). The intravenous injection of larger doses of SRBC (10^6-10^9) led to a precipitous decline in DTH (it had long been known that the induction of DTH is exquisitely sensitive to blocking by antigen if adjuvant is not used [3]), and this was associated with a progressive increase in the generation of specific antibody. When mice were inoculated with SRBC subcutaneously, peak delayed-type hypersensitivity responses were achieved with a dose of SRBC 100 times greater than that required to produce an optimal response on intravenous challenge. The important point is that, although small quantities of antigen infused intravenously may prime for DTH, larger doses of antigen (i.e., SRBC) stimulated antibody production and decreased DTH. This inverse rela-

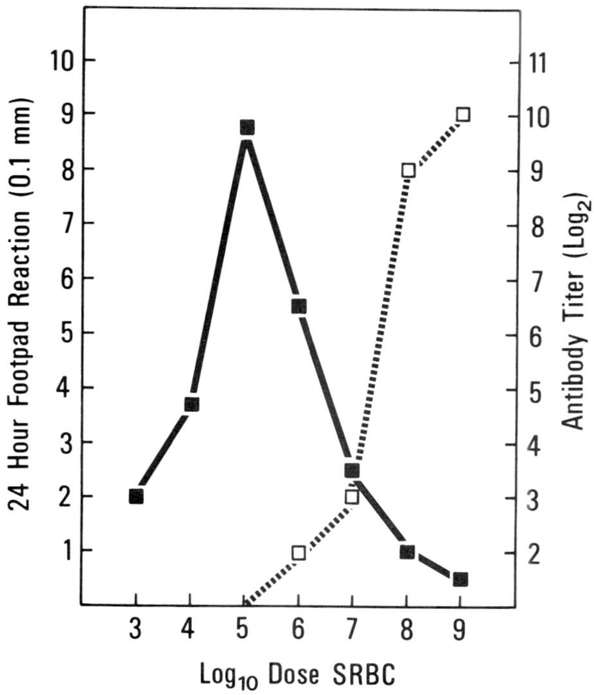

FIGURE 1 Illustrating mean levels of delayed-type hypersensitivity (■) and anti-SRBC antibody (□) assessed on day 4 following intravenous immunization with indicated doses of SRBC. Larger intravenous inocula of SRBC are seen to be associated with the generation of antibody and a reciprocal suppression of delayed-type hypersensitivity. (Figure drawn based on data presented in Reference 124.)

tionship between antibody titer and prevailing level of DTH suggested a direct inhibitory effect of antibody on the production or function of specifically sensitized lymphocytes responsible for DTH.

The inverse correlation between antibody and DTH just noted is in fact a frequent observation. We have recently reported [119] that a reciprocal relationship exists between specific antibody and DTH to a heterologous (sheep) immunoglobulin in an experimental nephritis model system. The clinical relevance of these observations will be clarified in the following pages as we critically review the transfusion effect in renal transplantation and discuss our new understanding of the role of DTH in allograft rejection.

Effect of Splenectomy on the Induction of DTH

Splenectomy was noted to have a profound effect on the induction of DTH. Whereas normal mice exhibited peak DTH following intravenous sensitization with 10^5 SRBC and were suppressed with larger inocula, greater numbers of SRBC (10^9 versus 10^5) were required for optimal sensitization for DTH by the intravenous route in splenectomized animals, and a suppressive effect of excess antigen could not be documented. Although this observation is of inherent interest, since it has been noted that enhancement is more difficult in splenectomized animals [46,174], the principal importance of this finding is that it pointed to a central effect (i.e., the role of the spleen) in antibody-mediated immunosuppression (see below).

Suppression of Delayed-Type Hypersensitivity by Antibody and Role of the Spleen

As noted, intravenous infusion of large doses of SRBC resulted in a brisk humoral response but suppressed DTH. Immune sera drawn 4 days following the intravenous infusion of large blocking doses of SRBC (10^9) were tested for blocking activity in mice that had been immunized by a footpad injection of 10^8 sheep red blood cells, a highly sensitizing dose when given by this route. Such blocking sera, designated S4, given 12 hr prior to footpad sensitization, partially suppressed DTH reactions to SRBC in this model system. Additional studies revealed that even if these blocking sera were absorbed repeatedly with SRBC to reduce the hemagglutinating titer, the sera (designated AS4) remained highly active in inhibiting induction of DTH. These studies suggested that DTH was in fact being inhibited by a product of the antigen-antibody interaction. Continuing, these authors demonstrated that these absorbed day 4 sera did not interfere with the lymphoproliferative response in the contiguous popliteal lymph nodes in mice sensitized with SRBC in the footpad but did abolish the generation of a state of delayed-type hypersensitivity that is a normal accompaniment of these responses, therefore suggesting that the intravenous infusion of AS4 acted by blocking effector cell dissemination. Further, these authors have demonstrated that when mice were rendered anergic by large intravenous doses of sheep erythrocytes, their inability to mount a DTH reaction was not due to absence of mediator cells, for these cells could be detected in the spleen by cell transfer. Such blocking factors were unable to inactivate the mediators of delayed-type hypersensitivity in vitro, nor did they suppress DTH when introduced locally into the reaction site. These blocking factors were, however, active when given intravenously to systemically sensitized mice, providing that the sensitized animals had an intact spleen. If the spleen had been removed prior to cell transfer, the blocking factors were no longer able to suppress a DTH reaction.

MacKaness and Lagrange and colleagues, in a series of reports [106,107,124,125], provided convincing experimental data to support their thesis that suppression of DTH in animals undergoing a vigorous antibody response is due to diversion of antigen-reactive cells (ARC) from the circulation and trapping of ARC in the spleen to undertake an alternate role in antibody formation. Though their contribution is seldom acknowledged, their findings in fact would appear to provide the foundation for the ARCO hypothesis, to be discussed, and our present concept of the mechanism of enhancement.

In conclusion, studies in early immunology definitively demonstrate that antibody can suppress both immediate (humoral immunity) and delayed-type hypersensitivity.

ENHANCEMENT AND MODULATION OF THE ALLOIMMUNE RESPONSE IN EXPERIMENTAL TRANSPLANTATION

Placement of a homograft initiates a brisk humoral immune response and the development of cellular immunity, the latter consisting of the generation of cytotoxic effector cells (Tc) and the appearance of delayed-type hypersensitivity. Although the contribution of these various components of the alloimmune response to rejection of allogeneic tissues remains somewhat controversial, as will be discussed, in this section some of the available experimental data on the effect of various enhancement protocols on the alloimmune response in experimental transplantation are reviewed.

Immunomodulation in Experimental Transplantation by Passive Enhancement

The administration of hyperimmune alloantisera with specificity for the organ donor markedly diminishes but does not completely abrogate the humoral component of the alloimmune response (reviewed in Reference 26). The generation of cytotoxic T cells, however, is but mildly depressed, as detected by ^{51}Cr release lymphocyte mediated cytotoxicity (LMC) assays using mononuclear effector cells recovered either from the recipient spleen or from the graft (reviewed in References 26 and 138). A number of reports have suggested that the peak of cytolytic activity is delayed by 2-4 days in enhanced organ allograft recipients [14,159,184]. Both humoral and cellular immune responses wane within the first few weeks posttransplant and are usually not detected in recipients with long-surviving renal allografts [204]. Data on the effect of passive enhancement on the development of DTH in experimental organ transplantation are virtually nonexistent. Brent and Medawar did note, however, that passively transferred antibody could decrease DTH to extracts of allogeneic cells [19].

Alloimmune Responses in Actively Enhanced Experimental Organ Allograft Recipients

There are comparatively few studies on the effect of active enhancement on alloimmune responses in experimental organ allograft recipients. Such data as are available [26], however, are quite similar to those obtained with passive enhancement. Humoral immune responses are blunted, but the generation of cytotoxic T cells is relatively unchanged. Splenocytes of actively enhanced LEW recipients of (LEW × BN) F_1 renal allografts remain normally reactive in GVH assays, demonstrating that tolerance has not been induced [146].

Combined Active and Passive Enhancement in Experimental Transplantation

In 1968, Stuart et al. [187] reported significantly prolonged survival of rat renal allografts by treatment with alloantigen and/or alloantibody. Transplantation was performed across differences at the major histocompatibility locus (RT1) in the rat. LEW rats served as recipients of (LEW × BN) F1 hybrid kidneys. Combined treatment with alloantigen and antibody was noted to be superior in promoting graft survival to the use of either antigen or antibody alone. It is of interest that the rationale for the treatment with both antigen and antiserum was provided by the observation of Axelrad [7] that delayed-type hypersensitivity could be suppressed by antigen and antibody more effectively than by either alone. Experimental renal allograft recipients prepared by combined antigen and antibody pretreatment, administered days 11 and 10 prior to grafting, manifest markedly diminished humoral immune responses. In contrast to the results obtained in animals prepared by treatment with either antibody or antigen alone, animals prepared for renal transplantation by combined antigen-antibody pretreatment lacked detectable cytotoxic T cells in the spleen in the posttransplant period [188].

A brief perusal of the data on the effect of various enhancement protocols on the alloimmune response in experimental renal transplantation reveals that humoral immune responses are generally diminished and only the combined active and passive pretreatment protocol inhibits the generation of cytotoxic effectors in the spleen. Few data are available on the effect of various enhancement protocols on the development of DTH to alloantigen following placement of a vascularized organ allograft, DTH being somewhat difficult to assess in the rat, the species in which most of this work has been performed.

Neither cytotoxic effector cells nor specific antibody are, in general, detectable in long-surviving renal allograft recipients [208]. It is important to note, however, that at no point do these animals appear to be "tolerant." Spleen cells from rats prepared for renal transplantation by antigen and/or antibody are normally reactive in mixed lymphocyte cultures (MLC) and in graft-versus-host assays [45,146,208]. Even in recipients prepared for transplantation by combined antigen and antibody pretreatment, that lack cytolytic effector cells in their spleens in the early posttransplant period, there remain specifically antigen reactive cells in their spleens as evidenced by the generation of cytotoxic T cells in MLC when splenic mononuclear cells from such animals are stimulated in vitro by donor strain lymphoid cells [185,186].

MECHANISM OF ENHANCEMENT

Theories of the Site of Action of Enhancing Antibody

Inherent in the definition of enhancement, presented in the introduction to this chapter, is the suggestion that enhancement, both active and passive, is antibody mediated. Numerous theories have been advanced to explain how the presence of antibody in the graft recipient might promote graft survival. Three alternate possibilities were formulated by Brent and Medawar [19] in a tentative analysis of the mechanism(s) of enhancement. These are briefly as follows.

Afferent Blockade Theory

Antibody coats the relevant alloantigens in the graft and thereby prevents the host from recognizing the graft as foreign. Numerous pieces of evidence [72] suggest that this hypothesis is incorrect, and these include the following: (1) enhancement was noted to occur even if the injection of enhancing antiserum was administered 1 week after grafting of sarcoma I tumor into C57 BL/K, a time when the homograft rejection was already "full-blown"; (2) even minute doses of specific antibody are effective in promoting graft survival, and these are likely inadequate to coat all the alloantigens presented by the graft (this specific criticism is open to question since only a limited number of cells within the graft, dendritic cells, may be responsible for stimulating the host alloimmune response); (3) it has been noted that intact IgG, not the $F(ab')_2$ digest, is active in enhancement, and an afferent blockade theory would offer no explanation for this observation (see below). However, since it is now suspected that only a limited number of dendritic cells are responsible for stimulating the best alloimmune response, it is conceivable that specific antibody may modulate the relevant antigens on such cells, thereby promoting graft survival.

Central Theory

The presence of antibody in the recipient at the time of grafting blocks the host's alloimmune response through a central mechanism. The central theory, originally favored by Brent and Medawar [19], appears to be compatible with most of the known observations on enhancement and accordingly will be discussed more completely below.

Efferent Blockade Theories

The presence of specific antibody in the circulation somehow blocks immune effector mechanisms, activated in response to the graft, from producing their expected injurious effects. Gorer, in 1961, noted [72] that walling off of antigen by passively administered antibody was not a likely explanation since this would be expected to produce only a slight delay in regression and in fact even a small dose of enhancing antisera could lead to fatal tumors. Further, quantitative changes in the host's immune response are induced in the host by contact with both antigen and/or antibody.

Central Blockade and the Mechanism of Enhancement

A central blockade theory, to provide for the mechanism of enhancement and the known effects of enhancing protocols on the various aspects of the alloimmune response recounted above, must provide explanations for the reduced antibody formation, suppression of DTH, and impaired cytotoxic T-cell generation.

Antibody-Mediated Suppression of Humoral Immunity

It is well recognized that humoral immune responses to alloantigen are T-cell dependent, and clearly, therefore, the diminution of such responses through antibody-induced immunosuppression might be mediated by effects on T cells at the level of T-cell-B-cell interaction, or on B cells themselves. Experimental data reported by Sinclair and Chan [175] and others suggested that antibody may inhibit antibody production at the level of the mature B cell, leading to specific B-cell tolerance. Specifically, having demonstrated that IgG was more effective in suppressing a specific humoral immune response than the Fab portion of the same immunoglobulin, these authors suggested that, following antigen binding to the B-cell antigen receptor (i.e., cell surface immunoglobulin), the Fab portion of antibody with specificity for other epitopes on this antigen may bind to antigen, allowing the Fc portion of the immunoglobulin to interact with the Fc receptor. It was suggested that bridge formation between antigen and Fc receptor, via specific antibody, suppresses B-cell activation through an as yet undefined mechanism. Although there is no doubt that the phenomenon of pure B-cell tolerance does exist [1,104], its importance in antibody-mediated immunosuppression has not been established.

Experimental data to support a novel theory of the mechanism of T-B interaction has recently been reported by Lanzavecchia [108]. Briefly, this investigator has shown that immunoglobulin on the B-cell surface is involved in the uptake and concentration of antigen, which is in turn internalized, processed, and presented to T cells in association with class II alloantigens, in an MHC-restricted manner, analogous to the mechanism of antigen presentation by more classic antigen-presenting cells (APC), that is, monocytes and dendritic cells. The analogy between B cells and classic APC is heightened by the demonstration that Epstein-Barr (EB) virus-transformed human B cells liberate interleukin-1-like activity [173]. Little is known at present, however, of just how such T-B cell interaction promotes specific antibody generation. Further insight into the mechanism of antibody-induced immunosuppression at the level of T-B interaction must clearly await further conceptual advances in this field. The "feedback" effects of antibody on the provision of T-cell "help" is discussed below.

Suppression of Cellular Immunology by Antibody

Prior to considering the suppression of cellular immune responses by antibody we must note that comparatively recent data suggest that helper (Th) and cytotoxic/suppressor (Tc/s) T-cell subsets are preferentially reactive with class II and class I MHC-encoded alloantigens, respectively [191]. Such preferential reactivity of Th and Tc/s for class II and class I alloantigens, respectively, appears to be related not to major differences in the antigen receptors of these two functional T-cell subsets [169] but rather may well be linked to the function of T4, T8 T-cell differentiation antigens in stabilizing interaction with class II, class I restricting elements [2]. Although it was thought that the T-helper cell subset was primarily responsible for mediating delayed-type hypersensitivity and contact sensitivity [200], there is recent evidence that the cytotoxic/suppressor T-cell subset may indeed be responsible for delayed-type hypersensitivity to class I alloantigens and mediate contact sensitivity restricted by class I alloantigens [189,192]. Similarly, although the cytotoxic effector cell was thought to have specificity for class I alloantigens, cytotoxic T cells with specificity for class II alloantigens have been described and these have been shown to bear the helper phenotype [134].

How, then, can immunologic enhancement protocols give rise to a relative paralysis of both alloreactive "helper" and "cytotoxic" T-cell subsets through a central mechanism? Considerable insight into possible central mechanisms whereby antibody may blunt cellular immune responses was, in fact, provided by the studies of MacKaness, Miller, and Lagrange. It may be useful to recall that they noted an inverse correlation between DTH and specific antibody production. Further, specific antibody and/or antibody-antigen complexes were shown to reduce demonstrable delayed-type hypersensitivity by an effect exerted in the circulation. They suggested that, by as yet undetermined mechanisms, antigen and/or a combination of antigen and antibody caused anergy by trapping specifically sensitized cells in the spleen. The presence of specifically sensitized cells in the spleen was demonstrated by adoptive transfer. Such a central mechanism of antibody-mediated immunosuppression has also been proposed and embellished by Hutchinson and Zolla (reviewed in Reference 87), who hypothesized that antigen-reactive cell opsonization is responsible for enhancement (the ARCO hypothesis). Specifically, they suggest that antigen-reactive cells bind antigen and in the presence of specific antibody reactive with other determinants on the same antigens, such complexes of *antigen-reactive cell, antigen, and antibody* are trapped by the reticuloendothelial system through the interaction of the Fc piece of the immunoglobulin with the Fc receptor on macrophage. Central to this theory is the observation of Nagy et al. [140], reported in 1976, that specific K (class I) and I (class II) region products of the mouse H-2 complex bind to activated thymus-derived T cells belonging to different Ly subclasses (i.e., Tc and Th, respectively). The superior enhancement achieved by pretreating prospective recipients with both antigen and antibody, as opposed to either antigen or antibody alone in inducing enhancement [187], also fits with the concept that the antigen-antibody complexes are in fact responsible for opsonizing antigen-reactive T cells. This theory clearly provides an explanation for the importance of the Fc component of enhancing immunoglobulin [22,23,41,212].

Hutchinson et al. suggested that antigen-reactive cells are diverted to the liver in the presence of antigen and antibody and thus specifically and permanently eliminated [87]. The fate of opsonized antigen-reactive T cells envisaged by the proponents of the ARCO hypothesis differs from that previously suggested by MacKaness et al., who in fact proposed that antigen-reactive cells are trapped in the spleen in the presence of specific antibody where they collaborate with B cells in the development of humoral immunity. Support for this latter thesis was provided by the demonstration, by MacKaness et al., that antigen-reactive T cells are indeed present in the spleen and are able to adoptively transfer cellular immunity. Clearly, however, both splenic entrapment and hepatic elimination of antigen-reactive T cells may occur and together account for the quantitative effects of antibody on cellular immunity. It is also conceivable that the partial elimination of specific antigen-reactive T cells (hepatic entrapment) would also decrease provision of T-cell help for T-B interaction and so decrease antibody production.

In summary, therefore, current thought about the mechanism of antibody-mediated suppression of cellular immunity appears to be limited to the following hypothesis: specific antigen-reactive cells, that is, cells with helper or cytotoxic phenotypes, become trapped within the reticuloendothelial (RE) system, following binding of specific antigen (class II or class I, respectively), in the presence of specific antibody. It is noted that within the framework of this theory class I reactive cells, bearing the cytotoxic/suppressor phenotype, whoud be diverted to the RE system in the presence of antibody to the class I alloantigen, but cells with the phenotype of the helper cell subset would be entrapped in the presence of antibody to class II alloantigen. Presumably, antigen-reactive cells with specificity for minor histocompatibility antigens would be entrapped in the presence of antibody to the minor histocompatibility antigens in question, although there are conceptual difficulties with this formulation.

We have reviewed on a fairly superficial level some observations that would support the hypothesis that antigen-reactive cells may localize in the RE system in the presence of specific antibody. Some of the data from early studies that would support this thesis were presented in detail. Numerous pieces of experimental evidence from various enhancement models are also consistent with this hypothesis. Specifically, in the various enhancement models studied to date, antigen-reactive cells capable of responding in mixed lymphocyte culture and graft-versus-host assays and with the capacity to generate into active cytotoxic effectors following in vitro stimulation with the relevant alloantigens have indeed been identified in the spleen.

One could ask how the entrapment of antigen-reactive cells in the spleen might lead to prolonged allograft survival. The simplest answer would be that, for antigen-reactive cells to injure an allograft, they must traverse the peripheral circulation to reach the graft itself, and since antigen is presumably being released continuously from the graft in the presence of low titers of specific antibody, the process of opsonization would continue. The numbers of antigen-reactive cells reaching the graft would, we suggest, be quantitatively reduced and likely, therefore, insufficient to cause rejection. The observation that there may be cytotoxic effector cells in the grafts of passively enhanced experimental renal allograft recipients despite maintenance of good graft function [14,184] may be related to the observation that the transferred alloantisera used in such experiments contain primarily anti-class II antibody [67,133], and as such the opsonization of class I-reactive cytotoxic T cells may be relatively incomplete.

PATHOGENESIS OF ALLOGRAFT REJECTION

Since a discussion of immunologic enhancement would seem somewhat deficient were it not to include at least passing reference to the immunologic processes responsible for allograft rejection, we propose to briefly outline the evolution of thought about the mechanism of graft rejection from the time that Medawar first recognized that graft rejection was immunologically mediated. In early studies graft rejection was attributed to delayed-type hypersensitivity and antibody was considered relatively unimportant since graft rejection was readily induced by adoptive transfer of cells but not serum [135]. Brent and Medawer, in 1961, stated: "Homografts of all kinds excite the formation of humoral antibodies but the part played by antibodies with rejection of homografts is still uncertain" [19]. In the early 1970s, graft rejection was generally attributed to the function of cytotoxic T cells and cell-mediated cytolysis [26,138,188]. Cytotoxic T cells were readily detected (4-hr ^{51}Cr release LMC assay) in the recipient spleen as well as the graft at the time of rejection [185]. Some investigators also speculated that antibody may be playing a major role in the rejection of experimental vascularized organ allografts, since immunoglobulin and complement were seen in the walls of affected vessels [161,184].

In the late 1970s, there developed a progressive disenchantment with antibody [65] and cytotoxic T cells as the sole effectors of allograft rejection. Cytotoxic T cells were not uniformly detected in rejecting organ allografts. Enhancement protocols in rats leading to indefinite survival of renal allografts frequently only mildly delayed the generation of cytotoxic T cells. Further, the rejection of skin grafts mismatched for a single antigen (H-Y) in mice occurred even in strains that failed to develop cytotoxic T cells to the mismatched antigen, and in fact, graft rejection was best correlated with DTH [86]. Although, as noted, some investigators suggested that antibody may play a significant pathogenetic role in the rejection of experimental vascularized organ allografts [26], adoptive transfer studies definitively demonstrated that antibody was not required for the rejection of vascularized cardiac allografts in the rat [75,118].

In 1981, Loveland et al. [111] reported that mice rendered immunocompetent by adult thymectomy, lethal irradiation, and bone marrow reconstitution (AT × BM) would reject skin allografts when reconstituted with T-helper cells, that is, lymphoid inocula depleted of cytotoxic T cells and their precursors by treatment with anti-Ly 23 antisera plus complement. Since T-helper cells in mice had previously been shown to be exclusively responsible for adoptive transfer of delayed-type hypersensitivity [200], the observation of Loveland et al. provided the first concrete experimental data linking DTH with graft rejection in the modern era.

The development of monoclonal antibodies to helper and cytotoxic T-cell subsets in rats [20,131] provided the necessary tools to explore the role of diverse T-cell subsets in organ allograft rejection, primary vascular anastomosis, being excessively difficult to carry out in the mouse. Lowry et al. [116] demonstrated that T-helper cells in rats (W3/25$^+$, OX8$^-$) were exclusively responsible for the adoptive transfer of delayed-type hypersensitivity to alloantigen and phenotypically distinct and separable (fluorescent-activated cell sorter) from cytotoxic T cells and their precursors (W3/25$^-$, OX8$^+$), and this has been independently confirmed [123].

Experimental adoptive transfer studies in rats demonstrated that heart [116] and kidney grafts [73,121] bearing a full haplotype disparity (WF → LEW) were rejected when sublethally irradiated recipients were reconstituted with sensitized syngeneic spleen cells depleted of cells positive for surface immunoglobulin, as well as cytotoxic T cells and their precursors. Immunologic monitoring studies confirmed that graft rejection in such recipients proceeded in the absence of both specific antibody and cytotoxic T-cell generation [116]. Further, as might have been expected, T-helper cells were shown to be independently capable of effecting rejection of heart grafts transplanted across isolated MHC-encoded class II disparities (RT1B/D in rats, analogous to HLA-D/DR in humans) in the absence of cytotoxic T cells or alloantibody [115]. The independent pathogenic potential of T-helper cells in rat organ allograft rejection has been confirmed [76,81] in a variety of model systems since that time and is, we believe, now generally accepted.

Though such studies have been frequently criticized on the grounds that they ignore the potential contribution of the irradiated host to cytotoxic T-cell generation, Lowry et al. [116] and Hall et al. [77] have shown that allospecific cytotoxic T cells present in the spleen and grafts of sublethally irradiated recipients, reconstituted with unfractionated immune spleen cells, were derived exclusively from the reconstituting inoculum and not from the irradiated recipient. Conversely, a number of laboratories [116,128] have shown that the majority of cells infiltrating rejecting organ allografts in sublethally irradiated recipients reconstituted with sensitized syngeneic inocula are, in fact, of host origin, suggesting that the majority of infiltrating cells have been secondarily recruited through immunologically nonspecific mechanisms.

None of the data reviewed above exclude the possibility that the cytotoxic T-cell subset may also play an independent pathogenic role in allograft rejection. Adoptive transfer studies carried out across a full haplotype disparity clearly demonstrated that brisk rejection may also be mediated by the cytotoxic/suppressor subset (OX8$^+$, W3/25$^-$), provided that appropriate numbers of specifically sensitized cells are transferred to the recipient [116]. Additional investigation carried out by Lowry et al. [120] has also shown that, although the noncytotoxic class II-reactive T-helper-DTH subset (W3/25$^+$, OX8$^-$) plays a critical independent effector role in the rejection of isolated class II disparate grafts, rejection of isolated class I disparate heart grafts required the presence of the cytotoxic/suppressor subset (OX8$^+$, W3/25$^-$). The class I disparate heart grafts were promptly rejected when sublethally irradiated recipients were reconstituted with unfractionated immune spleen cells, but such grafts survived virtually indefinitely when the reconstituting inocula were depleted of Tc and their precursors. The latter data are in agreement with the observations that the cytotoxic/suppressor T-cell subset is primarily responsible for the rejection of H-2D disparate split heart grafts in mice [158] and for the rejection of cultured endocrine allografts that express primarily class I alloantigens [89].

Whether class I-reactive cells induce rejection primarily through direct cell-mediated cytotoxicity or release of lymphokines is at present unclear. Prowse et al. [166] recently suggested that the rejection of cultured pancreatic islets by cloned cells bearing the cytotoxic phenotype may be related to lymphokine release (i.e., DTH). Specifically, his group observed that cyclosporin A, which inhibits lymphokine released by these cells but not direct lymphocytic toxicity, is capable of preventing allograft rejection by the cloned cytotoxic T-cell lines in vivo. Conversely, Lowry et al. [120] have obtained data that suggest that the pivotal role of the cytotoxic T cell in allograft rejection may indeed be related to direct lymphocytotoxicity. Specifically, heart grafts bearing isolated class I disparities, from F1 hybrid donors, survived indefinitely in semiallogeneic F1 hybrid recipients, but parental heart grafts bearing the same class I disparity were promptly rejected. The prolonged survival of class I disparate heart grafts from F1 hybrid donors, despite an equivalent alloimmune response, was shown to correlate with a reduced susceptibility of lymphoid cells of the F1 hybrid donor to lysis by cytotoxic effectors with specificity for the relevant class I disparity, which effected significant lysis of parental lymphoid cells bearing the same class I disparity. Since the efficacy with which cytotoxic cells produced target lysis is proportional to target antigen density [61], these data might suggest that the pivotal role of cytotoxic/suppressor T-cell subset in the rejection of class I disparate heart grafts is related to direct cell-mediated cytolysis. Immunoelectron microscopic studies carried out in collaboration with Forbes have demonstrated [122] the presence of a conspicuous accumulation of T-cytotoxic cells ($OX8^+$) within the allograft interstitium, as well as in close apposition to both normal and irreversibly altered cardiac myofibers, and this is compatible with the data suggesting that direct cell-mediated cytolysis may occur in the process of rejection. Additional studies are, however, required to definitively define the role of cytotoxic T cells in graft rejection in vivo.

Having reviewed recent conceptual advances on the pathogenesis of allograft rejection, it is appropriate now to critically examine whether antibody-induced immunosuppression might really be expected to modulate the alloimmune response processes responsible for allograft destruction. Studies in both classic and transplant immunology have clearly demonstrated that antibody-induced immunosuppression is clearly capable of severely limiting or reducing DTH. In the preceding paragraphs, we have demonstrated that graft rejection effected independently by the helper T-cell subset, if not also the cytotoxic/suppressor subset, is likely linked to DTH. Accordingly, it is clear that specific antibody, provided passively or generated in response to active immunization, may limit DTH to alloantigen and so effectively interfere with what has come to be seen as one of the principle effector mechanisms in allograft rejection.

Enhancement protocols have been readily shown to decrease the generation of specific antibody in response to challenge with an allogeneic graft. The present data suggest that the critical effects of antibody in allograft rejection are likely limited to the causation of hyperacute rejection of vascularized organ allografts when high titers of specific antibody are present at the time of transplantation [194], and there is little if any hard evidence that antibody is playing any major role in either acute or chronic rejection. Indeed, serial ultrastructural tracer studies using an administered colloidal carbon and horseradish peroxidase in an adoptive transfer model of rat cardiac allograft rejection have revealed that a humoral antibody response is not essential for microvascular endothelial damage, which is a characteristic feature of fulminant acute cardiac allograft in the rat [62,63,118]. These data are in agreement with other morphologic investigations that have provided evidence that vascular injury in rejecting allografts is directly induced by T-lymphocyte-dependent immune mechanisms [6].

Enhancement protocols vary in their ability to reduce the generation of cytotoxic effector cells. The significance of this observation is uncertain since the role of cytotoxic effector cells in allograft rejection is at present unclear and recent reports have indicated that the rejection of allografts bearing isolated class I disparities, in which the cytotoxic/suppressor T-cell subset would be expected to play a pivotal role [120], is frequently indolent [117,165].

RELATIONSHIP OF IMMUNOLOGIC ENHANCEMENT TO CLINICAL TRANSPLANTATION

Specific Immunologic Enhancement in Human Renal Transplantation: Preliminary Trials

There have been few documented attempts to induce specific immunologic enhancement in human renal transplantation. Kelly, in 1967, was likely the first to report such an attempt [101]. Although there was no evidence of any ensuing deleterious effects, at the same time there was little evidence that such attempts at immunologic enhancement led to improved graft survival [10,64,101]. Two controlled clinical trials of immunologic enhancement in human renal transplantation using alloreactive sera obtained from postpartum females (retroplacental blood) or from hypersensitized dialysis patients [211] have been reported. In the latter study the immunoglobulin contained in the serum was isolated and submitted to pepsin digestion and the $F(ab')_2$ fragment infused into renal allograft recipients both prior to and following transplantation. No statistically significant benefit was seen to be derived in the latter study. Although it is now recognized that Fab fragments, per se, are not active in enhancement, additional immunochemical analysis did demonstrate the presence of some intact immunoglobulin in the preparation.

Given the paucity of demonstrable beneficial effect in the various attempts at inducing enhancement of organ allografts in most mammalian species other than the rat [93,130,132,168,182,201], it is hardly surprising that more clinical trials have not been attempted. One possible reason for the poor results obtained in attempting to reproduce the dramatic immunologic enhancement of organ allografts obtained in rats is thought to be related to the greater susceptibility of other mammalian tissue grafts to the deleterious effect of antibody plus complement [132].

In the human, both class I and II MHC alloantigens are expressed (immunohistologic assessment) on vascular endothelium, but such antigens are undetectable on vascular endothelium of the rat [79,80,206]. Accordingly, human organ allografts would be more susceptible than rodent grafts to injury by "enhancing" antibody. Even in early studies it was recognized that grafts that were more susceptible to the deleterious effect of specific antibody (presumably related to complement-mediated injury) were less likely to be promoted by passively administered enhancing antibody [71,98]. Certainly the observation by Hirshberg et al. [84] that human endothelial cells could be killed with antibody to class II (DR) alloantigens in the presence of complement would suggest that organ grafts in humans might be injured by the presence of anti-DR antibody if present in adequate titer at the time of transplantation. Accordingly, it is clear that if anti-class II and/or class I alloantibodies are going to play any role in enhancing renal allograft survival in humans, the titers of antigraft antibody at the time of transplantation would have to be exceedingly low and consequentially any potential beneficial effect attributable to antibody-mediated immunosuppression may be expected to be quite subtle. Clearly, also, the detection of such antigraft antibody at the time of transplantation may well require more sensitive diagnostic techniques than the usual pretransplant cross-match (i.e., flow cytometry [69], an indirect rosette microassay [88], or in vivo donor (B) lymphocyte migration studies).

Promotion of Renal Allograft Survival in Humans by Pretransplant Transfusion

Although Dossetor et al. [43] suggested in 1967 that pretransplant transfusion may promote renal allograft survival, we saw in the early 1970s a deliberate attempt in numerous transplant centers to avoid transfusion if at all possible in the hope of reducing the potential deleterious effects of sensitization. The "transfuse only if absolutely required" policy was associated with a general decline (i.e., 1968-1974) in renal allograft survival around the world [4] even while patient survival was improving. In the mid-1970s, reports appeared, based initially on retrospective studies and more recently on prospective multicenter studies [17,21,55,56,66,105,139,148-150,152,154,156,179], that have conclusively demonstrated that pretransplant transfusion promotes renal allograft survival. Intraoperative transfusion was seen to be of lesser, if any, benefit on subsequent renal allograft survival [153].

The number of transfusions required to produce a beneficial effect in clinical renal transplantation remains somewhat controversial. Although Opeltz et al. are in agreement that a single transfusion confers significant benefit, these investigators have repeatedly reported an increased benefit with larger numbers (most recently optimal results have been achieved with six to ten transfusions) [151,156]. Conversely, other investigators have reported that, indeed, optimal results may be obtained with a single random transfusion [54,163,164,210] or a single transfusion of donor-specific blood [9]. Certainly, experimental studies in rodents as well as larger mammals have documented that a single third-party transfusion can promote skin and organ allograft survival [100,147,201]. The debate about the optimal number of transfusions continues to this day, the protagonists continuing to remind us that the risks of broad presensitization and/or infection with viral agents may well increase with increasing numbers of transfusions [21,105,155,163, 179].

The mechanisms whereby pretransplant transfusions exert a favorably beneficial effect in clinical renal transplantation are uncertain. In the pages that follow evidence will be presented that would support the thesis that the transfusion effect is linked to the phenomenon of enhancement.

Is the Beneficial Effect of Pretransplant Transfusion Related to the Phenomenon of Enhancement?

Opelz [155], writing recently on the beneficial effects of pretransplant transfusion, ascribes the beneficial effect of transfusion on renal allograft survival to the generation of suppressor cells and/or the formation of anti-idiotypic antibody. Since the evidence that would support either of these two conclusions is not totally compelling, I would like to present some of the data that would support a link between enhancement and the transfusion effect in clinical transplantation.

The Transfusion Effect: Analogy with Tumor Promotion Phenomena and Enhancement of Experimental Organ Allografts

As reviewed earlier in this chapter, Kaliss was the first to relate tumor promotion phenomena to the presence of antigraft antibody, generated in response to prior inoculation with tumor. He demonstrated that the passive transfer of serum from animals that had been inoculated with tumor in a manner that would lead to tumor promotion would promote survival of tumor allografts if transferred to naive hosts at the time of inoculation with live tumor. Similar studies in rats and guinea pigs have documented that antibody is likewise generated in response to active immunization for the purpose of enhancing kidney and skin allografts, and this can be passively transferred and promote allograft survival in naive recipients [141,146]. There is no doubt, therefore, that antibody generated in the recipient as a result of active inoculation is able to serve in the induction of the enhanced state, as demonstrated by passive transfer experiments. When seeking to explain the transfusion effect it would seem promising to consider the possibility that the promotion of graft survival in transfused patients may be related to the presence of antibody, albeit in low titers, serving to effect enhancement as is so readily demonstrated in tumor promotion and experimental organ allograft studies. Although it remains to be answered whether active immunization, in fact, induces the generation of additional immunologic mechanisms capable of suppressing a host's immune response to an allograft, that is, suppressor cells or autoanti-idiotypic antibody, it is our belief that no other potential mediator capable of suppressing the host immune responses to tissue allografts in clinical or experimental transplantation has been as convincingly and scientifically validated as the phenomena of antibody-induced immunosuppression. This is not to deny the possibility that additional immunosuppressive modalities, that is, suppressor cells, may, with time, develop in *successfully enhanced* recipients and serve an important role in permitting the long-term survival of the allograft, as has been demonstrated experimentally [78,82,144].

The parallels between the planned transfusion of patients awaiting renal transplantation for the purpose of promoting allograft survival and the enhancement protocols employed in tumor promotion and experimental organ transplantation studies in rodents are striking. Such similarities are all the more obvious when one considers the clinical protocols that employ donor-specific transfusion (DST) in recipients of haploidentical living related organ grafts. In the initial report, DST (i.e., three donor-specific transfusions) were seen to increase 1-year survival of MLC-reactive haploidentical living related donor renal allografts from approximately 56% in historical controls to over 94% [171]. The principal drawback of DST was that it resulted in approximately a 30% incidence of presensitization (a positive cross-match) to the prospective donor [156,172]. Although a positive T-cell cross-match is, in general, an absolute contraindication to transplantation, in some instances the positive cross-match has disappeared on longer follow-up and such donor-recipient combinations have been successfully transplanted (i.e., References 9 and 70). A number of recent reports suggest, however, that three transfusions of random blood are as beneficial as DST in promoting survival of MLC-reactive haploidentical allografts from related donors and do not carry the same risk of presensitization [156]. Accordingly, although the beneficial effect of DST may look like specific immunologic enhancement, the favorable response to a small number of random transfusions would be hard to explain on this basis. However, additional data will be presented below that we believe strongly supports the notion that sensitization with lymphocyte cells from a third party may also induce specific immunologic enhancement.

Biologic Significance of a Positive Pretransplant Cross-Match

In 1966, Kissmeyer-Neilson et al. [103] reported that a positive pretransplant cross-match (i.e., complement-mediated killing of donor lymphocytes by antibodies present in recipient serum) was associated with a high incidence (approximately 80%) of hyperacute rejection of the allograft, and this was quickly confirmed by Williams et al. [209] and Patel et al. in 1977 [160]. Hyperacute rejection appeared to be related to presensitization since it occurred with increased frequency in multiparous women as well as in patients who had rejected previous grafts in an accelerated manner. Further, the rapidity of graft loss and the presence of characteristic pathologic changes in early biopsies (microvascular thrombosis and polymorphonuclear leukocyte infiltration) suggested, by analogy with the kinetics and histopathologic appearance of grafts lost following inadvertant transplantation across an ABO blood group incompatibility, that humoral immune mechanisms were indeed responsible for hyperacute rejection of kidneys transplanted across a positive lymphocyte cross-match.

As a result of these observations, transplant physicians became acutely sensitized to the threat posed by preexistent humoral immunity, a pretransplant cross-match came to be performed routinely prior to renal transplantation and patients were not knowingly transplanted in the presence of antidonor antibody.

Following the report by Stuart et al. [187] that diverse enhancement protocols could induce indefinite survival of rat renal allografts, cautious attempts were made to reproduce these results in clinical transplantation. Since it was well recognized that active immunization could give rise to both transplant immunity (capable of leading to accelerated rejection of the graft) and an enhanced state (capable of leading to increased survival of the graft), the technique of passive enhancement was adopted to initial clinical trials. $F(ab')_2$ fragments of appropriate alloantibodies were employed because of fears of precipitating vascular injury and hyperacute rejection if intact IgG were administered intravenously. As noted earlier in this chapter, such trials were largely inconclusive. In view of the fact that it was extremely difficult to obtain the large amounts of appropriate alloimmune serum required and since a number of reports appearing in the mid- to late 1970s suggested that intact IgG, not $F(ab')_2$; was active in enhancement, further attempts at inducing specific immunologic enhancement in clinical renal transplantation were abandoned. Since that time, however, there has been an ongoing re-evaluation of the significance of a positive cross-match, as will be discussed below.

In 1973, van Leeuwen et al. [202] reported the detection of the serologic equivalents (HLA-DR) of the predominant mixed lymphocyte reaction (MLR) stimulating antigens on a subset of (10-15%) of peripheral blood mononuclear cells (i.e., B cells and monocytes). Since it was thought, at least in some circles [23,42,91,180,183], that anti-class II antibody was more important than antibody to class I alloantigens in facilitating (enhancing) allograft survival, the report by Ettenger et al. in 1976 [47] that patients could be successfully transplanted across a positive cross-match employing B-enriched lymphocyte preparations led to a brief resurgence of interest in enhancement in clinical transplantation. With but a few exceptions [5,8,13,136,176,190], subsequent studies confirmed that the presence of antibody reactive with donor B cells in pretransplant sera [complement-dependent cytotoxicity; erythrocyte antibody rosette inhibition (EAI)] does not exert a deleterious effect on graft survival [92,110,137]. A limited number of studies have indeed suggested that the presence of B-cell-reactive (class II reactive?) antibody prior to transplantation may be beneficial [38,49,90,126,157].

In an attempt to resolve the ensuing controversy over the biologic significance of a positive B-cell cross-match, attempts were made to delineate the target specificities recognized by such B-cell-reactive sera. Some sera with preferential B-cell reactivity were shown to contain antibodies to HLA A and B [129,167], and this was likely due to the fact that B cells express three times as many HLA antigens as do peripheral T lymphocytes [58,162]. In the majority of instances, such antibodies have been associated with early graft loss. Other B-cell-reactive antibodies were shown either to be autoreactive [157] or to be reactive with cell surface immunoglobulin [35], and it is now recognized that both of these are benign [196]. Although some investigators have found it useful to divide B-cell-reactive antibodies into those predominantly reactive at 4 or 37°C (i.e., Reference 90), the value of such distinctions has been questioned [39].

The consequences of a positive B-cell cross-match due to antibody to MHC-encoded class II alloantigens (i.e., HLA-DP, DQ, and DR) remains unresolved, and this is due, at least in part, to the fact that few such B-cell cytotoxins have clear-cut reactivity with defined class II alloantigens of panel cells [39]. Two papers have appeared, however, that purport to demonstrate that anti-DR antibodies may be implicated in the causation of "immediate" rejection [13,136]. These and the few other reports suggesting that B-cell-positive, T-cell-negative cross-matches lead to early rejection are, however, subject to the criticism that they either demonstrated high-titered antibody (i.e., Reference 136) or failed to indicate that the sera were platelet absorbed to exclude the possibility that a weak HLA-A, B antibody may be present (i.e., References 5, 13, 25, and 176). There is little if any evidence that antibody to the class II alloantigens of the donor may precipitate hyperacute rejection of the graft [27]. The validity of attributing graft rejection 39 and 130 days posttransplantation (i.e., Reference 136) [or up to 6 weeks posttransplant (i.e., Reference 190)] to the pre-existence of antibody (i.e., anti-class II) is questionable [194]. Among patients awaiting renal transplantation (transfusion history not specified), serologic reactivity to a B-cell panel has been shown to be highly correlated ($p < 0.0001$) with rejection of a previous graft [48], and this is in accordance with reports that anti-class II B-cell cytotoxic antibodies frequently appear de novo at the time of graft rejection [48,136,181]. Accordingly, the inclusion of highly sensitized patients, many of whom have rejected previous grafts in an accelerated manner, in studies of the biologic significance of a positive B-cell cross-match, may at times have led to the possibly erroneous conclusion that antibody to donor class II alloantigens inherently has a deleterious effect on the graft [25,136,196]. Although the intravenous infusion of antigen may tend to favor enhancement, it was noted earlier in this chapter that presensitization with a solid organ graft tended to favor immunization and rejection of the subsequent graft. Cellular immune mechanisms, previously reported [44,102] to induce accelerated or even hyperacute renal allograft rejection in the absence of detectable antibody, may indeed be responsible for the early loss of grafts, transplanted across a B-cell-positive, T-cell-negative cross-match, in the sensitized recipient.

Although there is no direct proof that the pretransplant presence of antibody to class II alloantigens of the donor may promote kidney graft survival in humans, one group of investigators [126] has consistently reported excellent results when transplantation is performed in the presence of a positive B-cell cross-match [erythrocyte antibody rosette inhibition assay (EAI)]. Previous studies in rodents have linked EAI with antibody to MHC-encoded class II [Ia] antigens (reviewed in Reference 180), but formal demonstration that EAI developing in transfused patients awaiting renal transplantation detects antibody with specificity for MHC-encoded alloantigens was not available. Accordingly, it is of considerable interest to note that serologic B-cell reactivity detected by EAI, developing after donor-specific transfusion, has been linked to the major histocompatibility complex [127]. These latter data, therefore, provide some credence for the thesis that anti-class II alloantibody may indeed facilitate survival of renal allografts in humans.

Since, as reviewed above, the majority of evidence indeed suggests that a positive B-cell cross-match is benign and may even be associated with superior graft survival, and since patients may be inappropriately denied a graft on the basis of positive cross-match due to the presence of B-cell cytotoxins, we undertook to determine whether a negative pure T-

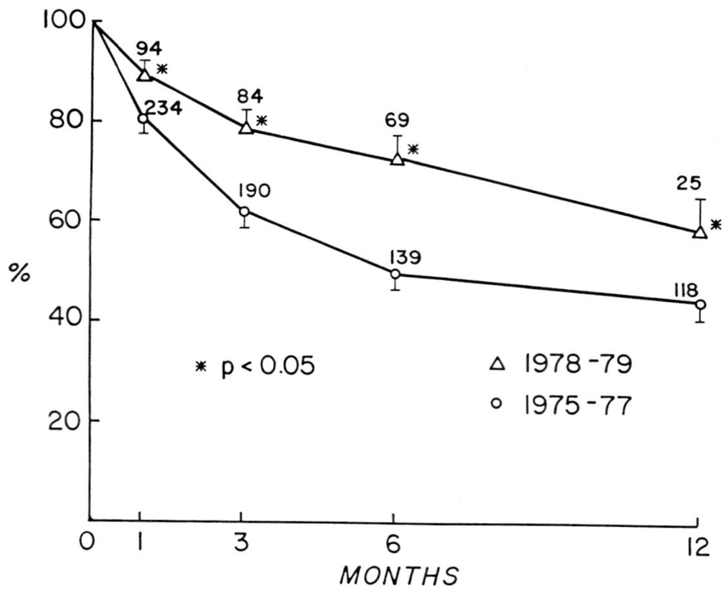

FIGURE 2 Survival of cadaveric renal allografts transplanted on the basis of a negative cross-match versus nylon wool-purified donor T lymphocytes (1978-1979) in one hospital center was significantly ($p < 0.05$) greater than that obtained in a historical control group transplanted on the basis of a negative cross-match versus unseparated donor mononuclear leukocytes (1975-1977). All allograft loss, with the exception of kidneys removed due to technical problems (n = 4, 1978-1979) is included in the actuarial survival curves. These data suggest that a negative T-cell cross-match is adequate for successful transplantation.

cell cross-match is indeed adequate to permit successful renal transplantation. Some of the results of this study have been previously published [112]. A total of 98 cadaveric renal allografts were transplanted (1978-1979) on the basis of a negative cross-match versus purified donor T lymphocytes. T- and B-cell separation was performed using nylon wool columns as described [113]. As illustrated in Figure 2, cumulative renal allograft survival at 1, 3, 6, and 12 months was significantly ($p < 0.05$) greater than obtained in an historical control group, that is, patients transplanted between 1975 and 1977 (n = 234). B-cell cross-matches were performed in 29 of the 98 patients included in this study at 4 and 37°C incubation. Warm reactive B-cell antibodies were detected in 7 patients (platelet absorbed sera) and cold reactive antibodies in 4. A single patient had antibody cytotoxic to donor B cells at both 4 and 37°C. Cumulative graft survival in patients with donor-specific B-cell cytolytic antibody (warm or cold reactive) pretransplant had a cumulative renal allograft survival insignificantly different from those lacking such activity (Figure 3). The superior renal allograft survival documented in this study of patients transplanted on the basis of a negative T-cell cross-match is compatible with the thesis that B-cell cytotoxins are indeed benign. It should be noted that the adequacy of the pure T-cell cross-match has withstood the test of time and continues to be used to this day at the center in which its use was first established, as well as in others [27].

Although the evidence that the presence in the recipient, at the time of transplantation, of antibody to class II determinants born by the specific graft promotes allograft sur-

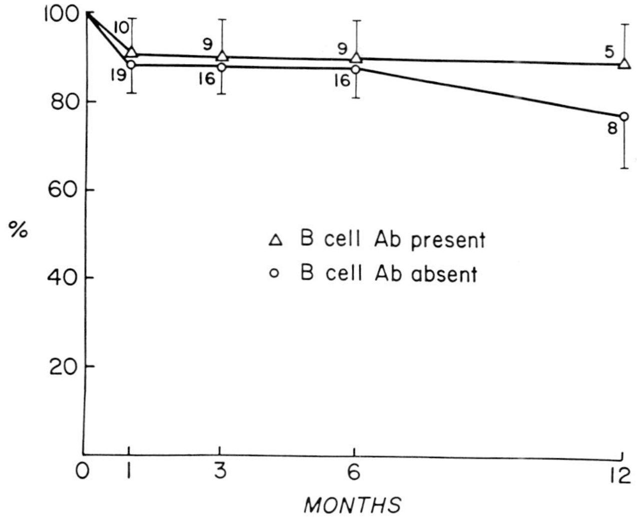

FIGURE 3 Actuarial graft survival of patients transplanted on the basis of a negative T-cell cross-match in the presence or absence of B-cell cytotoxins. The presence of a positive B-cell cross-match at the time of transplant appears to be benign.

vival may be somewhat tenuous, it is of note that patients who make antibody reactive with >20% of the panel on screening have been reported [143] to demonstrate superior graft survival (100%) when compared with patients producing antibody reactive with between 3 and 20% of the panel (72%). Graft survival at 1 year in patients who produced antibody to less than 3% of the panel was only 22%. These data are in agreement with the previously published observation that patients who produce antibody following transfusion have good graft survival after transplantation [16,139,154]. The potential importance of these observations are made even more significant by the recent observation that a positive cross-match using remote serum does not necessarily preclude transplantation if the immediate pretransplant cross-match is negative against donor T cells by the standard complement-dependent cytotoxicity assay or flow cytometry [24]. Based on currently available data, it appears that the presence of antibody with specificity for donor B cells in a low titer (i.e., anti-class II alloantibody) likely does not have an immediate deleterious effect on survival of the allograft and may even facilitate graft survival. Conversely, although anti-class I alloantibody has been reported to be effective in enhancing experimental organ allograft survival, there are few or no data that the presence of anti-class I alloantibody (i.e., anti-HLA-A, B) is other than deleterious in clinical transplantation.

The Transfusion Effect and Altered Alloreactivity in Humans

It is now generally conceived that alloreactivity is a cross-reactive by-product of the molecular mechanism of antigen and self-recognition mediated by a single T-cell receptor [170]. One of the more elegant studies documenting this concept is the recent demonstration by Kaye and Janeway [99] that the Fab fragment of a directly activating monoclonal antibody, which precipitates a disulfide-linked heterodimer from a mouse helper T-cell clone, blocks activation by either allogenic Ia(I-A^b) or antigen (ovalbumin) and self-Ia (I-A^k).

Discounting the possibility that the beneficial effect of pretransplant transfusion may be due to the selective eliminative of "high responders" from the pool of patients awaiting renal transplantation [156], let us briefly consider the principal alternate theses that have been advanced to account for the blunting of alloreactivity by pretransplant transfusion, that is, suppressor cell induction and the generation of autoanti-idiotypic antibody.

Suppressor Cells Suppressor cells have been identified at various times following transplantation in successfully enhanced recipients of heterotopic cardiac allografts in the inbred rat. Hall [78] has recently demonstrated the presence of suppressor cells in the spleens of (passively enhanced) rats that did not reject their cardiac allograft for 75 days, by cotransfer of splenic mononuclear cells, together with limiting numbers of spleen cells from unmodified rats, to sublethally irradiated syngeneic graft recipients. Hendry et al. [82] demonstrated the presence of suppressor cells in the thymus of cardiac allograft recipients, enhanced by pretreatment with both antigen and alloantibody, on day 6 posttransplantation. These latter investigators demonstrated that it was indeed essential to perform cardiac transplantation in order to demonstrate suppressor cells. Suppressor cells were not induced by antigen-antibody pretreatment alone. Experimental DST in a rat model also leads to striking graft prolongation, and this is due initially to the presence of antigraft antibody in the serum at the time of transplantation (i.e., active enhancement), but subsequently prolonged survival is likely due to the emergence of suppressor cells 30 days later [144]. I would like to emphasize that in these three studies *suppressor cells are seen to appear following transplantation in successfully enhanced recipients.*

The use of DST in humans has provided a unique opportunity to determine whether pretransplant transfusion leads to the generation of suppressor cells at the time of transplantation. Preliminary studies in this setting have provided conflicting evidence for suppressor cell induction prior to transplantation. More specifically, reduced mixed lymphocyte reactivity has not been uniformly observed and suppression of the MLR in admixture experiments has been variable [18,34,193,197]. The possible role of suppressor cells in renal transplantation is discussed more extensively elsewhere in this volume (Chapter 7).

Autoanti-idiotypic Antibody If DST were to lead to the generation of autoanti-idiotypic antibody (Chapter 6), it is hypothesized that the presence of such antibodies in recipient serum at the time of transplantation should suppress the ability of recipient lymphoid cells to respond to the specific donor if the cultures are conducted in recipient serum. The results of recent experiments designed to test this hypothesis have been equivocal [18,34,193,197].

The author would conclude, therefore, that there is no convincing evidence, at present, that the beneficial effect of pretransplant transfusion may be attributed to either suppressor cell induction or to the generation of autoanti-idiotypic antibody.

Enigmatic Success of a Single Pretransplant Transfusion with Blood from a Random Donor

One of the principal observations that has deterred some individuals from considering specific antibody-mediated enhancement as the immunologic mechanism underlying the apparently nonspecific beneficial effect of transfusion in clinical transplantation has been the surprising efficacy of a single random blood transfusion in promoting allograft survival

TABLE 1 Serologically Defined Public and Private B-cell (Ia) Alloantigen Specificities (RT1.B RT1.D) in the Rat[a]

		Ia								
RT1 haplotype	Strain	1	2	3	4	5	6	14	15	16
l	LEW	1	-	-	-	-	-	-	-	-
lvl	F233	1	-	-	-	-	-	14	-	-
n	BN	-	-	3	-	-	-	14	15	-
u	WF	-	2	-	-	-	-	14	-	16
b	BUF	-	-	-	-	-	6	-	15	16

[a]A system of public and private B-cell specificities were defined in the rat by ^{51}Cr release complement-dependent cytotoxicity assay using selectively absorbed hyperimmune alloantisera [114]. Data are presented in the text that strongly suggest that prolongation of organ allograft survival following immunization with lymphoid cells of a third party represents specific immunologic enhancement mediated by antibody to public "Ia" alloantigen specificities.

(i.e., References 21, 85, 127, and 144). How can a single transfusion from a random donor (or multiple transfusions from the same donor) generate antibody with specificity for the kidney that is eventually transplanted? This very question aroused the curiosity of the author, and this led to an exploration of the "specificity" of alloimmune responses in inbred rats. Briefly, Lowry et al. [114] observed that immunization of inbred LEW rats with fully allogeneic BN lymphoid cells led to the generation of antibody cytotoxic to nylon wool-enriched B-lymphocyte preparations, all available MHC disparate strains, including F344 ($RT1^{lvl}$); BN ($RT1^{n}$), WF (RT^{u}), and BUF ($RT1^{b}$). Similarly, hyperimmune sera raised in LEW by immunization with BUF lymphoid cells were cytotoxic to B lymphocytes of all strains listed above, except F344. For reasons to be clarified below, it is important to note that LEW anti-BUF hyperimmune serum was exclusively cytotoxic to BN B cells and was not reactive with BN T cells either in complement-dependent cytotoxicity assays or by indirect immunofluorescence. A population of (LEW × BN) F_2 rats was used to demonstrate that the target specificity recognized by LEW anti-BUF hyperimmune sera on B-enriched lymphocyte preparations from BN rats was linked to the major histocompatibility locus (RT-1). Further support for the developing thesis that the cross-reactivity of LEW anti-BUF on BN was directed at BN class II MHC (Ia) alloantigens was derived from the observation that LEW anti-BUF hyperimmune sera would inhibit LEW lymph node cells from proliferating in mixed lymphocyte reactions on stimulation with irradiated BN lymphoid cells. Extending these studies further, Lowry et al. were able to define a system of public and private class II alloantigens in available rat strains, as indicated in Table 1. It is noted that these studies were performed prior to definition of a second class II locus in the rat, RT1-D, and thus it was not possible to determine on which MHC locus the specificities noted in Table 1 are encoded. Since that time, however, we have learned that both loci, RT1.B and RT1.D, encode public (Ia-like) specificities (Cramer, personal communication; International Rat Workshop, Montreal, Canada, 1984).

Additional studies were subsequently performed to determine whether public class II alloantigens may play a role in enhancement. LEW rats were sensitized to BUF allogantigens. Preimmunization with BUF was shown to enhance the survival of bilaterally nephrecto-

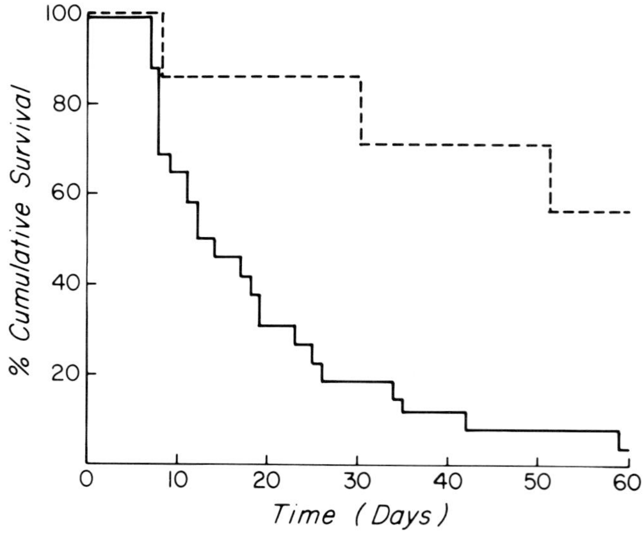

FIGURE 4 Cumulative survival of bilaterally nephrectomized LEW recipients of (LEW × BN) F_1 renal allografts is significantly greater ($p < 0.005$ by log rank analysis) in LEW hosts preimmunized with BUF (— — —) (n = 7) than in unmodified controls (——) (n = 26). Data are presented in the text to suggest that improved renal allograft survival following immunization with lymphoid cells from a third party is related to specific immunologic enhancement. (Figure reproduced from Reference 114 with the consent of the publishers.)

mized LEW recipients of (LEW × BN) F_1 renal allografts ($p < 0.005$ by log rank analysis) when compared with the survival of unsensitized controls (Figure 4). This difference in survival was associated with the production of anti-"Ia" alloantibodies against public "Ia" specificity(ies) shared between BUF and BN. These data are, in fact consistent with previous reports. Passive enhancement of skin allografts by antibody to public Ia antigens has been previously reported in the mouse [214]. Cross-reacting alloantisera have been shown on other model systems to have enhancing activity [31,183].

It is of interest to note that broadly reactive antibodies of ill-defined specificity (attributed either to antigen sharing or cross-reactivity) has previously been observed in humans as well as rodents [53]. Numerous published reports are indeed compatible with the thesis that antibody to public determinants generated by active immunization with blood or lymphoid cells from a third party (i.e., References 40,100,144, and 201) may lead to enhancement. It is certainly conceivable, therefore, that a single random transfusion may promote organ allograft survival in clinical transplantation through generation of antibody to shared antigens, or, more likely, cross-reactive antibodies to public specificities on antigens, encoded by the MHC (i.e., specific immunologic enhancement).

Components of a Whole-Blood Transfusion Required to Promote Renal Allograft Survival

It is currently recommended that whole blood or packed cells be administered to prospective renal allograft recipients to promote the survival of the subsequent graft. Frozen washed red cells, which contain few viable mononuclear leukocytes, appear to be entirely ineffective [16,150]. The efficacy of platelets, which bear class I but not class II alloantigens, in promoting allograft survival is controversial. Recent studies (i.e., Reference 33) have not supported the early observation that pretransplant platelet transfusion may promote renal allograft survival in humans. These data stand somewhat in contrast to reports of recent excellent studies in rodents that have convincingly demonstrated that prior inoculation with platelets may promote the survival of islet allografts that express primarily class I alloantigens [207] and numerous other reports suggesting that inoculation with purified red cells [213], which in a rodent express isolated class I alloantigens, or platelets [12], may lead to prolonged organ allograft survival. Our interpretation of the experimental data is that in some strain combinations prior inoculation with particulate antigen-bearing class I alloantigens may suffice, whereas in others, cells bearing class II alloantigens may be required since it is now apparent that helper and cytotoxic/suppressor T-cell subsets demonstrate independent pathogenic potential in allograft rejection. Clearly, in the presence of an isolated class I disparity, it may only be necessary to modulate the activity of class I-reactive cells. In other model systems, that is, in the presence of an isolated class II disparity, Ia-bearing cells may need to be included in the sensitizing inoculum in order to activate those immune mechanisms that may serve in the modulation of class II-reactive T cells. In the context of the thesis being presented in this chapter, it should be recognized that mononuclear leukocytes appear largely responsible both for inducing the transfusion effect in human renal transplantation as well as active enhancement in experimental organ transplantation.

CONCLUSIONS

Attempts at inducing specific immunosuppression by passive enhancement were unsuccessful, and in retrospect likely ill conceived (it is now recognized that intact IgG and not $F(ab')_2$ is active in enhancement), but data were presented that strongly support the thesis that pretransplant transfusion promotes renal allograft survival by a mechanism akin to active enhancement. We have reviewed the historical evolution of the concept of enhancement. Enhancement phenomena were first documented in early studies in tumor systems and subsequently reproduced in organ transplantation. Enhancement was seen to be mediated by antigraft antibody through a central mechanism involving opsonization of alloreactive cells, resulting in a quantitative reduction in specific immune reactivity. Although the beneficial effects observed clinically and experimentally following immunization with lymphoid elements from a third party might have suggested that the transfusion effect was entirely nonspecific, data were presented that demonstrate that sensitization with lymphoid cells from a third party may indeed induce specific immunologic enhancement mediated by antibody reactive with shared (public) antigenic specificities expressed on both the sensitizing inoculum (i.e., the transfused blood) and the specific graft.

Although not previously discussed in this chapter, we should point out that synergism has frequently been noted between specific immunologic enhancement and pharmacologic immunosuppression. To this end it is interesting to note that the beneficial effect of transfusion is noted even in patients treated with the potent new immunosuppressive agent, cyclosporin A, following renal transplantation [156].

Although the transfusion effect looks very much like active enhancement, formal proof that the two are indeed synonymous is lacking. Numerous factors, including antigeneic disparity, prior sensitization and the mode of sensitization, the age and sex of the recipient, and the immunosuppressive therapy employed posttransplant, are all likely critical determinants of the fate of a transplanted graft. It is important to recognize that the primary value of the pretransplant cross-match is limited to detection of pre-existent humoral immunity. Transplantation is not performed in the presence of a positive T-cell cross-match and likely should not be performed in the presence of high titers (> 1:4) of B-cell cytotoxins. At present there is no way of determining the level of pre-existent cellular immunity to the specific allograft prior to transplantation [194]. Accordingly, given that numerous factors may affect survival of an allograft, it would be simplistic to imagine that the presence of antigraft (enhancing) antibody in an appropriate titer would of necessity translate into permanent survival of the transplanted organ.

Pretransplant transfusion is now recognized to be one of the most important single determinants affecting renal allograft survival in humans. With the advent of improved diagnostic tools (i.e., the fluorescent-activated cell sorter) for the detection of antigraft antibody it is our hope that questions about the relationship between immunologic enhancement and clinical transplantation may soon be laid to rest. Clearly, however, this will not be easy and much work remains to be done.

ACKNOWLEDGMENTS

Supported in part by grants from the Medical Research Council of Canada and the Kidney Foundation of Canada. The excellent secretarial assistance of Ms. E. Milne and Ms. E. Cacolyris is gratefully acknowledged.

REFERENCES

1. Abbas, A. K. Two distinct mechanisms of B cell tolerance. *Cell. Immunol.* 46:178-183, 1979.
2. Acuto, O., and Reinherz, E. L. The human T cell receptor; structure and function. *N. Engl. J. Med.* 312:1100-1111, 1985.
3. Adler, F. L. Studies on mouse antibodies. I. The response to sheep red cells. *J. Immunol.* 95:26-38, 1965.
4. Advisory Committee to the Renal Transplant Registry. The 13th report of the human renal transplant registry. *Transplant Proc.* 9:9-26, 1977.
5. Albrechtsen, D., Arnesen, E., Solheim, B. G., and Thorsby, E. Significance of HLA-DR matching and of B cell crossmatch tests in vitro and in cadaver renal transplantation. *Transplant. Proc.* 11:743-747, 1979.
6. Anderson, N. D., Wyllie, R. G., and Shaker, I. J. Pathogenesis of vascular injury in rejecting rat renal allografts. *Johns Hopkins Med. J.* 141:135-147, 1977.
7. Axelrad, M. A. Suppression of delayed type hypersensitivity by antigen and antibody. Is a common precursor cell responsible for both delayed hypersensitivity and antibody formation. *Immunology* 15:159-171, 1968.
8. Ayoub, G., Park, M. S., Terasaki, P. I., Iwaki, Y., and Opelz, G. B cell antibodies and crossmatching. *Transplantation* 29:227-229, 1980.
9. Barry, J. M., Norman, D. J., Bohannon, L. L., Wetzsteon, P., and Fisher, S. Comparison of two donor specific transfusion protocols. *Transplant. Proc.* 17:1072-1074, 1985.
10. Batchelor, J. R., Ellis, F., French, M. E., Bewick, M., Cameron, J. S., and Ogg, C. S. Immunologic enhancement of human kidney graft. *Lancet* 2:1007-1010, 1970.
11. Batchelor, J. R., and Welsh, K. I. Mechanisms of enhancement of kidney allograft survival. A form of an operational tolerance. *Br. Med. Bull.* 32:113-117, 1976.
12. Batchelor, J. R., Welsh, K. I., and Burgos, H. Immunologic enhancement. *Transplant. Proc.* 9:931-936, 1977.

13. Berg, B., and Möller, E. Immediate rejection of a HLA-A,B compatible HLA-DR incompatible kidney with a positive donor-recipient B cell crossmatch. *Scand. J. Urol. Nephrol. (Suppl.)* 54:36, 1980.
14. Biesecker, J. L., Fitch, F. W., Rowley, D. A., and Stuart, F. P. Cellular and humoral immunity after allogenic transplantation in the rat. III. The effect of passive antibody on cellular and humoral immunity after allogenic renal transplant. *Transplantation* 16:432-440, 1973.
15. Billingham, R. E., and Sparrow, E. M. Studies on the nature of immunity to homologous grafted skin with special reference to the use of pure epidermal grafts. *J. Exp. Biol.* 31:16-39, 1954.
16. Birtch, A. G., McConnachie, P. R., and Finch, W. T. Pretransplant transfusion—a panacea. *Transplant. Proc.* 14:305-307, 1982.
17. Bore, P. J., Sells, R. A., Jamieson, V., and Burrows, K. Transfusion induced renal allograft prolongation. *Transplant. Proc.* 11:148-151, 1979.
18. Braun, W. E., Zachary, A. A., Novick, A. C., Steinmuller, D. R., Cunningham, R. J., Streem, S. B., Buszta, C., and Protiva, D. Humoral and cellular responses to donor specific transfusions. *Transplant. Proc.* 17:1062-1065, 1985.
19. Brent, L., and Medawar, P. B. Quantitative studies on tissue transplantation immunity. V. The role of antiserum in enhancement and desensitization. *Proc. R. Soc.* 155:392-416, 1961.
20. Brideau, R. J., Carter, P. B., McMaster, W. R., Mason, D. W., and Williams, A. F. Two subsets of rat T lymphocytes defined by monoclonal antibodies. *Eur. J. Immunol.* 10:609-615, 1980.
21. Burrows, L., Schanzer, H., Feingold, R., Miller, C., Giannone, G., Curtis, A., Rubenstein, P., and Fotino, M. The use of repeated, third party, small aliquot HLA-defined blood transfusions in renal recipients. *Transplant. Proc.* 15:956-961, 1983.
22. Capel, P. J. A., Tamboer, W. P. M., de Waal, R. M. W., Jansen, J. L. J., and Koene, R. A. P. Passive enhancement of mouse skin allograft by alloantibodies is Fc dependent. *J. Immunol.* 122:421-425, 1979.
23. Capel, P. J. A., de Waal, R. M. W., Démant, P., and Koene, R. A. P. Enhancement and antibody-mediated rejection of mouse skin allografts with anti-H-2K, H-2D, H2L antibodies. *Transplant. Proc.* 13:649-653, 1981.
24. Cardella, C. J., Falk, J. A., Nicholson, M. I., Harding, M., and Cook, G. T. Successful renal transplantation in patients with T-cell reactivity to donor. *Lancet* 2:1240-1242, 1982.
25. Cardella, C. J., and Falk, J. A. Graft outcome in patients with antibody reactive with donor T and B cells. *Transplant. Proc.* 15:1142-1144, 1983.
26. Carpenter, C. B., D'Apice, A. J. F., and Abbas, A. K. The role of antibodies in the rejection and enhancement of organ allograft. *Adv. Immunol.* 22:1-65, 1976.
27. Carpenter, C. B., and Milford, E. L. Immunologic monitoring before transplantation. In *Renal Transplantation: Principles and Practice,* P. J. Morris, ed. Grune & Stratton, New York, 1984, pp. 181-197.
28. Casey, A. E. Experimental enhancement of malignancy in the Brown-Pearce rabbit tumor. *Proc. Soc. Exp. Biol. Med.* 29:816-818, 1932.
29. Casey, A. E. A species limitation of an enhancing material derived from a mammalian tumor. *Proc. Soc. Exp. Biol. Med.* 30:674-677, 1933.
30. Casey, A. E. Specificity of enhancing materials from mammalian tumors. *Proc. Soc. Exp. Biol. Med.* 31:663-665, 1934.
31. Catto, G. D. R., Carpenter, C. B., Strom, T. B., and Williams, R. M. Passive enhancement of rat renal allografts by antibodies to a non-SD (Ag-B) locus analogous to Ia and demonstration of linkage to the MHC. *Transplant. Proc.* 9:957-960, 1977.
32. Chambers, H., and Scott, G. M. Experiments on immunity to tumor growth. *Br. J. Exp. Pathol.* 5:1-12, 1924.

33. Chapman, J. R., Fisher, M., Ting, A., and Morris, P. J. Platelet transfusions before renal transplantation in man. *Transplant. Proc.* 17:1038-1040, 1985.
34. Cheigh, J. S., Suthanthiran, M., Riggio, R. R., Stubenbord, W. L., Kaplan, M., Fotino, M., Evelyn, M., Schechter, N., Stenzel, K. H., and Rubin, A. L. Induction of immune alterations and successful renal transplantation with a simplified method of donor specific blood transfusion. *Transplant. Proc.* 17:1075-1076, 1985.
35. Cicciarelli, J. C., Chia, D., and Terasaki, P. I. IgM anti-IgM cold lymphocytotoxins to B cells. *Transplant. Proc.* 11:1950-1953, 1979.
36. Clarke, C. A., Donohoe, W. T. A., McConnell, R. B., Woodrow, J. C., Finn, R., Krevans, J. R., Kluke, W., Lehane, D., and Sheppard, P. M. Further experimental studies on the prevention of Rh hemolytic disease. *Br. Med. J.* 1:979-984, 1963.
37. Crowle, A. J., and Hu, C. C. Inhibition of the development of delayed type hypersensitivity with antiserum. *J. Immunol.* 94:555-562, 1965.
38. D'Apice, A. J. F., and Tait, B. D. Improved survival and function of renal transplants with positive B cell crossmatches. *Transplantation* 27:324-328, 1979.
39. D'Apice, A. J. F., and Tait, B. D. Most positive B cell crossmatches are not caused by anti-HLA-DR antibodies. *Transplantation* 30:382-383, 1980.
40. Davies, D. A. L., and Alkins, B. J. What abrogates heart transplant rejection in immunologic enhancement? *Nature* 247:294-297, 1974.
41. de Waal, R. M. W., Cornelissen, I. M. H. A., Capel, P. J. A., and Koene, R. A. P. Passive enhancement of mouse tumor allografts by alloantibodies is Fc dependent. *J. Immunol.* 123:1353-1355, 1979.
42. de Waal, R. M. W., Capel, P. J. A., and Koene, R. A. P. The role of anti-H-2K and H-2D alloantibodies in enhancement and acute antibody-mediated rejection of mouse skin allografts. *J. Immunol.* 124:719-723, 1980.
43. Dossetor, J. B., MacKinnon, K. J., Gault, M. H., and MacLean, L. D. Cadaver kidney transplants. *Transplantation* 5:844-853, 1967.
44. Eichwald, E. J., Craven, C. M., Spellman, C., and Dolberg, M. L. The cell type mediating hyperacute rejection of allogeneic mouse skin grafts. *Cell. Immunol.* 33:219-223, 1977.
45. Elkins, W. L., Hellström, I., Hellström, K. E. Transplantation tolerance and enhancement. Concepts and questions. *Transplantation* 18:38-45, 1974.
46. Enomato, K., and Lucci, Z. J. Immunologic enhancement of renal allografts in the rat. III. Role of the spleen. *Transplantation* 15:8-16, 1973.
47. Ettinger, R. B., Terasaki, P. I., Opelz, G., Malekzadeh, M., Pennisi, A. J., Uittenbogaart, C., and Fine, R. Successful renal allografts across a positive cross-match for donor B-lymphocyte alloantigens. *Lancet* 2:56-58, 1976.
48. Ettenger, R. B., Terasaki, P. I., Ting, A., Malekzadeh, M. H., Pennisi, A. J., Uittenbogaart, C., Garrison, R., and Fine, R. N. Anti-B lymphocytotoxins in renal-allograft rejection. *N. Engl. J. Med.* 295:305-309, 1976.
49. Ettenger, R. B., Terasaki, P. I., Ting, A., Malekzadeh, M. H., Pennisi, A. J., Uittenbogaart, C. H., and Fine, R. H. Role of antibodies to B lymphocytes in renal transplantation. *Transplant. Proc.* 9:751-753, 1977.
50. Ettenger, R. B., Robinson, B. J., Uittenbogaart, C. H., Hacker, T. A., Pennisi, A. J., Malekzadeh, M. H., and Fine, R. N. Antibodies to donor B lymphocyte and autoantibodies in renal transplantation. *Transplant. Proc.* 11:401-403, 1979.
51. Fabre, J. W., and Morris, P. J. Dose response studies in passive enhancement of rat renal allografts. *Transplantation* 15:397-403, 1973.
52. Fabre, J. W., and Morris, P. J. Passive enhancement of homozygous renal allografts in the rat. *Transplantation* 18:429-435, 1974.
53. Fabre, J. W., Bishop, M., Sen, T., McKenzie, J., Williams, K. A., Denton, T. G., Millard, P. R., and Morris, P. J. A study of three protocols of blood transfusion before renal transplantation in the dog. *Transplantation* 26:94-98, 1978.

54. Feduska, N. J., Amend, W. J., Vincenti, F., Duca, R., and Salvatierra, O. Blood transfusions before and on the day of transplantation: Effect on cadaver graft survival. *Transplant. Proc.* 14:302-304, 1982.
55. Fehrman, I., Groth, C. G., Lundgren, C. Y., Magnusson, G., and Möller, E. Pretransplant blood transfusion—correlation with cadaver kidney graft survival. *Transplant. Proc.* 11:152-155, 1979.
56. Fehrman, I., Ringdén, O., Öst, L., and Groth, C. G. The long term effect of pretransplant blood transfusions on cadaveric kidney graft and patient survival rates. *Transplant. Proc.* 17:1080-1082, 1985.
57. Feldmann, J. D. Immunological enhancement: A study of blocking antibodies. *Adv. Immunol.* 15:167-214, 1972.
58. Ferrara, G. B., Tosi, R. M., Azzolina, G., Carminati, G., and Kissmeyer-Nielsen, F. The production of anti HL-A cytotoxic antisera through planned immunization by intravenous injections of small aliquots of whole blood. *Tissue Antigens* 2:359-373, 1972.
59. Finkelstein, M. S., and Uhr, J. W. Specific inhibition of antibody formation by passively administered 19S and 7S antibody. *Science* 146:67-69, 1964.
60. Flexner, S., and Jobling, J. W. On the promoting influence of heated tumor emulsions on tumor growth. *Proc. Soc. Exp. Biol. Med.* 4:156-157, 1907.
61. Flores, R. V., and Gilmer, P. J. Differential recognition and lysis of EL4 target cells by cytotoxic T cells. Differences in H-2K^b antigenic density and cytoskeletal proteins. *J. Immunol.* 132:2767-2774, 1984.
62. Forbes, R. D. C., Guttmann, R. D., Gommersall, M., and Hibberd, J. A controlled renal ultrastructural tracer study of first set cardiac allograft rejection in the rat: Evidence that the microvascular endothelium is the primary target of graft destruction. *Am. J. Pathol.* 111:184, 1983.
63. Forbes, R. D. C., Lowry, R. P., Gommersall, M., and Blackburn, J. Comparative immunohistologic studies in an adoptive transfer model of acute rat cardiac allograft rejection. *Transplantation* (in press).
64. French, M. E., and Batchelor, J. R. Enhancement of renal allografts in rats and man. *Transplant. Rev.* 13:115-141, 1972.
65. French, M. E. The early effects of alloantibody and complement on rat kidney allografts. *Transplantation* 13:447-451, 1972.
66. Fuller, T. C., Delmonico, F. L., Cosimi, A. B., Huggins, C. E., King, M., and Russel, P. S. Effects of various types of RBC transfusions on HLA alloimmunization and renal allograft survival. *Transplant. Proc.* 9:117-119, 1977.
67. Gallico, G. G., and Mason, D. W. Correlation between an aberrant serological response to transplantation antigens and renal allograft enhancement in allogenic recipients. *Transplantation* 26:46-51, 1978.
68. Gallico, G. G., Butcher, G. W., and Howard, J. C. The role of subregion of the rat major histocompatibility complex in the rejection and passive enhancement of renal allografts. *J. Exp. Med.* 149:244-253, 1979.
69. Garovoy, M. R., Reinschmidt, M. A., and Bigos, M., Perkins, H., Colombe, B., Feduska, N., and Salvatierra, O. Flow cytometry analysis: A high technology crossmatch technique facilitating transplantation. *Transplant. Proc.* 15:1939-1944, 1983.
70. Garovoy, M. R., Colombe, B. W., Melzer, J., Feduska, N., Shields, C., Cross, D., Amens, W., Vincenti, F., Hopper, S., Duca, R., and Salvatierra, O. Flow cytometry crossmatching for donor-specific transfusion recipients and cadaveric transplantation. *Transplant. Proc.* 17:693-695, 1985.
71. Gorer, P. A., and Kaliss, N. The effect of isoantibodies in vivo on three different transplantable neoplasms in mice. *Cancer Res.* 19:824-830, 1959.
72. Gorer, P. A. The antigenic structure of tumors. *Adv. Immunol.* 1:345-393, 1961.
73. Gurley, K. E., Lowry, R. P., and Forbes, R. D. C. Immune mechanism in organ allo-

graft rejection. II. T helper cells, delayed type hypersensitivity and rejection of renal allografts. *Transplantation* 36:401-405, 1983.

74. Haaland, M. The contrast in the reactions to the implantation of cancer after the inoculation of living and mechanically disintegrated cells. *Proc. R. Soc.* [*B*] 82:293-298, 1910.
75. Hall, B. M., Dorsch, S., and Roser, B. The cellular basis of allograft rejection in vivo. I. The cellular requirement for first set rejection of heart grafts. *J. Exp. Med.* 148: 878-889, 1978.
76. Hall, B. M., de Saxe, I., and Dorsch, S. E. The cellular basis of allograft rejection in vivo. III. Restoration of first set rejection of heart grafts by T helper cells in irradiated rats. *Transplantation* 36:700-705, 1983.
77. Hall, B. M., Gurley, K. E., and Dorsch, S. E. Do T helper-inducer cells mediate rejection without T cytotoxic-suppressor cells? *Transplant. Proc.* 17:233-234, 1985.
78. Hall, B. M. Mechanism maintaining enhancement of allografts. I. Demonstration of a specific suppressor cell. *J. Exp. Med.* 161:123-133, 1985.
79. Hart, D. N. J., and Fabre, J. W. Major histocompatibility complex antigens in rat kidney, ureter and bladder. Localization with monoclonal antibodies and demonstrate of Ia-positive dendritic cells. *Transplantation* 31:318-325, 1981.
80. Hart, D. N. J., Fuggle, S. V., Williams, K. A., Fabre, J. W., Ting, A., and Morris, P. J. Localized of HLA-ABC and DR antigens in human kidney. *Transplantation* 31: 428-433, 1981.
81. Heidecke, C. D., Kupiec-Weglinski, J. W., Abbud-Filho, M., Araujo, J. L., Lear, P. A., Strom, T. B., and Tilney, N. L. T helper and T cytotoxic/suppressor cells and lymphokines are critical in acute organ graft rejection in B rats. *Transplant. Proc.* 17:866-868, 1985.
82. Hendry, W. S., Tilney, N. L., Baldwin, W. M., Graves, M. J., Milford, E., Strom, T. B., and Carpenter, C. B. Transfer of specific unresponsiveness to organ allografts by thymocytes. *J. Exp. Med.* 149:1042-1055, 1979.
83. Heslop, B. F. Immunological enhancement of skin allografts in rats following pretreatment of the recipient with nonviable allogeneic cells. *Transplantation* 4:32-47, 1966.
84. Hirshberg, H., Moen, T., and Thorsby, E. Specific destruction of human endothelial cell monolayers by anti-DRw antisera. *Transplantation* 28:116-120, 1979.
85. Hunsicker, L. G., Oei, L. S., Freeman, R. M., Thompson, J. S., and Corry, R. J. Effect of blood transfusions on cadaveric renal allograft survival. *Transplant. Proc.* 11:156-159, 1979.
86. Hurme, H., Chandler, P. R., Hetherington, C. M., and Simpson, E. Cytotoxic T cell responses to H-Y: Correlation with the rejection of syngeneic male skin grafts. *J. Exp. Med.* 147:768-775, 1978.
87. Hutchinson, I. V. Antigen-reactive cell opsonization (ARCO) and its role in antibody mediated immune suppression. *Immunol. Rev.* 49:167-197, 1980.
88. Indiveri, F., Fagiolo, U., Pellegrino, M. A., and Ferrone, S. Uremic patients immunized with planned blood transfusions: Detection of HLA antibodies with the cytotoxic test and an indirect rosette microassay. *Transplant. Proc.* 11:167-170, 1979.
89. Isakov, N., Biel, L. W., and Bach, F. H. Induction of class I antigen-disparate pancreatic islet graft rejection by in vivo administration of cloned helper-independent cytolytic T lymphocytes. *Transplant. Proc.* 17:727-728, 1985.
90. Iwaki, Y., Park, M. S., Terasaki, P. I., and Billing, R. Enhancement of human kidney allografts by cold B-lymphocyte cytotoxins. *Lancet* 1:1228-1229, 1978.
91. Jansen, J. L. J., Koene, R. A. P., von Kamp, G. J., Hagemann, J. F. H. M., and Wijdeveld, P. G. A. B. Hyperacute rejection and enhancement of mouse skin grafts by antibody with a distinct specificity. *J. Immunol.* 115:392-394, 1975.

92. Jeannet, M., Benzonana, G., and Arni, I. Donor-specific B and T lymphocyte antibodies and kidney graft survival. *Transplantation* 31:160-163, 1981.
93. Jeekel, J., Obertop, H., Vriesendorp, H. M., McDicken, I., and Westbroek, D. L. Effect of anti-donor serum (ADS) and donor cells on renal allograft survival on DL-A tissue typed littermate beagles. *Transplant. Proc.* 7:435-438, 1975.
94. Jeekel, J., van Dongen, J., Majoor, G., and Harder, F. Enhancement of rat renal allograft with antibodies against erythrocyte associated antigens (EAA). *Transplant. Proc.* 9:969-972, 1977.
95. Kaliss, N., and Snell, G. D. The effects of injections of lyophilized normal and neoplastic mouse tissues on the growth of tumor homoiotransplant in mice. *Cancer Res.* 11:122-126, 1951.
96. Kaliss, N. The survival of homografts in mice pretreated with antisera to mouse tissues. *Ann. N.Y. Acad. Sci.* 64:977-993, 1957.
97. Kaliss, N. Immunological enhancement of tumor homografts in mice. A review. *Cancer Res.* 18:992-1003, 1958.
98. Kaliss, N. The elements of immunologic enhancement, a consideration of mechanisms. *Ann. N.Y. Acad. Sci.* 101:62-79, 1962.
99. Kaye, J., and Janeway, C. A. The Fab fragment of a directly activating monoclonal antibody that precipitates a disulfide-linked heterodimer from a T helper cell clone blocks activation by either allogeneic Ia or antigen and self Ia. *J. Exp. Med.* 159: 1397-1412, 1984.
100. Kelley, S. E., and Cory, R. J. Prolongation of mouse heart allografts survival by prior administration of nonspecific blood. *Transplant. Proc.* 13:518-522, 1981.
101. Kelly, W. D., Lillehie, R. C., Aust, J. B., Varco, R. L., Leonard, A. S., Griffin, W. O., Markland, C., Herdman, R. C., Vernier, R. L., Michael, A. F., and Levitt, J. Kidney transplantation. Experiences at the University of Minnesota Hospitals. *Surgery* 62: 704-720, 1967.
102. Kirkman, R. L., Flye, M. W., Williams, G. M., Colvin, R. B., and Sachs, D. H. Evidence for cellular immune mechanisms in hyperacute rejection of renal allografts in miniatrue swine. *Transplant. Proc.* 11:790-792, 1979.
103. Kissmeyer-Nielson, F., Olsen, S., Peterson, V. P., and Fjeldborg, O. Hyperacute rejection of kidney allografts associated with preexisting antibodies against donor cells. *Lancet* 1:662-665, 1966.
104. Klaus, G. G. B., and Abbas, A. K. Antigen receptor interactions in the induction of B-lymphocyte unresponsiveness. *Curr. Top. Microbiol. Immunol.* 78:22-68, 1977.
105. Klintmalm, G., Brynger, H., Flatmark, A., Frödin, L., Husberg, B., Thorsby, E., and Groth, C. G. The blood transfusion, DR matching and mixed lymphocyte culture effects are not seen in cyclosporine-treated renal transplant recipients. *Transplant. Proc.* 17:1026-1031, 1985.
106. Lagrange, P. H., MacKaness, G. B., and Miller, T. E. Influence of dose and route of antigen on the immunological induction of T cells. *J. Exp. Med.* 139:528-542, 1974.
107. Lagrange, P. H., and MacKaness, G. B. Site of action of factors that block delayed type hypersensitivity in mice. *J. Exp. Med.* 148:235-245, 1978.
108. Lanzavecchia, A. Antigen-specific interaction between T and B cells. *Nature* 314: 537-539, 1985.
109. Leitch, A. Experimental diminution of resistance to mouse cancer. *Lancet* 1:991-992, 1910.
110. Lobo, P. I., Westervelt, F. B., and Rudolf, L. E. Kidney transplantation across a positive cross-match. Crossmatch assays and distribution of B lymphocytes in donor tissues. *Lancet* 1:925-927, 1977.
111. Loveland, B. E., Hogarth, P. M., Ceredig, R. H., and McKenzie, I. F. C. Cells mediating graft rejection in the mouse. I. Lyt-1 cells mediate skin graft rejection. *J. Exp. Med.* 153:1044-1057, 1981.

112. Lowry, R. P., Myrberg, S., Goguen, J. E., Carpenter, C. B., Cho, S., Garovoy, M. R., and the Interhospital Organ Bank of New England, Inc. A negative T cell crossmatch is adequate to permit successful renal transplantation. *Proc. Dial. Transplant. Forum* 9:201-204, 1979.
113. Lowry, R. P., Goquen, J., Carpenter, C. B., Strom, T. B., and Garovoy, M. R. Improved B cell typing for HLA-DR using nylon wool enriched B lymphocyte preparations. *Tissue Antigens* 1:325-330, 1979.
114. Lowry, R. P., and Carpenter, C. B. Public B cell alloantigen determinants (Ia) and active enhancement of renal allografts in the rat. *Transplantation* 30:347-353, 1980.
115. Lowry, R. P., and Gurley, K. E. Immune mechanisms in organ allograft rejection. III. Cellular and humoral immunity in rejection of organ allografts transplanted across MHC subregion disparity RT1.B (RT1.D). *Transplantation* 36:405-411, 1983.
116. Lowry, R. P., Gurley, K. E., and Forbes, R. D. C. Immune mechanisms in organ allograft rejection. I. Delayed type hypersensitivity and lymphocytotoxicity in heart graft rejection. *Transplantation* 36:391-401, 1983.
117. Lowry, R. P., and Blackburn, J. K. Studies on rejection of heart grafts bearing isolated RT1.A-encoded Class I disparities. *Transplant. Proc.* 16:1118-1123, 1984.
118. Lowry, R. P., and Forbes, R. D. C. The nonessential role of a humoral antibody response in acute rat cardiac allograft rejection: An ultrastructural tracer study in an adoptive transfer model. *Transplantation* 37:182-187, 1984.
119. Lowry, R. P., Forbes, R. D. C., and Blackburn, J. H. Immune reactivity and immunosuppressive intervention (TLI) in experimental nephritis. I. Immunopathologic correlates in the accelerated autologous form of nephrotoxic serum nephritis. *J. Immunol.* 132:1001-1006, 1984.
120. Lowry, R. P., Forbes, R. D. C., Blackburn, J., and Marghesco, D. The pivotal role of cytotoxic T cells in the rejection of heart grafts bearing isolated class I disparities. *Transplant. Proc.* 17:227-230, 1985.
121. Lowry, R. P., Blackburn, J., and Marghesco, D. Immune mechanisms in organ allograft rejection. VI. Delayed-type hypersensitivity and lymphotoxin in renal allograft rejection. *Transplantation* 40, 1985.
122. Lowry, R. P., Forbes, R. D. C., Blackburn, J., and Marghesco, D. Immune mechanisms in organ allograft rejection. V. Pivotal role of the cytotoxic-suppressor T-cell subset in the rejection of heart grafts bearing isolated class I disparities. *Transplantation* 1985 (in press).
123. Hunt, H. D., and Luboroff, D. M. Interaction of T lymphocyte subpopulation bearing the RT6 alloantigen. *Transplant. Proc.* 17, 1861-1863, 1985.
124. MacKaness, G. B., Lagrange, P. H., Miller, T. E., and Ishibashi, T. Feedback inhibition of specifically sensitized lymphocytes. *J. Exp. Med.* 139:543-559, 1974.
125. MacKaness, G. B., and Lagrange, P. H. Restoration of cell-mediated immunity to animals blocked by a humoral response. *J. Exp. Med.* 140:865-870, 1974.
126. MacLeod, A. M., Mason, R. J., Stewart, K. N., Power, D. A., Shewan, W. G., Edward, N., and Catto, G. R. D. Fc-receptor-blocking antibodies develop after blood transfusions and correlate with good graft outcome. *Transplant. Proc.* 15:1019-1021, 1983.
127. MacLeod, A., Catto, G., Mather, A., Manson, R., Stewart, K., Power, D., Shewan, G., and Urbaniak, S. Beneficial antibodies in renal transplantation developing after blood transfusions: Evidence for HLA linkage. *Transplant. Proc.* 17:1057-1058, 1985.
128. MacPherson, G. G., and Christmas, S. E. The role of the macrophage in cardiac allograft rejection in the rat. *Immunol. Rev.* 77:143-166, 1984.
129. Majsky, A. Evidence of anti-HLA-A cytotoxins with only B lymphocytes. *Tissue Antigens* 13:75-76, 1979.
130. Marquet, R. L., van Es, A. A., Heystek, G. A., van Leersum, R. H., and Balner, H.

Attempts to induce immunological enhancement for kidney allografts in Rhesus monkeys. I. Effect of various alloantisera, including B cell antisera. *Transplantation* 25:188-192, 1978.
131. Mason, D. W., Brideaw, R. J., MacMasler, W. R., Webb, M., While, R. A., and Williams, A. F. Monoclonal antibodies that define T lymphocyte subsets in the rat. In *Monoclonals,* G. I. Ada and R. R. Porier, eds. Plenum Press, New York, 1980, p. 251.
132. McDowall, R. A. W., Batchelor, J. R., and French, M. E. Hyperacute rejection and enhancement of rabbit-kidney allografts. *Lancet* 1:797-801, 1973.
133. McKenzie, J. L., Fabre, J. W., and Morris, P. J. Studies on the cross-reactivity of allosera for kidney graft enhancement in rats. *Transplantation* 30:9-13, 1980.
134. Meuer, S. C., Schlossman, S. F., and Reinherz, E. L. Clonal analysis of human cytotoxic T lymphocytes: $T4^+$ and $T8^+$ effector T cells recognize products of different histocompatibility complex regions. *Proc. Natl. Acad. Sci. USA* 79:4395-4399, 1982.
135. Mitchison, N. A., and Phil, D. Studies on the immunological response to foreign tumor transplants in the mouse. *J. Exp. Med.* 102:157-177, 1955.
136. Mohanakumar, T., Rhodes, C., Mendez-Picon, G., Goldman, M., Moncure, C., and Lee, H. Renal allograft rejection associated with presensitization to HLA-DR antigens. *Transplantation* 31:93-95, 1981.
137. Morris, P. J., Ting, A., Oliver, D. O., Bishop, M., Williams, K., and Dunnill, M. S. Renal transplantation and a positive serologic crossmatch. *Lancet* 1:1288-1291, 1977.
138. Morris, P. J. Suppression of rejection of organ allografts by alloantibody. *Immunol. Rev.* 49:93-125, 1980.
139. Murray, S., Dewar, P. J., and Uldall, P. R., Wilkinson, R., Kerr, D. N. S., Taylor, R. M. R., and Swinney, J. Some important factors in cadaver-donor kidney transplantation. *Tissue Antigens* 4:548-557, 1974.
140. Nagy, Z., Elliott, B. E., and Nabholz, M. Specific binding of K- and I-region products of the H-2 complex to activated thymus-derived (T) cells belonging to different Ly subclasses. *J. Exp. Med.* 144:1545-1553, 1976.
141. Nelson, D. S. Enhancement of skin homografts in guinea pigs. *Transplant. Bull.* 28: 26-27, 1961.
142. Nelson, D. S. Immunological enhancement of skin homografts in guinea pigs. *Br. J. Exp. Pathol.* 43:1-11, 1962.
143. Norman, D. J., Barry, J. M., Boehne, C., and Wetzsteon, P. Natural history of patients who make cytotoxic antibodies following prospective fresh blood transfusions. *Transplant. Proc.* 17:1041-1043, 1985.
144. Ochiai, T., Nagata, M., Nakajima, K., Asano, T., Gunji, Y., Uematsu, T., and Sato, H. The role of Ia-positive cells and the mechanism of the additive effect of simultaneous administration of cyclosporine and donor specific transfusion in cardiac allotransplantation in the rat. *Transplant. Proc.* 17:1097-1100, 1985.
145. Ockner, S. A., Guttmann, R. D., and Lindquist, R. R. Renal transplantation in the inbred rat. XIII. Modification of rejection by active immunization with bone marrow cells. *Transplantation* 9:30-38, 1970.
146. Ockner, S. A., Guttmann, R. D., and Lindquist, R. R. Renal transplantation in the inbred rat. XIV. Mechanism of the modified rejection produced by bone marrow cell pretreatment. *Transplantation* 9:39-48, 1970.
147. Okazaki, H., Maki, T., Wood, M. L., and Monaco, A. P. Effect of blood transfusion on skin allograft survival in immunosuppressed mice. *Transplant. Proc.* 13:515-517, 1981.
148. Okazaki, H., Takahashi, H., Miura, K., Ishizaki, M., Oguma, S., and Taguchi, Y. Effect of buffy coat transfusion in living related and cadaveric renal transplantation. *Transplant. Proc.* 17:1034-1037, 1985.

149. Opelz, G., Sengar, D. P. S., Mickey, M. R., and Terasaki, P. I. Effect of blood transfusions on subsequent kidney transplants. *Transplant. Proc.* 5:253-259, 1973.
150. Opelz, G., and Terasaki, P. I. Poor kidney-transplant survival in recipients with frozen-blood transfusions or no transfusions. *Lancet* 2:696-698, 1974.
151. Opelz, G., and Terasaki, P. I. Enhancement of kidney graft survival by blood transfusions. *Transplant. Proc.* 9:121-122, 1977.
152. Opelz, G., and Terasaki, P. I. Dominant effect of transfusions on kidney graft survival. *Transplantation* 29:153-158, 1980.
153. Opelz, G., and Terasaki, P. I. Importance of preoperative (not peroperative) transfusions for cadaveric kidney transplants. *Transplantation* 31:106-108, 1981.
154. Opelz, G., and Terasaki, P. I. International study of histocompatibility in renal transplantation. *Transplantation* 33:87-95, 1982.
155. Opelz, G. Blood transfusion and renal transplantation. In *Kidney Transplantation: Principles and Practice,* P. J. Morris, ed. Grune & Stratton, London, 1984, pp. 324-334.
156. Opelz, G., for the Collaborative Transplant Study. Current relevance of the transfusion effect in renal transplantation. *Transplant. Proc.* 17:1015-1022, 1985.
157. Park, M. S., Terasaki, P. I., and Bernoco, D. Autoantibody against B lymphocytes. *Lancet* 2:465-467, 1977.
158. Park, M. M., Davis, W. C., and Burger, D. The role of T cell subpopulations in rejection and enhancement of heart grafts. *Fed. Proc. Am. Soc. Exp. Biol.* 39:354, 1980.
159. Park, M. M., and MacDonald, T. L. Effect of enhancing antibodies on the generation of cytotoxic T cells, in vivo and in vitro. *Transplantation* 30:314-317, 1980.
160. Patel, R., and Terasaki, P. I. Significance of a positive crossmatch test in renal transplantation. *N. Engl. J. Med.* 280:735-739, 1969.
161. Pedersen, N. C., and Morris, B. The role of humoral antibody in the rejection of primary renal allografts in sheep. *J. Exp. Med.* 140:619-630, 1974.
162. Pellegrino, M. A., Belvedere, M., Pellegrino, A. G., and Ferrone, S. B peripheral lymphocytes express more HLA antigens than T peripheral lymphocytes. *Transplantation* 25:93-95, 1978.
163. Persijn, G. G., Cohen, B., Lansbergen, Q., and van Rood, J. J. Retrospective and prospective studies on the effect of blood transfusions in renal transplantation in the Netherlands. *Transplantation* 28:396-401, 1979.
164. Persijn, G. G., van Leeuwen, A., Parlevliet, J., Cohen, B., Lansbergen, Q., D'Amaro, J., and van Rood, J. J. Two major factors influencing kidney graft survival in Eurotransplant: HLA DR matching and blood transfusion(s). *Transplant. Proc.* 13:150-154, 1981.
165. Pescovitz, M. D., Thistlethwaite, J. R., Auchincloss, H., Ildstad, S. T., Sharp, T. G., Terrill, R., and Sachs, D. H. Effect of class II antigen matching on renal allograft survival in miniature swine. *J. Exp. Med.* 160:1495-1508, 1984.
166. Prowse, S. J., Lafferty, K. J., and Sellins, K. Cytotoxic T cell-mediated graft rejection is lymphokine dependent. *Transplant. Proc.* 17:1552-1554, 1985.
167. Richardi, P., Diotallevi, P., Meteje, T., Carbonara, A. O., and Curtoni, E. S. HLA antibodies cytotoxic only for B lymphocytes. *Tissue Antigens* 10:323-329, 1979.
168. Rowinski, W., Ryffa, T., Ruke, M., Wasowska, B., Tilney, N. L., and Olszewski, W. L. Platelet induced donor-specific unresponsive to kidney allografts in mongrel dogs treated with ALG. *Transplant. Proc.* 13:586-588, 1981.
169. Royer, H. D., Bensussan, A., Acuto, O., and Reinherz, E. L. Functional isotypes are not encoded by the constant region genes of the β subunit of the T cell receptor for antigen/major histocompatibility complex. *J. Exp. Med.* 160:947-952, 1984.
170. Saito, H., Kranz, D. M., and Takagaki, Y., Hayday, A. C., Eisen, H. N., and Tonegawa, S. Complete primary structure of a heterodimeric T-cell receptor deduced from cDNA sequences. *Nature* 309:757-762, 1984.

171. Salvatierra, O., Amend, W., Vincenti, F., Potter, D., Iwaki, Y., Opelz, G., Terasaki, P., Duca, R., Hanes, D., Cochrum, K. C., Hopper, S., and Feduska, N. J. Pretreatment with donor specific blood transfusion of haploidentical recipients with high MLC.
172. Salvatierra, O., Vincenti, F., Amend, W., Potter, D., Iwaki, Y., Opelz, G., Terasaki, P., Duca, R., Cochrum, K., Hanes, D., Stoney, R. J., and Feduska, N. J. Deliberate donor-specific blood transfusions prior to living related renal transplantation. *Ann. Surg.* 192:543-552, 1980.
173. Scala, G., Kuang, Y. D., Hall, R. E., Muchmore, A. V., and Oppenheim, J. J. Accessory cell function of human B cells. I. Production of both interleukin I-like activity and an interleukin I inhibitory factor by an EBV-transformed human B cell line. *J. Exp. Med.* 159:1637-1652, 1984.
174. Shelby, J., Wakely, E., and Corry, R. J. Splenectomy abrogates the improved graft survival achieved by donor-specific transfusion. *Transplant. Proc.* 17:1083-1086, 1985.
175. Sinclair, N. R. St. C., and Chan, P. L. Regulation of the immune response. IV. The role of the Fc fragment in feedback inhibition by antibody. In *Morphologic and Functional Aspects of Immunity,* K. Lindahl Kiessling, G. Alm, and M. G. Hanna, eds. Plenum Press, New York, 1971, p. 609.
176. Sirchia, G., Mercuriali, F., Scalamogna, M., Secondo, V. R. D. S., Pizzi, C., and Poli, F. The cadaver kidney transplant programme of Milano: Immunological report. *Transplantation* 23:391-395, 1977.
177. Smith, T. Active Immunity produced by so-called balanced or neutral mixtures of diphtheria toxin and antitoxin. *J. Exp. Med.* 11:241-256, 1909.
178. Snell, G. D. The enhancing effect (or actively acquired tolerance) and the histocompatibility-2 locus in the mouse. *J. Natl. Can. Inst.* 15:665-675, 1954.
179. Solheim, B. G., Flatmark, A., Jervell, J., and Arnesen, E. Influence of blood transfusions on kidney transplant and uremic patient survival. *Scand. J. Urol. Nephrol.* (*Suppl.*) 42:65-69, 1977.
180. Soulillou, J. P., Carpenter, C. B., D'Apice, A. J., and Strom, T. B. The role of nonclassical Fc receptor-associated, Ag-B antigen (Ia) in rat allograft enhancement. *J. Exp. Med.* 143:405-421, 1976.
181. Soulillou, J. P., Peyrat, M. A., and Guenel, J. Association between treatment-resistant kidney allograft rejection and post-transplant appearance of antibodies to donor B-lymphocyte alloantigens. *Lancet* 1:354-356, 1978.
182. Soulillou, J. P., Keribin, D., Lecoquic, D., Decoquic, G., and Robine-Leon, S. Attempts to enhance kidney allografts in DLA-identical dogs with specific anti-Ia-like sera. *Transplantation* 29:314-319, 1980.
183. Staines, N. A., Guy, K., and Davies, D. A. L. The dominant role of Ia antibodies in the passive enhancement of H-2-incompatible skin grafts. *Eur. J. Immunol.* 5:782-789, 1975.
184. Strom, T. B., Carpenter, C. B., Garovoy, M. R., Abbas, A. K., Corson, J. M., Bear, R. A., and Soulillou, J. P. Modification of the rat alloimmune response by enhancing antibodies and the role of blocking factors in the survival of renal grafts. *Transplantation* 20:368-380, 1975.
185. Strom, T. B., Tilney, N. L., Paradysz, J. M., Banceqicz, J., and Carpenter, C. B. Cellular components of allograft rejection: Identity, specificity and cytotoxic function of cells infiltrating acutely rejecting allografts. *J. Immunol.* 118:2020-2026, 1977.
186. Stuart, F. P., McKearn, T. J., Weiss, A., and Fitch, F. W. Suppression of rat renal allograft rejection by antigen and antibody. *Immunol. Rev.* 49:127-165, 1980.
187. Stuart, F. P., Saito, T., and Fitch, F. W. Rejection of renal allografts: Specific immunologic suppression. *Science* 160:1463-1465, 1968.
188. Stuart, F. P., Scollard, D. M., McKearn, T. J., and Fitch, F. W. Cellular and humoral

immunity after allogenic renal transplantation in the rat. V. Appearance of anti-idiotypic antibody and its relationship to cellular immunity after treatment with donot spleen cells and alloantibody. *Transplantation* 22:455-466, 1976.

189. Sunday, M. E., and Dorf, M. E. Hapten-specific T cell response to 4-hydroxy-3-nitrophenyl acetyl. X. Characterization of distinct T cell subsets mediating cutaneous sensitivity responses. *J. Immunol.* 127:766-768, 1981.
190. Suthanthiran, M., Gailiunas, P., St. Louis, G., Fagan, G., Carpenter, C. B., and Garovoy, M. R. Presensitization to donor B cell ("Ia") antigens is associated with early graft failure. *Transplant. Proc.* 9:1807-1809, 1977.
191. Swain, S. T cell subsets and the recognition of MHC class. *Immunol. Rev.* 74: 129-142, 1983.
192. Tagart, V. Cytotoxicity in picryl chloride-painted mice is enhanced by pretreatment with cyclophosphamide. *Transplantation* 23:287-289, 1977.
193. Takeuchi, H., Sakagami, K., Seki, Y., Tsuboi, K., Matsumoto, M., Miyazaki, M., and Orita, K. Anti-idiotypic antibodies and suppressor cells induced by donor-specific transfusion in potential kidney transplant recipients. *Transplant. Proc.* 17: 1059-1061, 1985.
194. Thorsby, E. On the antibody crossmatch controversies. *Transplant. Proc.* 17:1533-1536, 1985.
195. Tilney, N. L., and Bell, P. R. F. Studies on enhancement of cardiac and renal allografts in the rat. *Transplantation* 18:31-37, 1974.
196. Ting, A. HLA and renal transplantation. In *Kidney Transplantation: Principals and Practice,* P. J. Morris, ed. Grune & Stratton, New York, 1984, pp. 159-180.
197. Tyler, J. D., Anderson, C. B., Sicard, G. A., Murphy, M. K., Anderman, C. K., and Etheredge, E. E. Decreased mixed lymphocyte reactivity towards donor antigens following donor specific transfusion combined with azathioprine immunosuppression. *Transplant. Proc.* 17:1053-1056, 1985.
198. Uhr, J. W., and Baumann, J. B. Antibody formation. II. The specific amnestic antibody response. *J. Exp. Med.* 113:959-970, 1961.
199. Uhr, J. W., and Möller, G. Regulatory effect of antibody on the immune response. *Adv. Immunol.* 8:81-127, 1968.
200. Vadas, M. A., Miller, J. F. A. P., and McKenzie, I. F. C. Ly and Ia antigen phenotypes of T cells involved in delayed type hypersensitivity and in suppression. *J. Exp. Med.* 144:10-19, 1976.
201. van Es, A. A., Marguet, R. L., Von Rood, J. J., and Balner, H. Influence of a single blood transfusion on kidney allograft survival in unrelated Rhesus monkeys. *Transplantation* 26:325-330, 1978.
202. van Leeuwen, A., Schuit, H. R. E., and van Rood, J. J. Typing for MLC (LD). II. The selection of nonstimulator cells by MLC inhibition tests using SD-identical stimulator cells (MISIS) and fluorescence antibody studies. *Transplant. Proc.* 5: 1539-1542, 1973.
203. Voisin, G. A., Kinsky, R., and Maillard, J. Protection against homologous disease in hybrid mice by passive and active immunological enhancement-facilitation. *Transplantation* 6:184-202, 1968.
204. Voisin, G. A. Immunological facilitation, a broadening of the concept of the enhancement phenomenon. *Prog. Allergy* 15:328-485, 1971.
205. Voisin, G. A. Role of antibody classes in the regulatory facilitation reaction. *Im. munol. Rev.* 49:3-60, 1980.
206. von Willebrand, E., Lautenschlager, I., Inkinen, K., Lehto, V. P., Virtanen, I., and Häyry, P. Distribution of the major histocompatibility complex antigens in human and rat kidney. *Kidney Int.* 27:616-621, 1985.
207. Weber, C. J., Pernis, B., and Reemtsma, K. Donor specific platelet transfusion prolongs mouse islet allograft survival. *Transplant. Proc.* 17:116-117, 1985.

208. Weiss, A., Stuart, F. P., and Fitch, F. W. Immune reactivity of cells from long-term rat renal allograft survivors. *Transplantation* 26:346-352, 1978.
209. Williams, G. M., Hume, D. M., Hudson, R. P., Morris, P. J., Kano, K., and Milgrom, F. "Hyperacute" renal-homograft rejection in man, *N. Engl. J. Med.* 279:611-618, 1968.
210. Williams, K. A., Ting, A., Cullen, P. R., and Morris, P. Transfusions: Their influence on human renal graft survival. *Transplant. Proc.* 11:175-178, 1979.
211. Wilson, R. E., Garovoy, M. R., Strom, T. B., Lowry, R. P., Busch, G. J., Vineyard, G. C., and Tilney, N. L. Passive enhancement of cadaver renal allografts: A prospective randomized trial of $F(ab^1)_2$ therapy. *Transplant. Proc.* 13:531-532, 1981.
212. Winearis, C. G., Fabre, J. W., Millard, P. R., and Morris, P. J. A quantitative comparison of whole antibody and $F(ab^1)_2$ in kidney allograft enhancement. *Transplantation* 28:36-39, 1979.
213. Wood, K. J., and Morris, P. J. The blood transfusion effect: Suppress of renal allograft rejection in the rat with affinity-purified RBCs. *Transplant. Proc.* 17:1135-1136, 1985.
214. Zimmerman, B., and Feldmann, J. D. Enhancing antibody. II. Specificity and heterogeneity. *J. Immunol.* 103:383-385, 1969.

6

ROLE OF ANTI-IDIOTYPIC RESPONSES IN REGULATING ALLOGRAFT REJECTION

Frank P. Stuart and Brian W. Haag
University of Chicago, Chicago, Illinois

TERMINOLOGY

In the evolving lexicon of immunologists, any molecular protuberance that functions as an antigen or immunogen has come to be known as an *epitope.* The combining site on an antibody that reacts with an epitope is called a *paratope* (Figure 1). Being rather large molecules, antibodies have their own immunogenic protuberances, epitopes, scattered along the variable and constant amino acid sequences. Some of the epitopes found in the constant region of the antibody molecule are shared throughout a species and determine an antibody's class (IgG, IgM, IgE, and so on). Because these epitopes in the constant region are shared throughout the species, they are also referred to as allotopes. Collectively, the profile of allotopes on a particular antibody gives rise to its allotype. Hence, antibodies directed against allotopes are referred to as anti-allotypic antibodies.

Although epitopes in the immunoglobulin constant regions (allotopes) have been recognized for many years, epitopes were not suspected in variable regions until 1963 [19]. Because epitopes found in the variable region are more individually specific and are less widely shared within the species, they are referred to as idiotopes rather than allotopes. The set of immunogenic idiotopes in the variable regions of an antibody molecule comprise an idiotypic profile that can be recognized by the combining sites (paratopes) of other antibody molecules; these latter antibodies are referred to as anti-idiotypic. The terminology can be grasped more easily by assigning numbers to antibody responses. Thus, Ab1 is the response to a particular epitope (antigen), and Ab2 would be the response to Ab1. This secondary response, Ab2, is directed against idiotopes in the variable region of the Ab1 molecule. These idiotopes may be part of or immediately adjacent to the combining site (paratope) of Ab1, or they may be at a distance from it. In either case, the Ab2 response is an anti-antibody response directed against the idiotype of Ab1. The process can go on. That is, idiotopes on Ab2 can stimulate an Ab3 response. The end point for this cascade of internal responses is not clear.

An individual's B-cell receptor (immunoglobulin) and T-cell receptor directed at the same antigen may or may not share idiotopes [15,30]. Thus, an Ab2 response might react not only with Ab1, but also with T1 (T1 represents the T-cell response to the initiating antigen). A series of T1, T2, and T3 responses parallels the series of antibody responses.

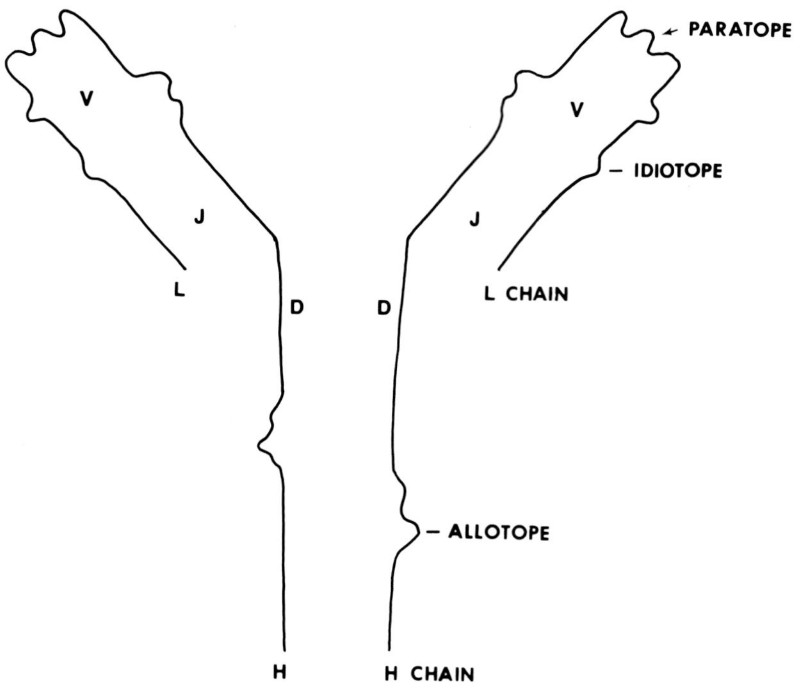

FIGURE 1 Schematic representation of immunoglobulin molecule showing heavy (H) and light (L) chains as well as variable (V), junctional (J) and constant (D) regions of the amino acid sequences.

Adding to the complexity of this system is the heterogeneity of idiotypes for a particular Ab1 or T1 response. There is a family of B-cell clones and T-cell clones capable of reacting with any particular antigen. These clones differ by the series of idiotopes on the immunoglobulin molecule or the T-cell receptor. Consequently, the Ab2 or T2 response is also heterogeneous; it is directed against the variety of idiotypes expressed in the initial Ab1 response to antigen. Despite the idiotypic heterogeneity of an Ab1 or T1 response, a few idiotypes are widely shared among individuals within a species for responses to particular antigens. For example, many individuals might express the same idiotopes on antibodies directed against a particular antigen (e.g., HLA-B5). Because of extensive sharing of idiotypes for the Ab1 response, the Ab2 response of one individual would be expected to cross-react with the Ab1 response of another person, as well as the individual's. In similar fashion, individuals may share T-cell idiotypes in their T1 response to a particular antigen.

THE IDIOTYPIC NETWORK THEORY

In his idiotypic network theory of how the immune system develops and operates, Jerne suggests that genes of the immune system have evolved to encode antibodies and perhaps T-cell receptors that recognize the self antigens of the species [15]. He assumes that evolution, in order to counter stimulation of these undesirable B and T cells, has favored the emergence of genes that encode complementary elements (anti-idiotypic B and T cells). In ontogeny, self antigens will induce the production of anti-self Ig molecules and T cells. But these B1 (Ab1) and T1 responses binding to self then invoke the production of B2 (Ab2) and T2 anti-idiotypic responses.

According to Jerne, the repertoire of idiotopes in the initial anti-self responses is vast and mimics many antigens found in the outside environment. Consequently, the organism acquires much of its immunity against the outside world in the process of developing its Ab2 and T2 responses against self-reactive T and B cells. Also, V, D, and J gene segments can rearrange in innumerable ways; together with somatic mutation, this provides an antibody repertoire that has no upper limit except the number of functional lymphocytes. Occasionally gene rearrangements and somatic mutations will create an anti-self reactive cell. By binding to self, however, an anti-idiotypic response will again be evoked that can shut off this short-lived event. According to Jerne's view, the evolutionary pressures on the shaping of V genes are the self antigens of the species, and the anti-idiotypic reflection against anti-self. Viruses and bacteria that multiply in the body cannot escape because of the ever-renewed repertoire. Microbes that can either mimic self or that survive in spite of an antagonistic immune system are difficult to control because they mimic the "self" situation and continue to evoke the formation of anti-idiotypic antibodies to the antibodies directed against them. In addition, a small fraction of lymphocytes that react to self may escape idiotypic suppression and cause disease.

Jerne reviews evidence that significant numbers of lymphocytes and immunoglobulin molecules are long-lived, perhaps as old as the individual. These long life spans suggest that the immune system possesses stable repertoires. The rapid disappearance of antibody molecules from the blood after an immune response can be viewed as the rejection of these immunoglobulin structures to which the stable system accords only short life spans.

Anti-idiotypic antibodies have been shown to be potent enhancers or inhibitors of the expression of antibodies of the corresponding idiotype [30,33]. In experiments in which mice are immunized with Ab1, the usual response is formation of a complementary antibody. Occasionally, however, Ab2 "looks like" the antigen and even mimics the antigen functionally. Striking examples of this are anti-idiotypic antibodies against various hormone-specific antibodies. Subsets of such anti-idiotypic antibodies have been shown to mediate hormone-specific effects [36]. Whether Ab2 enhances or suppresses an Ab1 response may depend on whether it looks like and mimics an antigen, that is, whether it is the internal image of an external antigen. For the most part, Ab3 was similar or identical to Ab1 in experiments in which mice were immunized with Ab2 [30]. These findings lead to the dualistic idea that one feature of the idiotypic network is the occurrence of pairs of antibodies, preferred partners. But, in that case, mutual idiotypic recognition would be different from the recognition by antibodies of epitopes presented on molecules other than immunoglobulins. The classic antibody response to foreign antigens is characterized by the production, usually, of several hundreds of different antibody molecules [10]. Idiotopes, therefore, would not be just epitopes, and the rules of the idiotypic network would have to be so formulated to allow for a distinction between idiotopes and epitopes, or perhaps rather a distinction between a certain set of *germline* encoded idiotypes and the universe of *other* idiotopes and epitopes.

In summary, Jerne's network theory likens the immune system to a series of mirrors. The immune system first reflects ourselves (anti-self). Then it produces a reflection of this reflection (the Ab2 anti-idiotypic response). Finally, it reflects the outside world as mutations and gene rearrangements in the first and second mirror images permit recognition of nonself. The mirror images of the outside world, however, do not have permanence in the genome. Each individual must start with self.

GENETIC BASIS OF THE IDIOTYPIC REPERTOIRE ON B AND T CELLS

Where are idiotopes localized structurally within the variable (V) region of immunoglobulin? Chain reassociation experiments have shown that idiotypic determinants usually require both heavy (H) and light (L) chains for full expression, although in certain instances some reactivity of isolated chains with the anti-idiotypic antibody is found [9]. Interaction of idiotope and anti-idiotope cannot be attributed to a single stretch of amino acids; sequences in V, D, and J segments of the immunoglobulin seem to be involved in various combinations.

Despite the complex structure of idiotopes, very small changes in primary sequence can cause drastic changes in idiotypic specificity. In an example cited by Rajewski, exchange of a single amino acid in the D sequence of an immunoglobulin led to modification of one idiotope and the loss of seven others from the parent molecule [30]. Yet, the variant antibody fully retained its binding specificity for the immunogen. Thus, idiotypic determinants appear to be complex structures to which both H and L chains usually contribute. Within a chain more than a single region (V, J, and D for heavy chains; V and J for light chains) is involved. Idiotopes may be distant from or closely associated with an antigen-binding site of the antibody. But even an idiotope invariably associated with antibodies of a given antigen specificity and recognized by an antigen (epitope) inhibitable anti-idiotope does not necessarily coincide with the antigen combining site (paratope).

The expression of idiotypes at the level of antibodies induced against selected haptens reveals two types of idiotypic markers, private (minor) idiotypes, expressed irregularly in some individuals of a given species or strain, and recurrent (major; cross-reactive) idiotypes that regularly appear in certain immune responses in members of a certain species or strain or even several species [30]. Molecular analysis of several murine immune responses dominated by recurrent idiotypes showed that each of these responses is based on the expression of a single or very few V_H and a single or very few V_L genes in the germ line. This is true for the response of mice to arsonate, dextran, phosphorylcholine, and nitrophenyl. In these four systems the antibody response is known to consist of one or a few antibody families, each of which is characterized by the expression of a single V_H gene in combination with several D and J_H segments and of one or a few V_L and J_L genes. Thus, at least in responses to certain epitopes, the V-region repertoire is controlled and limited by a few germ line genes, despite extensive somatic mutation. A simple interpretation of the phenomenon of recurrent and private idiotypes in antigen-induced immune responses is that recurrent idiotypes are markers of those germ line V genes from which antibodies in the corresponding immune response are derived; private idiotypes are characteristic for somatic mutants. In this view, recurrent idiotopes are markers of germ line V (and possibly D) genes and idiotopes specific for somatic variants are expressed irregularly and are thus private.

IMMUNOGLOBULIN IDIOTYPES ON T CELLS

After the initial findings by Eichmann and Rajewsky [8] that anti-idiotypic antisera could specifically induce idiotype-bearing T-helper cells and by Binz and Wigzell [1] that alloantibodies shared idiotypes with alloreactive T cells, much additional experimental evidence has confirmed the expression of recurrent antibody idiotypes on functional T cells and antigen-binding factors of T-cell origin [2,29].

Almost without exception, idiotype expression in the mouse is exclusively under the control of the IgH locus. However, most evidence argues against the idea that V, D, and J genes that control antibody structure are also expressed in T cells. There is no evidence that V_L genes participate in encoding T-cell receptors for antigen or that they are involved in idiotype expression by T cells. The V_H genes may take part in the encoding of T-cell receptors and idiotopes, but available evidence argues against the notion that the *same* V_H genes that encode antibody V regions are expressed in T cells [20,35].

SHARING OF IDIOTYPES BY B AND T CELLS

Clearly, T cells express idiotypes and anti-idiotypic specificities; they are partners along with B cells and immunoglobulin in the idiotypic network. But, if T-cell idiotypes are not encoded by antibody V genes, how does one explain the idiotypic polymorphism that develops in parallel in the B- and T-cell compartments? Rajewski suggests that T cells are selected in the immune system in ontogeny such that their receptors idiotypically resemble that of B-cell receptors [30]. He suggests further that the T-cell repertoire might be selected in ontogeny not only for recognition of self-histocompatibility (major histocompatibility complex; MHC) antigens but also for self B-cell idiotypes. This hypothesis would explain idiotype sharing between T and B cells by idiotypic interactions between these cells leading to the selection of a T-cell receptor repertoire complementary to that of B-cell receptors. Because the latter contain complementary receptors and because anti-idiotypic T cells selected for B-cell idiotypes might in turn expand idiotypic T cells, a situation would result in which efficient idiotypic T-B cell interactions would be guaranteed. Also, the receptor repertoire of T cells would be idiotypically and anti-idiotypically similar, although not identical [4,16,24,28].

ROLE OF THE IDIOTYPIC NETWORKS

Lymphocytes expressing complementary receptors do coexist in the immune system. At the level of B cells, anti-idiotypic antibodies can be induced in animals known to possess B-cell precursors expressing the corresponding idiotype [9]. In the course of an immune response, animals often produce anti-idiotypic antibodies against idiotypic determinants of their own antibodies, although usually in low concentration [7,18,23]. At the T-cell level, idiotype-bearing and anti-idiotypic T-helper and suppressor cells can be induced in animals that express similar idiotypes and anti-idiotypes at the B-cell level. Thus, there is no question that self-recognition at the level of receptor idiotopes is possible within the immune system. From the standpoint of Jerne's hypothesis, the coexistence of idiotypes and anti-idiotypes is an essential feature of the immune system [13-15]. Cells with complementary binding sites interact with each other, and an equilibrium of idiotypes and anti-idiotypes is established. Immune response are seen as disturbances of this equilibrium and attempts of the system to re-equilibrate.

When considering the functional role of idiotypic interactions in the immune system, one should bear in mind that the anti-idiotype may control the expression of the idiotope-bearing antibody as well as the reverse. Anti-idiotypic antibody will induce the production of two types of complementary antibodies, namely, (1) antibodies carrying the idiotype defined by the anti-idiotype used for immunization, and (2) anti-anti-idiotypes. The usual serologic assays used for idiotype titration do not distinguish between these two types of molecules. In general, anti-idiotype, when given in native form, does not directly induce synthesis of idiotypic molecules. Rather, its effect appeared to be a long-lasting modification of the functional idiotypic repertoire, but the effect may be related to dose [34]. Injection of 10-100 ng of anti-idiotope into an adult mouse enhanced, whereas 10 μg suppressed the expression of the target idiotope in immune responses induced 4-8 weeks later [30]. Anti-idiotypes of all classes (IgG1, IgG2a, and IgG2b) enhanced idiotope expression in nanogram doses and were suppressive in microgram doses. A single microgram of monoclonal anti-idiotope injected into a newborn mouse was sufficient for essentially complete idiotope suppression for several months. The enhancement by nanogram doses is not at the level of effector functions, such as high-rate antibody production, but presumably it involves mainly the recruitment of T and B cells expressing complementary binding sites. Rajewski suggests that the enhancing effect of exogenous low doses of antibody may reflect a fundamental driving force in the immune system in the sense of a network hypothesis. Low-level natural antibody production could accompany and promote interactions between diverse sets of cells with complementary receptors. However, once the concentration of antibody-binding sites is above a certain threshold (microgram range), for example, when the system engages in an active immune response, a different set of mechanisms is set in motion. Microgram quantities of anti-idiotypic antibody shut off in the bone marrow the production of cells with complementary (idiotypic) receptors; suppressor T cells suppressing the activation of such cells in the periphery are induced. The system stabilizes the expression of those binding sites (in this case, the anti-idiotype) to which it has committed itself. This is strikingly demonstrated by the finding that idiotype can facilitate the expression of the same idiotype (idiotypic memory).

The central issue for idiotypic networks is whether idiotypic interactions are the natural way for T cells to communicate with each other and with B cells. As already mentioned, T and B cells see similar but not necessarily identical idiotopes on antibodies [12, 16,28]. Regulatory idiotopes might be those that T cells are able to see [27]. The B cell appears to be an ideal target for T cells: it expresses class I and class II MHC antigens on its surface and also a unique structure, the immunoglobulin idiotype. Moreover, a close structural similarity of immunoglobulin domains and the domains of class I and class II antigens is increasingly apparent [21]. This similarity has led to speculation that Ig domains as well as MHC antigens might function as restriction elements for T cells [17], and that V regions could have been selected in evolution for structural similarity with MHC antigens.

TOLERANCE AND CHIMERISM

In a recent review, Nossal described three prevailing attitudes toward cellular mechanisms of immunologic tolerance [25]. First was that there is nothing so special about self antigens, and that avoidance of autoimmunity depends on myriad immunoregulatory and feedback mechanisms, none of which is uniquely important to self-recognition and all of which may apply in particular circumstances to foreign antigens as well. The second considers suppressor T lymphocytes as central to immunologic tolerance. In this view, the repertoire of immunocytes is perfectly competent to recognize self antigens, but the capacity to threaten health by actually switching on these immunocytes is thwarted by a powerful activation of the appropriate suppressors. The third attitude sees the most important bulwark against autoreactivity as some purging of the immunologic dictionary. Effector precursors with receptors for self are either destroyed or inactivated in some way. Miller stresses that these three major approaches are not mutually exclusive, nor are the conceptual demarcations between them as rigid as might first appear. Given the importance of avoiding uncontrolled autoimmunity, it makes sense to buttress a repertoire-purging mechanism with a suppressor system that acts as a fail-safe device. The thought that an anti-idiotypic suppressor T cell might stop a particular response is not so far from the thought that idiotype is silenced by clonal purging of the cell bearing it. Finally, a selective immune system geared to react to the unknown must be degenerate and redundant. Otherwise, the repertoire of unispecific cellular elements would have to be infinitely large. A necessary consequence of this is that the affinity of antibodies varies greatly and that cross-reactivities among unrelated antigens and antibodies are common. Thus, the number and diversity of self antigens must be very large, and clonal deletion of all cells with any reactivity to any self antigen cannot be absolutely correct because there would be a real risk of deleting the total repertoire. It appears, then, that immunologic tolerance cannot be described or explained simplistically or in isolation from immune responses as a whole. Miller concludes that the complex processes of self-tolerance and chimerism are probably an amalgam of repertoire purging, suppression, sequestration of self antigens, and blockade of receptors by monovalent, nonimmunogenic self molecules and other regulatory loops, including anti-idiotype networks.

In a recent study, Glazier provides strong support for the notion that self-tolerance is maintained by an active suppressor mechanism [11]. This group demonstrated that irradiated rats, repopulated with syngeneic or even autologous marrow cells and given cyclosporine daily for several weeks, develop a lethal systemic autoimmune disease soon after treatment with cyclosporine is discontinued. Symptoms and findings are similar to allogeneic graft-versus-host disease (GVHD). Further studies by this group indicated that (1) this autoimmune disease is adoptively transferable to irradiated syngeneic recipients by T-cell populations from diseased donors, and (2) normal rats are refractory to autoimmune disease either following transfer of these same autoimmune cell populations or after withdrawal of cyclosporine treatment. Evidently, normal rats possess an active tolerance-maintaining mechanism that suppresses disease-causing anti-self clones. Cyclosporine is a highly fat soluble, 11-amino acid cyclopolypeptide. It acts at the level of T cells entering the proliferative cycle, and it inhibits development of cytolytic T cells. Wilson suggests that the pool of down-regulating T-suppressor cells in Glazier's experiments might be an actively proliferating population, thereby vulnerable to and depleted by cyclosporine, while the anti-self reactive clones are in a resting state; they become activated later by self antigens in the absence of the Ts population when cyclosporine treatment is discontinued [44].

Wilson makes an analogy between Glazier's system and one involving systemic graft versus host disease and specifically induced resistance to GVHD that has been studied extensively in rats. Normal F_1 hybrid rats of MHC disparate matings (A/B), given large numbers (10^9) of parental strain lymphocytes, routinely succumb to lethal GVHD with symptoms very similar to those already described for the autoimmune model; for lightly irradiated animals (100-750 R), the lethal dose of parental strain cells is much less ($1 - 3 \times 10^7$). Thus, there exists in the normal rat a radiosensitive mechanism that prevents the activation of donor T-cell clones by MHC antigens and the onset of allogeneic GVHD. Wilson points out that the system of induced resistance to allogeneic GVHD may relate to Glazier's self-tolerance/autoimmunity model in two ways. First, anti-MHC receptors appear to be highly conserved in different rat strains. It follows that cross-reactive idiotypic determinants expressed on anti-MHC^b receptors of T cells from strains A, C, D, and E are also expressed in strain B and A/B F_1 animals as well, and if T cells expressing these receptors were not restrained in some way, the result would be autoimmunity. Second, one interesting feature of the GVH resistance model is that it is very rapidly induced. The F_1 rats immunized with small numbers of parental T cells and then irradiated, even as soon as 1 day later, demonstrate specific GVH resistance to subsequent challenge with T cells from the same parental strain. Thus, the onset of the GVH resistance mechanism becomes radioresistant very rapidly. This finding suggests that a normal A/B rat already has clones of lymphocytes with specificity for the anti-MHC^b receptors on donor T cells; these can be rapidly primed and become radioresistant; they behave as a population already expressing immunologic memory. If this is so, what is the internal self antigen in the A/B F_1 rat that drives them? Wilson believes it is most likely that these self antigens are the receptor molecules present on anti-self MHC^b reactive T cells in the F_1 rat, the same cells that cause autoimmune disease in the cyclosporine-treated rats. One component of this circuit is the clones of T cells bearing receptor molecules specific for self histocompatibility antigens. In the normal animal these self MHC-reactive clones stimulate suppressive responses by the second component of this circuit, T cells with specificity for anti-MHC receptors, which comprise the self-tolerance maintenance mechanism.

IDIOTYPIC NETWORKS AND PREGNANCY

Survival during pregnancy of a fetus that possesses antigens foreign to the mother remains an enigma. There is considerable evidence that a maternal cellular and humoral immune response to fetal antigens occurs. But, despite HLA incompatibility between mother and fetus, only 30% of multiparous women show anti-HLA antibodies at the time of delivery. Both the apparent absence of anti-HLA immunity in the remaining 70% of multipara and the tolerance to the fetus displayed by alloimmunized multiparous mothers are unexplained. Suciu-Foca suggests that these paradoxes might be explained in part by anti-anti-HLA antibodies found in sera of 20 of 21 primipara at the time of delivery [42]. These anti-idiotypic antisera (Ab2) specifically inhibited the anti-HLA activity of maternal sera reacting with the father's class I or class II antigens. Although 20 of 21 exhibited anti-idiotypic activity, only 7 of them had direct anti-HLA activity against paternal cells. The Ab2 is therefore present in sera both with and without HLA antibodies. This suggests that serum anti-HLA activity merely reflects the prevalence of Ab1 (anti-HLA) or Ab2 (anti-anti-HLA). Suciu-Foca has found that Ab2 appears in maternal blood as early as month 5 of pregnancy. The Ab2 activity was measured by the capacity of its $F(ab')_2$ portion to block the binding of autologous Ab1 found in placental serum to activated T lymphoblasts from fathers. This anti-idiotypic $F(ab')_2$ also inhibited, to various degrees, the anti-HLA activity of sera from other individuals against paternal antigens; this latter observation suggests broad sharing of idiotypes for specific anti-HLA responses among various individuals. Because alloantisera contain a heterogeneous population of antibody molecules and a wide array of Ab2 are expected to develop in response to Ab1, it is surprising and remarkable that a single individual's anti-idiotypic antibodies can inhibit not only the corresponding autologous idiotypic anti-HLA antibodies, but also those found in alloantisera of other individuals. Thus, human anti-idiotypic antibodies to HLA may recognize in alloantisera certain public idiotypes that are expressed on the products of highly conserved germ line genes.

The finding that alloimmunization via pregnancy leads to the development of autoantibodies against T-cell receptors for allogeneic HLA-DR antigens implies that receptor for self and non-self DR antigens must be different. If the receptors were the same, then autoanti-idiotypic antibodies developing after alloimmunization would block the T-cell recognition system. This would imply that pregnant women fail to recognize T-cell-dependent antigens (that alloimmunization leads to T-cell deficiency), which is certainly not the case.

Two sets of observations suggest that the repertoire of idiotypic receptors for HLA-DR are relatively limited. First, sera from two women who had been alloimmunized through pregnancy against the same haplotype were capable of binding autologous as well as each other's lymphoblasts; their receptor for the immunizing allogeneic DR antigen and their anti-receptor antibodies were cross-reacting. Second, a serum tested for the presence of anti-idiotypic antibodies against anti-HLA-DR2 antibodies and found to react with autologous lymphocytes primed against DR2 also inhibited the lymphocytotoxic activity of two anti-HLA-DR2 alloantisera. The anti-anti-HLA receptors expressed by T and B lymphocytes therefore seem to share common determinants and to display little variability from one individual to another.

Suciu-Foca found anti-idiotypic antibodies are to be present both in women who developed anti-HLA antibodies and in those who did not. The capacity of anti-idiotypic antibodies to inhibit the anti-HLA antibody activity of earlier sera from the same donor was documented, suggesting that responsiveness versus unresponsiveness to histocompatibility antigens might reflect the balance between anti-HLA and anti-anti-HLA antibodies [41]. When the former dominate, the presence of the latter will be overlooked; when the anti-anti-HLA antibodies prevail, the balance will swing to what appears to be unresponsiveness to alloantigens. This phenomenon could account for the absence of HLA antibodies in allosensitized individuals.

ANTI-IDIOTYPIC RESPONSES AFTER BLOOD TRANSFUSION AND KIDNEY TRANSPLANTATION

In 1974, Opelz and Terasaki reported a beneficial effect of pregraft transfusions on subsequent kidney allograft survival [26]. In part, the transfusion effect is achieved by selection. Some patients react to blood transfusions by mounting vigorous anti-HLA responses. A few become reactive to almost the entire population and are of course very unlikely to receive a kidney transplant because they will have a positive cross-match with almost any donor. Others develop anti-HLA antibodies to a segment of the population but usually do well when they finally receive a kidney from a cross-match-negative donor. Most individuals do not develop anti-HLA antibodies after transfusion and do quite well after kidney transplantation with only the usual immunosuppressive regimens. But selection of the relatively small group (less than 20%) of vigorous anti-HLA responders away from transplantation could not explain all of the beneficial effect of transfusions, which added about 40 percentage points to 1-year kidney allograft survival from cadaver donors. It was suspected early that part of the transfusion effect might be induction of specific immunosuppression, perhaps via anti-idiotypic responses. Several groups have now shown in both mice and humans that blood transfusions do induce both anti-anti-HLA and anti-HLA responses [6,32,37,54]. In most cases the presence of anti-idiotypic antibodies in these sera was investigated using a mixed leukocyte culture (MLC) inhibition test in which spleen cells from normal mice were tested for proliferative responses to x-irradiated allogeneic stimulator cells (same strain as blood transfusion donor) in the presence of sera from transfused mice. Sera from transfused mice caused significant and specific inhibition of MLC responses. In mouse strain combinations disparate for the entire H-2 region, anti-idiotypic antibodies developed after a single transfusion [22].

Reed has investigated the development of anti-anti-HLA (Ab2) antibody in recipients who, following three transfusions, have not developed anti-HLA antibodies against their respective haploidentical transfusion donors and subsequently received this donor's kidney. The Ab2 occurred 2 weeks following the first transfusion in five patients and 2 weeks following the third transfusion in one [32]. The presence of Ab2 was detected by (1) the ability of $F(ab')_2$ fragments to inhibit the lymphocytotoxic effect of reference alloantisera, and (2) the ability to inhibit the autologous MLC in which the patient's own T lymphocytes are cultured with autologous T lymphoblasts that had been alloactivated in a 5-day MLC against the immunizing donor. All had significant Ab2 4 weeks after the last transfusion when they received kidney transplants; no rejection has occurred. It is known from other reports that donor-specific transfusions according to this protocol lead to 95% graft function 1 year after transplantation of kidneys from related donors.

An additional three patients who were HLA-DR identical to the DST donor and successfully transplanted were tested for Ab2 activity against alloantisera that detected the class I antigens for which they were mismatched. None of these patients showed any detectable Ab1 activity in their own sera. Moreover, their sera failed to inhibit reference anti-class I antisera that reacted with donor lymphocytes [31]. Although this suggested that HLA-DR-matched patients do not develop Abl or Ab2 against the mismatched class I antigens of the donor, it is quite possible that the reference sera used for testing contained idiotypic antibodies not formed by the patient.

For about 15 years it has been the practice of most transplant centers to rule out the use of a donor whose lymphocytes gave a positive cross-match with any serum from the intended donor. Thus, a positive cross-match on a serum 1 and 2 years old would rule out acceptance of a particular kidney even though cross-match with a current serum from the intended recipient might be negative. But, during the past 2 or 3 years, several groups have suggested that historical positive cross-matches could be ignored without jeopardizing graft survival [5]. Such an apparent paradox could be explained only if these antibodies were directed against non-HLA antigens, in which case they may not affect the graft, or if their disappearance was accounted for by the development of Ab2. Reed has reported studying the presence of Ab2 in sequential samples of Ab1-negative sera obtained from two patients who lost their anti-HLA antibodies 1 year prior to transplantation. The Ab1-negative sera were tested for their capacity to inhibit earlier autologous sera that contained antibodies against the cadaveric donor. In both patients the disappearance of Ab1 was associated with development of Ab2, which remained present in the serum during the year until transplantation. Rejection has occurred in neither patient.

Reed has also searched for Ab1 and Ab2 in patients with acute and chronic rejection. As might be expected, several patterns emerged. In one patient with acute rejection, anti-HLA antibodies appeared after transplant nephrectomy but Ab2 could not be detected in any sera, either before or after nephrectomy. In another patient with acute rejection, anti-HLA antibodies also appeared after transplant nephrectomy; in this case, Ab2 coexisted against some but not all the Ab1 against HLA antigens present in the donor but absent from the recipient. In a patient with chronic rejection, anti-HLA antibodies appeared prior to loss of all renal function, but the sera showed no Ab2 activity. Suciu-Foca and Reed and colleagues believe that alloimmunity in transfused and transplanted patients is down regulated by development of anti-idiotypic antibodies. Absence of Ab1 in recipients was usually associated with the presence of Ab2. In instances in which the patients had neither Ab1 nor Ab2, Reed suspects that Ab3 has appeared; if so, Ab3 may predominate over Ab2 and obscure its presence. Studies are underway to test this hypothesis.

In clinical organ transplantation, massive immunosuppression is required during the first few weeks and months to prevent rejection. Regimens include azathioprine, cyclosporine, antilymphocyte globulin, and steroid hormones. Gradually, some of the immunosuppressive drugs are discontinued or their doses are reduced, usually without triggering rejection. Eventually some recipients take only small doses of a single immunosuppressive drug; a few discontinue immunosuppressive drugs altogether without losing the graft. What are the mechanisms that permit such drastic reduction of immunosuppression? In part, the graft becomes less immunogenic as passenger hemopoietic cells of donor origin disappear from the microcirculation and interstitial spaces of the graft [39]. Yet, vascular endothelial cells and parenchymal cells of the grafted organ continue to express donor class I and class II histocompatibility antigens. In several experimental models, long-term rat kidney transplants retain their ability to trigger graft rejection; they are rejected if transferred from their long-term host to a new host syngeneic with the first [38]. Peripheral blood and spleen lymphocytes from long-term recipients (both humans and experimental animals) usually retain their ability to proliferate in mixed leukocyte culture against cells from the original donor. Such cultures can usually generate cytolytic T-cell responses against the donor, but the kinetics of the responses may be more characteristic of primary than of a secondary or memory response [43].

Detection of anti-idiotypic responses in long-term recipients requires complicated assays and meticulous attention to detail. Even after such responses have been identified, it is difficult to know whether they are the cause or the effect of a good result. Nevertheless, anti-idiotypic responses do appear to be associated with the stable homeostatic immune response that permits long-term graft acceptance without rejection. Anti-idiotypic responses may be useful as prognostic indicators; they may help to pinpoint the time when immunosuppressive drugs can be safely reduced or withdrawn.

THERAPEUTIC IMPLICATIONS OF ANTI-IDIOTYPIC RESPONSES

Passive Immunization

During the past two decades the sera of postpartum women have been a valuable source of anti-HLA antibodies for tissue typing. It now appears that such sera will be an equally rich source of anti-anti-HLA (Ab2) antibodies. Suciu-Foca and colleagues have suggested that these antibodies might be useful as part of the early immunosuppressive regimen. We have been unsuccessful in our attempts to enhance the survival of rat kidney allografts with anti-idiotypic sera [40]. If anti-idiotypic antibodies are important for preventing graft rejection, they probably must be part of the recipient's own active immune response in order to take part in long-term homeostasis. Passive immunization with Ab2 might prevent or delay the recipient's own Ab2 response.

Active Immunization

Binz and Wigzell reported that immunization with autologous Ab1 led to prolonged skin allograft survival in mice [3]. The effect was modest and has been difficult to reproduce. A A second method of inducing an autoanti-idiotypic response before organ grafting is to immunize intended recipients with their own T cells that have been cultured in vitro with donor antigen. In effect, the in vitro culture provides an enriched source of autologous T cells engaging in the T1 response to donor alloantigen. By immunizing with T1 cells obtained in culture, one can stimulate the T2, Ab2 response in vivo without having to pass through the in vivo T1 response, which is so threatening to an allograft. However, this active approach also has usually led to only modest graft prolongation in experimental animals [34]. Perhaps the recipient switches to a T1 response of a secondary idiotype that was not expressed on the T cells obtained from in vitro culture. If this approach is to work, it may be necessary to immunize with a series of autologous T cells that express a significant proportion of the recipient's T1 idiotypes.

In summary, the role of anti-idiotype responses to organ allografts is not yet established. Improved assays for detecting these Ab2 and T2 responses should encourage the studies needed to determine what role the idiotypic network plays in down regulating allograft rejection.

REFERENCES

1. Binz, H., and Wigzell, H. Shared idiotypic determinants on B and T lymphocytes reactive against the same antigenic determinants. *J. Exp. Med.* 142:197-211, 1975.
2. Binz, H., and Wigzell, H. Antigen binding idiotypic T lymphocyte receptors. *Contemp. Top. Immunobiol.* 7:113-117, 1977.
3. Binz, H., Tarcsay, L., Wigzell, H., and Dukor, P. Specific impaired alloreactivity of mice immunized with syngeneic MLC T-lymphoblasts using muramylpeptides as adjuvant. *Transplant. Proc.* 13:566-573, 1981.
4. Bona, C. A., and Kohler, H. Anti-idiotypic antibodies and internal images. In *Monoclonal and Anti-idiotypic Antibodies: Probes for Receptor Structure and Function,* J. C. Venter, C. M. Fraser, and J. Lindstrom, eds. Alan R. Liss, Inc., New York, 1984.
5. Cardella, C. J., Falk, J. A., Halloran, P., Robinette, G., Arbus, G., and Bear, R. Transplantation can be performed with positive (non current) crossmatch. *Transplant. Proc.* 17:1530-1532, 1985.
6. Catto, G., MacLeod, A., Mather, A., Mason, R., Stewart, K., Power, D., Shewan, G., and Urbaniak, S. Beneficial antibodies in renal transplantation developing after blood transfusion: Evidence for HLA linkage. *Transplant. Proc.* 17:1057-1958, 1985.
7. Cerny, J., and Kelsoe, G. Priority of the anti-idiotypic response after antigen administration: Artefact or intriguing network mechanism? *Immunol. Today* 5:61-63, 1984.
8. Eichmann, K., and Rajewsky, K. Induction of T and B cell immunity by anti-idiotypic antibody. *Eur. J. Immunol.* 5:661-666, 1975.
9. Eichmann, K. Expression and function of idiotypes on lymphocytes. *Adv. Immunol.* 26:195-254, 1978.
10. Fazekas de St. Groth, S., Underwood, P. A., and Scheidegger, D. The repertoire of anti-influenza antibodies. In *Protides of the Biological Fluids,* H. Peeters, ed. Pergamon Press, Oxford, xxxx, pp. 559-563.
11. Glazier, A., Tutschka, P. J., Farmer, E. R., and Santos, G. W. Graft-versus-host disease in cyclosporin A-treated rats after syngeneic and autologous bone marrow reconstitution. *J. Exp. Med.* 158:1-8, 1983.
12. Gleason, K., and Kohler, H. Regulatory idiotypes. T helper cells recognize a shared V_H idiotope on phosphorylcholine-specific antibodies. *J. Exp. Med.* 156:539-549, 1982.
13. Jerne, N. K. Towards a network theory of the immune system. *Ann. Immunol.* 125C: 373-389, 1974.
14. Jerne, N. K. The immune system: A web of V-domains. *Harvey Lect.* 70:83-110, 1975.
15. Jerne, N. K. Idiotypic networks and other preconceived ideas. *Immunol. Rev.* 79:5-24, 1984.
16. Jorgensen, T., and Hannestad, K. Helper T cell recognition of the variable domains of a mouse myeloma protein. *J. Exp. Med.* 155:1587-1596, 1982.

17. Juy, D., Primi, D., Sanchez, P., and Cazenave, P. A. Idiotype regulation: Evidence for the involvement of Igh-c restricted T cells in the M-460 idiotype suppressive pathway. *Eur. J. Immunol.* 12:24-30, 1982.
18. Kelsoe, G., and Cerny, J. Reciprocal expansions of idiotypic and anti-idiotypic clones following antigen stimulation. *Nature* 279:333-334, 1979.
19. Kunkel, H. G., Mannik, M., and Williams, R. C. Individual antigenic specificity of isolated antibodies. *Science* 140:1218-1219, 1963.
20. Kurosawa, Y., von Boehmer, H., Haas, W., Sakano, H., Traunecker, A., and Tonegawa, S. Identification of D segments of immunoglobulin heavy chain genes and their rearrangement in T c lymphocytes. *Nature* 290:565-570, 1981.
21. Larhammar, D., Schenning, L., Gustafsson, K., Wiman, K., and Claesson, L. Complete amino acid sequence of an HLA-DR antigen-like B chain as predicted from the nucleotide sequence: Similarities with immunoglobulins and HLA-A, -B, -C antigens. *Proc. Natl. Acad. Sci. USA* 79:3687-3692, 1982.
22. Ludwin, D., Joseph, S., and Singal, D. P. MLC inhibiting antibodies in mice after blood transfusions. *Transplantation* (in press).
23. McKearn, T. J., Hamada, Y., Stuart, F., and Fitch, F. W. Anti-receptor antibody and resistance to graft-versus-host disease. *Nature* 251:648-650, 1974.
24. Nadler, P. I., Miller, G. G., Sachs, D. H., and Hodes, R. J. The expression and functional involvement of nuclease specific idiotype on nuclease primed helper T cells. *Eur. J. Immunol.* 12:113-120, 1982.
25. Nossal, G. J. V. Cellular mechanisms of immunological tolerance. *Ann. Rev. Immunol.* 1:33-62, 1983.
26. Opelz, G., and Terasaki, P. I. Poor kidney transplant survival in recipients with frozen blood transfusions or no transfusions. *Lancet* 1:696, 1974.
27. Paige, C. J., Kincade, P. W., and Ralph, P. Independent control of immunoglobulin heavy and light chain expression in a murine pre-B-cell line. *Nature* 292:631-633, 1981.
28. Pierce, S. K., Speck, N. A., Gleason, K., Gearhart, P. J., and Kohler, H. Balb/c T cells have the potential to recognize the TEPC15 prototype antibody and its somatic variants. *J. Exp. Med.* 154:1178-1187, 1981.
29. Rajewsky, K., and Eichmann, K. Antigen receptors of T helper cells. *Contemp. Top. Immunobiol.* 7:69-112, 1977.
30. Rajewsky, K., and Takemori, T. Genetics, expression, and function of idiotypes. *Annu. Rev. Immunol.* 1:569-607, 1983.
31. Reed, E., Bonagura, V., Kung, P., King, D. W., and Suciu-Foca, N. Anti-idiotypic antibodies to HLA-DR4 and DR2. *J. Immunol.* 131:2890-2894, 1983.
32. Reed, E., Hardy, M., Lalles, C., Brensiluer, J., McCabe, R., Reemtsma, K., and Suciu-Foca, N. Anti-idiotypic antibodies and their relevance to transplantation. *Transplant. Proc.* 17:735-738, 1985.
33. Rowley, D. A., Griffith, P., and Lorbach, I. Regulation by complementary idiotypes: Ig protects the clone producing it. *J. Exp. Med.* 153:1377-1390, 1981.
34. Schrieber, H. Idiotype network interactions in tumor immunity. *Adv. Cancer Res.* 41:291-321, 1984.
35. Shuler, W., Weiler, E., and Weiler, I. J. Biological and serological comparison of syngeneic and allogeneic anti-idiotypic antibodies. *Mol. Immunol.* 18:1095-1105, 1981.
36. Sege, K., and Peterson, P. A. Use of anti-idiotypic antibodies as cell-surface receptor probes. *Proc. Natl. Acad. Sci. USA* 75:2443-2447, 1978.
37. Singal, D. P., and Joseph, S. Blood transfusion, suppressor cells and anti-idiotypic antibodies. *Transplant. Proc.* 17:1104-1107, 1985.
38. Stuart, F. P., Fitch, F. W., and Rowley, D. A. Specific suppression of renal allograft rejection by treatment with antigen and antibody. *Transplant. Proc.* 2:483, 1970.
39. Stuart, F. P., McKearn, T. J., Weiss, A., and Fitch, F. W. Suppression of rat renal allograft rejection by antigen and antibody. *Immunol. Rev.* 49:127-165, 1980.

40. Stuart, F. P., Fitch, F. W., and McKearn, T. J. Enhancement of rat renal allografts with idiotypic and anti-idiotypic monoclonal alloantibodies. *Transplant. Proc.* 14: 313-315, 1982.
41. Suciu-Foca, N., Reed, E., Rohowsky, C., Kung, P., and King, D. W. Anti-idiotypic antibodies to anti-HLA receptors induced by pregnancy. *Proc. Natl. Acad. Sci. USA* 80:830-834, 1983.
42. Suciu-Foca, N., Reed, E., Rohowsky-Kochan, C., Popovic, M., Bonagura, V., King, D. W., and Reemtsma, K. Idiotypic network regulations of the immune response to HLA. *Transplant. Proc.* 17:716-719, 1985.
43. Weiss, A., Fitch, F. W., McKearn, T. J., and Stuart, F. P. Immunological memory is regulated in the enhanced rat renal allograft recipient. *Nature* 273:662, 1978.
44. Wilson, D. B. Idiotypic regulation of self-reactive and all-reactive T cells in autoimmunity and graft-versus-host disease. *Immunol. Today* 5:228-230, 1984.
45. Wood, M. L., Gottschalk, R., and Monaco, A. P. Immune response in mice transfused with blood from donors differing at defined regions of the H-2 complex. *Transplant. Proc.* 17:1108-1110, 1985.

7

SUPPRESSOR CELL REGULATION AND ALLOGRAFT POTENTIATION

James F. Burdick
The Johns Hopkins University School of Medicine, Baltimore, Maryland

Initial evidence for an active mechanism regulating the immune response was presented over a decade ago [17,106,318] by authors who have remained in the forefront of the innovative studies on this topic ever since. The older concept of tolerance as a deletion of specific clones was challenged by this evidence that suppression could be transferred adoptively as "infectious immunological tolerance" [105]. Overwhelming experimental evidence has now developed for the presence of suppressor T cells in many systems, and the sequence and variety of cell types and factors apparently involved has reached such a degree of sophistication that papers appear on the subject with no mention in the title, abstract, or introduction of the type of response under suppression. The topic is of fundamental importance in all of immunology. Indeed, it may be that our antigen-oriented view of immunity must defer to a concept that all responses represent perturbation in a set of balanced forces of complementary specificity [61] in which suppressor cell protection from the autologous immune response is of prime importance. In spite of the volumes of experimental data, however, practical application of suppressor cell concepts to understanding and treatment of experimental and clinical organ graft rejection has remained rudimentary. Suppressor cell effects are often invoked, but usually a compelling relationship to rejection or acceptance of a transplant is lacking, and the elegant systems described for defined antigens have not been related in detail to the allograft response. In this chapter I will consider why this should be, and what directions further work might take to better understand and manipulate the suppressor cell component of the allograft response. There are several excellent recent reviews on certain aspects of this topic (e.g., References 13, 73, 117, and 303). Here I shall selectively describe a fraction of the literally thousands of papers relevant to the subject of suppressor cell allograft regulation.

BIOLOGY OF SUPPRESSOR CELLS

Although presentation of an animal with foreign material generally induces immune mechanisms that can attack the immunizing antigens, a large number of circumstances have been found in which the antigen actually induces a net suppressive response. It may be, in fact, that any immune response, at least in vivo, involves concomitant suppressor induction, outweighed, in the case of stimulation of immunity, by the positive induction of immune effectors [21,51,59,102,250,253].

Induction of Suppressor Cells

The spleen is an important organ in the generation of suppressor cells. It has often been reported that intravenous or intraperitoneal, as opposed to subcutaneous, administration of antigen is most effective for the production of a predominant suppressor cell response [190,349]. It has been proposed that this is because antigen is predominantly encountered by the spleen, rather than lymph nodes, after intravenous or intraperitoneal injection [157, 222,298]. Although suppression may be generated by foot pad [275] or subcutaneous [179] injection, the spleen is the usual organ from which suppressor cells are obtained, even when they are not demonstrable elsewhere [275,339] and splenectomy can interfere with suppressor cell generation in some instances [16,179,314]. The presence of a thymus is also generally necessary for generation of suppressor cells [14,92].

A major factor cited in the past as an explanation for the induction of net suppression instead of a positive response has been encounter of antigen directly by lymphocytes, without the intermediary of macrophage processing [85,93,192,259,346]. That suppressor cells appear to recognize antigen without intrinsic H-2 restriction [316,321] and the observation by some that allogeneic stimulation by presentation of class I antigens after heat treatment to remove the class II stimulus induced suppression,seemed consistent with this [54,55,93]. However in other instances suppressor cells are induced against class II antigens [121,270] and incompatibility at the H-2 I region seems helpful in the generation of suppression against irradiated cells [191]. More recent experiments have indicated that macrophages are involved in the mechanism of induction of suppression, perhaps at several levels (Figure 1) [4,8,169,194,347].

The culture of lymphocytes in vitro with appropriate stimulators can induce cells that suppress further humoral [78,340] or cellular [137,150,245,272,296] in vitro responses. Suppressor cells may also be generated by cultures of lymphocytes using routine culture conditions in the absence of added antigen or mitogen [44,138]; this was believed to be due to a mitogenic effect of fetal calf serum for mouse cells. In murine experiments the alternative use of normal mouse serum is complicated by the powerful interleukin-2 inhibitor present [129]. However, since serum can be dispensed with completely in at least some cases of culture generation of suppressor cells, it may be that a process of maturation after release from a regulatory environment is responsible for the appearance of suppressor cells in culture [139].

The relationship between the antigenic site recognized on a molecule (epitope), the combining site to this induced on mediators of immunity (idiotype), and the combining site of other immunologic mediators for an idiotype (anti-idiotype), plays a key role in the development of suppressor cells. It was hoped that immunization with idiotypes to transplantation antigens would cause production of an immunosuppressive anti-idiotype response that would provide a generally useful way to actively prevent rejection [3,310]. However, it has become clear that the spontaneous regulatory response to the antigen itself involves a complex pattern of idiotype-anti-idiotype interactions [119], so that the results of idiotypic immunization are not as predictable as hoped. Treatment of primed T cells in vitro with anti-idiotypic antibody with or without antigen before adoptive transfer induces suppression of the response against the relevant antigen [38,161]. Conversely, injection of idiotypic antibody (=anti-idiotopic), particularly when coupled to

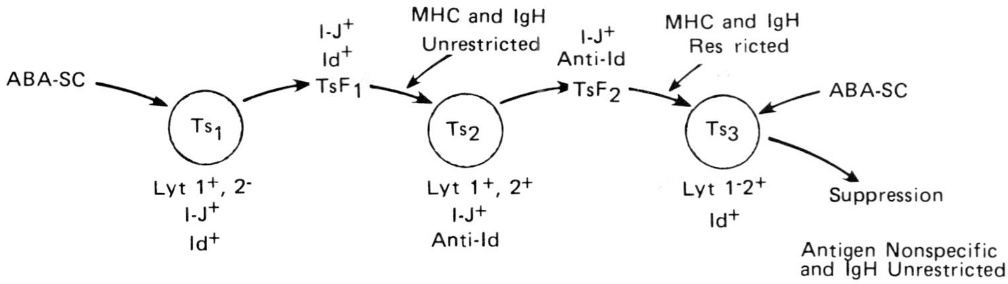

FIGURE 1 Suppressor pathway induced by *p*-azobenzenearsonate (ABA) coupled to syngeneic splenocytes. Note the idiotypic-anti-idiotypic pattern, the multiple factors and phenotypes, the need for antigen plus spleen cells for Ts3 activation, and the non-specific final suppressor factor. (From Ref. 22, used by permission.)

normal spleen cells, can induce suppression [72,100]. As will be described later in this chapter, the induction of suppression in defined antigen systems has been shown to involve induction of multiple cells and factors, in a process utilizing idiotypic-anti-idiotypic networks.

Some cloned suppressor cell lines were found to also have natural killer cell activity [244], and one function of natural killer cells might be to regulate antibody synthesis by suppressing activated B cells [230].

Tolerance due to suppressor cells may be induced to antigen presented via the gastrointestinal tract [204]. The suppressor cells develop in the gut-associated lymphoid tissue and apparently travel to the spleen, creating a net systemic unresponsiveness in the face of active immune protection in the gastrointestinal tract [203,350]. This is an intriguing possibility for graft potentiation, but oral tolerance has not been accomplished with histocompatibility antigens as yet [335].

Multiple Steps in the Suppressor Cell Cascade

Initial studies of immune suppression mediated by cells documented that this was generally due to T cells, and this suppressor T-cell subpopulation was identifiable in mice by its strong expression of Lyt 2, but not Lyt 1, antigen [48,150]. Cytotoxic T cells also express Lyt 2 strongly. The subsequent demonstration that all murine T cells do express Lyt 1 at least weakly [184] has not negated the practical usefulness of the strong Lyt 2 antigen expression. However, that both human [183] and murine [85,291] suppressor cells are difficult to distinguish from cytotoxic cells on the basis of surface antigen phenotype has caused a great deal of difficulty in analyzing graft rejection.

A second T-cell type involved in suppression of humoral [77] and cell-mediated [311] immunity was next discovered. Further murine studies with defined antigens, in some cases with strain-dependent cross-reactive idiotype responses that allowed analysis of the genetic origin of receptor coding [15,33,103,356], have revealed a remarkably complex system. Generally, the first cell (Ts_1) bears an idiotypic receptor, directed against a specific epitope of the antigen under study [72,162,355]. The second cell (Ts_2) [25,72,162,252,313,355] is anti-idiotypic and can be induced by appropriate presentation of idiotype-bearing antibody to animals that have never been exposed to the relevant antigen [72]. It seemed possible that this anti-idiotypic Ts2 could interact directly with the (idiotypic) antigen-binding site on the B cell or the (presumably idiotypic) helper or delayed-type hypersensitivity (DTH) effector T cells to produce suppression; the paradox in the case of the T cells, however, was that these target lymphocytes do not have detectable idiotype of this sort [313,315]. However, a third suppressor cell (Ts_3) was found for some systems, which does exhibit idiotype that therefore allows it to be acted upon by the Ts_2 [4,71,309,348]. Another characteristic that distinguishes the different suppressor cell types is that the first cell in the pathway is only effective during the initial induction of the immune response [219,237], whereas later suppressor cell stages can overcome the effector phase of the response [235,354]. It remains possible that B-cell responses may be directly suppressed by a two-cell system [209,242], and also generation of suppression of T-cell help for B-cell responses may be different, involving only two rather than three steps [23]. It should be noted that alternative nomenclatures have developed during the elucidation of these various systems, such as "suppressor-inducer" leading to "suppressor-effector(-acceptor)" leading to "suppressor-auxiliary." In this summary the numerical designation was used for simplicity. Scrutiny of the characteristics of this complicated cascade has been facilitated recently by the study of long-term cell lines or clones of different Ts types [8,25,28,95,164,220,232,308,320]. It must be borne in mind, however, that the correlation or absence of separate antigens or functions in clones could be due to a genetic artefact in that clone. In the human, co-operation between subsets of Leu 2/T8$^+$ (suppressor/cytotoxic) cells seems to be necessary for development of suppression [97,225]. However, an important fact to emphasize is that in many systems Lyt 1-positive, Lyt 2-negative [23,37,77,91,177,197,265, 315,369], or Leu 3/T4 positive, Leu 2/T8 negative [65,66,244,330], lymphocytes of the T-helper phenotype have been described as playing an important role in the development of T-cell-mediated suppression. This complicates attempts to study or manipulate graft rejection in terms of helper cells.

A major feature of two- and three-cell idiotypic networks is the degree of control over the immune response that it may afford. The effect of a given degree of cell activation at one stage may be regulated by the degree of subsequent activation at another stage, so that, for instance, in the absence of conditions leading to Ts_2 activation, primed Ts_3 cells produce no suppression [217,312]. Also, the antigen specificity of the suppression might be markedly altered by the abstraction of the actual antigenic structure represented by the anti-idiotypic Ts_2 intermediary. Furthermore, since the final mediator of suppression, at least in the case of cell-mediated immunity, may not be specific for the original antigenic epitope [95,311,315,320], accurate targeting of the suppressive effect is necessary to prevent damage to the host.

Suppressor Factors

Initially there were reports that suppressor cells acted by direct cell-to-cell contact [244, 242], but effects mediated by soluble proteins have been described in many suppressor cell systems [83,120,181,276,324,338]. The biologic relevance of the factors might be questioned when they have been obtained by cell disruption, but in many cases they have been extracted from culture supernatants, which suggests they are, in fact, secreted messengers. These factors have proven to be as numerous as the cells involved [201,235,237,368, 369] and have been designated where possible by their cell of origin, for example, as TsF_1, TsF_2, or TsF_3 (Figure 2). It may be that most suppressor cell actions, whether to induce the next cell in the pathway or to finally effect suppression, are mediated by soluble fac-

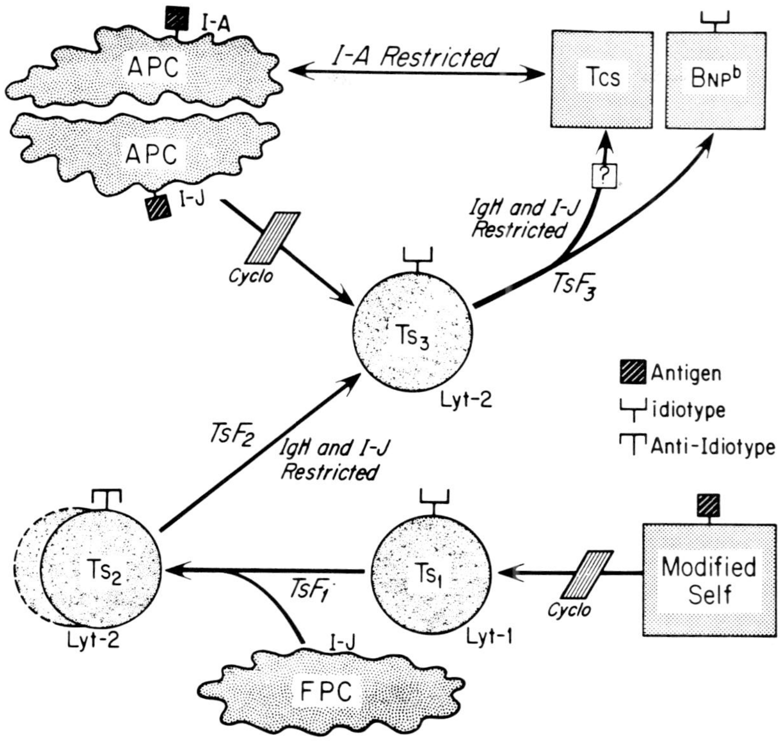

FIGURE 2 A summary of the NP suppressor cell cascade. Note the idiotype-anti-idiotype pattern and multiple factor-presenting and antigen-presenting cells. (Used by permission from ref. 4).

tors. Each factor in the suppressor cell cascade bears the idiotype or anti-idiotype of the cell producing it, which allows each factor to interact with the next cell in line [119,235].

Since they have been comparatively convenient to study, much of our present understanding of the complexities of T-cell-mediated suppression has derived from analyzing suppressor factors. Generally, suppressor factors are genetically restricted so that they only interact effectively with certain strains; typically, the idiotype-bearing TsF_1 and TsF_3 are restricted to interaction with other strains bearing the same allele for a gene linked to the immunoglobulin heavy chain gene complex [216,217,219,235,237,369], and the anti-idiotypic TsF_2 are restricted by an H-2 region compatibility requirement [71,219,319,370]. In some instances TsF_3 is also restricted by H-2 [217,235]. In the human, suppressor factor was reported that was restricted to interaction with HLA-D-identical cells [83].

Several suppressor factors consisting of one macromolecular chain (usually 28,000-90,000 daltons) have been reported [95,154,181]. As described in Mechanism of Action of Suppressor Cells, smaller molecular weight proteins have been described as involved in the final effector mechanism of suppression, sometimes as fragments derived from larger chains.

Some descriptions of TsF_3 involve two covalently linked chains secreted by the same cell [12,281,287,322,368]. In one case, one chain evidently bears the immuno-

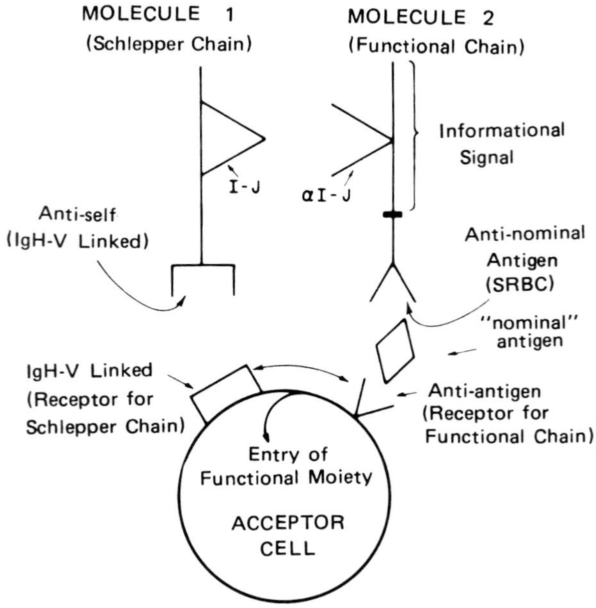

FIGURE 3 Composition and functional makeup of an antigen-specific suppressor factor. Note the I-J coordination between chains, the separate IgH-V and antigen receptor regions, and the antigen bridge. (Used by permission,from ref. 90.)

globulin gene-linked structure and the other, the antigen-binding moiety [368]. In a similar factor [323], a heavy chain responsible for antigen specificity and a light chain that produces major histocompatibility complex (MHC) restriction have been described. Alternatively, the two chains may be secreted by separate cells [90,91,258,377]; in this case, as in many of these suppressor factor and cellular interactions, the structure specified by I-J (see next section) is found to be important. The effect of the two separately secreted molecules is brought to bear on the appropriate target cell by a three-part interaction that includes involvement of the I-J determinant to coordinate the chain interaction, plus idiotypic and immunoglobulin-linked interactions similar to other descriptions, as depicted in Figure 3 [91]. The picture now envisioned for this mechanism is more complex, with as many as seven interactions envisioned [90,258]. Others have not found evidence for I-J-restricted interaction between chains [323].

The interaction of the final suppressor cell or factor with the cell toward which its suppression is targeted is of interest. Since in the cascades described this ingredient is idiotypic, it could not act directly with the target cell receptor, which also presumably bears idiotype. There is evidence in some systems that this is mediated by an "antigen bridge," so that the target of suppression and the factor jointly combine with the antigen [23,368]. This conceptual problem of how two structures with the same idiotypic receptor site bind to an individual molecule of natural antigen that has no repeating epitopes [23], is unsolved but might relate to a difference in the way the target cell antigen receptor and the combining site of the factor bind. Although these facts are often viewed as acting in an isolated fashion on the surfaces of the cells they influence, there is considerable evidence in some systems that macrophages or other antigen-presenting cells [4,218,260,347,348], designated in one case as "factor presenting cells" [4], are involved in the process (as depicted in Figure 2). It has been reported that the MHC restriction usually seen for factor activity is a requirement not for matching for the cell upon which the factor is acting, but rather restriction with regard to interaction of the factor with the adherent macrophage that presents the factor to the target cell [348].

I-J, the Antigen Receptor, and Other Structures Associated with the Suppressor Phenotype

In 1976, Murphy et al. [229] described an antigen that occurs on murine suppressor cells, and Tada et al. [317] found the same determinant on a suppressor factor. Based critically on the results with B10.A(3R) anti-B10.A(5R) antiserum, it was postulated that this specificity was due to a new locus in the I region of H-2, designated I-J. Anti-I-J reagents have since played a key role in the definition of suppressor cells and factors. The Lyt 2-positive suppressor cells in the mouse generally express the I-J antigen, allowing distinction in the mouse between these and cytotoxic T cells. As noted in a previous section, Lyt 1-positive cells have also been found in the cascade of cells leading to suppression in the mouse; some of these have been found to express I-J [23,91,177,221]. Also, adherent accessory cells necessary for suppression of induction may exhibit I-J [91,115]. Other structures expressed on suppressor cells include histamine receptors [293] and Qa1 [77,143]. Human suppressor cells may be identified by surface antigens as described in Identifying Characteristics of Human Suppressor Cells.

In many cases the function of I-J region determinants has seemed analogous in the generation of suppression to the role of the I-A region in the generation of help [217], so that whether a factor will produce suppression or help seems determined by whether it expresses I-J or I-A [287]. Similar to the stimulation of immunity against allogeneic tissue caused by I-A incompatibility, it was proposed that initiation of suppression against allogeneic cells is potentiated by I-J incompatibility [62]. Rich et al. [274] found that conconavalin A antigen-nonspecific suppressor factor responsible for suppression of mixed lymphocyte cultures was not restricted by I-J but rather by another H-2 locus, I-C, and suggested that antigen-specific factors are I-J restricted but nonspecific ones are I-C restricted. It may be that I-J is somewhat different on different types of suppressor cells [178,232,309,353].

In spite of the large number of studies employing anti-I-J antisera, the physiologic role of I-J has not been as easily defined as it was for I-A [178,218,348]. It has not been easily studied at the molecular level, unlike the other major histocompatibility loci and their products, although the practical usefulness of anti-I-J antiserum is unquestioned. It has been possible to influence responses in vitro and in vivo by anti-I-J antisera [91,208, 250]. The mechanism of this could be through steric hindrance or some other interference with the function of the cells and factors expressing I-J. The anti-I-J monoclonal antibodies that are now available [352] should be helpful in studying the role of I-J at the molecular level.

The immunologic world was startled when Hood and associates examined the region of DNA to which the I-J locus had been mapped and found the "I-J region" to be nonexistent, or at least less than 1 kb in length [141,173,302], which is too small to encode a protein. Klein et al. had previously been skeptical of I-J as a defined region of H-2 [168]. His editorial (Trouble in the J-Land) on the occasion of the report that I-J was unaccounted for suggested immunologists had fallen prey to an illusion [166]. Subsequent papers have emphasized that the reagents and tests employing I-J are undoubtedly real. The best evidence proposed to date for an explanation for this problem of a protein without a corresponding region of DNA to encode it is the report that B10.A(3R) and B10.A(5R), the pair of strains used for the original definition of the I-J specificity, differ for an additional residual gene on a different chromosome from that bearing H-2 [132], which might, as one possibility, govern glycosylation of a protein encoded by I-E. Whatever the explanation for the origin for I-J, it must take into account the relationship to H-2 that I-J seems to exhibit.

The antigen receptor on the suppressor T cell has occupied a great deal of attention. The fundamental characteristic of the T-cell receptor, which distinguishes it in general from the B-cell receptor and immunoglobulin, is its inability to recognize antigen in the absence of appropriate H-2 association. However, some experiments have indicated that the suppressor cell is unlike other T cells in its ability to attach to antigen in the absence of major histocompatibility determinants, presented, for instance, adherent to petri dishes in plating experiments [316,321]. In addition, the interactions of suppressor T cells and their factors are characterized by an interesting relationship to immunoglobulins. Strain-specific characteristic idiotypic components, which are similar or identical to those that characterize the immunoglobulin-binding sites against certain antigens, are found in suppressor T-cell responses [103,313], which suggested that the genes responsible for the T-cell receptor and the immunoglobulin-combining site are the same or similar. It seemed that the variable region of the immunoglobulin heavy chain might actually contribute to the T-cell receptor [236,313]. In the case of suppressor cell action this has been analyzed for the suppressor factors [91,368], and at least in some cases, it turns out that this determinant linked to the variable region of the heavy chain gene is separate from the specific antigen-binding site, as depicted in Figure 3. The other relationship with immunoglobulin is the presence on suppressor and helper T cells of allotypic determinants that are linked to the immunoglobulin allotype genes, although not identical with these [241,333,334], suggesting that immunoglobulin constant portion genes contribute to the T-cell receptor [313,316]. In fact, it has been suggested that a series of such suppressor cell isotypes occurs during differentiation of the different suppressor cell types [240]. If this close relationship with immunoglobulin were true, it would constitute a special situation for suppressor T cells, since the immunoglobulin genes in other T cells do not exhibit the rearrangement of the immunoglobulin gene complex required for differentiation of a specific antigen-binding structure [49].

Although the usual concept of immune response genes involves an inherited inability for potentiation of a response to a given hapten by major histocompatibility determinants, it also seems that a lack of responses to certain antigens in some strains is genetically determined by their selective capacity to induce active suppression in these strains [152,292]. It was suggested that suppressor T cells recognize antigen in the context of I-J rather than I-A determinants [217]. By this theory, whether net suppression or help was generated depended upon the capacity of I-J and I-A, respectively, to present antigen [147,287,316], and suppression against a given antigen would not occur (implying a strong positive response would be likely) if the I-J of a strain could not interact appropriately with that antigen and other cells necessary for the generation of suppression [21,167]. This seems consistent with many of the characteristics of I-J. An alternative genetic origin for "nonsuppressor" status that results in a positive response in certain strains is the congenital lack of a certain cell or factor in the cascade leading to suppression [188].

A related issue is whether I-J is part of the actual antigen receptor [236,316]. That this is unlikely is suggested by the experiments from Gershon's group [91] indicating that, at least on a suppressor factor, I-J is involved in a chain-chain interaction distinct from the antigen-combining site, as depicted in Figure 3. Also, F_1 cells express both I-J determinants [216], which seems hard to reconcile with involvement in the generation of a single unique antigenic receptor site. A role for I-J in the immune receptor, in a slightly different proposal, is that I-J represents a nonvariable portion (possibly subject to posttranscriptional modification) of the recognition site on the suppressor T-cell receptor, for an I-E plus antigen complex [22,178].

These issues may soon be clarified, since the elusive T-cell receptor has recently been identified; the variable, antigen-binding part (Ti) consists of a β chain [371] and an α chain [128]. This Ti complex has now been identified specifically for a suppressor T-cell line [27]. In spite of the above-noted differences in the recognition of antigen by suppressor T cell, the overall structure of this receptor does not seem markedly different from that on other T cells. Recently, evidence was presented that known major histocompatibility complex or immunoglobulin complex-controlled molecules, including I-J, are not present in the receptor of a suppressor T-cell hybridoma [174]. However, both the α and β chains of Ti are transcribed in a rearranged form very homologous to immunoglobulin [84]; this may be responsible for the homologies previously noted with the immunoglobulin heavy chain regions. Finally, as described in the next section, suppressor cells, unlike other T cells, react to stimulation of the antigen receptor with a 3-day lag of unresponsiveness, prior to evincing activation [27], which is another way in which suppressor T-cell interaction with antigen is unique.

Mechanism of Action of Suppressor Cells

The action of many suppressor cells, including the final Ts_3 suppressor cell, seems to be to inhibit the T-helper cell [9,10,23,36,95,118,135,170,298]; in some cases in which there is inhibition of antibody formation, the B cell may also be directly inhibited [209, 242]. Acquired unresponsiveness to histocompatibility antigens may involve the prevention of differentiation of cytotoxic T cells from stem cells [112,113,231] or the recruitment of fresh naive cells [280]. In early work it was suggested that cell-mediated suppression was not due to a separate suppressor cell but rather to "too much help" [262]. An inhibitory effect of high levels of help, or of antibody, was appealing as a feedback regulatory mechanism and seemed to tie in with the well-documented tendency for DTH responses to be inhibited by regimens that stimulated antibody formation effectively [262,263,359]. In fact, it seems that one possible mechanism of suppression in some cases may be absorption or inactivation of IL-2 [201]. It was recently shown that a balance between IL-2 production and IL-2 receptor concentration exists. It appears that during stimulation of T lymphocytes, IL-2 release induces the formation of more IL-2 receptors, which in a positive feedback manner induce more IL-2 production. However, an overshoot may occur so that at some point an excess of receptors absorbs all the available IL-2, producing a relative IL-2 deficiency that then damps the stimulation [79]. Although certain responses may be regulated in this way [123,193,243,326], the evidence for T-suppressor cells as an independent subpopulation [48,78,99,101,118], and that, in many systems, suppression is specific for some antigens but does not affect others in a culture [63] and is not otherwise demonstrably due to IL-2 consumption [56,67,154], argue against this as a dominant mechanism. Of course, an important effect of inhibition of helper T-cell activation due to any mechanism will be a decrease in the IL-2 present in the system.

The specificity of the final event at the end of the series of interactive steps leading to suppression may be different from the initial antigenic stimulus. Suppression for DTH may be directed against all antigens (epitopes) found on the immunogen, unlike suppression for antibody formation, which can be generated specifically for an isolated hapten on a complex immunogen [312]. It has even been reported that B cells can induce anticarrier inhibition by activating memory suppressor cells primed for the carrier [327]. The final mechanism is also commonly found to be nonspecific [11,119,258,298,315,375,376], although in at least one case a hybridoma suppressor-effector factor was found to be very antigen specific [232]. Papain may be used to split the factor in one report [95]; one of the two resultant fragments binds specifically to antigen, and the other produces suppression that is nonspecific when this portion is detached from the antigen-specific portion. A pair of smaller molecules (5000 and 35,000 daltons) have been described [281] that produce suppression nonspecifically after their release is induced by prostaglandin E_2. Another small factor is the inhibitory IgE-binding factor [151]. Mouse IgE nonresponder strains can develop antigen-specific suppressor T cells that inhibit glycosylation of IgE-binding factor, thereby preventing the binding factor from potentiating the IgE effect; this glycosylation-inhibiting factor is a fraction of lipomodulin, which is a phospholipase inhibitor. Based on the data in the IgE system, it has been suggested that the final suppressive event in all systems might be inhibition of phospholipases, which play a role in the activation of various cells. These changes in specificity between induction and the final action of suppression might be of great importance in the suppressor cell regulation of allograft rejection.

Of great interest in the analysis of the mechanism of active suppression is the temporal relationship between the stimulus for induction of immunosuppression and the evident effect. In the case of regimens or cells that are only effective when introduced early in the induction of the response, it has often been noted that 1-3 days may elapse before the suppression is manifest, even though the stimulus to suppression cannot be delayed for this time [27,249]. In the case of the suppressor cascade this may reflect the need to generate the sequential steps before actual interference with the response is possible, since certain suppressor steps are capable of inhibiting only the induction [25,112,113,215,222,231,280] or the effector [214,219,235] phase of the immune response. It also may be that later steps in the induction of a positive response becomes less sensitive to suppression [36,231,245], which would be consistent with differentiation beyond a suppression-sensitive proliferation step. Also, as mentioned in I-J, the Antigen Receptor, and Other Structures Associated with the Suppressor Phenotype, there are some fascinating recent observations concerning the status of the suppressor cell immediately following stimulation. Hu et al. [143] described incubation of an inducer cell population with antigen and macrophages; if this incubation was for longer than 3 days, then a phenotypic change involving the expression of Qa1 occurred and these cells would subsequently suppress the action of T-helper cells. This might be related to the results of recent experiments with the T-cell receptor. Most T cells, upon stimulation of either the Ti antigen-recognizing portion, or the T3 stimulus-triggering portion of the receptor, react by modulation of the receptor complex and a burst of activation; however, when a receptor on a suppressor T-cell line was thus stimulated, it was found to introduce a 3-day lag period of unresponsiveness, following which activation occurs [27]. It seems that this is a fundamental regulatory effect that allows net positive response to be initiated but also allows the induction of an eventual obligatory activation of suppression. Certainly, experiments on T-cell suppression must take these temporal factors into account.

Contrasuppression and Level 2 Suppression

It now appears that the regulatory mechanisms developed when the immune system is disturbed by an antigen are much more complex than described in the chapter thus far. The next layer of regulation discovered serves to limit the suppressor cell effect and has been dubbed "contrasuppression" by Gershon and associates [104]. This is a T-cell mechanism that potentiates a positive response. It is distinguishable from helper cell activity because contrasuppressor cells do not have any effect on their own [257], and they express I-J. In addition it was found that contrasuppressor cells adhere to *Vicia villosa* lectin, allowing this subpopulation to be separated from other T lymphocytes [116,148]. Special antigen-presenting cells may be responsible for activation of the contrasuppressor system [148]. Contrasuppressor cells also seem sensitive to cyclophosphamide, so that in one system it was found that suppression of an immune response was actually increased by cyclophosphamide due to decreased contrasuppression [39]. It may be that a report of a hybridoma factor that suppresses suppressor cells is related to the contrasuppressor system [146]. A mechanism has been described in the human that may be similar to murine contrasuppression [114, 331]. These additional levels of control presumably allow rapid immunoregulation and facilitate the generation of effective immune responses in required anatomic locations, while allowing the responses to be suppressed elsewhere in the body [2].

Finally, there is now an additional cellular regulatory layer postulated, called level 2 suppression. In the mouse, these cells have differing sensitivities to antiserum against Thy 1 and render suppression dominant when the appropriate interactive cells are present [115]. A recently published diagram of the relationships envisioned between level 1 suppression, contrasuppression, and level 2 suppression is reproduced in Figure 4.

The Effects of Immunosuppression on Suppressor Cells

Some of the first experiments indicating the existence of suppressor cells involved demonstrations that immune responses were heightened rather than depressed by treatment of animals with moderate doses of radiation [214] or antilymphocyte serum [17]. It was subsequently found that delayed-type hypersensitivity responses are heightened by administration of low doses of cyclophosphamide [107,179,300]. At least one suppressor cell subpopulation, Ts3, is not particularly sensitive to cyclophosphamide [235], but generally suppressor cells are quite sensitive compared with other T cells. The effect of cyclophosphamide in vitro has been studied using an active metabolite [156]. Why suppressor cells should exhibit this particular sensitivity to the DNA effects that constitute the mechanism of action of cyclophosphamide is unclear [294].

The sensitivity to cyclophosphamide is possibly related to the similar finding that suppressor cells are often found to be sensitive to treatment with irradiation or mitomycin C, suggesting that these subpopulations probably require cell division for their action [36,56,206,231]. Once the later stages of suppressor cell activation have been generated, they are not radiosensitive [36,56,153,206,254,342]. Suppressor cells may also be more sensitive to hydrocortisone than other cell subpopulations [158]. The effect of antilymphocyte serum is interesting. There is no reason to suspect a differential level of

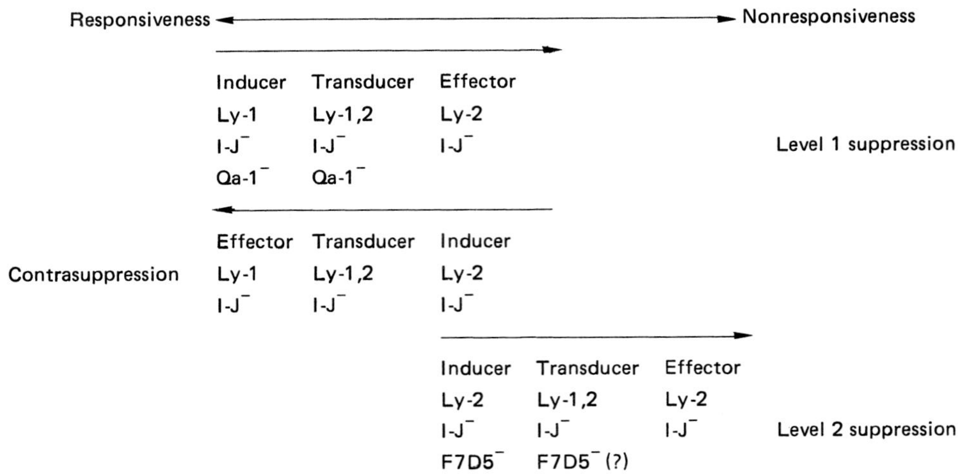

FIGURE 4 Proposed immunoregulatory pathways to immune responsiveness or nonresponsiveness. Note the different Lyt and I-J phenotypes. F7D5 distinguishes different levels of Thy-1-like antigen expression. (Used by permission, from ref. 115).

sensitivity of different types of lymphocytes to antilymphocyte serum, and yet, as described later in this chapter and in Chapter 17, it has been suggested that preferential formation of suppressor cells may be the explanation for long-term survival of grafts placed using temporary immunosuppression that includes antilymphocyte serum.

A major conceptual problem with immunosuppression employed clinically has been the presumed tendency to inhibition of suppressor cell activity as completely as the rest of the response. This dilemma has not been easily solved in view of the tendency already noted for a particular sensitivity on the part of many suppressor cell types to the available immunosuppressive agents. Cyclosporine may appear to be an exception; a striking lack of sensitivity to cyclosporine on the part of suppressor cells, compared with other lymphocyte types, appears to be an important aspect of the mechanism of action of this important new drug [125,136,145,182]. This may be because the mechanism of action of cyclosporine is largely due to interference with the interleukin-2 mechanism [76,80]. Presumably this lymphokine is not required for the generation of suppression, and so the elaboration of a strong capacity for suppression of helper cells can proceed unchecked while the interleukin-2 mechanism for generation of help is paralyzed. This presents the conceptual problem of how the helper/inducer phenotype cells that are important for the induction of suppression in many systems can perform in the presence of cyclosporine. Investigation of the detailed effect of the drug in one of the complex defined systems already described should be rewarding.

SUPPRESSOR CELLS AND RESPONSES TO EXPERIMENTAL TISSUE GRAFTS

Some of the experiments cited previously in this chapter dealt with suppression or responses against histocompatibility antigens, but most involved other types of specificities. This portion of the chapter will deal more specifically with transplantation antigens. It must be recognized that this distinction is artificial, to the extent that antialloantigen responses are experimental analogs of certain events during the processing of antigenic information in the natural immune response. However, because alloantigens represent an unusual stimulus for the immune apparatus, the extent to which the same regulatory mechanisms might exist warrants specific attention. Conceptually, hapten-modified lymphocytes may be similar to alloantigens as immunogens, and many experiments in this section involve haptenated cells. Mechanisms for graft potentiation that are apparently mediated by antibody, such as enhancement, direct anti-idiotype antibody inhibition, and antigen-reactive cell opsonization, are treated in other chapters of this book.

Classic Neonatal Tolerance and Self-Tolerance

The mechanism of induction of unresponsiveness to allogeneic tissue by neonatal inoculation may bear on the fundamental issue of avoidance of autoimmune reactions by the normal immune system and also might be a powerful method for creation of allograft unresponsiveness. Neonatal tolerance is characterized by an antigen-specific unreactivity to allografts, with no detectable proliferative response against the relevant alloantigens in vitro. Clonal deletion seemed the explanation for neonatal tolerance and protection from autoimmunity, but experiments suggesting an active inhibition of normal lymphocyte responses by lumphocytes of tolerant animals [40,112,113,121,130,204] and the ease of induction of self-reactive clones [28,195] have challenged this view. In addition to the apparent induction of suppressor cells in tolerance, it has been found that neonatal mice have cells spontaneously capable of inhibiting immune responses [227,304, 305]. These are antigen nonspecific [284] and may [5] or may not [305] express Lyt 1, or I-J [5]. This constitutive expression of antigen-nonspecific suppressor cells decreases with time, so that spontaneous suppressor cells are lacking in adults, in whom induction of specific suppression remains possible [40,224,284]. A possible mechanism for this change with age may be an increase in the effect of a regulatory population of macrophages [6].

In spite of these experiments indicating the presence of suppressor cells, it has not been easy to prove that they are important for neonatal or self-tolerance [303,304], since experiments employing the transfer of putative suppressor cells might include a minimal amount of unsuspected antigen in the inoculum, and also because the recipients of the transferred putative suppressor cells generally require a modest dose of radiation to demonstrate suppression. In one system, haptenated syngeneic cells were found to induce tolerance associated with suppressor T cells, whereas similarly treated allogeneic cells also induced tolerance, but without associated suppressor cells detected [212]. However, this result must be reconciled other experiments in which haptenated allogeneic cells did induce afferent suppression, whereas syngeneic cells inhibited the efferent portion of the response [214,215]. There are other cases in which the presence of demonstrable suppressor cells does not correlate with the tolerant state [57,113,140,314]. One possible explanation for these findings might be that suppressor cells can induce apparent clonal deletion by inhibiting stem cell proliferation for cells reactive against the relevant antigen, so that the animal appears to lack cells reactive against this specificity [112,113,304, 344].

Furthermore, there is a complex relationship between the development of tolerance and suppressor T cells. It has been suggested that a clonal deletion "phenotype" and a peripheral suppressor cell capable of preventing immune response generation by more differentiated cells may be complementary mutually reinforcing mechanisms for prohibiting anti-self responses [110,111,121,304]. In the radiation chimera model, it appears that a gradual change occurs from nonspecific suppressor cells to specific suppressor cells, then finally, at 2 years, to apparent clonal deletion [344,345]. In another case the clonal deletion appears before the suppressor cells become evident [213].

Maintenance of the tolerant state for alloantigens may be divided into chimeric and nonchimeric situations [124]. When animals that are tolerant for another strain are investigated carefully, live donor strain lymphocytes may be detected long after tolerance induction, at least in the spleen ("microchimerism"). There is evidence that the continued presence of antigen may be necessary, at least in some instances, for the maintenance of suppressor cell-associated tolerance [130,283], and the microchimeric cells could serve this function. However, in the definitive experiments by Dorsch and Roser, it appeared that the donor strain chimeric cells were actually the suppressor cells, reactive against the host antigraft idiotype [74,75]. With regard to maintenance of tolerance, evidence has been presented for suppressor memory cells, which would not be immediately evident in a long-term animal but are reactivated by new presentation of antigen [192].

An interesting paradox exists with regard to the tolerizing antigens. Guided by the paradigm that class II incompatibility generates help for responses against class I incompatibilities, it has seemed that incompatibility for class II should be quite detrimental to graft survival. However, Streilein has presented extensive evidence that it is much more difficult to break tolerance against class II antigens and that this is because suppressor cells are easily generated against class II, but not class I, antigens [304]. It was suggested that this is a second-order mechanism for the prevention of autoimmune attack of antigen-presenting cells that otherwise might be seen as foreign [121]. Perhaps the situation is different when immunosuppression is used [366], in view of the clinical observation that the HLA D-region incompatibility is detrimental to graft survival. It is also possible that the situation is different for primarily vascularized organ allografts, since class II incompatibility may exacerbate the rejection of primarily vascularized cardiac allografts in mice [43,60] and renal allograft rejection in miniature swine [325] in some cases.

Regulation of Allogeneic Responses in Vitro

There have been many studies of suppressor cell regulation of allogeneic responses in vitro. Prior to the availability of reagents for distinguishing lymphocyte subpopulations, it was found that the suppressor T cells responsible could be separated by density gradient sedimentation or centrifugation [101,271,341]. In the extensive studies by Rich and associates (e.g., References 271 and 273-277), the cells were antigen nonspecific when generated in vitro by mixed lymphocyte culture (MLC) or conconavalin A (ConA) stimulation but were specific in their capacity to suppress only cells bearing the I-C region in common. The generation of suppressors of lymphocyte stimulation involves cooperation between multiple cell types both in the mouse [24,25,98] and in the human [63,288]. Cells capable of suppressing mixed lymphocyte reactions may be antigen specific in some cases [63,140,290,339], and this may be related to the Lyt antigen phenotype of the suppressor cells in mice [131].

It is possible to induce suppression of the generation of mixed lymphocyte reactions or the generation of cytotoxic T cells in vivo [31,275,339]. In such experiments, attention to the time after the induction stimulus [96,122] and the anatomic source is important. As mentioned early in the chapter, suppressor cells are often found in the spleen. However, in one system a local lymph node reaction after foot pad injection produced suppressor cells not demonstrable systemically [360]. In some cases, suppression that is demonstrable in vivo is not evident in assays in vitro [31,86].

Suppression of mixed lymphocyte cultures generated by prior mixed lymphocyte or conconavalin A stimulation involves a suppressor factor [24,70,274]. In some systems, factors have been described that act to induce a second suppressor cell, which then leads to in vitro suppression [24,154].

The minimal degree to which minor antigens stimulate naive recipient cells in vitro has been puzzling in view of the strong graft rejection that they may produce and the strong in vitro responses developed after in vivo priming with minor antigens. This may be in part due to strong suppressor cell inhibition of responses against minor antigens [197,254]. The suppressor cell response to minor antigens seems to involve a prominent Lyt 1-positive cell and may be quite different from the cells regulating the response to major histoincompatibilities [254]. Miller, using a multiple culture technique, generated suppressor cells between strains identical at H-2 but incompatible for M1s and many other minor antigens [210].

It has been found that T cells react in mixed lymphocyte culture to autologous B cells and to activated or irradiated T cells [357]. This autologous mixed lymphocyte reaction appears to represent, at least in part, generation or reactivation of suppressor T cells [64,299,367], apparently responding to the receptors on the stimulating cells. Different subpopulations respond to different types of autologous cells [251], implying the existence of different types of suppressor cells.

Although the detailed scheme of regulatory levels reviewed in the first part of this chapter has not yet been similarly described specifically for alloantigens, there is evidence for mechanisms capable of regulating the suppressor system [114,251,331], perhaps similar to the contrasuppression described earlier for defined antigens.

A remarkable alternative cell-mediated mechanism for inhibition of allogeneic responses, which is apparently different from any other type of immunoregulation, has been described by Bevan and his colleagues. Veto cells apparently occur that are capable of confronting cytotoxic T cells directed against them and of preventing their action. Most intriguingly, this does not require recognition of the cytotoxic cells by the veto cells, only recognition by the cytotoxic cells of the veto cells, for these veto cells to produce their effect [87]. This device may prevent cytotoxic cells from destroying host-derived antigen-presenting cells that otherwise should be seen as foreign [88]. Veto cells are demonstrable as a powerful effect in vivo [261].

Suppressor Cell Regulation of Nonvascularized Grafts

Delayed-type hypersensitivity against allogeneic cells might be considered the simplest nonvascularized allograft. The numerous experiments with suppressor cell regulation of delayed-type hypersensitivity against allogeneic and syngeneic haptenated cells, and of contact sensitivity, have been included mainly in the first section of the chapter, since they constitute a major part of the work in which the complex regulatory mechanisms were delineated. Bone marrow transplantation constitutes a nonvascularized graft of major importance. Although the extensive literature in this field cannot be reviewed in this chapter, it was previously noted that suppressor cells may be found during the development of stable radiation chimeras [343]. Parental cells injected into F_1 animals may produce T cells that can abrogate anti-donor cytotoxic T-cell generation [295,301]. Protection from graft-versus-host disease may be in part due to suppressor cells [127] that inhibit the inductive part of the response [255], although in one opposite report, strong suppressor cell activity was correlated with fatal graft-versus-host disease [282]. The possibility that tumor graft survival might be influenced by suppressor cells has been studied but is beyond the scope of this chapter.

An enticing result was reported by Brent and colleagues in 1975 [160]. They found that mice rendered unresponsive to H-2-incompatible skin grafts by treatment with *Bordetella pertussis* vaccine, donor strain liver extract, and antilymphocyte serum had in their spleens a population of T cells that, when transferred to another strain, would significantly prolong skin graft survival. The authors noted that the transferred spleen cells were reactive in mixed lymphocyte culture and could mediate graft-versus-host disease, even though they produced this net suppression in vivo. In later work, it was shown that procarbazine plus anti-lymphocyte serum and liver extract can induce similar suppressor cells [41]. Donor blood can be substituted for liver extract [365], which enhances the potential for clinical application.

It was subsequently demonstrated by Wood and Monaco that mice treated with antilymphocyte serum plus donor strain bone marrow and then given a skin graft developed suppressor cells and also exhibited prolonged graft survival [362]. The animals proved to be microchimeric [198], and donor strain cells were found to be proliferating in the spleen [363]. Donor strain blood may be substituted for liver extract or bone marrow [364]. The specificities responsible are curious: third-party cells induce suppression for a strain incompatible only for class I and multiple minor antigens, whereas only donor-specific blood is effective in preconditioning for class I plus class II plus minor antigens on the subsequent skin graft [199,233,234]. Isolated class I is ineffective for preconditioning in these experiments, which requires class II incompatibility, at both I-A and I-J [233]. This is much like the requirements for class II incompatibility in the generation of suppressor cells described by Streilein (see Classic Neonatal Tolerance and Self-Tolerance). The relevance of suppressor cells to this graft potentiation is challenged by the observation that thymectomized animals have even more prolonged skin graft survival, but do not have demonstrable suppressor cells [361].

In another report, hyperimmunized mice were found to have cells that prolonged skin graft survival in vivo yet were cytotoxic in vitro [50]; it seems possible that quantitative differences in the effects of suppressor and cytotoxic cells in the different settings might explain this paradox. Monkeys treated with antilymphocyte serum had prolonged skin graft survival due to macrophagelike suppressor cells [328,329]. These cells suppressed mitogenesis in vitro nonspecifically, and their effect was abolished by indomethacin treatment. In several reports the effect of antilymphocyte serum seems to be to allow generation of nonspecific suppressor cells, perhaps due to a greater destruction of long-lived recirculating cells that are slower to repopulate than suppressor cells [362]. The suppressors are antigen specific if antigen is given and nonspecific if antilymphocyte serum alone is given [200].

Suppressor Cell Regulation of Vascularized Allografts

Long-term survival is generally more easily achieved with primarily vascularized allografts than with skin [124]. Primarily vascularized cardiac or renal allografts in the rat have been studied extensively. Prolonged survival can be produced in recipients, usually of F_1

grafts, that have been treated with some combination of donor antigen and antibody. Since such recipients were found to have transiently heightened in vitro reactivity against the donor strain [94], the mechanism was clearly different from neonatal tolerance. The effect was considered to be antibody-mediated enhancement, perhaps due to a central depression of the immune system from anti-idiotypic antibody [306]. Until recently it has not been possible to assess the incompatibilities in vascularized allografts in the rat with regard to the class I versus class II effect found by Streilein, and Wood and Monaco, to be important in the generation of suppressor cells for nonvascularized grafts in the mouse. However, recipients of enhanced skin grafts were not found to have suppressor cells [205], and doubt has also been expressed in the past that suppressor cells were responsible for the long-term survival of primarily vascularized organ grafts [19,126]. More recently, such recipients have been found to have thymocytes that transfer a modest prolongation of graft survival, but only when obtained at about 6-9 days posttransplant [134,332]; splenocytes produce a lesser prolongation. Batchelor et al., in a modification of an earlier opinion [20], and Marquet and Heystek [202] have found suppressor cells to be demonstrable in cells from long-term survivors administered to irradiated second hosts. Liver allotransplants in rats often enjoy prolonged survival with no immunosuppression, and suppressor cells have been implicated in this by some [81,142]. Using the minipigs with defined major histocompatibility loci that they have developed, Sachs and associates found evidence for suppressor cells capable of suppressing mixed lymphocyte cultures in class I-incompatible situations [246]. This is in opposition to the importance of class II for the generation of suppressor cells in neonatal tolerance noted above in the mouse, and more studies will be required in the pigs before this difference is clarified.

Alternatively, it is possible to begin looking at the effect of different H-2 regions on possible suppressor cell potentiation of primarily vascularized organ grafts in mice. Peripheral blood from long-surviving murine recipients of cardiac allografts has been examined for the presence of suppressor cells in limit-dilution assays, with the possible demonstration of suppressor cells in some cases [45]. This inconclusive answer was also obtained in our experiments with long-term B10.A recipients of primarily vascularized B10.BR cardiac allografts. Splenocytes from the recipients of these grafts, which are incompatible only for the portion of H-2 extending from "H-2 I-C" [168] through H-2 D, were highly reactive in mixed lymphocyte generation of cytotoxic lymphocytes during the first 2 weeks after grafting, but cells from recipients bearing successful long-term grafts were found to be capable of generating cytotoxicity to the same, or a slightly lesser degree than naive recipients. When these long-term splenocytes were added as third-party cells, a slight net depression of the generation of cytotoxicity was usually observed (Table 1). Therefore, suppressor cells seem to be present in such animals, but the determination of their biologic significance awaits a more subtle approach.

As described under The Effects of Immunosuppression on Suppressor Cells, the benefit of cyclosporine has been ascribed in part to sparing of suppressor cells. Long-term recipients of primarily vascularized allografts suppressed temporarily with cyclosporine have been found to harbor suppressor cells [145,175,372], and their immune status appears to be different from other states of transplant tolerance [125]. In one case a significant prolongation was transferrable from cyclosporine-treated recipients by lymphocytes bearing the suppressor/cytotoxic phenotype, but a prolongation almost as great (although not statistically significant), was noted with cells of the helper phenotype [35]. The effect in the adoptive transfer recipients of cells from cyclosporine-treated animals is always weak and never leads to long-term survival. However, evidence has been presented

TABLE 1 Testing for Suppressor Cells (Cs) from Long-Term Recipients[a]

Group	Suppressor to responder ratio	Normalized cytotoxicity[b]
1. Control	0	25
Splenocyte Cs	1:1	22
2. Control	0	32
Splenocyte Cs	1:1	17
Thymocyte Cs	1:1	29
3. Control	0	18
Splenocyte Cs	0.5:1	19
Thymocyte Cs	2:1	13
4. Control	0	25
Splenocyte Cs	0.5:1	25
Thymocyte Cs	2:1	21

[a]Splenocytes from long-term successful B10.A recipients of B10.BR primarily vascularized heart grafts were added in the indicated ratios as third-party cells in mixed lymphocyte reaction generation of cytotoxicity.
[b]Normalized cytotoxicity: the percentage of chromium-51 release at several E:T ratios was used to derive an average line, and then the value at E:T of 30:1 was determined

that treatment to abolish suppressor cells in long-term graft recipients will lead to rejection [176].

Antigen Nonspecific Cells and Factors in Immune Suppression

As already mentioned, the final suppressive mechanism may not be precisely specific for the inducing antigen. In some culture conditions, a polyclonal activation of multiple cells, each with a potentially demonstrable specificity, may in fact occur. However, there appear to be alterations in the specificity of the response generated that are intrinsic to suppressor cell induction. For instance, in addition to the final nonspecific suppressor factors that may mediate all suppressor T-cell activity (see Suppressor Factors), there are reports of primed suppressor cells capable of stimulation to activity by cells or factors derived from responses against different antigens [201,258]. Also, as noted above, the idiotype-anti-idiotype nature of suppressor cell cascades is likely to result in some alteration in the ultimate specificity of suppression; this may amplify the effect of a small number of initial clones specific for the antigen, to result in suppression against a much larger number of specificities [320]. Experiments supporting this must be viewed cautiously, however, since at least one cloned suppressor-effector line turned out to be very specific, and it was suggested that decreased specificity in some previous experiments might have stemmed from artefact [232]. With respect to transplantation, suppression induced against one specificity may subsequently involve related antigens on the challenge cells, even if the antigens are not too closely associated physically [29,30]. Whether these influences explain differences in specificity between helper and suppressor cells in allogeneic responses [122] remains to be fully investigated.

Macrophages probably play a role in the generation of suppression. The interaction of suppressor T cells with antigen-presenting cells has been described often [4,7,23,143, 169,187,252,260,297,347], although certain steps or systems are reportedly able to function in the absence of demonstrable antigen-presenting cells [63,66,67,70]. Since these macrophages, either nonspecific or perhaps bearing suppressor factors or processed antigen, might represent a rate-limiting step in certain culture conditions, the finding of a strong influence of their removal or inactivation [328] does not rule out the concomitant activity of specific suppressor T cells in the actual system in vivo. Ultraviolet irradiation can induce tumors in mice; their growth is potentiated by suppressor cells specific for this class of tumors, which may arise due to an irradiation-induced defect in the antigen-presenting cells [93,172]. On the other hand, macrophages also have the potential to produce a more general immunosuppression. Uterine macrophages are immunosuppressive [144]. Monocytes reportedly induce suppressor cells by prostaglandin E_2 secretion [56] and can produce paralysis of an inducer clone [143]. Recent evidence indicates that interferon can control this process: β interferon increases macrophage cytotoxic potential but decreases macrophage-induced suppression; γ interferon decreases suppression, but if employed only for a short time, stimulates IL-1 release but not development of cytotoxicity by macrophages [34]. A contrasting report describes hyporesponsiveness induced with macrophage-depleted immunizing allogeneic cells, whereas mixed lymphocyte reactions were increased if the macrophages were not depleted [286].

Artefacts Leading to the Appearance of Suppressor T-Cell Effects

Several possibilities exist for suppression of allogenic responses in culture in the absence of a special T cell devoted to regulation. As described under Mechanism of Action of Suppressor Cells, it was suggested that suppression, rather than due to an independent cell type, merely represented excess helper cell activity. In fact, interleukin-2 consumption can sometimes be shown to suppress responses; however, this probably is not usually an artefactual source of apparent suppressor cell activity.

The development of cytotoxic T cells so efficient that, when added as third-party cells to secondary cultures, they destroy the antigen before it effectively stimulates the naive cells to respond, could produce the appearance of suppressor cell effect. Articles invoking destruction of antigenic cells as at least a contributing mechanism of suppression have appeared [89,137,264,307,373]. However, in many more systems this mechanism has been carefully sought and ruled out as an alternative to actual suppressor T cells [1,56,66,67,96,112,113,122,131,211,245,255,271,275,291,296,339,341], generally on the basis of kinetics, specificity, or the absence of demonstrable cytotoxicity in cells able to suppress.

Consumption of interleukin-2, antibody or B-cell-mediated inhibition, destruction of antigen by cytotoxic T cells, the inhibitory effect of natural killer cells, stimulation of macrophage activity, and veto cell regulation, all represent important possible mechanisms of immune inhibition to be considered as alternatives in any purported demonstration of suppressor T cells. However, neither singly nor in concert do these appear to be a satisfactory explanation for most suppressor cell-regulated events.

SUPPRESSOR CELLS IN HUMAN IMMUNE RESPONSES

Evidence for Regulation in Human Immunity

There are several diseases in which abnormalities of suppressor cells may play a role. Since experimental autoimmune diseases have been found to be associated with alterations in regulation by suppressor T cells [18,32,47,239,256], this has been evaluated clinically. In rheumatoid arthritis, patients have increased levels of suppressor T cells inducible by concanavalin A or thymosin [374]. Patients with multiple sclerosis have increased numbers of T8-positive cells of the suppressor/cytotoxic phenotype [269]. Infectious mononucleosis cells undergo a phenotypic change with time, having predominantly a suppressor/cytotoxic phenotype early during the acute phase, which later progresses to T4 helper/inducer predominance [187,267,289]. During the acute phase, suppressor cells are demonstrable as functionally distinct from cytotoxic cells [69,171,337]. These can be shown to nonspecifically suppress activated B-cell proliferation, whereas serologically positive individuals a long time after infection have suppressor cells specific for B cells proliferating due to Epstein-Barr virus (EBV) infection [133,336]. Development of the late sequelae of polyclonal B-cell activation or agammaglobulinemia may occur if the suppressor T-cell activity becomes too low or too high [351]. Histiocytosis X is a disorder characterized by multiple immunodeficiencies. Depressed levels of histamine-binding T-suppressor cells are restored to normal in some patients with this disease by treatment with thymosin, and in these patients the clinical problems resolve, suggesting a return to a normal state of suppressor cell regulation [238]. Patients with chronic graft-versus-host disease after bone marrow transplantation have histamine-binding cells that suppress PHA stimulation, and these suppressor cells disappear coincidently with the development of acute graft-versus-host disease [268]. The desensitization of allergy patients may depend in part upon the induction of suppressor mechanisms [155] regulated by histamine-sensitive suppressor T cells [279]. It is likely that suppressor cells contribute to the immunosuppression that occurs after trauma [177,228]. Specific anergy to the offending organism may be due to suppressor cells in lepromatous leprosy [207] and in diffuse cutaneous leishmaniasis [247].

Immunoregulatory events must be important in the maternal-fetal relationship [149]. An interesting series of experiments documented the existence, in a multiparous mother, of suppressor T cells that would suppress proliferation of HLA-D-matched lymphocytes against paternal antigens [206], associated with production of a suppressor factor [83]. The cells could be studied conveniently as third-party additions to mixed lymphocyte cultures since their suppressive capacity remained intact after 1000 rad of irradiation, a dose sufficient to abrogate their capacity to proliferate. Unfortunately, six other multiparous women examined had no demonstrable cells of this sort [82]. Suppressor cells associated with pregnancy in experimental animals are only evident after multiple pregnancies [52], raising the question of how important they are biologically. However, it could be that the cells are less evident early but are required to be greatly expanded in effect or number with time.

Others have studied suppressor cells in experimental human immune reactions [46, 108,358]. In one report, class II cells had to be rendered "nonimmunogenic" for stimulation of suppressor cells rather than cytotoxic cells to occur [109]. In another report, different cell types were induced to become suppressor cells against class I, compared with class II, antigens, but the result in both cases involved specificity for class II [270]. Aldomet has been reported to potentiate development of auto-red cell antibody by raising cyclic AMP levels, which apparently interferes with suppressor cell development [163].

Identifying Characteristics of Human Suppressor Cells

It is well-known that human suppressor cells generally express the cell membrane specificity recognized by Leu 2 and OKT8 monoclonal antibodies [42,56,66,67,97]. Whether a distinction between these and cytotoxic cells that also bear this antigen is possible has been a problem. It may be that T8 has only certain epitopes directed toward cytotoxicity, but it is likely that it is the same structure on both cell types. Other antigens have been reported to occur only on cells in the suppressor circuit, including the "juvenile rheumatoid arthritis antigen" [226], "D12" [58,180], "TQ1" [225], and the "Fc-gamma" receptor [223]. Also, the antigen 9.3 is found only on the cytotoxic, not the suppressor, fraction of the Leu 2/OKT8-positive cells [63,68,196]. Suppressor cells seem to be characterized by prominent expression of histamine receptors [26,278,279], although these may occur in a low number on all human lymphocytes [285]. The DR antigens are apparently expressed by suppressor T cells at certain points during differentiation [97,266], and these may vary with the activity of the cells in ways that have just begun to be studied [187]. Recently, I-J-like determinants have been reported on a subset of T8-positive human lymphocytes [185]. None of these identifying characteriistics have been applied in a widespread fashion as yet, but they may help to distinguish various suppressor cells from cytotoxic cells more clearly in future studies.

In addition, as with mouse T-cell subsets, the helper phenotype (recognized by Leu 3 and OKT4 in the human), is often found on some cells in the suppressor circuit [56, 63,65,66,67,97,109,226,244,270,330,331]. These helper-type lymphocytes required for generation of suppression are often inducer phase cells, with differentiation into effector suppressors accompanied by a change to, or induction of cells with, the Leu 2/OKT8 phenotype [56,63,66,67,97,331]. When incubated with normal lymphocytes, T-lymphoblast leukemia cells can be induced to develop into suppressor cells capable of inhibiting B-cell proliferation [42], indicating that multiple cell types may be involved in the generation of human suppressor cells, as would be predicted from the experiments in mice. Other evidence of cell collaboration in the development of the suppressor cell effect in the human includes the requirement for a TQ1-positive, a TQ1-negative population in the generation of suppression effect [225] and the differences in subpopulations that respond to differences in the autologous mixed lymphocyte reaction as described above. Also, contrasuppressorlike cells have been reported [114,331] and may be distinguished by streptococcal antigen binding [186].

Suppressor Cells, Blood Transfusions, and Renal Allografts

Patients with chronic renal failure probably have immune abnormalities. Evidence has been presented that the concanavalin A generation of cells capable of suppressing mixed lymphocyte cultures is increased in hemodialysis patients, perhaps because of altered lipid metabolism leading to an increase in these cells [266]. At least two groups have obtained evidence that the blood transfusion effect is associated with suppressor cells. One experimental approach involves the apparent decrease in short-lived suppressor cells, allowing increased proliferation to concanavalin A after 24 hr in culture, so that an increase in the degree of stimulation when mitogen is added at 24 hr, versus at time 0, is evidence for suppressor cells. Using this assay in pretransplant dialysis patients, evidence was found that, during the first 14 days after transfusion, adherent mononuclear cells were causing suppression, and later on suppressor T cells became evident [189]. This approach does not assess suppressor function in an easily interpretable way. In a more functional approach, it was found that, after receiving blood transfusions, patients have cells that can cause nonspecific inhibition of mixed lymphocyte cultures [165]. In another report on functionally identified suppressor cells, peripheral blood lymphocytes from patients who had received greater than five blood transfusions were able to decrease mixed lymphocyte cultures by about 50% when added as third-party cells [159].

Several experimental results mentioned in previous sections bear on the possible involvement of suppressor cells in the effect of blood transfusions (e.g., Reference 364). A particularly troublesome question is how a small number of transfusions could induce suppression against a sufficient number of antigens to enable prevention of rejection against some individual specificity present on the graft but not on any of the transfusions. The complete lack of apparent specificity in some systems described above might contribute to this. However, it seems more likely that the decreased specificity at the effector end of the suppressor cell cascade described earlier in the chapter would blanket associated antigens without being totally nonspecific; from these experiments it might be predicted that, if *any* of the specificities seen on the graft had been present in the blood, suppression for *all* of the antigens on the graft would be produced. The continued requirement for antigen to maintain suppressor T cells in many systems would seem to indicate a need for continued replacement of antigen; such a need for continued reintroduction of antigen, rather than total amount or volume per se, might be part of the reason that increasing numbers of transfusions seem to improve the effect.

Charpentier and colleagues have used frozen pretransplant recipient cells to provide a uniform population of responders against which to test third-party cells for suppression. They found that some stable transplant patients have developed cells that can suppress mixed lymphocyte culture responses of pretransplant cells, but these are not demonstrable in patients with rejection [53]. Pfeffer similarly reported a capacity of cells from successful one-haplotype living donor transplant recipients to inhibit generation of cell-mediated cytotoxicity as third-party cells [248].

SUPPRESSOR CELLS: STATUS AND PROSPECTS

Viewing the complexities described above with an eye toward the principles important for graft rejection, several points are evident.

1. Simple concepts of the relationship of a lymphocyte subpopulation bearing a given surface antigen to suppression or induction of a positive response are certainly no longer tenable in the mouse, and to the extent that data exist in the human, probably not justified clinically.
2. Just as evidence for the involvement of suppressor cells needs thoughtful scrutiny in each case, data indicating that suppressor cells are not important in a given state of decreased responsiveness must be viewed with caution, in view of the evidence for their fundamental importance in immunology and the various subtypes that might only be manifest under certain experimental conditions.
3. A given degree of apparent potentiation or suppression of graft rejection in vivo could correspond, in different situations, to far different regulatory situations, which, for instance, might respond quite differently to a change in immunosuppression.

4. A far better capacity to monitor the activities of different types of lymphocytes is required before useful interpretations and manipulations of suppressor cell activity will be generally possible. In the cumbersome allograft situation it may be that the use of hybridoma cell lines or their factors, which would produce certain known effects only on populations primed in a certain way, would be a promising approach to circumventing the complexities.
5. In an even greater leap over the complexities of the suppressor cell mechanism, the antigen-nonspecific final effect of suppressor cell generation should be studied intensely, since it might be very successfully exploited for immunosuppression.

ACKNOWLEDGMENTS

Supported in part of PHS grants RO1 AI15081 and PO1 AI19373. Stimulating discussion with Dr. Kimishige Ishizaka and excellent secretarial assistance from Ms. Pamela Creevey are gratefully acknowledged.

REFERENCES

1. Al Adra, A. R., and Pilarski, L. M. Antigen-specific suppression of cytotoxic T cell responses in mice. I. Suppressor T cells are not cytotoxic cells. *Eur. J. Immunol.* 8: 504-511, 1978.
2. Altmann, D. M., and Blyth, W. A. Lipopolysaccharide-induced suppressor cells for delayed-type hypersensitivity to herpes simplex virus—nature of suppressor cell and effect on pathogenesis of herpes simplex. *Immunology* 53:473-480, 1984.
3. Andersson, L. C., Aguet, M., Wight, E., Andersson, R., Binz, H., and Wigzell, H. Induction of specific immune unresponsiveness using purified mixed leukocyte culture-activated T lymphoblasts as autoimmunogen. I. Demonstration of general validity as to species and histocompatibility barriers. *J. Exp. Med.* 146:1124-1137, 1977.
4. Aoki, I., Minami, M., and Dorf, M. E. A mechanism responsible for the induction of H-2-restricted second-order suppressor T cells. *J. Exp. Med.* 157:1726-1735, 1983.
5. Argyris, B. F. Nature of neonatal splenic suppressor cells in the mouse. *Cell. Immunol.* 66:352-359, 1982.
6. Argyris, B. F. Mechanism by which adult mouse peritoneal macrophages affect neonatal suppressor cell activity. *Transplantation* 36:328-333, 1983.
7. Argyris, B. F., and Cotellessa, A. Absorption of suppressor cell activity on mouse macrophage monolayers. *Transplantation* 28:372-376, 1979.
8. Asano, Y., and Hodes, R. J. T cell regulation of B cell activation. I-A-restricted T suppressor cells inhibit the major histocompatibility complex-restricted interactions of T helper cells with B cells and accessory cells. *J. Exp. Med.* 157:1867-1884, 1983.
9. Asano, Y., and Hodes, R. J. T cell regulation of B cell activation: Cloned Lyt-1^+2^- T suppressor cells inhibit the major histocompatibility complex-restricted interaction of T helper cells with B cells and/or accessory cells. *J. Exp. Med.* 158:1178-1190, 1983.
10. Asano, Y., and Hodes, R. J. T cell regulation of B cell activation. T cells independently regulate the responses mediated by distinct B cell subpopulations. *J. Exp. Med.* 155: 1267-1276, 1982.
11. Asherson, G. L., Dorf, M. E., Colizzi, V., Zembala, M., and James, B. M. B. Equivalence of conventional anti-picryl T-suppressor factor in the contact sensitivity system and monoclonal anti-NP TsF3—their final non-specific effect via the T-acceptor cell. *Immunology* 53:491-497, 1984.
12. Asherson, G. L., Watkins, M. C., Zembala, M. A., and Colizzi, V. C. Two-chain structure of T-suppressor factor: Antigen-specific T-suppressor factor occurs as a single

molecule and as separate antigen-binding and I-J+ parts, both of which are required for biological activity. *Cell. Immunol.* 86:448-459, 1984.
13. Asherson, G. L., and Zembala, M. Suppressor T cells in cell-mediated immunity. *Br. Med. Bull.* 32:158-164, 1976.
14. Asherson, G. L., Zembala, M., Maghew, B., and Goldstein, A. Adult thymectomy: Prevention of the appearance of suppressor T cells which depress contact sensitivity to picryl chloride and reversal of adult thymectomy effect by thymus extract. *Eur. J. Immunol.* 6:699-703, 1976.
15. Bach, B. A., Greene, M. I., Benacerraf, B., and Nisonoff, A. Mechanisms of regulation of cell-mediated immunity. IV. Azobenzenearsonate-specific suppressor factor(s) bear cross-reactive idiotypic determinants the expression of which is linked to the heavy-chain allotype linkage group of genes. *J. Exp. Med.* 149:1084-1098, 1979.
16. Bach, B. A., Sherman, L., Benacerraf, B., and Greene, M. I. Mechanisms of regulation of cell-mediated immunity. II. Induction and suppression of delayed-type hypersensitivity to azobenzene arsonate-coupled syngeneic cells. *J. Immunol.* 121:1460-1468, 1978.
17. Baker, P. J., Barth, R. F., Stashak, P. W., and Amsbaugh, D. F. Enhancement of Ab response to type 3 pneumococcal polysaccharide in mice treated with antilymphocyte serum. *J. Immunol.* 104:1313-1315, 1970.
18. Bartholomaeus, W. N., Reed, W. D., and Joske, R. A. Autoantibody to liver-specific lipoprotein in the mouse: Regulation by naturally occurring autoantigen specific suppressor cells. *Clin. Exp. Immunol.* 58:307-316, 1984.
19. Batchelor, J. R., Brent, L., and Kilshaw, P. J. Absence of suppressor cells from rats bearing passively enhanced kidney allografts. *Nature* 270:522-524.
20. Batchelor, J. R., Phillips, B. E., and Grennan, D. Suppressor cells and their role in the survival of immunologically enhanced rat kidney allografts. *Transplantation* 37: 43-46, 1984.
21. Baxevanis, C. N., Ikezawa, Z., Klein, J., and Nagy, Z. Mechanisms involved in the IR-gene control of T suppressor cell response to lactate dehydrogenase B. *J. Mol. Cell. Immunol.* 1:201-210, 1984.
22. Baxevanis, C. N., Ishii, N., Nagy, Z. A., and Klein, J. Role of the E^k molecule in the generation of suppressor T cells in response to LDH_B. *Scand. J. Immunol.* 16:25-31, 1982.
23. Baxevanis, C. N., Ishii, N., Nagy, Z. A., and Klein, J. H-2-controlled suppression of T cell response to lactate dehydrogenase B. Characterization of the lactate dehydrogenase B suppressor pathway. *J. Exp. Med.* 156:822-833, 1982.
24. Beckwith, M., and Rich, S. S. Suppressor-target interaction in alloantigen induced responses: Induction of a second cell in the suppressive pathway. *J. Immunol.* 128: 791-796, 1982.
25. Beckwith, M., and Rich, S. Suppressive mechanisms in alloantigen-induced T cell responses. *J. Exp. Med.* 158:1853-1867, 1983.
26. Beer, D. J., and Rocklin, R. E. Histamine-induced suppressor-cell activity. *J. Allergy Clin. Immunol.* 73:439-452, 1984.
27. Bensussan, A., Acuto, O., Hussey, R. E., Milanese, C., and Reinherz, E. L. T3-Ti receptor triggering of T8+ suppressor T cells leads to unresponsiveness to interleukin-2. *Nature* 311:565-567, 1984.
28. Bensussan, A., Meuer, S. C., Schlossman, S. F., and Reinherz, E. L. Delineation of an immunoregulatory amplifier population recognizing autologous Ia molecules. *J. Exp. Med.* 159:559-576, 1984.
29. Bianchi, A. T., Bril, H., and Benner, R. Alloantigen-specific suppressor T cells can also suppress the in vivo immune response to unrelated alloantigens. *Nature* 301:614-616, 1983.

30. Bianchi, A. T. J., Hussaarts-Odijk, L. M., and Benner, R. Antigen-specific suppressor T cells suppress in vivo the cellular immune response to unrelated "bystander" antigens. *Transplant. Proc.* 15:760-764, 1983.
31. Bitter-Suermann, H., and Shevach, E. M. Induction of transplantation tolerance in guinea pigs by spleen allografts. III. Transfer of tolerance to normal hosts. *Transplantation* 36:161-165, 1983.
32. Bogen, S., Mazes, E., and Fuchs, S. Induction of acetylcholine receptor-specific suppression. An in vitro model of antigen-specific immunosuppression in myasthenia gravis. *J. Exp. Med.* 159:292-304, 1984.
33. Bona, C., Hooghe, R., Cazenave, P. A., Leguern, C., and Paul, W. E. Cellular basis of regulation of expression of idiotype. II. Immunity to anti-MOPC-460 idiotype antibodies increases the level of anti-trinitrophenyl antibodies bearing 460 idiotypes. *J. Exp. Med.* 149:815-823, 1979.
34. Boraschi, D., Censini, S., and Tagliabue, A. Interferon-γ reduces macrophage-suppressive activity by inhibiting prostaglandin E_2 release and inducing interleukin 1 production. *J. Immunol.* 133:764-768, 1984.
35. Bordes-Aznar, J., Kupiec-Weglinski, J. W., Duarte, A. J. S., Milford, E. L., Strom, T. B., and Tilney, N. L. Function and migration of suppressor lymphocytes from cyclosporine A-treated heart graft recipients. *Transplantation* 35:185-190, 1983.
36. Borkowsky, W., and Valentine, F. T. The proliferative response of human lymphocytes to antigen is suppressed preferentially by lymphocytes precultured with the same antigen. *J. Immunol.* 122:1867-1873, 1979.
37. Bottomly, K., Kaye, J., Jones, B., Jones, F. III, and Janeway, C. A., Jr. A cloned, antigen-specific, Ia-restricted Lyt-1^+, 2^- T cell with suppressive activity. *J. Mol. Cell. Immunol.* 1:42-49, 1983.
38. Bottomly, K., Mathieson, B. J., and Mosier, D. E. Anti-idiotype induced regulation of helper cell function for the response to phosphorylcholine in adult BALB/c mice. *J. Exp. Med.* 148:1216-1227, 1978.
39. Braley-Mullen, H. Regulation of the antibody response to type III pneumococcal polysaccharide by contrasuppressor T cells. *J. Exp. Med.* 160:42-54, 1984.
40. Brent, L., Brooks, C. G., Medawar, P. B., and Simpson, E. Transplantation tolerance. *Br. Med. Bull.* 32:101-106, 1976.
41. Brent, L., and Opara, S. C. Specific unresponsiveness to skin allografts in mice. V. Synergy between donor tissue extract, procarbazine hydrochloride, and antilymphocyte serum in creating long-lasting unresponsiveness mediated by suppressor T cells. *Transplantation* 27:120-126, 1979.
42. Broder, S., Uchiyama, T., Muul, L. M., Goldman, C., Sharrow, S., Poplack, D. G., and Waldman, T. A. Activation of leukemic pro-suppressor cells to become suppressor-effector cells. Influence of cooperating normal T cells. *N. Engl. J. Med.* 304:1382-1387, 1981.
43. Burdick, J. F., and Clow, L. W. Rejection of murine cardiac allografts: relative roles of major and minor antigens. *Transplantation* in press, 1986.
44. Burns, F. D., Marrack, P. C., Kappler, J. W., and Janeway, C. A., Jr. Functional heterogeneity among the T-derived lymphocytes of the mouse. IV. Nature of spontaneously induced suppressor cells. *J. Immunol.* 114:1345-1347, 1975.
45. Burton, R. C., Fortin, J. L., and Russell, R. S. T cell responses to alloantigens. I. Studies of in vivo and in vitro immunologic memory and suppression by limit dilution analysis. *J. Immunol.* 124:2936-2943, 1980.
46. Callard, R. E., Winger, C. M., and Tiernan, S. L. Antigen-specific suppression of human antibody responses by allogeneic T cells. I. Frequency and antigen specificity of allogeneic suppressor T cells and their role in major histocompatibility complex-controlled genetic restriction. *J. Exp. Med.* 159:1225-1237, 1984.
47. Cantor, H., McVay-Boudreau, L., Hugenberger, J., Naidorf, K., Shen, F. W., and

Gershon, R. K. Immunoregulatory circuits among T-cell sets. II. Physiologic role of feedback inhibition in vivo: Absence in NZB mice. *J. Exp. Med.* 147:1116-1125, 1978.

48. Cantor, H., Shen, F. W., and Boyse, E. A. Separation of helper T cells from suppressor T cells expressing different Ly components. II. Activation by antigen: After immunization, antigen-specific suppressor and helper activities are mediated by distinct T-cell subclasses. *J. Exp. Med.* 143:1391-1440, 1976.
49. Cayre, Y., Palladino, M. A., Marcu, K. B., and Stavnezer, J. Expression of an antigen receptor on T cells does not require recombination at the immunoglobulin JH-C mu locus. *Proc. Natl. Acad. Sci. USA* 78:3814-3818, 1981.
50. Chang, A. E., and Sugarbaker, P. H. Assessment of T cell function with a skin allograft assay. *Transplantation* 29:381-387, 1980.
51. Chen, B. P. P., and Splitter, G. A. Transplant tolerance: Lyt-1^+2^- helper T cells require a second proliferation signal to overcome Lyt-1^-2^+ suppressor T cell activity. *J. Immunol.* 131:57-63, 1983.
52. Chaouat, G., and Voisin, G. A. Regulatory T cell subpopulations in pregnancy. I. Evidence for suppressive activity of the early phase in MLR. *J. Immunol.* 122:1383-1388, 1979.
53. Charpentier, B. M., Lang, P., Martin, B., and Fries, D. Specific recipient-donor unresponsiveness mediated by a suppressor cell system in human kidney allograft tolerance. *Transplantation* 33:470-477, 1982.
54. Chiu, K. M., Faanes, R. B., and Choi, Y. S. Suppression of the in vivo cytotoxic T lymphocyte response with heat-treated allogeneic cells. *Transplantation* 29:159-160, 1980.
55. Chiu, K. M., Faanes, R. B., and Choi, Y. S. Activation of specific suppressor cells with heat-treated allogeneic tumor cells. *Cell. Immunol.* 49:283-292, 1980.
56. Chouaib, S., Chatenoud, L., Klatzmann, D., and Fradelizi, D. The mechanisms of inhibition of human IL 2 production. II. PGE_2 induction of suppressor T lymphocytes. *J. Immunol.* 132:1851-1857, 1984.
57. Claman, H. N., Miller, S. D., Conlon, P. J., and Moorhead, J. W. Control of experimental contact sensitivity. *Adv. Immunol.* 30:121-157, 1980.
58. Clement, L. T., Dagg, M. K., and Landay, A. Characterization of human lymphocyte subpopulations: Alloreactive cytotoxic T-lymphocyte precursor and effector cells are phenotypically distinct from Leu 2^+ suppressor cells. *J. Clin. Immunol.* 4:395-402, 1984.
59. Colizzi, V., Doria, G., and Adorini, L. Immunoregulation of lysozyme-specific suppression. I. Induction and suppression of delayed-type hypersensitivity to hen egg-white lysozyme. *Eur. J. Immunol.* 14:820-825, 1984.
60. Corry, R. J., Winn, H. J., and Russell, P. S. Primarily vascularized allografts of hearts in mice. The role of H-2D, H-2K, and non-H-2 antigens in rejection. *Transplantation* 16:343-350, 1973.
61. Coutinho, A., Forni, L., Holmberg, D., Ivars, F., and Vaz, N. From an antigen-centered, clonal perspective of immune response to an organism-centered, network perspective of autonomous activity in a self-referential immune system. *Immunol. Rev.* 79:151-168, 1984.
62. Czitrom, A. A., Sunshine, G. H., and Mitchison, N. A. Suppression of the proliferative response to H-2D by IJ subregion gene products. *Immunogenetics* 11:97-102, 1980.
63. Damle, N. K., and Engleman, E. G. Immunoregulatory T cell circuits in man. Alloantigen-primed inducer T cells activate alloantigen-specific suppressor T cells in the absence of the initial antigenic stimulus. *J. Exp. Med.* 158:159-173, 1983.
64. Damle, N. K., and Gupta, S. Autologous mixed lymphocyte reaction in man. V.

Functionally and phenotypically distinct human T-cell subpopulations respond against non-T and activated T cells in autologous mixed lymphocyte reaction. *Scand. J. Immunol.* 16:59-68, 1982.

65. Damle, N. K., and Gupta, S. Heterogeneity of concanavalin A-induced suppressor T cells in man defined with monoclonal antibodies. *Clin. Exp. Immunol.* 48:581-588, 1982.
66. Damle, N. K., Mohagheghpour, N., and Engleman, E. Activation of antigen-specific suppressor T lymphocytes in man involves dual recognition of self class I MHC molecules and LEU-4/T3-associated structures on the surface of inducer T lymphocytes. *J. Immunol.* 133:1235-1240, 1984.
67. Damle, N. K., Mohagheghpour, N., and Engleman, E. G. Soluble antigen-primed inducer T cells activate antigen-specific suppressor T cells in the absence of antigen-pulsed accessory cells: Phenotypic definition of suppressor-inducer and suppressor-effector cells. *J. Immunol.* 132:644-650, 1984.
68. Damle, N. K., Mohagheghpour, N., Hansen, J. A., and Engleman, E. G. Alloantigen-specific cytotoxic and suppressor T lymphocytes are derived from phenotypically distinct precursors. *J. Immunol.* 131:2296-2300, 1983.
69. De Waele, M., Thielemans, C., and Van Camp, B. K. Characterization of immunoregulatory T cells in EBV-induced infectious mononucleosis by monoclonal antibodies. *N. Engl. J. Med.* 304:460-462, 1981.
70. Dennison, D. K., Rich, S. S., and Rich, R. R. Cellular and antigenic requirements for production of mixed leukocyte reaction suppressor factor. *J. Immunol.* 127:2176-2182, 1981.
71. Dietz, M. H., Sy, M. S., Benacerraf, B., Nisonoff, A., Greene, M. I., and Germain, R. N. Antigen- and receptor-driven regulatory mechanisms. VII. H-2-restricted anti-idiotypic suppressor factor from efferent suppressor T cells. *J. Exp. Med.* 153:450-463, 1981.
72. Dohi, Y., and Nisonoff, A. Suppression of idiotype and generation of suppressor T cells with idiotype-conjugated thymocytes. *J. Exp. Med.* 150:909-918, 1979.
73. Dorf, M. E., and Benacerraf, B. Suppressor cells and immunoregulation. *Annu. Rev. Immunol.* 2:127-157, 1984.
74. Dorsch, S., and Roser, B. Suppressor cells in transplantation tolerance. I. Analysis of the suppressor status of neonatally and adoptively tolerized rats. *Transplantation* 33:518-524, 1982.
75. Dorsch, S., and Roser, B. Suppressor cells in transplantation tolerance. II. Identification and probable mode of action of chimeric suppressor T cells. *Transplantation* 33:525-529, 1982.
76. Dos Reis, G. A., and Shevach, E. M. Effect of cyclosporin A on T cell function in vitro: The mechanism of suppression of T cell proliferation depends on the nature of the T cell stimulus as well as the differentiation state of the responding T cell. *J. Immunol.* 129:2360-2367, 1982.
77. Eardley, D. D., Hugenberger, J., McVay-Boudreau, L., Shen, F. W., Gershon, R. K., and Cantor, H. Immunoregulatory circuits among T-cell sets. I. T-helper cells induce other T-cell sets to exert feedback inhibition. *J. Exp. Med.* 147:1106-1115, 1978.
78. Eardley, D. D., Staskawicz, M. O., and Gershon, R. K. Suppressor cells: Dependence on assay conditions for functional activity. *J. Exp. Med.* 143:1211-1219, 1976.
79. Eastman, A. Y., and Lawrence, D. The allogeneic effect: The mechanism of allosuppression by Lyt-1, Ia^- T cells. *J. Immunol.* 133:1155-1162. 1984.
80. Elliott, J. F., Lin, Y., Mizel, S. B., Bleackley, R. C., Harnish, D. G., and Paetkau, V. Induction of interleukin 2 messenger RNA inhibited by Cyclosporin A. *Science* 226: 1439-1441, 1984.
81. Engemann, R., Ulrichs, K., Thiede, A., Muller-Ruchholtz, W., and Hamelmann, H.

A mechanism of tolerance in arterialized rat liver transplantation. *Transplant. Proc.* 15:729-733, 1983.

82. Engleman, E. G., McMichael, A. J., Batey, M. E., and McDevitt, H. O. A suppressor T cell of the mixed lymphocyte reaction in man specific for the stimulating alloantigen. Evidence that identity at HLA-D between suppressor and responder is required for suppression. *J. Exp. Med.* 147:137-146, 1978.
83. Engleman, E. G., McMichael, A. J., and McDevitt, H. O. Suppression of the mixed lymphocyte reaction in man by a soluble T-cell factor. Specificity of the factor for both responder and stimulator. *J. Exp. Med.* 147:1037-1043, 1978.
84. Fabbi, M., Acuto, O., Smart, J. E., and Reinherz, E. L. Homology of Ti α-subunit of a T-cell antigen-MHC receptor with immunoglobulin. *Nature* 312:269-271, 1984.
85. Feldmann, M., Beverly, P. C., Woody, J., and McKenzie, I. F. C. T-T interaction in the induction of suppressor and helper T cells: Analysis of membrane phenotype of precursor and amplifier cells. *J. Exp. Med.* 145:793-801, 1977.
86. Finberg, R., Burakoff, S. J., Benacerraf, B., and Greene, M. I. The cytolytic T lymphocyte response to trinitrophenyl-modified syngeneic cells. II. Evidence for antigen-specific helper T cells. *J. Immunol.* 123:1210-1214, 1979.
87. Fink, P. J., Rammensee, H-G, Benedetto, J. D., Staerz, U. D., Lefrancois, L., and Bevan, M. J. Cloned cytolytic T cells can suppress primary cytotoxic responses directed against them. *J. Immunol.* 133:1775-1781, 1984.
88. Fink, P. J., Rammensee, H-G., and Bevan, M. J. Studies on the mechanism of suppression of primary cytotoxic responses by cloned cytotoxic T lymphocytes. *J. Immunol.* 133:1769-1774, 1984.
89. Fitch, F. W., Engers, H. D., Cerottini, J.-C., and Bruner, K. T. Generation of cytotoxic T lymphocytes in vitro. VII. Suppressive effect of irradiated MLC cells on CTL response. *J. Immunol.* 116:716-723, 1976.
90. Flood, P. M., Yamauchi, K., and Gershon, R. K. Analysis of the interactions between two molecules that are required for the expression of Ly-2 suppressor cell activity. Three different types of focusing events may be needed to deliver the suppressive signal. *J. Exp. Med.* 156:361-371, 1982.
91. Flood, P. M., and Louie, D. S. Mechanism of Ly2 suppressor cell activity: Activation of an Ly1 I-J$^+$ cell is required to transduce the suppressive signal. *J. Exp. Med.* 159: 1413-1428, 1984.
92. Folch, H., and Waksman, B. H. The splenic suppressor cell. II. Suppression of the mixed lymphocyte reaction by thymus-dependent adherent cells. *J. Immunol.* 113: 140-144, 1974.
93. Fox, I. J., Sy, M. S., Benacerraf, B., and Greene, M. I. Impairment of antigen-presenting cell function by ultraviolet radiation. II. Effect of in vitro ultra-violet irradiation on antigen-presenting cells. *Transplantation* 31:262-265, 1981.
94. French, M. E., and Batchelor, J. O. R. Enhancement of renal allografts in rats and man. *Transplant. Rev.* 13:115-141, 1972.
95. Fresno, M., McVay-Boudreau, L., and Cantor, H. Antigen-specific T lymphocyte clones. III. Papain splits purified T suppressor molecules into two functional domains. *J. Exp. Med.* 155:981-993, 1982.
96. Gascoigne, N. R. J., and Crispe, I. N. Suppression of the cytotoxic T cell response to minor alloantigens in vivo. *Eur. J. Immunol.* 14:210-215, 1984.
97. Gatenby, P. A., Kotzin, B. L., Kansas, G. S., and Engleman, E. G. Immunoglobulin secretion in the human autologous mixed lymphocyte reaction. Definition of a suppressor-amplifier circuit using monoclonal antibodies. *J. Exp. Med.* 156:55-67, 1982.
98. Gautam, S. C., Beckman, K. D., Wong, H. L., and Battisto, J. R. Characterization of two suppressor cells that together prevent in vivo development of cytolytic T cells to hapten-altered self. *Cell. Immunol.* 87:23-34, 1984.

99. Gautum, S. C., Hilfiker, M. L., and Battisto, J. R. In vivo development of cytolytic T lymphocytes (CTL) to hapten-altered self: Mls-disparate cells facilitate the response by neutralizing IL 2 inhibitor. *J. Immunol.* 130:533-537, 1983.
100. Geha, R. S. Current concepts in immunology: Regulation of the immune response by idiotypic-antiidiotypic interactions. *N. Engl. J. Med.* 305:25-28, 1981.
101. Gerber, N. L., and Steinberg, A. D Physical separation of "suppressor" from "helper" thymocytes. *J. Immunol.* 115:1744-1745, 1975.
102. Germain, R. N., and Benacerraf, B. A single major pathway of T lymphocyte interactions in antigen-specific immune suppression. *Scand. J. Immunol.* 13:1-10, 1981.
103. Germain, R. N., Ju, S. T., Kipps T. J., Benacerraf B., and Dorf, M. E. Shared idiotypic determinants on antibodies and T-cell-derived suppressor factor specific for the random terpolymer L-glutamic acid^{60}-L-alanine^{30}-L-tyrosine^{10}. *J. Exp. Med.* 149: 613-622, 1979.
104. Gershon, R. K., Eardley, D. D., Durun, S., Green, D. R., Shen, F. W., Yamauchi, K., Cantor, H., and Murphy, D. B. Contrasuppression: A novel immunoregulatory activity. *J. Exp. Med.* 153:1533-1546, 1982.
105. Gershon, R. K., and Kondo, K. Infectious immunological tolerance. *Immunology* 21:903-914, 1971.
106. Gershon, R. K., and Kondo, K. Cell interactions in the induction of tolerance: The role of thymic lymphocytes. *Immunology* 18:723-737, 1970.
107. Gill, H. K., and Liew, F. W. Regulation of delayed-type hypersensitivity. III. Effects of cyclophosphamide on the suppressor cells for delayed-type hypersensitivity to sheep erythrocytes in mice. *Eur. J. Immunol.* 8:172-176, 1978.
108. Gluckman, J-C., Klatzmann, D., Brisson, E., and Chapries, F. Mixed lymphocyte culture suppressor cells can be induced by non-HLA differences in man. *Cell. Immunol.* 89:242-249, 1984.
109. Goeken, N. E. Human suppressor cell induction in vitro: Preferential activation by class I MHC antigen. *J. Immunol.* 132:2291-2299, 1984.
110. Good, M. F., and Nossal, G. J. V. Functional clonal deletion and suppression as complementary mechanisms operative in adult hapten-induced cytotoxic T cell tolerance. *J. Immunol.* 131:2662-2669, 1983.
111. Gorczynski, R. M., and Chang, M. P. Peripheral (somatic) expansion of the murine cytotoxic T lymphocyte repertoire. II. Comparison of diversity in recognition repertoire of alloreactive T cells in spleen and thymus of young or aged DBA/2J mice transplanted with bone marrow cells from young or aged donor. *J. Immunol.* 133:2381-2389, 1984.
112. Gorczynski, R. M., and MacRae, S. Suppression of cytotoxic response to histoincompatible cells. I. Evidence for two types of T lymphocyte-derived suppressors acting at different stages in the induction of a cytotoxic response. *J. Immunol.* 122: 737-746, 1979.
113. Gorczynski, R. M., and MacRae, S. Suppression of cytotoxic response to histoincompatible cells. II. Analysis of the role of two independent T suppressor pools in maintenance of neonatally induced allograft tolerance in mice. *J. Immunol.* 122: 747-752, 1979.
114. Green, D. R. T8$^+$ augmenting cells: Contrasuppression in man? *J. Mol. Cell. Immunol.* 1:111-113, 1984.
115. Green, D. R., Chue, B., and Gershon, R. K. Discrimination of 2 types of suppressor T cells by cell surface phenotype and by function. *J. Mol. Cell. Immunol.* 1:19-28, 1983.
116. Green, D. R., Eardley, D. D., Kimura, A., Murphy, D. B., Yamauchi, K., and Gershon, R. K. Immunoregulatory circuits which modulate responsiveness to suppressor cell signals: Characterization of an effector cell in the contrasuppressor circuit. *Eur. J. Immunol.* 11:973-980, 1981.

117. Green, D. R., Flood, P. M., and Gershon, R. K. Immunoregulatory T-cell pathways. *Annu. Rev. Immunol.* 1:439-463, 1983.
118. Green, D. R., Gershon, R. K., and Eardley, D. D. Functional deletion of different Ly-1 T-cell-inducer subset activities by Ly-2 suppressor T lymphocytes. *Proc. Natl. Acad. Sci. USA* 78:3819-3823, 1980.
119. Greene, M. I., Nelles, M. J., Sy, M. S., and Nisonoff, A. Regulation of immunity to the azobenzenearsonate hapten. *Adv. Immunol.* 32:253-300, 1982.
120. Greene, M. I., Pierres, A., Dorf, M. E., and Benacerraf, B. The I-J subregion codes for determinants on suppressor factor(s) which limit the contract sensitivity response to picryl chloride. *J. Exp. Med.* 146:293-296, 1977.
121. Gruchalla, R. S., Strome, P. G., and Streilein, J. W. Analysis of neonatally induced tolerance of H-2 alloantigens. III. Ease of abolition of tolerance of class I, but not class II, antigens with infusions of syngeneic, immunocompetent cells. *Transplantation* 36:318-323, 1983.
122. Gualde, N., Weinberger, O., Rafnofsky, S., Benacerraf, B., and Burakoff, S. J. In vitro generation of helper T cells and suppressor T cells that regulate the cytolytic T lymphocyte response to trinitrophenyl-modified syngeneic cells. *Transplantation* 33:422-426, 1982.
123. Gunther, J., Haas, W., and Von Boehmer, H. Suppression of T cell responses through completion for T cell growth factor. *Eur. J. Immunol.* 12:247-249, 1982.
124. Hall, B. M. Mechanisms of specific unresponsiveness to allografts. *Transplant. Proc.* 16:938-943, 1984.
125. Hall, B. M., Jelbart, M. E., and Dorsch, S. E. Suppressor T cells in rats with prolonged cardiac allograft survival after treatment with cyclosporine. *Transplantation* 37:595-600, 1984.
126. Hall, B. M., Roser, B. J., and Dorsch, S. E. A model for study of the cellular mechanisms that maintain long-term enhancement of cardiac graft survival. *Transplant Proc.* 11:958-961, 1979.
127. Halle-Pannenko, O., Pritchard, L. L., and Rappaport, H. Alloimmunization-activated suppressor cells. I. Abrogation of lethal graft-versus-host reaction directed against non-H-2 antigens. *Transplantation* 36:60-68, 1983.
128. Hannum, C. H., Kappler, J. W., Trowbridge, I. S., Marrack, P., and Freed, J. H. Immunoglobulin-like nature of the α-chain of a human T-cell antigen/MHC receptor. *Nature* 312:65-67, 1984.
129. Hardt, C., Rollinghoff, M., Pfizenmaier, K., Mosmann, H., and Wagner, H. Lyt-23$^+$ cyclophosphamide-sensitive T cells regulate the activity of an interleukin 2 inhibitor in vivo. *J. Exp. Med.* 154:262-274, 1977.
130. Harris, D. E., Cairns, L., Rosen, F. S., and Borel, Y. A natural model of immunologic tolerance. Tolerance to murine C5 is mediated by T cells, and antigen is required to maintain unresponsiveness. *J. Exp. Med.* 156:567-584, 1982.
131. Hathcock, K. S., and Hodes, R. J. Regulatory mechanisms in cell-mediated immune response. V. Distinct Lyt subsets mediate antigen-specific and antigen-nonspecific suppression. *Transplantation* 36:298-303, 1983.
132. Hayes, C. E., Klyczek, K. K., Krum, D. P., Whitcomb, R. M., Hullet, D. A., and Cantor, H. Chromosome 4 Jt gene controls murine T cell surface I-J expression. *Science* 223:559-563, 1984.
133. Haynes, B. F., Schooley, R. T., Payling-Wright, C. R., Grouse, J. E., Dolin, R., and Fauci, A. S. Emergence of suppressor cells of immunoglobulin synthesis during acute Epstein-Barr virus-induced infectious mononucleosis. *J. Immunol.* 123:2095-2101, 1979.
134. Hendry, W. S., Tilney, N. L., Baldwin, W. M. 3rd, Graves, M. J., Milford, E., Strom, T. B., and Carpenter, C. B. Transfer of specific unresponsiveness to organ allografts

by thymocytes. Specific unresponsiveness by thymocyte transfer. *J. Exp. Med.* 149:1042-1055, 1979.

135. Herzenberg, L. A., Okumura, K., Cantor, H., Sato, V. L., Shen, F-W., Boyse, E. A., and Herzenberg, L. A. T-cell regulation of antibody responses: Demonstration of allotype-specific helper T cells and their specific removal by suppressor T cells. *J. Exp. Med.* 144:330-344, 1976.

136. Hess, A. D., and Tutschka, P. J. Effect of cyclosporin A on human lymphocyte responses in vitro. I. CsA allows for the expression of alloantigen-activated suppressor cells while preferentially inhibiting the induction of cytolytic effector lymphocytes in MLR. *J. Immunol.* 124:2601-2608, 1980.

137. Hirano, T., and Nordin, A. A. Cell-mediated immune response in vitro. I. The development of suppressor cells and cytotoxic lymphocytes in mixed lymphocyte cultures. *J. Immunol.* 116:1115-1122, 1976.

138. Hodes, R. J., and Hathcock, K. S. In vitro generation of suppressor cell activity: Suppression of in vitro induction of cell-mediated cytotoxicity. *J. Immunol.* 116: 167-177, 1976.

139. Hodes, R. J., and Hathcock, K. S. Regulatory mechanisms in cell-mediated immune responses. IV. Evidence for the spontaneous generation of suppressor cells in vitro. *Transplantation* 28:430-432, 1979.

140. Hodes, R. J., Nadler, L. M., and Hathcock, K. S. Regulatory mechanism in cell-mediated immune responses. III. Antigen specific and nonspecific suppressor activities generated during MLC. *J. Immunol.* 119:961-967, 1977.

141. Hood, L., Steinmetz, M., and Malissen, B. Genes of the major histocompatibility complex of the mouse. *Annu. Rev. Immunol.* 1:529-568, 1983.

142. Houssin, D., Charpentier, B., Gugenheim, J., Baudot, P., Tamisier, D., Lang, D., Gigou, M., and Bismuth, H. Spontaneous long-term acceptance of RT-1-incompatible liver allografts in inbred rats. Analysis of the immune status. *Transplantation* 36:615-620, 1983.

143. Hu, S. K., Eardley, D. D., Gershon, R. K., and Cantor, H. Acquisition of paralytic activity by inducer cells. *J. Mol. Cell. Immunol.* 1:91-98, 1984.

144. Hunt, J. S., Manning, L. S., and Wood, G. W. Macrophages in murine uterus are immunosuppressive. *Cell. Immunol.* 85:499-510, 1984.

145. Hutchinson, I. F., Shadur, C. A., Duarte, J. S., Strom, T. B., and Tilney, N. L. Cyclosporin A spares selectively lymphocytes with donor-specific suppressor characteristics. *Transplantation* 32:210-216, 1981.

146. Ikezawa, Z., Arden, B., Nagy, Z. A., and Klein, J. Feedback regulation of immune suppression by a suppressor factor. *Eur. J. Immunol.* 14:681-686, 1984.

147. Ishii, N., Baxevanis, C. N., Nagy, Z. A., and Klein, J. Selection of H-2 molecules for the context of antigen recognition by T lymphocytes. *Immunogenetics* 14: 283:292, 1981.

148. Iverson, M., Tpak, W., Green, D. R., and Gershon, R. K. Role of contrasuppression in the adoptive transfer of immunity. *J. Exp. Med.* 158:982-987, 1983.

149. Jacoby, D. R., Olding, L. B., and Oldstone, M. B. Immunologic regulation of fetal-maternal balance. *Adv. Immunol.* 35:157-208, 1984.

150. Jandinski, J., Cantor, H., Tadakuma, T., Peavy, D. L., and Pierce, C. W. Separation of helper T cells from suppressor T cells expressing different Ly components. I. Polyclonal activation: Suppressor and helper activities are inherent properties of distinct T-cell subclasses. *J. Exp. Med.* 143:1382-1390, 1976.

151. Jardiere, P., Ude, T., and Ishizaka, K. IGE-binding factors from mouse T lymphocytes. III. Role of antigen-specific suppressor T cells in the formation of IgE-suppressive factor. *J. Immunol.* 133:3266-3273, 1984.

152. Kapp, J. A., Pierce, C. W., Schlossman, S., and Benacerraf, B. Genetic control of

immune responses in vitro. V. Stimulation of suppressor T cells in nonresponder mice by the terpolymer L-glutamic acid^{60}-L-alanine^{30}-L-tyrosine^{10} (GAT). *J. Exp. Med.* 140:172-184, 1974.

153. Kapp, J. A., Pierce, C. W., Theze, J., and Benacerraf, B. Modulation of immune responses by suppressor T cells. *Fed. Proc.* 37:2361-2364, 1978.
154. Kasakura, S., Taguchi, M., Murachi, T., Uchino, H., and Hanaoka, M. A new mediator (suppressor cell induction factor) activating T cell-mediated suppression: Characterization of suppressor cells, kinetics of their generation, and mechanisms of their action. *J. Immunol.* 131:2307-2315, 1983.
155. Katz, D. H., Chen, S. S., Liu, F. T., Bogowitz, C. A., and Katz, L. R. Biologically active molecules regulating the IgE antibody system: Biochemical and biological comparisons of suppressive factor of allergy and enhancing factor of allergy. *J. Mol. Cell. Immunol.* 1:157-166, 1984.
156. Kaufmann, S. H., Hahn, H., and Diamantstein, T. Relative susceptibilities of T cell subsets involved in delayed-type hypersensitivity to sheep red blood cells to the in vitro action of 4-hydroperoxycyclophosphamide. *J. Immunol.* 125:1104-1108, 1980.
157. Kaymakcalan, Z., Nitecki, D. E., Lewis, G. K., and Goodman, J. W. Differential induction of help and suppression in mice by bifunctional antigens administered via different routes. *Mol. Immunol.* 21:529-536, 1984.
158. Kedar, E., and Avraham, Y. Amplification by hydrocortisone of the induction of cytotoxic response in vitro to syngeneic murine leukemias. *Transplantation* 29:169-171, 1980.
159. Kerman, R. H., Agastino, G., Van Buren, C. T., Payne, W., Flechner, S., Conley, S., Brewer, E., and Kahan, B. D. Effect of blood transfusions on graft survival and immune responsiveness. *Transplant. Proc.* 15:1022-1025, 1983.
160. Kilshaw, P. J., Brent, L., and Pinto, M. Suppressor T cells in mice made unresponsive to skin allografts. *Nature* 255:489-491, 1975.
161. Kim, B. S. Mechanisms of idiotype suppression. I. In vitro generation of idiotype-specific suppressor T cells by anti-idiotype antibodies and specific antigen. *J. Exp. Med.* 149:1371-1378, 1979.
162. Kim, B. S., and Greenberg, J. A. Mechanisms of idiotype suppression. IV. Functional neutralization in mixtures of idiotype-specific suppressor and hapten-specific suppressor T cells. *J. Exp. Med.* 154:809-820, 1981.
163. Kirtland, H. H., III, Mohler, D. N., and Horwitz, D. A. Methyldopa inhibition of suppressor-lymphocyte function: A proposed cause of autoimmune hemolytic anemia. *N. Engl. J. Med.* 302:825-832, 1980.
164. Kitamura, K., Nakauchi, H., Koyasu, S., Yahara, I., and Tada, O. K. Characterization of an antigen-specific suppressive factor derived from a cloned suppressor effector T cell line. *J. Immunol.* 133:1371-1378, 1984.
165. Klatzmann, D., Gluckman, J. C., Foucault, C., Bensussan, A., Assabga, U., and Duboust, A. Suppression of lymphocyte reactivity by blood transfusions in uremic patients. I. Proliferative responses. *Transplantation* 35:332-338, 1983.
166. Klein, J., and Nagy, Z. A. Trouble in the J-land. *Nature* 300:12-13, 1982.
167. Klein, J. What causes immunologic non-responsiveness? *Immunol. Rev.* 81:177-202, 1984.
168. Klein, J., Juretic, A., Baxevanis, C. N., and Nagy, Z. A. The traditional and a new version of the mouse H-2 complex. *Nature* 291:455-460, 1981.
169. Knop, J., Malorny, U., and Macher, E. Selective induction of delayed hypersensitivity T-effector and T-suppressor lymphocytes in vitro by haptenized bone-marrow-derived macrophages. *Cell. Immunol.* 88:411-420, 1984.
170. Kontiainen, S., and Feldmann, M. Suppressor cell induction in vitro. I. Kinetics of induction of antigen-specific suppressor cells. *Eur. J. Immunol.* 6:296-301, 1976.

171. Koszinowski, U. H., and Kramer, M. Selective inhibition of T suppressor-cell function by a monosaccharide. *Nature* 289:181-184, 1981.
172. Kripke, M. Immunological unresponsiveness induced by ultraviolet radiation. *Immunol. Rev.* 80:87-102, 1984.
173. Kronenberg, M., Steinmetz, M., Kabori, J., Kraig, E., Kapp, J. A., Pierce, C. W., Sorensen, C. M., Suzuki, G., Tada, T., and Hood, L. RNA transcripts for I-J polypeptides are apparently not encoded between the I-A and I-E subregions of the murine major histocompatibility complex. *Proc. Natl. Acad. Sci. USA* 80:5704-5708, 1983.
174. Kumagai, Y., Okumura, K., and Tada, T. Photoaffinity-labeled hapten-binding T-cell receptor on a suppressor T-cell hybridoma. *Mol. Immunol.* 21:545-559, 1984.
175. Kupiec-Weglinski, J. W., Filko, M. A., Strom, T. B., and Tilney, N. L. Sparing of suppressor cells: A critical action of cyclosporine. *Transplantation* 38:97-101, 1984.
176. Kupiec-Weglinski, J. W., Lear, P. A., Bordes-Aznar, J., Tilney, N. L., and Strom, T. B. Acute rejection in cyclosporin A-treated graft recipients occurs following abrogation of suppressor cells. *Transplant. Proc.* 15:531-534, 1983.
177. Kupper, T. S., and Green, D. R. Immunoregulation after thermal injury: Sequential appearance of I-J+, Ly1 T suppressor inducer cells and Ly-2 T suppressor effector cells following thermal trauma in mice. *J. Immunol.* 133:3047-3053, 1984.
178. Kurata, A., Yamauchi, K., Watanabe, T., Nonaka, M., Abe, R., Okumura, K., and Tada, T. Is there multiplicity in I-J subregion products? *J. Mol. Cell. Immunol.* 1: 267-277, 1984.
179. Lagrange, P. H., and Mackaness, G. B. Site of action of serum factors that block delayed-type hypersensitivity in mice. *J. Exp. Med.* 148:235-245, 1978.
180. Landay, A., Gartland, G. L., and Clement, L. T. Characterization of a phenotypically distinct subpopulation of Leu-2$^+$ cells that suppresses T cell proliferative responses. *J. Immunol.* 131:2757-2761, 1983.
181. Lau, C. Y., Budz-Tymkewycz, S., Wang, E. Y., and Ishaque, A. A mutant human T-cell line producing immunosuppressive factors. *Cell. Immunol.* 87:35-52, 1984.
182. Leapman, S. B., Filo, R. S., Smith, E. J., and Smith, P. G. In vitro effects of cyclosporin A on lymphocyte subpopulations. I. Suppressor cell sparing by cyclosporin A. *Transplantation* 30:404-408, 1980.
183. Ledbetter, J. A., Evans, R. L., Lipinski, M., Cunningham-Rundles, C., Good, R. A., and Herzenberg, L. A. Evolutionary conservation of surface molecules that distinguish T lymphocyte helper/inducer and cytotoxic/suppressor subpopulations in mouse and man. *J. Exp. Med.* 153:310-323, 1981.
184. Ledbetter, J. A., Rouse, R. R., Micklem, H. S., and Herzenberg, L. A. T cell subsets defined by expression of Lyt-1,2,3 and Thy-1 antigens. Two parameter immunofluorescence and cytotoxicity analysis with monoclonal antibodies modifies current views. *J. Exp. Med.* 152:280-295, 1980.
185. Lehner, T., Brines, R., Jones, T., and Avery, J. Detection of cross-reacting murine I-J like determinants on a human subset of T8$^+$ antigen binding, presenting and contrasuppressor cells. *Clin. Exp. Immunol.* 58:410-419, 1984.
186. Lehner, T., and Jones, T. A comparative study of streptococcal antigen-binding human T8$^+$ cells and monocytes, in relation to the HLA-DRw6 locus and the helper, suppressor and contrasuppressor functions. *Immunology* 53:215-226, 1984.
187. Lehner, T., and Jones, T. Role of MHC class II antigenic determinants in the function of human antigen binding T8$^+$ cells, monocytes and helper and suppressor factors. *Clin. Exp. Immunol.* 56:683-693, 1984.
188. Lei, H.-Y., and Waltenbaugh, C. Regulation of immune responses by I-J gene products. IV. Distinct suppressor factors derived from "nonsuppressor" a strain mice. *J. Immunol.* 133:1723-1729, 1984.

189. Lenhard, V., Massen, G., Seifert, P., Johannsen, R., and Grosse-Wilde, H. Characterization of transfusion-induced suppressor cells in prospective kidney allograft recipients. *Transplant. Proc.* 14:329-332, 1982.
190. Liew, F. Y. Regulation of delayed-type hypersensitivity. I. T suppressor cells for delayed-type hypersensitivity to sheep erythrocytes in mice. *Eur. J. Immunol.* 7: 714-718, 1977.
191. Liew, F. Y. Regulation of delayed-type hypersensitivity. VII. The role of I-J subregion gene products in the inhibition of delayed-type hypersensitivity to major histocompatibility antigens by specific suppressor T cells. *Eur. J. Immunol.* 11:883-888, 1981.
192. Loblay, R. H., Fazekas de St. Groth, B., Pritchard-Briscoe, H., and Basten, A. Suppressor T cell memory. II. The role of memory suppressor T cells in tolerance to human gamma globulin. *J. Exp. Med.* 157:957-973, 1983.
193. Lomnitzer, R., Phillips, R., and Rabson, A. R. Suppression of interleukin-2 production by human concanavalin A-induced suppressor cells. *Cell. Immunol.* 86:362-370, 1984.
194. Lowy, A., Tominaga, A., Drebin, J. A., Takaoki, M., Benacerraf, B., and Greene, M. I. Identification of an I-J$^+$ antigen-presenting cell required for third order suppressor cell activation. *J. Exp. Med.* 157:353-358, 1983.
195. Lukic, M. L., and Mitchison, N. A. Self- and allo-specific suppressor T cells evoked by intravenous injection of F protein. *Eur. J. Immunol.* 14:766-768, 1984.
196. Lum, L. G., Orcutt-Thordarson, N., Seigneuret, M. C., and Hansen, J. A. In vitro regulation of immunoglobulin synthesis by T-cell subpopulations defined by a new human T-cell antigen. *Cell. Immunol.* 72:122-129, 1982.
197. Macphail, S., and Stutman, O. Suppressor T cells activated in a primary in vitro response to non-major histocompatibility alloantigens. *J. Exp. Med.* 156:1398-1414, 1982.
198. Maki, T., Gottschalk, R., Wood, M. L., and Monaco, A. P. Specific unresponsiveness to skin allografts in anti-lymphocyte serum-treated, marrow-injected mice: Participation of donor marrow-derived suppressor T cells. *J. Immunol.* 127:1433-1438, 1981.
199. Maki, T., Okazaki, H., Wood, M. L., and Monaco, A. P. Suppressor cells in mice bearing intact skin allografts after blood transfusions. *Transplantation* 32:463-466, 1981.
200. Maki, T., Simpson, M., and Monaco, A. P. Development of suppressor T cells by antilymphocyte serum treatment in mice. *Transplantation* 34:376-381, 1982.
201. Malkovsky, M., Asherson, G. L., Stockinger, B., and Walkins, M. C. Nonspecific inhibitor released by T acceptor cells reduces the production of interleukin-2. *Nature* 300:652-655, 1982.
202. Marquet, R. L., and Heystek, G. A. Induction of suppressor cells by donor-specific blood transfusions and heart transplantation in rats. *Transplantation* 31:272-274, 1981.
203. Mattingly, J. A. Immunologic suppression after oral administration of antigen. II. Activation of suppressor-inducer cells in the Peyer's patches. *Cell. Immunol.* 86: 46-52, 1984.
204. Mattingly, J. A., and Waksman, B. H. Immunologic suppression after oral administration of antigen. I. Specific suppressor cells formed in rat Peyer's patches after oral administration of antigen. I. Specific suppressor cells formed in rat Peyer's patches after oral administration of sheep erythrocytes and their systemic migration. *J. Immunol.* 121:1878-1883, 1978.
205. McCullough, C. S., Sugarbaker, P. H., and Matthews, W. Effects of passive enhancement on graft and host. *Transplantation* 37:91-96, 1984.

206. McMichael, A. J., and Sasazuki, T. A suppressor T cell in the human mixed lymphocyte reaction. *J. Exp. Med.* 146:368-380, 1977.
207. Mehra, V., Mason, L. H., Rothman, W., Reinherz, E., Schlossman, S. F., and Bloom, B. R. Delineation of a human t cell subset responsible for lepromin-induced suppression in leprosy patients. *J. Immunol.* 125:1183-1188, 1980.
208. Meruelo, D., Flieger, N., Smith, D., and McDevitt, H. O. In vivo or in vitro treatments with anti-I-J alloantisera abolish immunity to AKR leukemia. *Proc. Natl. Acad. Sci. USA* 77:2178-2182, 1980.
209. Milburn, G. L., and Lynch, R. G. Immunoregulation of murine myeloma in vitro. II. Suppression of MOPC-315 immunoglobulin secretion and synthesis by idiotype-specific suppressor T cells. *J. Exp. Med.* 155:852-862, 1982.
210. Miller, J., Clark, C., Sigmon, E., and Azar, M. Development of suppressor cells as a second generation mixed lymphocyte culture phenomenon in mls and non-H-2-disparate inbred mice. *Transplantation* 26:308-314, 1978.
211. Miller, S. D., and Butler, L. D. T-cell responses induced by the parenteral injection of antigen-modified syngeneic cells. III. Dissociation of primed cytolytic T-cell and efferent suppressor-T-cell activity following intravenous injection of trinitrophenol-modified syngeneic spleen cells. *Cell. Immunol.* 86:308-316, 1984.
212. Miller, S. D., Sy, M. S., and Claman, H. N. H-2 restriction of suppressor T cell induction by hapten-modified lymphoid cells in tolerance to 1-fluoro-2,4-dinitrobenzene contact sensitization. *J. Exp. Med.* 145:1071-1076, 1977.
213. Miller, S. D., Sy, M. S., and Claman, H. N. The induction of hapten-specific T cell tolerance using hapten-modified lymphoid cells. II. Relative roles of suppressor T cells and clone inhibition in the tolerant state. *Eur. J. Immunol.* 7:165-170, 1977.
214. Miller, S. D., Sy, M. S., and Claman, H. N. Suppressor T cell mechanisms in contact sensitivity. I. Efferent blockade by syninduced suppressor T cells. *J. Immunol.* 121:265-273, 1978.
215. Miller, S. D., Sy, M. S., and Claman, H. N. Suppressor T cell mechanisms in contact sensitivity. II. Afferent blockade by alloinduced suppressor T cells. *J. Immunol.* 121:274-280, 1978.
216. Minami, M., Aoki, I., Honji, N., Waltenbaugh, C., R., and Dorf, M. E. The role of I-J and IgH determinants on F_1 derived suppressor factor in controlling restriction specificity. *J. Exp. Med.* 158:1428-1443, 1983.
217. Minami, M., Furusawa, S., and Dorf, M. E. I-J restrictions on the activation and interaction of parental and F_1-derived Ts_3 suppressor cells. *J. Exp. Med.* 156:465-479, 1982.
218. Minami, M., Honji, N., and Dorf, M. E. Mechanisms responsible for the induction of I-J restriction on Ts_3 suppressor cells. *J. Exp. Med.* 156:1502-1515, 1982.
219. Minami, M., Okuda, K., Furusawa, S., Benacerraf, B., and Dorf, M. E. Analysis of T cell hybridomas. I. Characterization of H-2 and Igh-restricted monoclonal suppressor factors. *J. Exp. Med.* 154:1390-1402, 1981.
220. Minami, M., Okuda, K., Furusawa, S., and Dorf, M. E. Analysis of T cell hybridomas. IV. Characterization of inducible suppressor cell hybridomas. *J. Exp. Med.* 157:1379-1395, 1983.
221. Monroe, J. G., Lowy, A., Granstein, R. D., and Greene, M. I. Studies of immune responsiveness and unresponsiveness to the p-azabenzenearsonate (ABA) hapten. *Immunol. Rev.* 80:103-131, 1984.
222. Moorhead, J. W. Tolerance and contact sensitivity to DNFB in mice. VI. Inhibition of afferent sensitivity by suppressor T cells in adoptive tolerance. *J. Immunol.* 117:802-806, 1976.
223. Moretta, L., Webb, S. R., Grossi, C. E., Lydyard, P. M., and Cooper, M. D. Functional analysis of two human T-cell subpopulations: Help and suppression of B-

cell responses by T cells bearing receptors for IgM or IgG. *J. Exp. Med.* 146:184-200, 1977.

224. Morikawa, S., Baba, M., Harada, T., and Mitsuoka, A. Studies on delayed-type hypersensitivity in mice. III. Evidence for suppressive regulatory T-cell population in delayed hypersensitivity. *J. Exp. Med.* 145:237-248, 1977.
225. Morimoto, C., Distaso, J. A., Cheney, J. J., Reinherz, E. L., and Schlossman, S. F. Cellular interaction between subsets of T8 population for maximal suppression of antigen-specific antibody response. *Cell. Immunol.* 88:75-84, 1984.
226. Morimoto, C., Reinherz, E. L., Borel, Y., and Schlossman, S. F. Direct demonstration of the human suppressor inducer subset by anti-T cell antibodies. *J. Immunol.* 130:157-161, 1983.
227. Mosier, D. E., and Johnson, B. M. Ontogeny of mouse lymphocyte function. II. Development of the ability to produce antibody is modulated by T lymphocytes. *J. Exp. Med.* 141:216-226, 1975.
228. Munster, A. M. Post-traumatic immunosuppression is due to activation of suppressor T cells. *Lancet* 1:1329-1330, 1976.
229. Murphy, D. B., Herzenberg, L. A., Okumura, K. O., Herzenberg, L. A., and McDevitt, H. O. A new I subregion (I-J) marked by a locus controlling surface determinants on suppressor T lymphocytes. *J. Exp. Med.* 144:699-712, 1976.
230. Nabel, G., Allard, W. J., and Cantor, H. A cloned cell line mediating natural killer cell function inhibits immunoglobulin secretion. *J. Exp. Med.* 156:658-663, 1982.
231. Nadler, L. M., and Hodes, R. J. Regulatory mechanisms in cell-mediated immune responses. II. Comparison of culture-induced and alloantigen-induced suppressor cells in MLR and CML. *J. Immunol.* 118:1886-1895, 1977.
232. Nakauchi, H., Ohno, I., Kim. M., Okumura, K., and Tada, T. Establishment and functional analysis of a cloned, antigen-specific suppressor effector T cell line. *J. Immunol.* 132:88-94, 1984.
233. Okazaki, H., Maki, T., Wood, M. L., Jones, S., and Monaco, A. P. Prolongation of skin allograft survival in H-2 K and I region-incompatible mice by pretransplantation blood transfusion. *Transplantation* 32:111-115, 1981.
234. Okazaki, H., Maki, T., Wood, M., and Monaco, A. P. Effect of a single transfusion of donor-specific and nonspecific blood on skin allograft survival in mice. *Transplantation* 30:421-424, 1980.
235. Okuda, K., Minami, M., Furusawa, M., and Dorf, M. E. Analysis of T cell hybridomas. II. Comparisons among three distinct types of monoclonal suppressor factors. *J. Exp. Med.* 154:1838-1851, 1981.
236. Okuda, K., Minami, M., Ju, S. T., and Dorf, M. E. Functional association of idiotypic and I-J determinants on the antigen receptor of suppressor T cells. *Proc. Natl. Acad. Sci. USA* 78:4557-4561, 1981.
237. Okuda, K., Minami, M., Sherr, D. H., and Dorf, M. E. Hapten-specific T cell responses to 4-hydroxy-3-nitrophenyl acetyl. XI. Pseudogenetic restrictions of hybridoma suppressor factors. *J. Exp. Med.* 154:468-479, 1981.
238. Osband, M. E., Lipton, J. M., Lavin, P., Levey, R., Vawter, G., Greenberger, J. S., McCaffrey, R. P., and Parkman, R. Histiocytosis X. Demonstration of abnormal immunity. T-cell histamine H2-receptor deficiency and successful treatment with thymic extract. *N. Engl. J. Med.* 304:146-153, 1981.
239. Osband, M. E., and Parkman, R. The control of autoreactivity. I. Lack of autoreactivity in murine spleens is due to concomitant presence of suppressor and autocytotoxic lymphocytes. *J. Immunol.* 121:179-185, 1978.
240. Owen, F. L. Products of the IgT-C region of chromosome 12 are maturational markers for T cells. Sequence of appearance in immunocompetent T cells parallels ontogenetic appearance of Tthyd, Tindd, and Tsud. *J. Exp. Med.* 156:703-718, 1982.

241. Owen, F. L., Finnegan, A., Gates, E. R., and Gattlieb, P. D. A mature T lymphocyte subpopulation marker closely linked to the Ig-1 allotype Ch locus. *Eur. J. Immunol.* 9:948-955, 1979.
242. Owen, F. L., Ju, S. T., and Nisonoff, A. Presence on idiotype-specific suppressor T cells of receptors that interact with molecules bearing the idiotype. *J. Exp. Med.* 145:1559-1566, 1977.
243. Palacios, R., and Moller, G. T cell growth factor abrogates concanavalin A-induced suppressor cell function. *J. Exp. Med.* 153:1360-1365, 1981.
244. Pawelec, G., Schneider, M. E., and Piter, W. Cloned human T lymphocytes with lymphostimulatory capacity preferentially activate suppressor cells. *Eur. J. Immunol.* 14:335-340, 1984.
245. Peavy, D. L., and Pierce, C. W. Cell-mediated immune responses in vitro. I. Suppression of the generation of cytotoxic lymphocytes by concanavalin A and concanavalin A-activated spleen cells. *J. Exp. Med.* 140:365-369, 1974.
246. Pescovitz, M. D., Auchincloss, H., Jr., Thistlethwaite, J. R., Jr., and Sachs, D. H. Transplantation in miniature swine: Acceptance of class I antigen mismatched renal allografts. *Transplant. Proc.* 15:1124-1126, 1983.
247. Petersen, E. A., Neva, F. A., Oster, C. N., and Bogaert Diaz, H. Specific inhibition of lymphocyte-proliferation responses by adherent suppressor cells in diffuse cutaneous leishmaniasis. *N. Engl. J. Med.* 306:387-392, 1982.
248. Pfeffer, P. F., Thorsby, E., and Hirschberg, H. Donor-specific decreased cell-mediated cytotoxicity in recipients of well functioning, one HLA haplotype-mismatched kidney allografts. *Transplantation* 35:156-160, 1983.
249. Pierce, C. W., Peavy, D. L., and Tadakuma, T. Suppressor T cells as regulators of lymphocyte functions. *Ann. N.Y. Acad. Sci.* 256:365-374, 1975.
250. Pierres, M., Germain, R. N., Dorf, M. E., and Benacerraf, B. In vivo effects of anti-Ia alloantisera. I. Elimination of specific suppression by in vivo administration of antisera specific for I-J controlled determinants. *J. Exp. Med.* 147:656-666, 1978.
251. Pierri, I., Rogna, S., Pende, D., Viglione, D., Scudeletti, M., Barabino, A., and Indiveri, F. Role of normal adherent cells in the regulations of the autologous mixed lymphocyte reaction in humans. *J. Clin. Immunol.* 4:197-201, 1984.
252. Pilarski, L. M., and Gibney, D. J. Control by positive and negative regulatory cells of the generation of antigen-specific suppressor T cells that inhibit cytotoxic T cell responses to alloantigens. *Transplantation* 38:55-62, 1984.
253. Pilarski, L. M., and Krowka, J. F. Regulation of the induction of cytotoxic T cells by antigen-specific T cell factors. In *Recognition and Regulation of Cell-Mediated Immunity,* J. D. Watson and J. Marbrook, eds. New York, Marcel Dekker, 1985, p. 367.
254. Pilarski, L. M., and McKenzie, I. F. Lyt antigens on the T cells specific for minor histocompatibility antigens: Suppression by a Lyt $1^{+}2^{-}$ regulator. *Transplantation* 32:363-367, 1981.
255. Pritchard, L. L., and Halle-Pannenko, O. Alloimmunization-activated suppressor cells. II. In vitro activity of suppressor cells implicated in the abrogation of lethal graft-vs-host reaction. *Transplantation* 36:310-318, 1983.
256. Prud'homme, G. J., Fuks, A., Colle, E., Seemayer, T. A., and Guttman, R. A. Immune dysfunction in diabetes-prone BB rats. Interleukin 2 production and other mitogen-induced responses are suppressed by activated macrophages. *J. Exp. Med.* 159:463-478, 1984.
257. Ptak, W., Bereta, M., Marcinkiewicz, J. O., Gershon, R. K., and Green, D. R. Production of antigen-specific contrasuppressor cells and factor, and their use in augmentation of cell-mediated immunity. *J. Immunol.* 133:623-628, 1984.
258. Ptak, W., Gershon, R. K., and Flood, P. M. Mechanisms of suppression in the

transfer of contact sensitivity: Analysis of an I-J$^+$ molecule required for Ly2 suppressor cell activity. *J. Exp. Med.* 158:1822-1835, 1983.
259. Ptak, W., Rozycka, D., Askenase, P. W., and Gershon, R. K. Role of antigen-presenting cells in the development and persistence of contact hypersensitivity. *J. Exp. Med.* 151:362-375, 1980.
260. Ptak, W., Zembala, M., and Gershon, R. K. Intermediary role of macrophages in the passage of suppressor signals between T-cell subsets. *J. Exp. Med.* 148:424-434, 1978.
261. Rammensee, H.-G., Fink, P. J., and Bevan, M. J. Functional clonal deletion of class I-specific cytotoxic T lymphocytes by veto cells that express antigen. *J. Immunol.* 133:2390-2396, 1984.
262. Ramshaw, I. A., Bretscher, P. A., and Parish, C. R. Regulation of the immune response. I. Suppression of delayed-type hypersensitivity by T cells from mice expressing humoral immunity. *Eur. J. Immunol.* 6:674-679, 1976.
263. Ramshaw, I. A., Bretscher, P. A., and Parish, C. R. Regulation of the immune response. II. Repressor T cells in cyclophosphamide-induced tolerant mice. *Eur. J. Immunol.* 7:180-185, 1977.
264. Rao, A., Faas, S. J., Miller, L. J., Riback, P. S., and Cantor, H. Lysis of inducer T cell clones by activated macrophages and macrophage-like cell lines. *J. Exp. Med.* 158:1243-1258, 1983.
265. Rao, V. S., Bennett, J. A., Shen, F. W., Gershon, R. K., and Mitchell, M. S. Antigen-antibody complexes generate Lyt 1 inducers of suppressor cells. *J. Immunol.* 125: 63-67, 1980.
266. Raskova, J., Ghobrial, I., Shea, S., Eisinger, R., and Raska, K. Suppressor cells in end-stage renal disease. *Am. J. Med.* 76:847-853, 1984.
267. Reinherz, E. L., O'Brien, C., Rosenthal, P., and Schlossman, S. F. The cellular basis for viral-induced immunodeficiency: Analysis by monoclonal antibodies. *J. Immunol.* 125:1269-1274, 1980.
268. Reinherz, E. L., Parkman, R., Rappeport, J., Rosen, F. S., and Schlossman, S. F. Aberrations of suppressor T cells in human graft-versus-host disease. *N. Engl. J. Med.* 300:1061-1068, 1979.
269. Reinherz, E. L., Weiner, H. L., Hauser, S. L., Cohen, J. A., Distaso, J. A., and Schlossman, S. F. Loss of suppressor T cells in active multiple sclerosis. Analysis with monoclonal antibodies. *N. Engl. J. Med.* 303:125-129, 1980.
270. Ress, S. R., Strassmann, G., and Bach, F. H. The phenotype of antigen-specific suppressor T cells generated in human mixed leucocyte culture depends on the nature of the major histocompatibility regions recognized. *Hum. Immunol.* 10:41-55, 1984.
271. Rich, R. R., Chu, L., and Rich, S. S. Fractionation of lymphocyte subpopulations which regulate mixed lymphocyte reactions. *J. Immunol.* 118:1252-1258, 1977.
272. Rich, R. R., and Rich, S. S. Biological expressions of lymphocyte activation. IV. Concanavalin A-activated suppressor cells in mouse mixed lymphocyte reactions. *J. Immunol.* 114:1112-1115, 1975.
273. Rich, S. Regulatory mechanisms in cell-mediated immune responses. Role of I-J and I-C determinants in the activation of H-2I and H-2K/D alloantigen-specific suppressor T cells. *J. Exp. Med.* 158:738-751, 1983.
274. Rich, S. S., David, C. S., and Rich, R. R. Regulatory mechanisms in cell-mediated immune responses. VII. Presence of I-C subregion determinants on mixed leukocyte reaction suppressor factor. *J. Exp. Med.* 149:114-126, 1979.
275. Rich, S. S., and Rich, R. R. Regulatory mechanisms in cell mediated immune responses. I. Regulation of mixed lymphocyte reactions by alloantigen-activated thymus-derived lymphocytes. *J. Exp. Med.* 140:1588-1603, 1974.

276. Rich, S. S., and Rich, R. R. Regulatory mechanisms in cell-mediated immune responses. II. A genetically restricted suppressor of mixed lymphocyte reactions released by alloantigen-activated spleen cells. *J. Exp. Med.* 142:1391-1402, 1975.
277. Rich, S. S., and Rich, R. R. Regulatory mechanisms in cell-mediated immune responses. III. I-region control of suppressor cell interaction with responder cells in mixed lymphocyte reactions. *J. Exp. Med.* 143:672-677, 1976.
278. Rocklin, R. E., and Habarek-Davidson, A. Pharmacologic modulation in vitro of human histamine-induced suppressor cell activity. *Int. J. Immunopharmacol.* 6: 179-186, 1984.
279. Rocklin, R. E., Sheffer, A. L., Greineder, D. K., and Melmon, K. L. Generation of antigen-specific suppressor cells during allergy desensitization. *N. Engl. J. Med.* 302:1213-1219, 1980.
280. Rode, H. N., Uotila, M., and Gordon, J. Regulation of the mixed leukocyte culture reaction by suppressor cells. *Eur. J. Immunol.* 8:213-216, 1978.
281. Rogers, T. J., Nowowiejski, I., and Webb, D. R. Partial characterization of prostaglandin-induced suppressor factor. *Cell. Immunol.* 50:82-93, 1980.
282. Rolink, A. G., Radaszkiewicz, T., Pals, S. T., van der Meer, W. G., and Gleichmann, E. Allosuppressor and allohelper T cells in acute and chronic graft-vs-host disease. I. Alloreactive suppressor cells rather than killer T cells appear to be the decisive effector cells in lethal graft-vs-host disease. *J. Exp. Med.* 155:1501-1522, 1982.
283. Roser, B. J., Herbert, J., and Godden, U. The role of suppressor cells in transplantation. *Transplant. Proc.* 15:698-703, 1983.
284. Ross, C. A., and Pilarski, L. M. Suppressor T cells derived from early postnatal murine spleen inhibit cytotoxic T-cell responses. *Cell Immunol.* 58:345-355, 1981.
285. Ruby, J. C., Martin, C. L., and Muller, H. K. Flow cytometric detection of histomine binding to lymphocytes. *Int. Arch. Allergy Appl. Med.* 73:198-204, 1984.
286. Ryan, J. J., Gress, R. E., Hathcock, K. S., and Hodes, R. J. Recognition and response to alloantigens in vivo. II. Priming with accessory cell-depleted donor allogeneic splenocytes: Induction of specific unresponsiveness to foreign major histocompatibility complex determinants. *J. Immunol.* 133:2343-2350, 1984.
287. Saito, T., and Taniguchi, M. Chemical features of an antigen-specific suppressor T cell factor composed of two polypeptide chains. *J. Mol. Cell. Immunol.* 1:137-144, 1984.
288. Sasportes, M., Carosella, E., Bensussan, A., Mihaesco, C., and Dausset, J. Regulation of the human allogeneic proliferative response in vitro. II. Production of soluble suppressor factors by suppressor T cells and evidence in favor of "acceptor" cells for suppression among unprimed lymphocytes. *Immunogenetics* 14:117-127, 1981.
289. Schulof, R. S., Chorba, T. L., and Ney, A. B. Are the suppressor cells suppressing in infectious mononucleosis (letter)? *N. Engl. J. Med.* 304:1492-1493, 1981.
290. Schwartz, A., and Gershon, R. K. Regulation of in vitro cytotoxic T lymphocytes generation. III. Interactions of regulatory T cell subsets in suppressor and target populations. *J. Mol. Cell. Immunol.* 1:237-249, 1984.
291. Schwartz, A., Sutton, S. L., and Gershon, R. K. Regulation of in vitro cytotoxic T lymphocyte generation. II. Demonstration of non-cytotoxic alloantigen-specific suppressor T lymphocytes. *Eur. J. Immunol.* 12:380-386, 1982.
292. Schwartz, M., Waltenbaugh, C., Dorf, M., Cesla, R., Sela, M., and Benacerraf, B. Determinants of antigenic molecules responsible for genetically controlled regulation of immune responses. *Proc. Natl. Acad. Sci. USA* 73:2862-2866, 1976.
293. Segal, S., Melmon, K. L., and Weinstein, Y. Isolation of suppressor T lymphocytes adherent to histamine conjugated albumin and their role in suppression of IgG response to SRBC. *Cell Immunol.* 59:171-180, 1981.
294. Shand, F. L., and Liew, F. Y. Differential sensitivity to cyclophosphamide of helper

T cells for humoral responses and suppressor T cells for delayed-type hypersensitivity. *Eur. J. Immunol.* 10:480-483, 1980.

295. Shearer, G. M., and Polisson, R. P. Mutual recognition of parental and F_1 lymphocytes. Selective abrogation of cytotoxic potential of F_1 lymphocytes by parental lymphocytes. *J. Exp. Med.* 151:20-31, 1980.
296. Sheehy, M. J., Mawas, C., and Charmot, D. Specific inhibition of human lymphocyte responses by primed autologous lymphocytes. I. Evaluation of MLR inhibition as a model for suppression. *J. Immunol.* 122:2198-2203, 1979.
297. Sherr, D. H., Benacerraf, B., and Dorf, M. E. Immune suppression in vivo with antigen-modified syngeneic cells. V. Interacting T cell subpopulations in the suppressor pathway. *J. Immunol.* 125:1862-1868, 1980.
298. Sherr, D. H., Heghinian, K. M., Benacerraf, B., and Dorf, M. E. Immune suppression in vivo with antigen-modified syngeneic cells. III. Distinctions between T cell tolerance and T cell mediated suppression. *J. Immunol.* 123:2682-2688, 1979.
299. Smith, J. B., and Knowlton, R. P. Activation of suppressor T cells in human autologous mixed lymphocyte culture. *J. Immunol.* 123:419-422, 1979.
300. Smith, F., and Miller, J. F. Delayed type hypersensitivity to allogeneic cells in mice. I. Requirements for optimal sensitization and definition of the response. *Int. Arch. Allergy Appl. Immunol.* 58:285-294, 1979.
301. Smith, F. I., and Miller, J. F. Suppression of T cells specific for the nonthymic parental H-2 haplotype in thymus-grafted chimeras. *J. Exp. Med.* 151:246-251, 1980.
302. Steinmetz, M., Minard, K., Horvath, S., McNicholas, J., Srelinger, J., Wake, C., Long, E., Mach, B., and Hood, L. A molecular map of the immune response region from the major histocompatibility complex of the mouse. *Nature* 300:35-42, 1982.
303. Steinmuller, D. Suppressor cells and transplantation tolerance. *Transplantation* 26:2-3, 1978.
304. Streilein, J. W., Gruchalla, R. S., Wood, P., and Strome, P. Active clonal deletion in neonatal H-2 tolerance. *Ann. N.Y. Acad. Sci.* 392:276-290, 1982.
305. Strober, S., Okada, S., and Oseroff, A. Role of natural suppressor cells in allograft tolerance. *Fed. Proc.* 43:263-265, 1984.
306. Stuart, F. P., Scollard, D. M., McKearn, T. J., and Fitch, F. W. Cellular and humoral immunity after allogeneic renal transplantation in the rat. V. Appearance of anti-idiotypic antibody and its relationship to cellular immunity after treatment with donor spleen cells and alloantibody. *Transplantation* 22:455-466, 1976.
307. Sugarbaker, P. H., and Matthews, W. Cytotoxic cells suppress in vitro generation of cellular immunity by stimulator cell lysis. *Cell Immunol.* 57:124-135, 1981.
308. Sumida, T., Takei, I., and Taniguchi, M. Activation of acceptor-suppressor hybridoma with antigen-specific suppressor T cell factor of two-chain type: Requirement of the antigen and the I-J restricting specificity. *J. Immunol.* 133:1131-1136, 1984.
309. Sunday, M. E., Benacerraf, B., and Dorf, M. E. Hapten-specific T cell responses to 4-hydroxy-3-nitrophenyl acetyl. VIII. Suppressor cell pathways in cutaneous sensitivity responses. *J. Exp. Med.* 153:811-822, 1981.
310. Sunday, M. E., Weinberger, J. Z., Wolff, S., and Dorf, M. E. Anti-receptor antibody-induced suppression of murine H-Y specific delayed-type hypersensitivity responses. *Eur. J. Immunol.* 11:626-631, 1981.
311. Sy, M. S., Bach, B. A., Brown, A., Nisonoff, A., Benacerraf, B., and Greene, M. I. Antigen- and receptor-driven regulatory mechanisms. II. Induction of suppressor T cells with idiotype-coupled syngeneic spleen cells. *J. Exp. Med.* 150:1229-1240, 1979.
312. Sy, M. S., Bach, B. A., Dohi, Y., Nisonoff, A., Benacerraf, B., and Greene, M. I. Antigen- and receptor-driven regulatory mechanisms. I. Induction of suppressor T cells with anti-idiotypic antibodies. *J. Exp. Med.* 150:1216-1228, 1979.

313. Sy, M. S., Dietz, M. H., Germain, R. N., Benacerraf, B., and Greene, M. I. Antigen- and receptor-driven regulatory mechanisms. IV. Idiotype-bearing I-J^+ suppressor T cell factors induce second-order suppressor T cells which express anti-idiotypic receptors. *J. Exp. Med.* 151:1183-1195, 1980.
314. Sy, M. S., Miller, S. D., Kowach, H. B., and Claman, H. N. A splenic requirement for the generation of suppressor T cells. *J. Immunol.* 119:2095-2099, 1977.
315. Sy, M. S., Nisonoff, A., Germain, R. N., Benacerraf, B., and Greene, M. I. Antigen- and receptor-driven regulatory mechanisms. VIII. Suppression of idiotypic-negative p-azobenzenearsonate-specific T cells results from the interaction of an anti-idiotypic second-order T suppressor cell with a cross-reactive-idiotype-positive, p-azobenzenearsonate-primed T cell target. *J. Exp. Med.* 153:1415-1425, 1981.
316. Tada, T., Hayakawa, K., Okumura, K., and Taniguchi, M. Coexistence of variable region of immunoglobulin heavy chain and I region gene products on antigen-specific suppressor T cells and suppressor T cell factor. A minimal model of functional antigen receptor of T cells. *Mol. Immunol.* 17:867-875, 1980.
317. Tada, T., Taniguchi, M., and David, C. S. Properties of the antigen-specific suppressive T-cell factor in the regulation of antibody response of the mouse. IV. Special subregion assignment of the gene(s) that codes for the suppressive T-cell factor in the H-2 histocompatibility complex. *J. Exp. Med.* 144:713-725, 1976.
318. Tada, T., Taniguchi, M., and Okumura, K. Regulation of homocytotropic antibody formation in the rat. II. Effect of X-irradiation. *J. Immunol.* 106:1012-1018, 1971.
319. Takaoki, M., Sy, M. S., Tominaga, A., Lowy, A., Tsurufuji, M., Finberg, R., Benacerraf, B., and Greene, M. I. I-J-restricted interactions in the generation of azobenzenearsonate-specific suppressor T cells. *J. Exp. Med.* 156:1325-1334, 1982.
320. Takei, I., Sumida, T., and Taniguchi, M. Acceptor-suppressor T cell hybridoma with a receptor recognizing antigen-specific suppressor factor. *J. Exp. Med.* 158:1912-1923, 1983.
321. Taniguchi, M., and Miller, J. F. Enrichment of specific suppressor T cells and characterization of their surface markers. *J. Exp. Med.* 146:1450-1454, 1977.
322. Taniguchi, M., Saito, T., Takei, I., and Tokuhisa, T. Presence of interchain disulfide bonds between two gene products tha compose the secreted form of antigen-specific suppressor factor. *J. Exp. Med.* 153:1672-1677, 1981.
323. Taniguchi, M., Tokuhisa, T., Itoh, T., and Kanno, M. Functional roles of two polypeptide chains that compose an antigen-specific suppressor T cell factor. *J. Exp. Med.* 159:1096-1104, 1984.
324. Theze, J., Waltenbaugh, C., Germain, R. N., and Benacerraf, B. Immunosuppressive factor(s) specific for L-glutamic acid^{50}-L-tyrosine^{50}. IV. In vitro activity and immunochemical properties. *Eur. J. Immunol.* 7:705-710, 1977.
325. Thistlethwaite, J. R., Jr., Auchincloss, H., Jr., Lunney, J. K., Pennington, L. R. Pescovitz, M. D., and Sachs, D. H. Transplantation in miniature swine: In vitro testing and renal allograft survival in SLA-D matched swine. *Trans. Proc.* 15:151-155, 1983.
326. Thoman, M. L., and Weigle, W. O. Interleukin 2 induction of antigen-nonspecific suppressor cells. *Cell. Immunol.* 85:215-224, 1984.
327. Thomas, D. B., and Kennedy, M. W. Feedback control of the secondary antibody response. I. A suppressor, suppressor-inducer mechanism from the interaction of B-memory cells with Lyt 2^- T cells. *Immunology* 50:289-295, 1983.
328. Thomas, J. M., Carver, F. M., Haisch, C. E., Fahrenbruch, G., Deepe, R. M., and Thomas, F. T. Suppressor cells in rhesus monkeys treated with antithymocyte globulin. *Transplantation* 34:83-89, 1982.
329. Thomas, J., Thomas, F., Hoffmann, S., Johns, C., and Lee, H. M. Macrophage-

related suppressor cells in human renal transplant recipients. *Surgery* 86:266-274, 1979.

330. Thomas, Y., Rogozinski, L., Irigoyen, O. H., Friedman, S. M., Kung, P. C., Goldstein, G., and Chess, L. Functional analysis of human T cell subsets defined by monoclonal antibodies. IV. Induction of suppressor cells within the $OKT4^+$ population. *J. Exp. Med.* 154:459-467, 1981.
331. Thomas, Y., Rogozinski, L., Rabbani, L., Chess, A., Goldstein, G., and Chess, L. Functional analysis of human T cell subsets defined by monoclonal antibodies. *J. Mol. Cell. Immunol.* 1:103-110, 1984.
332. Tilney, N. L., Graves, M. J., and Strom, T. B. Prolongation of organ allograft survival by syngeneic lymphoid cells. *J. Immunol.* 121:1480-1482, 1978.
333. Tokuhisa, T., Komatsu, Y., Uchida, Y., and Taniguchi, M. Monoclonal antibodies specific for the constant region of T cell antigen receptors. *J. Exp. Med.* 156:888-897, 1982.
334. Tokuhisa, T., and Taniguchi, M. Two distinct allotypic determinants on the antigen-specific suppressor and enhancing T cell factors that are encoded by genes linked to the immunoglobulin heavy chain locus. *J. Exp. Med.* 155:126-139, 1982.
335. Tomasi, T. B., Jr. Oral tolerance. *Transplantation* 29:353-356, 1980.
336. Tosato, G., Magrath, I. T., and Blaese, R. M. T cell-mediated immunoregulation of Epstein-Barr virus (EBV) induced B lymphocyte activation in EBV-seropositive and EBV-seronegative individuals. *J. Immunol.* 128:575-579, 1982.
337. Tosato, G., Pike, S. E., and Blaese, R. M. Reversal of infectious mononucleosis-associated suppressor T cell activity by D-mannose. *J. Exp. Med.* 158:1048-1060, 1983.
338. Truitt, G. A., Dennison, D. K., Rich, R. R., and Rich, S. S. Interactions between T cells and non T-cells in suppression of cytotoxic lymphocyte responses. *J. Immunol.* 123:745-750, 1979.
339. Truitt, G. A., Rich, R. R., and Rich, S. S. Regulation of cytotoxic lymphocyte responses in vitro by alloantigen-activated spleen cells. *J. Immunol.* 119:31-37, 1977.
340. Tse, H., and Dutton, R. W. Separation of helper and suppressor T lymphocytes on a Ficoll velocity sedimentation gradient. *J. Exp. Med.* 143:1199-1210, 1976.
341. Tse, H. Y., and Dutton, R. W. Separation of helper and suppressor T lymphocytes. III. Positive and negative effects of mixed lymphocyte reaction-activated T cells. *J. Immunol.* 120:1149-1152, 1978.
342. Tse, H. Y., and Dutton, R. W. Separation of helper and suppressor T lymphocytes. II. Ly phenotypes and lack of DNA synthesis requirement for the generation of concanavalin A helper and suppressor cells. *J. Exp. Med.* 146:747-758, 1977.
343. Tutschka, P. J., Hess, A. D., Beschorner, W. E., and Santos, G. W. Suppressor cells in transplantation tolerance. I. Suppressor cells in the mechanism of tolerance in radiation chimeras. *Transplantation* 32:203-209, 1981.
344. Tutschka, P. J., Hess, A. D., Beschorner, W. E., and Santos, G. W. Suppressor cells in transplantation tolerance. III. The role of antigen in the maintenance of transplantation tolerance. *Transplantation* 33:510-514, 1982.
345. Tutschka, P. J., Ki, P. F., Beschorner, W. E., Hess, A. D., and Santos, G. W. Suppressor cells in transplantation tolerance. II. Maturation of suppressor cells in the bone marrow chimera. *Transplantation* 32:321-325, 1981.
346. Unanue, E. R. The regulatory role of macrophages in antigenic stimulation. Part two: symbiotic relationship between lymphocytes and macrophages. *Adv. Immunol.* 31:1-136, 1981.
347. Usui, M., Aoki, I., Sunshine, G. H., and Dorf, M. E. A role for macrophages in suppressor cell induction. *J. Immunol.* 132:1728-1734, 1984.
348. Usui, M., Aoki, I., Sunshine, G. H., and Dorf, M. Requirements for suppressor T cell activation. *J. Immunol.* 133:1137-1141, 1984.

349. Van der Kwast. T. H., Bianchi, A. T., Bril, H., and Benner, R. Suppression of antigraft immunity by preimmunization. I. Kinetic aspects and specificity. *Transplantation* 31:79-85, 1981.
350. Vines, J., Parks, D. E., and Weigle, W. O. Immunologic unresponsiveness after gastric administration of human γ-globulin: Antigen requirements and cellular parameters. *J. Immunol.* 125:1811-1816, 1980.
351. Waldmann, T. A., Durm, M., Broder, S., Blackman, M., Blaese, R. M., and Strober, W. Role of suppressor T cells in pathogenesis of common variable hypogammaglobulinemia. *Lancet* 2:609-613, 1974.
352. Waltenbaugh, C. Regulation of immune responses by I-J gene products. I. Production and characterization of anti-I-J monoclonal antibodies. *J. Exp. Med.* 154: 1570-1583, 1981.
353. Waltenbaugh, C., and Lei, H.-Y. Regulation of immune responses by I-J gene products. V. Heterogeneity of I-J gene products as detected by anti-I-J monoclonal antibodies. *J. Immunol.* 133:1730-1734, 1984.
354. Weinberger, J. Z., Benacerraf, B., and Dorf, M. E. Hapten-specific T cell responses to 4-hydroxy-3-nitrophenyl acetyl. III. Interaction of effector suppressor T cells is restricted by H-2 and Igh-V genes. *J. Exp. Med.* 151:1413-1423, 1980.
355. Weinberger, J. Z., Germain, R. N., Benacerraf, B., and Dorf, M. E. Hapten-specific T cell responses to 4-hydroxy-3-nitrophenyl acetyl. V. Role of idiotypes in the suppressor pathway. *J. Exp. Med.* 152:161-169, 1980.
356. Weinberger, J. Z., Germain, R. N., Jr, S. T., Greene, M. I., Benacerraf, B., and Dorf, M. E. Hapten-specific T-cell responses to 4-hydroxy-3-nitrophenyl acetyl. II. Demonstration of idiotypic determinants on suppressor T cells. *J. Exp. Med.* 150: 761-776, 1979.
357. Weksler, M. E., Moody, C. E., and Kozak, R. W. The autologous mixed-lymphocyte reaction. *Adv. Immunol.* 31:271-312, 1984.
358. Welte, K., Platzer, E., Wang, C. Y., Rinnooy Kan, E. A., Moore, M. A. S., and Mertelsmann, R. OKT8 antibody inhibits OKT3-induced IL 2 production and proliferation in $OKT8^+$ cells. *J. Immunol.* 131:2356-2361, 1983.
359. Whisler, R. L., and Stobo, J. D. Suppression of humoral and delayed hypersensitivity responses by distinct T cell subpopulations. *J. Immunol.* 121:539-542, 1978.
360. Wong, H. L., and Battisto, J. R. In vivo regulation of the cytolytic T cell response to hapten-altered self: Suppressor T cells induced in the regional lymph nodes by exposure to syngeneic spleen cells. *Eur. J. Immunol.* 14:629-633, 1984.
361. Wood, M. L., Gottschalk, R., and Monaco, A. P. Suppressor cells in specific unresponsiveness to skin allografts in thymectomized, ALS-treated, marrow-injected mice. *Transplantation* 28:387-388, 1979.
362. Wood, M. L., and Monaco, A. P. Suppressor cells in specific unresponsiveness to skin allografts in ALS-treated, marrow-injected mice. *Transplantation* 29:196-200, 1980.
363. Wood, M. L., and Monaco, A. P. Induction of unresponsiveness to skin allografts in adult mice disparate at defined regions of the H-2 complex. I. Effect of donor-specific bone marrow in ALS-treated mice. *Transplantation* 37:35-39, 1984.
364. Wood, M. L., and Monaco, A. P. Induction of unresponsiveness to skin allografts in adult mice disparate at defined regions of the H-2 complex. II. Effect of pregraft donor-specific blood transfusions in ALS-treated mice. *Transplantation* 37: 39-42, 1984.
365. Wood, P., Horsburgh, T., and Brent, L. Specific unresponsiveness to skin allografts in mice. VI. Graft survival in mice pretreated with blood. *Transplantation* 31:8-14, 1981.
366. Wood, P. J., and Streilein, J. W. Immunogenetic basis of acquired transplantation tolerance. *Transplantation* 37:223-226, 1984.

367. Yamashita, U., Ono, S., and Nakamura, H. The syngeneic mixed leukocyte reaction in mice. II. The I region control of suppressor T cell activity induced in the syngeneic mixed leukocyte reaction. *J. Immunol.* 128:1010-1017, 1982.
368. Yamauchi, K., Chao, N., Murphy, D. B., and Gershon, R. K. Molecular composition of an antigen-specific, Ly-1 T suppressor-inducer factor. One molecule binds antigen and is I-J^-; another is I-J^+, does not bind antigen, and imparts an IgH-variable region-linked restriction. *J. Exp. Med.* 155:655-665, 1982.
369. Yamauchi, K., Murphy, D., Cantor, H., and Gershon, R. K. Analysis of antigen-specific, Ig restricted cell-free material made by I-J^+ Ly1 cells (Ly-1 TsiF) that induces $Ly2^+$ cells to express suppressive activity. *Eur. J. Immunol.* 11:905-912, 1981.
370. Yamauchi, K., Murphy, D., Cantor, H., and Gershon, R. K. Analysis of an antigen-specific, H-2 restricted cell free products made by "I-J^-" Ly2 cells that suppresses Ly2 cell-depleted spleen cell activity. *Eur. J. Immunol.* 11:913-918, 1981.
371. Yashikai, Y., Anatoniou, D., Clark, S. P., Yanagi, Y., Sangster, R., Van der Elsen, P., Terhorst, C., and Mak, T. W. Sequence and expression of transcripts of the human T-cell receptor B-chain genes. *Nature* 312:521-524, 1984.
372. Yasumura, T., and Kahan, B. D. Prolongation of rat kidney allografts by pretransplant administration of donor antigen extract or whole blood transfusion combined with a short course of cyclosporine. *Transplantation* 36:603-609, 1983.
373. Zamoyska, R., and Waldmann, H. Allosuppression: Evidence for the involvement of both "noncytotoxic" and cytotoxic T cells. *Eur. J. Immunol.* 14:645-651, 1984.
374. Zatz, M. M., Hatcher, J., Goldstein, A. L., Novak, C., and Jacobs, R. P. Suppressor cell responses in patients with rheumatoid arthritis: The effect of thymosin. *Thymus* 6:205-218, 1984.
375. Zembala, M. A., Asherson, G. L., James, B. M., Stein, V. E., and Watkins, M. C. Antihaptene T suppressor factor acts through an I-J^+, Ly-1^-2^+, T acceptor cell that releases a nonspecific inhibitor of the transfer of contact sensitivity when exposed to antigen. *J. Immunol.* 129:1823-1829, 1982.
376. Zembala, M. A., Colizzi, V., Asherson, G. L., and Watkins, M. D. Non-specific inhibitor made by T-acceptor cells inhibits both the afferent and efferent stage of the contact sensitivity reaction. *Immunology* 52:599-606, 1984.
377. Sembala, M., Watkins, M., Colizzi, V., and Asherson, G. L. T suppressor factor activity is due to two separate molecules. The Lyt-1^-2^+I-J^+ cells. *Cell. Immunol.* 87: 240-251, 1984.

DIAGNOSIS OF REJECTION

8

PATHOLOGY OF ALLOGRAFT REJECTION

T. Steen Olsen
University Institute of Pathology, Municipal Hospital, Aarhus, Denmark

The pathology of the human renal allograft is a very broad subject since the graft can be affected by virtually all diseases that may occur in the native kidney. The aim of this chapter is to discuss lesions due to immunologic incompatibility between graft and host. Thus, the chapter deals with the pathology of rejection as it manifests itself in various clinical presentations. For several reasons it is, however, inexpedient to keep strictly to this definition of the subject matter. The main reason is that this chapter is written to serve as a practical guide in the interpretation of histopathologic lesions in the allograft removed surgically or at the autopsy or studied in biopsy material. In order to discuss differential diagnostic problems, brief references to lesions due to causes other than immunologic incompatibility will therefore be added. I have not attempted to discuss in detail the interpretation of the morphology in terms of pathogenesis.

The text is based partly on relevant literature and partly on personal experience from participation, for 20 years, as the pathologist member of a team engaged in clinical renal transplantation. The material in the files of the author consists of tissue specimens from more than 500 renal allotransplantations.

CLASSIFICATION AND NOMENCLATURE OF RENAL ALLOGRAFT REJECTION

Following a tradition developed during the two decades in which clinical renal transplantation has been performed, morphologic types of rejection have been defined and classified in accordance with clinical presentations. The three types that have been described are hyperacute, acute, and chronic rejection. Although this categorization is useful, it should be realized that mixed forms and transitions exist, which often make it difficult to fit a given case within this rigid framework. Thus, acute rejection in a sensitized patient may take on many of the characteristics of hyperacute rejection. Similarly, acute rejections occurring in later phases of the posttransplant course present with a histologic picture of acute rejection lesions on a background of alterations typical for chronic rejection.

Since the simplified classification into three main conditions has practical advantages, mainly of a didactic nature, it has been adhered to in the present survey. Following each presentation, the pathology of other conditions that may give rise to a similar clinical picture will be added.

HYPERACUTE REJECTION

Hyperacute rejection is characterized clinically by rapid cessation of urine flow, a mottled cyanotic color, and a flabby consistency of the graft occurring typically a few minutes after opening of the vascular anastomoses. Occasionally, the acute loss of function may set in later, but probably not later than 48 hr after the transplantation. Serologically, preformed circulating antibodies against donor antigen may be detected [18,35,37]. Pathologically, there is an early initial stage of a few minutes' duration with leukostasis in the glomerular and peritubular capillaries as the sole histopathologic change. This is followed by extensive microthrombosis in glomerular capillaries and juxtaglomerular arterioles (Fig. 1). Thrombi may also occur in other vessels, for instance, veins and peritubular capillaries. There is no interstitial cellular infiltration. Within 1 or 2 days, extensive tubular necrosis develops. The medulla is preserved, and if the graft is removed some days after transplantation, it will display the picture of cortical necrosis very similar to bilateral cortical necrosis in native kidneys occurring as a sequel to disseminated intravascular coagulation and in the experimental models of the Shwartzman reaction (Fig. 2).

Hyperacute rejection is caused by the action of preformed, circulating antibodies occurring in the host, often as a consequence of immunization by multiple pregnancies or blood transfusions. These may be HLA-system antibodies, but ABO antibodies and others may give rise to the same syndrome. Some cases occur in the absence of antibodies detectable by a direct cross-match, indicating that other factors may be operative.

Other conditions that may give rise to immediate acute graft failure or loss of function during the initial 48 hr are primary graft anuria, occlusion of the main vessels of the graft and ureteral obstruction. Perfusion injury is discussed in Chapter 9. Acute rejection will generally not occur in this early period, and the same applies to drug-induced damage to the graft.

Primary graft anuria ("acute tubular necrosis" of the graft; ischemic damage during the organ harvesting) is considered to be caused by factors operative during the warm and cold ischemic period due to the interruption of the blood supply in the period between removal of the kidney from the donor and opening of the vascular anastomoses in the recipient. Conditions present in the terminal phase of the donor's life (for instance, hypotension and infections) may, however, also influence the graft.

In primary graft anuria, no urine is produced after opening of the anastomoses in spite of good perfusion and normal tension and color of the graft. This anuric state may last a few days, but longer periods of several weeks are not rare. Acute renal failure is frequent in cadaver grafts but rare if a kidney from a living donor has been used. Experience at our institution indicates that the condition in itself does not seem to affect graft survival, and a satisfactory graft function after resumption of urine production usually occurs even following long periods of anuria. The most important problem associated with this state is the difficulty of diagnosing an acute rejection episode or other complications during the anuric period.

There have been no systematic investigations of the morphology of the graft in primary graft anuria, and the following description of the light microscopic (LM) picture as well as the appearance on electron microscopy (EM) is based on personal experience [3,39]. By LM, tubular lumina may be dilated and they often contain periodic acid-Schiff (PAS)-posi-

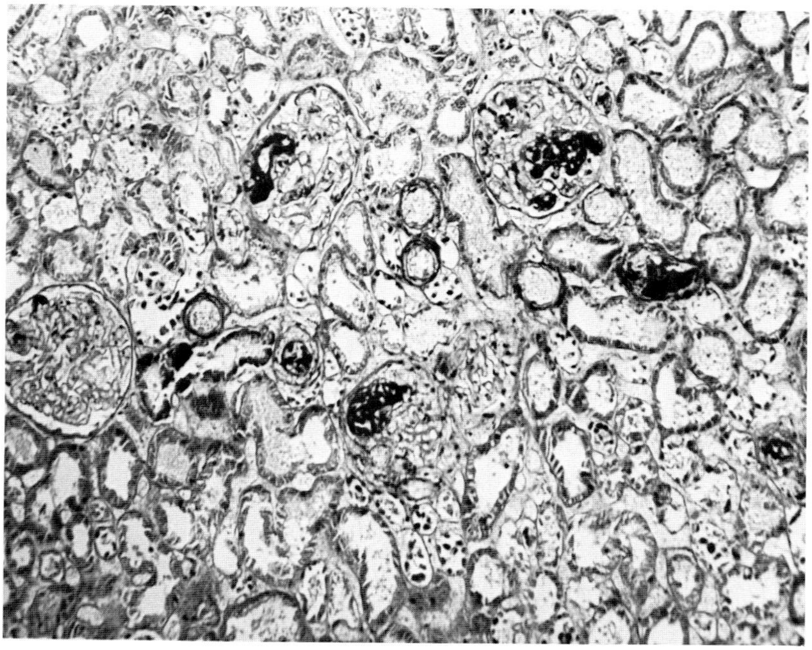

(A)

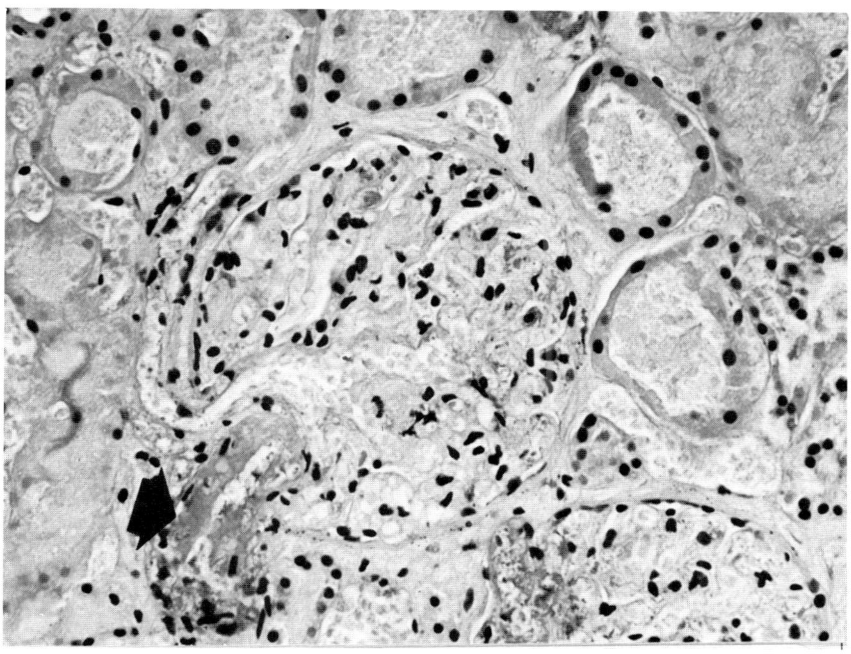

(B)

FIGURE 1 Hyperacute rejection. (A) Microthrombosis is present in glomerular capillaries (PTAH). (B) Thrombosis in juxtaglomerular arteriole (arrow). (H&E.)

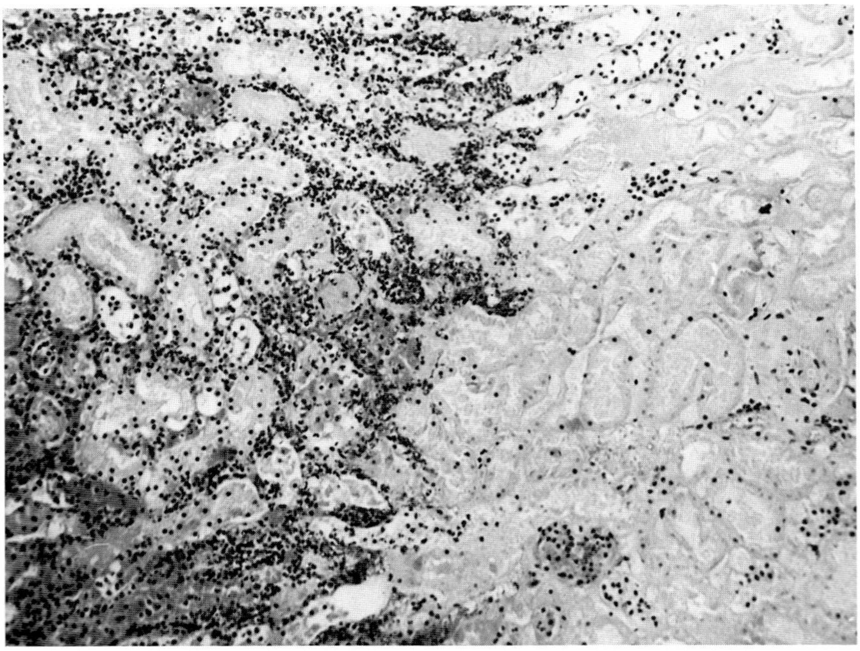

(A)

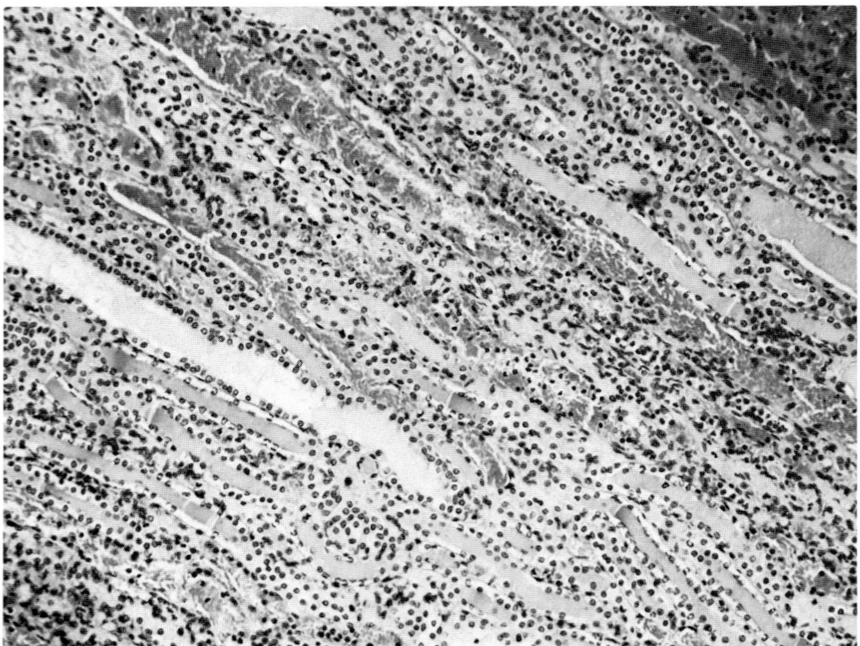

(B)

FIGURE 2 Hyperacute rejection. (A) The cortex is necrotic. Infiltration with leukocytes forms a narrow subcapsular demarcation zone (left) (H&E). (B) The medulla is not necrotic (H&E). The graft was removed 3 days after transplantation.

tive casts. Tubular cells may show nonspecific, degenerative changes and vacuolization. Single cell necrosis or more extended confluent epithelial necrosis may be present. Distal tubules are generally better preserved than proximal, but necrosis may also occur here. In later stages, tubular calcification may occur under conditions that make it probable that these calcium deposits have been laid down in cells that became necrotic during acute renal failure. By EM, anoxic epithelial changes (dilatation of endoplasmic reticulum, lysosomal and mitochondrial swelling, and large vacuoles) and necrotic cells may be seen.

The problem with the interpretation of these changes is that they may be present in well-functioning grafts, too, and that some of the EM changes may be due to fixation artefacts. Furthermore, many of the biopsies in which these changes have been seen were from periods more than 5-6 days posttransplant, in which the possibility of acute rejection cannot be excluded, at least as partly responsible.

The conditions following which acute graft anuria occur have quite naturally given rise to the view that this graft disease must be analogous to ischemic acute renal failure in the native kidney ("shock-kidney"; "acute tubular necrosis"). There is, however, need for careful and controlled investigations of renal graft biopsies from patients with primary graft anuria, including evaluation of the tubular cell surface alterations (loss of proximal brush border; reduction of basolateral infoldings) so characteristic of ischemic acute renal failure in the native kidney [16,27].

A special cause of primary graft anuria is damage due to *machine perfusion* of the graft during the ischemic period. This syndrome is clinically as well as histopathologically similar to that of hyperacute rejection [8]. (See Chapter 9.)

Occlusion of the main artery and/or vein may occur early or late. A biopsy performed during the first few days is of less value for this differential diagnosis since the histologic signs of necrosis will not have developed yet. If the graft is removed after a few days, it will be totally necrotic, in contradistinction to hyperacute rejection, in which the necrosis involves the cortex only, at least during the first week. Later in hyperacute rejection, main vessel occlusion may complicate the situation and the graft may become totally necrotic.

Ureteric obstruction due to kinking as well as ureteral wall necrosis may lead to failure of the graft function in the early posttransplant period. Tubular dilatation and enlarged Bowman's capsules may be present, but these changes are inconstant, and the diagnosis is difficult to make from a biopsy. The presence of PAS-positive casts in dilated lymphatics may possibly be helpful [38]. They are probably identical with the lakes of Tamm-Horsfall's protein seen in dilated lymphatics in hydronephrosis in native kidneys. In the final analysis, the diagnosis of urinary obstruction rests mainly on methods other than a graft biopsy.

ACUTE REJECTION

The pathology of acute rejection in the immunosuppressed human recipient much resembles acute rejection seen in experimental allografts in nonimmunosuppressed animals. It occurs suddenly and may set in a few days after transplantation, but usually not earlier than 7 days. It may also occur later on and may complicate the situation at any time during the whole life of the transplant if immunosuppression is suddenly stopped. Clinically, there is swelling of the graft, which becomes painful. There may be fever and proteinuria as the graft function decreases. Complete anuria may occur. Histologically, there are interstitial, vascular, and glomerular changes (Figs. 3-8).

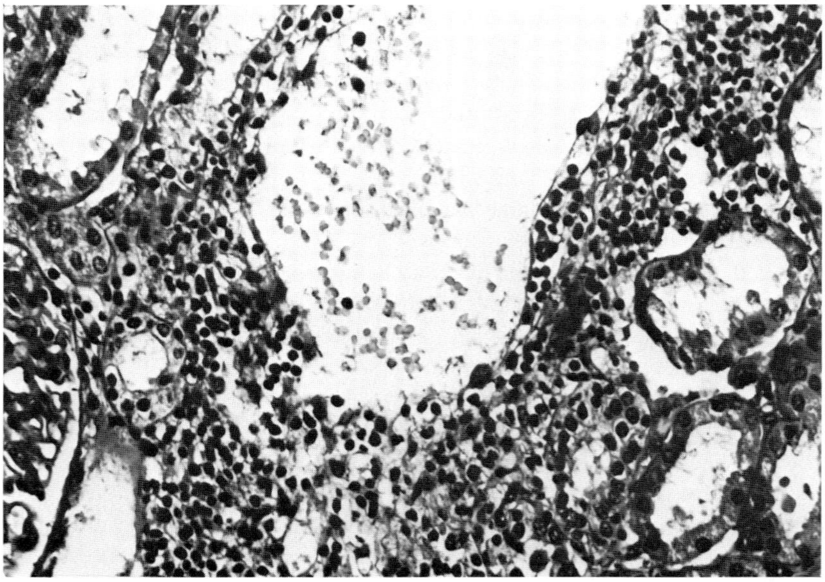

(A)

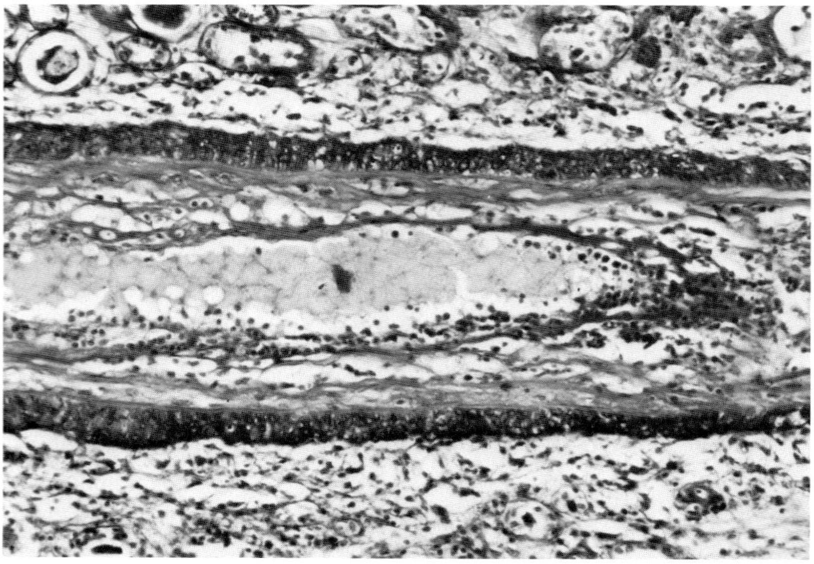

(B)

FIGURE 3 Acute rejection. (A) Severe interstitial infiltration with mononuclear cells around a dilated venule (PAS-hematoxylin). (B) Small artery (cut at length) with edematous intima containing lymphocytes (PAS-hematoxylin).

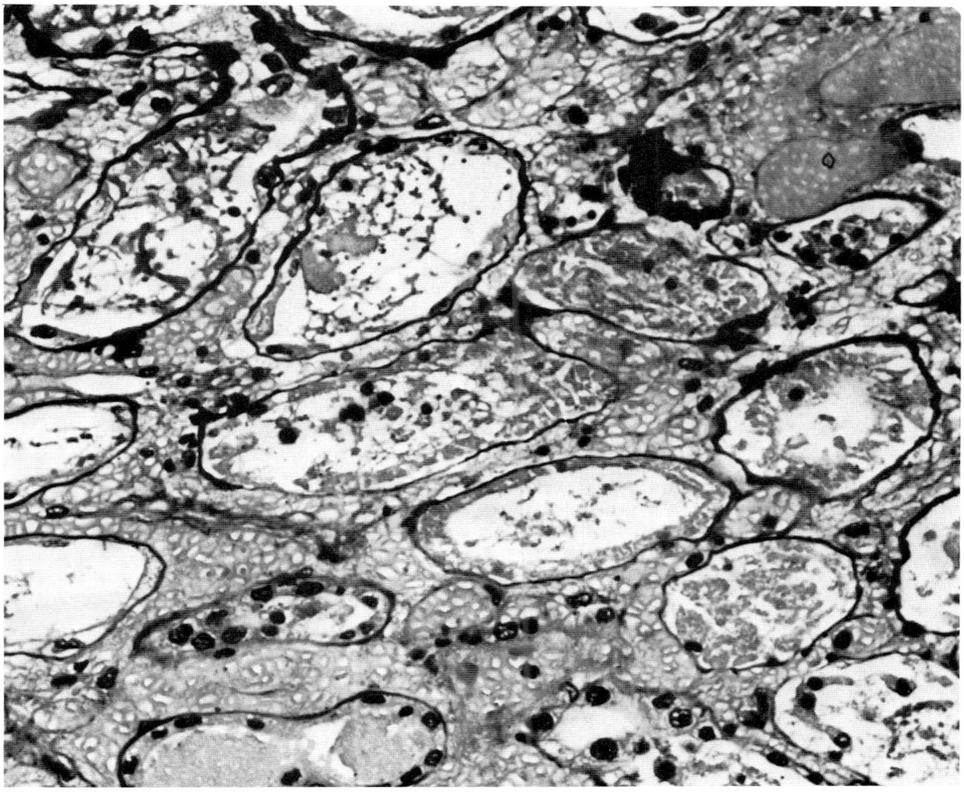

FIGURE 4 Acute rejection. A group of necrotic tubules and interstitial hemorrhage. These changes predict a poor prognosis for graft survival. (H&E.)

Interstitial infiltration with mononuclear cells has been regarded as one of the most important and characteristic lesions in graft rejection (Fig. 3). This lesion was well-known from experimental transplantation work before clinical renal transplantation became common, and it was at an early time interpreted as an indication of the importance of cellular ("delayed") immunity for the fate of the allograft. Although it has been demonstrated that some degree of interstitial infiltration may occur in the autograft [21] and in nonrejection graft biopsies [36] (see Chapter 10), and that the degree of infiltration is unrelated to the fate of the graft [19], this lesion has still kept its place as a characteristic allograft lesion occurring both in the presence and in the absence of clinical rejection.

Analysis of the cellular infiltrate on EM shows that it consists of about 50% lymphocytes (small, medium, and large), 25% macrophages, and 12% plasma cells [23]. Plasma cells and large lymphocytes (lymphoblasts) are rich in ribosomes and are strongly pyroninophilic by LM. The relative number of large ("blastlike") lymphocytes is particularly high in early rejection. Close contact is often found between the mononuclear cells. Monocytes, plasma cells, and lymphocytes (large as well as small) may be seen in passage through the capillary wall (Fig. 6). They usually pass between adjacent endothelial cells rather than through them, and EM photomicrographs leave the impression that the vessel wall closes

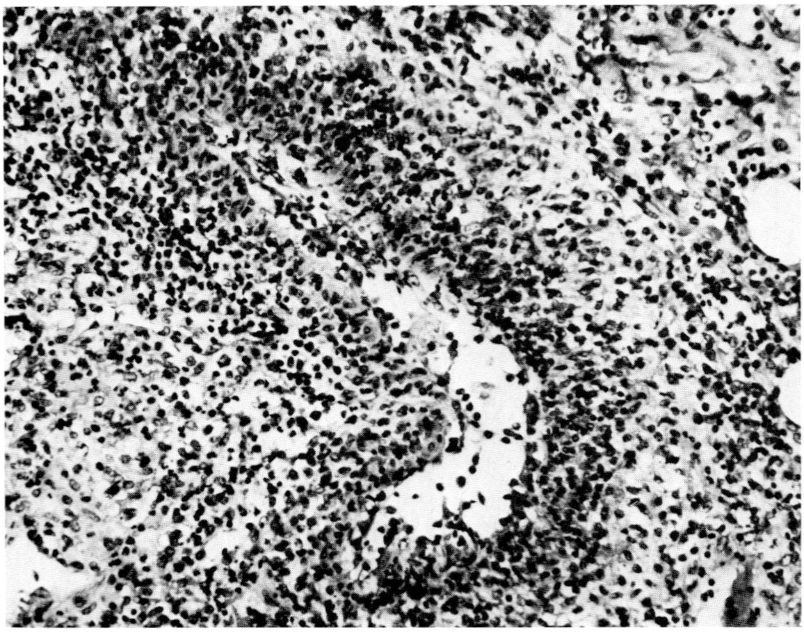

FIGURE 5 Acute rejection. Small artery with necrosis of the wall and severe transmural inflammation. This is a comparatively rare phenomenon, which can be seen, for example, in accelerated acute rejection or if immunosuppressive treatment has been discontinued before graftectomy. (H&E.)

after their passage, without any serious damage to the wall. Large defects of the capillary wall, including its basement membrane, may occur, however, and we have seen polymorphonuclear leukocytes with extrusion of granules near such defects [25]. We regard it as probable that this serious damage to the vessels may be due to enzymatic digestion. The defects may contribute to the hemorrhage and interstitial deposition of fibrin seen in severe rejection (Fig. 7).

Interstitial mononuclear infiltration is often most marked around small veins. The cell population has been characterized functionally by surface markers [6] and, more recently, by monoclonal antibodies in tissue sections [2] (see Chapter 10). It constituted a heterologous composition of T and B lymphocytes and macrophages. By immunofluorescence microscopy on frozen sections, immunoglobulins or complement can be demonstrated in only a few cells [20]. The severity of the interstitial infiltrate depends on the degree of histoincompatibility and on the effect of immunosuppressive treatment. The most intense infiltration can be seen in allografts removed following discontinuation of the treatment.

Credit should be given to Porter et al. [30], who in 1963 gave the first careful description of obliterative vascular changes in human renal allotransplants and interpreted them as due to immunologic mechanisms, thus categorizing these lesions with the interstitial cellular infiltration already known to occur from the experimental work that preceded clinical transplantation. Several later studies demonstrated the importance and severity of this group of allograft lesions [5,12,17,31].

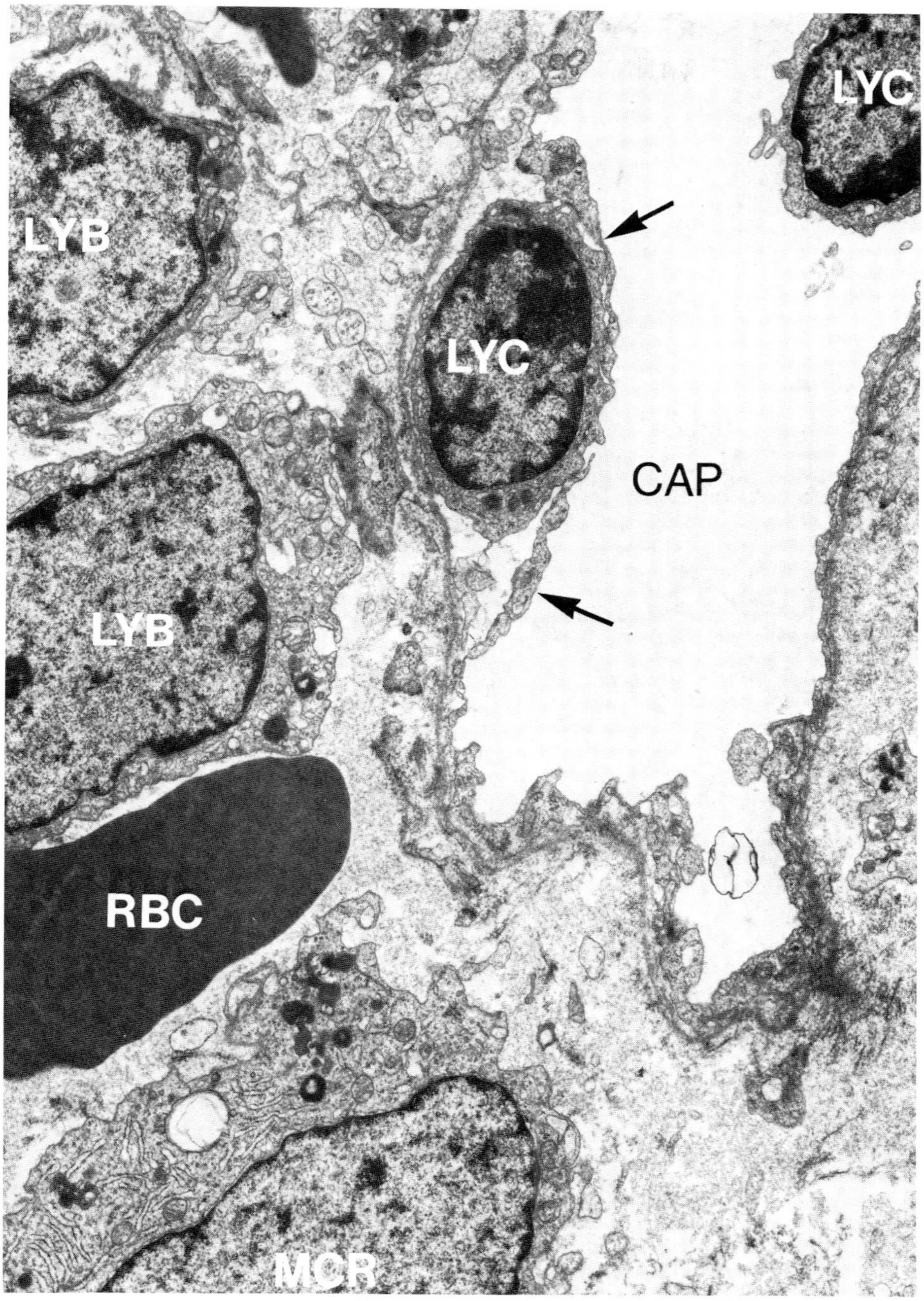

FIGURE 6 Acute rejection. Electron micrograph showing infiltrating cells and a capillary with lymphocytes, one of them in the process of wandering through the capillary wall. It has insinuated itself between the endothelium (arrows) and the capillary basement membrane; LYC, lymphocyte; LYB, lymphoblast; MCR, macrophage; CAP, capillary lumen. (X8000.)

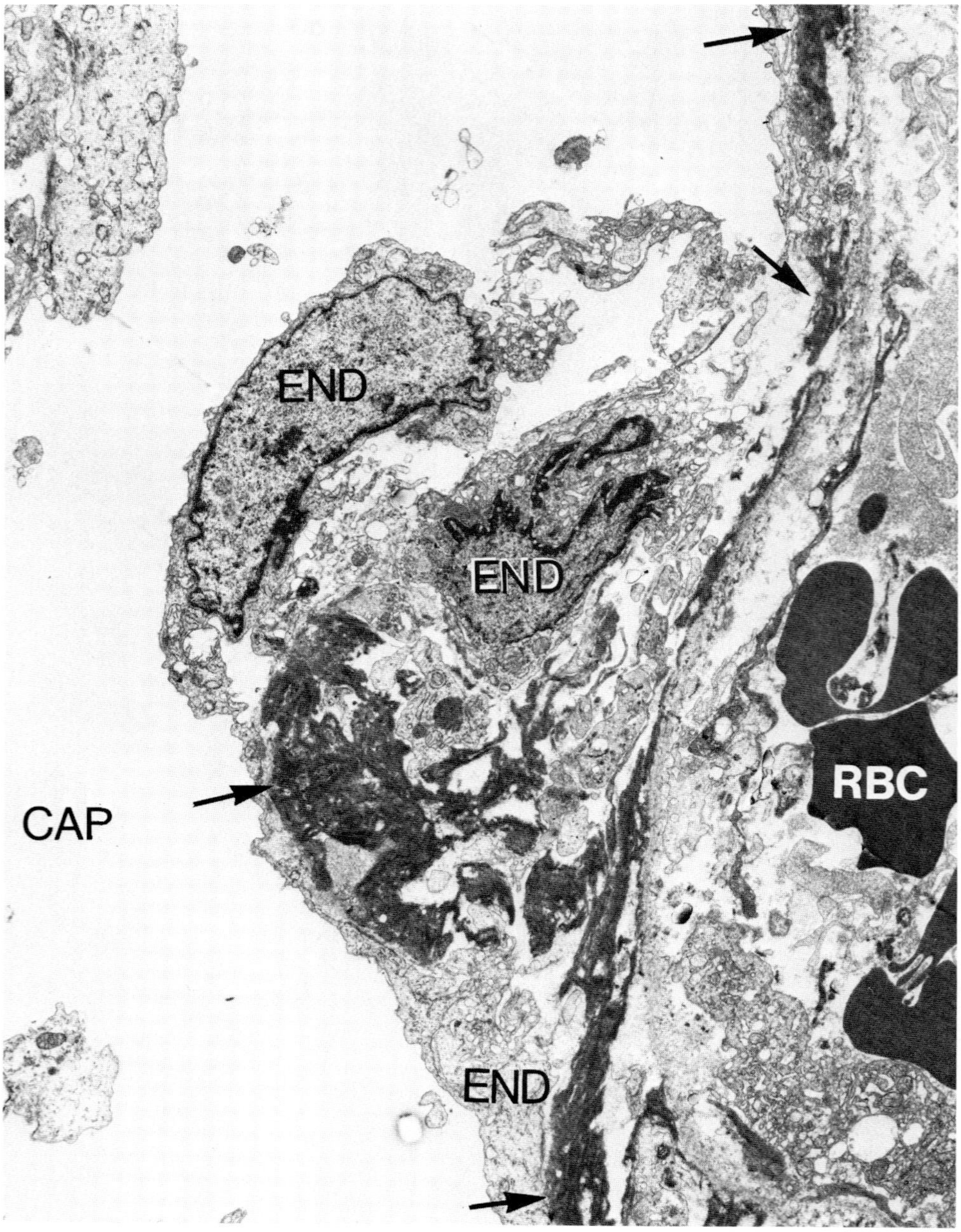

FIGURE 7 Acute rejection. Electron micrograph showing dilated capillary with loosening of the endothelial cells and deposition of fibrin (arrows). There is pericapillary hemorrhage; CAP, capillary lumen; END, endothelial cells; RBC, red blood corpuscles. (X8000.)

The most prominent vascular lesions are located in the arterial intima (Fig. 3B). Intimal thickening, that occurs in grafts rejected during the first few weeks after transplantation, is due to edema and infiltration with mononuclear cells of the same types as those constituting the interstitial infiltrate (see above). Endothelial cell proliferation may occur, but what has been interpreted as such is probably most often simulated by hyperplasia of other cells in the intima (e.g., fibroblasts) or by subendothelial infiltration with mononuclear cells. The intercellular matrix of the intima shows accumulation of acid mucopolysaccharides as demonstrated by Alcian Blue staining. Fibrin may also occur on the endothelium in denuded intimal areas as well as subendothelially.

Changes of the media mainly occur in accelerated rejection. The cells may show degeneration with hyperstainability or an uneven stainability with vacuoles. A more severe change is medial necrosis with nuclear pyknosis and fragmentation. It is usually associated with fibrin exudation ("fibrinoid necrosis") and infiltration with polymorphonuclear leukocytes, thus resembling the picture of a real arteritis (Fig. 5). (The term "arteritis" has also been used for the intimal changes described above, without transmural inflammation. This is only a matter of definition.) Medial necrosis involves the inner and outer elastic lamina, which become fragmented.

Immune deposits demonstrated by immunofluorescence microscopy are often present in the arteries displaying the changes described above. IgM, IgG, and C3 are most common. They are usually located in the intima but may also sometimes be demonstrated in the media, particularly in accelerated rejections.

By EM [5,25,32], the endothelial cells are enlarged and vacuolated. The intima is focally denuded due to endothelial defects. Fibrin deposits are very frequent, even in cases in which no fibrin can be seen by light microscopy. The thickened intima consists of increased amounts of ground substance and basement membrane-like material, probably forerunners of the collagen fibrils that are common in later stages. Fibrin may also be present in the media. Electron-dense, finely granular deposits may also occasionally be found. The cells of the thickened intima are lymphocytes, plasma cells, and macrophages with large polymorphous lysosomes. Modified smooth muscle cells ("myofibroblasts") are often abundant. Arterioles show similar alterations. In severe rejection, diffuse arteriolar necrosis may resemble the picture seen in malignant hypertension. Peritubular capillary thrombosis may occur. In severe acute rejection, vascular thrombosis is widespread and gives rise to a large number of small infarcts in the cortex. The thrombosis may involve the main vessels, with eventual development of total graft necrosis.

Glomerular changes are common but they are usually of slight degree [5,33]. Some cases show a more marked acute intracapillary glomerulitis, which may be diffuse and global or focal and segmental. The capillary lumina are stuffed with cells that may be of endothelial origin or monocytes. Some neutrophils may also be present. This picture has been reported to be characteristic of cytomegalovirus infection with viremia [34], but this association has not been evident in our series. Intracapillary glomerulitis occurs as frequently in patients who had glomerulonephritis in their native kidney as it does in patients with nonglomerular disease, and I am inclined to interpret this glomerular reaction as due to rejection.

On EM, an expanded electron-lucent space is often present between the lamina densa of the capillary basement membrane and the endothelial cells. A flocculent material with fine fibrils may be present in this space (Fig. 8). Immunoglobulins (G and M) and C3 can be demonstrated in a linear pattern by immunofluorescence microscopy.

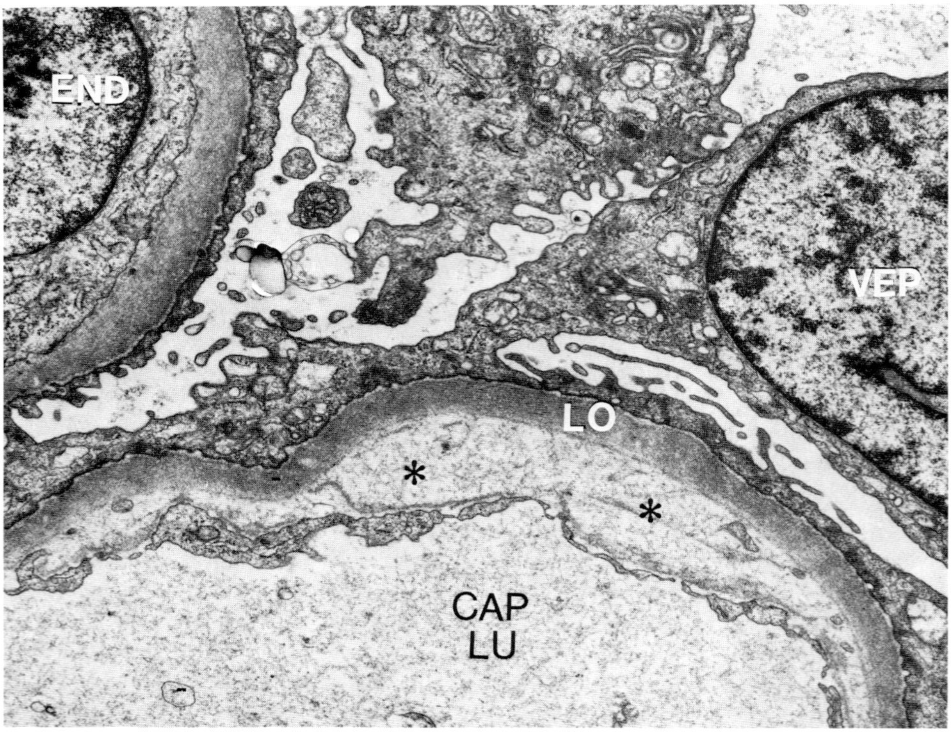

FIGURE 8 Acute rejection. Glomerular capillary showing accumulation of electron-lucent substance (abnormal basement membrane material, type 1) in subendothelial location (asterisk). This substance, which is usually more ample in chronic rejection, may also occur early in the graft; LD, lamina densa of the capillary basement membrane; VEP, visceral epithelial cell; END, endothelial cell. (X11,000.)

Several differential diagnostic possibilities have to be considered in acute graft failure occurring during the first few weeks posttransplant. Acute ischemic renal failure (which has been discussed above) usually presents as primary anuria but may rarely occur after initial function of the graft. The morphology of ureteral obstruction and main vessel occlusion has also been discussed.

A graft biopsy is often performed in early graft failure and may be of considerable help for the clinician. Its evaluation is, however, difficult and involves several pitfalls.

Interstitial mononuclear cell infiltration is not specific for rejection, and it may occur in slight or even moderate degree in grafts that are functioning well, without clinical evidence of rejection, as well as in grafts with primary graft anuria [36] (see Chapter 10). The typical arterial intimal lesion is regarded as specific by some authors [36], and this is probably true for practical purposes, although it should be recalled that intimal changes have occasionally been observed in experimental renal *autografts* [21].

If capillary thrombosis is very extensive in clinical acute rejection, it may give rise to a picture resembling that of hyperacute rejection with cortical necrosis. Thrombotic lesions of other vessels are, of course, not specific for acute rejection. They may occur in the main artery and vein as a sequel to mechanical lesions due to surgery or to infections in the area of anastomosis with subsequent thrombosis. They may spread to lesser vessels in the renal parenchyma. Total graft necrosis may thus be due to rejection as well as to other factors not associated with histoincompatibility. It can be difficult to determine the precise diagnosis, but even in a totally necrotic graft, it is often possible to discern arterial lesions typical of rejection. Stains for elastin are recommended for this purpose.

The possibility of acute pyelonephritis in the graft must also be considered. This diagnosis rests on the presence of polymorphonuclear leukocytes in the interstitium and on leukocyte casts in the tubular lamina. The differential diagnosis of glomerular lesions are discussed below. Graft failure due to the action of cyclosporin A is very difficult to distinguish from rejection changes [10]. This subject has been treated in other chapters of this book (see Chapters 10, 19, and 20).

A biopsy from a graft with early impaired function may give valuable prognostic information [11,13,14]. We found in a blinded semiquantitative study [19] that the presence in a graft biopsy of infarcts, glomerular thrombosis, or arterial or arteriolar thrombosis predicted graft loss within 1 year with 100% certainty. The presence of one or more of these lesions in a biopsy thus argues strongly for graft nephrectomy. Interstitial hemorrhage and hyperemia were also ominous. These data are somewhat in conflict with those of Solez et al. [36] (see Chapter 10), who found thromboses and infarcts in well-functioning grafts. However, it is clear from reviewing the material of Solez et al. that their infarcts date from the time of transplantation, whereas the infarcts we observed were more recent in appearance because they were brought about by a rejection episode. Our studies also showed that the severity of interstitial mononuclear cell infiltration has no influence on the fate of the graft [19], and this was also the finding of Herbertson et al. [13].

CHRONIC REJECTION

The functioning graft may suffer gradual loss of glomerular filtration, or the function may decrease discontinuously due to the effect of several episodes of acute rejection without complete restoration of the glomerular filtration. The situation may be complicated by slight or severe proteinuria, which may be so heavy as to produce the nephrotic syndrome. This clinical presentation is called chronic rejection.

The time span during which this deterioration of the graft evolves is quite variable. It may lead to uremia, requiring maintenance dialysis, or a new transplant within a couple of months, or it may develop very slowly, permitting reasonable function for many years before the graft becomes functionless. The most prominent lesions of this graft disease are vascular and glomerular.

The arterial changes present in acute rejection and as described above change gradually to those characteristic of the chronic rejection (Fig. 9) [4]. Later stages of the intimal thickening are characterized by the formation of collagen fibrils leading to relatively acellular fibrous scar tissue. The staining for acid mucosubstances usually persists into the late scarred stages. Accumulations of foam cells and deposition of calcium are late phenomena. Defects of the internal elastic membrane are probably residues from earlier episodes of graft arteritis. The internal elastic layer may also appear multilayered. The intimal changes lead to a progressive obliteration of the arteries and arterioles. Depending on the degree of this change, graft function may decrease or be totally abolished.

The late phase of intimal thickening on EM is characterized by increased amounts of basement membrane material and collagen as well as ingrowth of macrophages and fibromyocytes. Foam cells appear as macrophages with abundant vacuoles and lipid in-

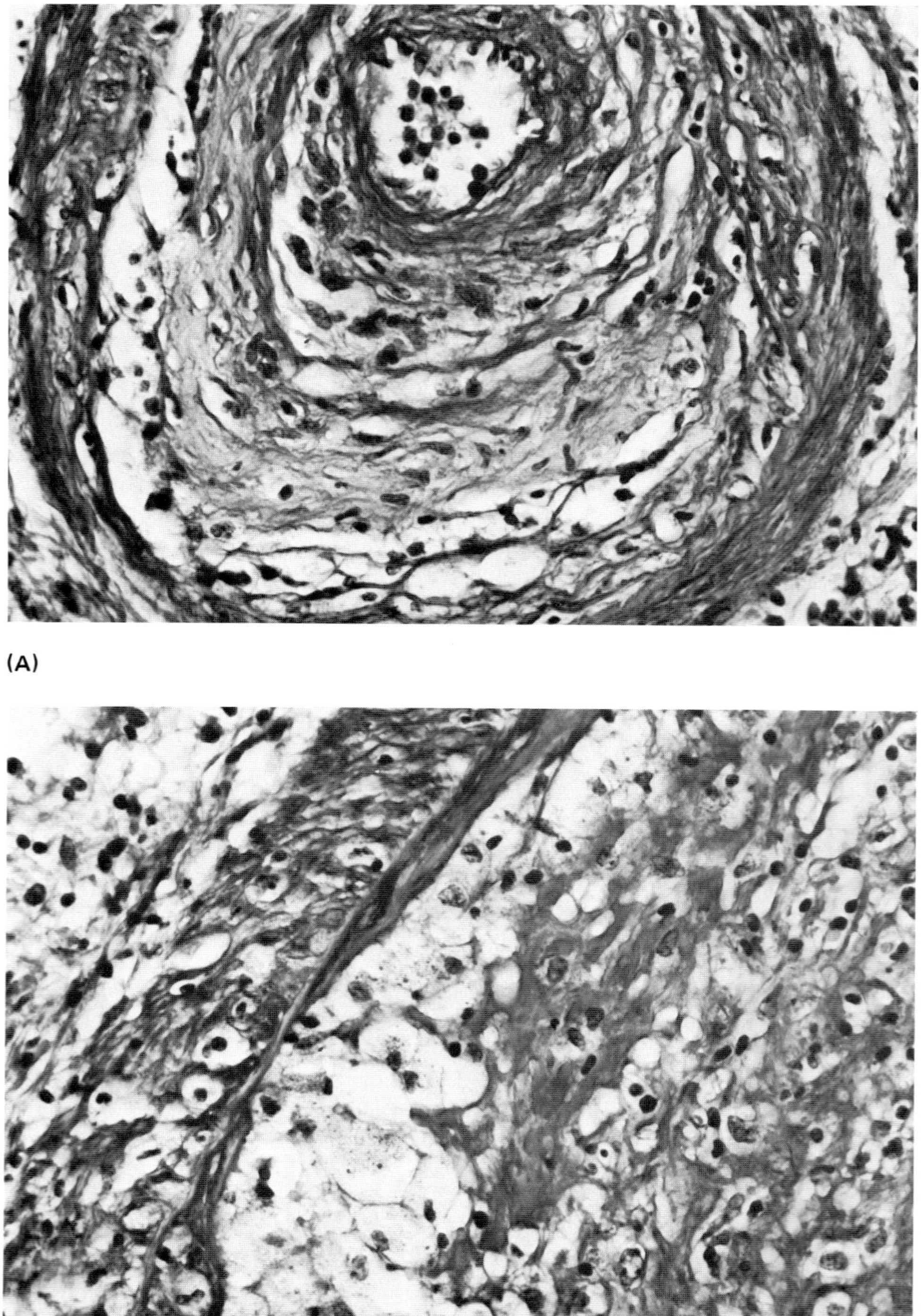

(A)

(B)

FIGURE 9 Chronic rejection. (A) Artery with severe fibrous intimal thickening. (B) Lipid containing foam cells in the thickened intima. This change is a late phenomenon that usually occurs more than 1 year posttransplant.

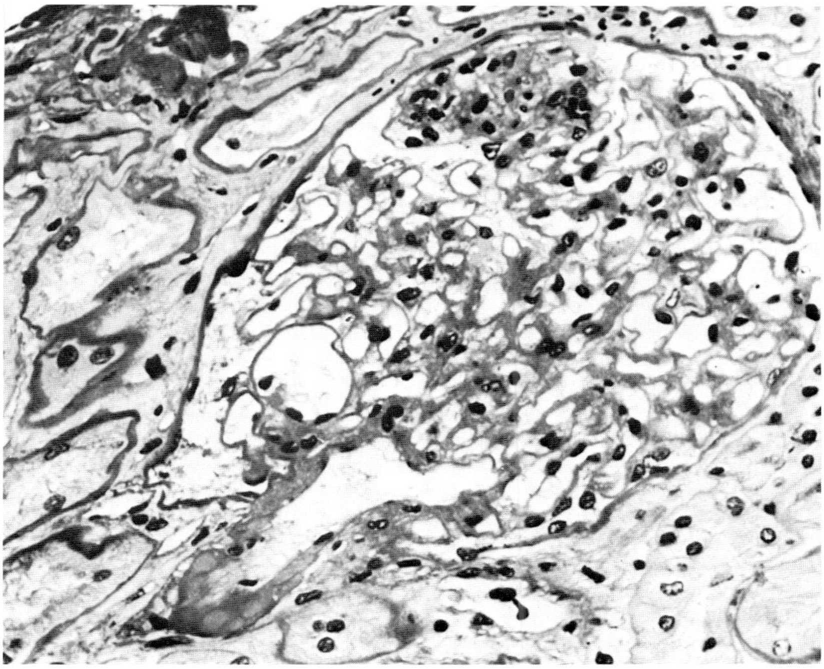

FIGURE 10 Chronic rejection of glomerular type. Glomerulus with moderate, segmental mesangial proliferation. (H&E.)

clusions. The elastic membranes may be ruptured or calcified. In late stages the media may consist of fibroblasts and collagen fibrils with few surviving myocytes.

As a consequence of the general vascular obliteration, the tubules become atrophic, the glomeruli become densely packed, and there may be interstitial fibrosis.

Glomerular changes in chronic rejection with heavy proteinuria (transplant glomerulopathy) are severe and heterogeneous [4,5,15,22,24,29]. Figures 10-14 illustrate the spectrum of glomerular changes that occur in chronic rejection associated with marked proteinuria. By light microscopy, transplant glomerulopathy is characterized by hypercellularity of endothelial and mesangial cells, which may be diffuse and global or focal and segmental. The mesangial areas are often broadened, and there may be peripheral mesangial interposition. Moderate or slight epithelial proliferation is common, typically present near adhesions between the capillary tuft and Bowman's capsule. A few typical crescents may also be found. Rarely, silver-stained sections may reveal spikes on the epithelial side of the capillary basement membrane. The lesions differ in severity and type, and the various components described above may be combined. It is therefore difficult to compare the picture with known types of native glomerulonephritis.

By immunofluorescence microscopy, there is strong glomerular staining for IgM, IgG, C3, and fibrinogen. Weak reactions for IgA may also be present. The pattern of the immune deposits is fine or coarsely granular in the peripheral capillary walls and sometimes also in the mesangial regions. Confluence of small granules may mimic a thick linear pattern, but the thin linear pattern typical of antibasement membrane glomerulonephritis is not seen.

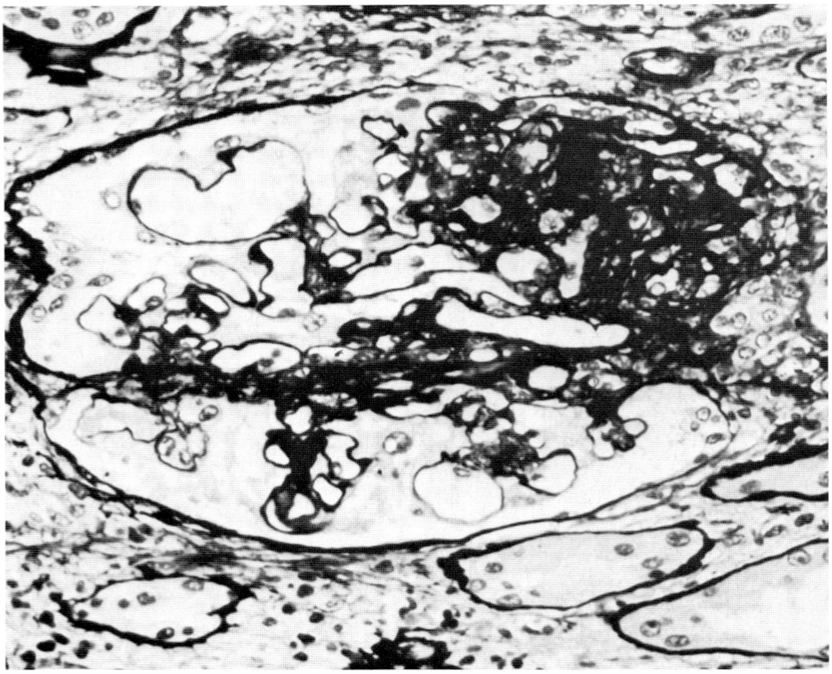

FIGURE 11 Chronic rejection of glomerular type. Segmental sclerosis. (Silver-methenamine-hematoxylin.)

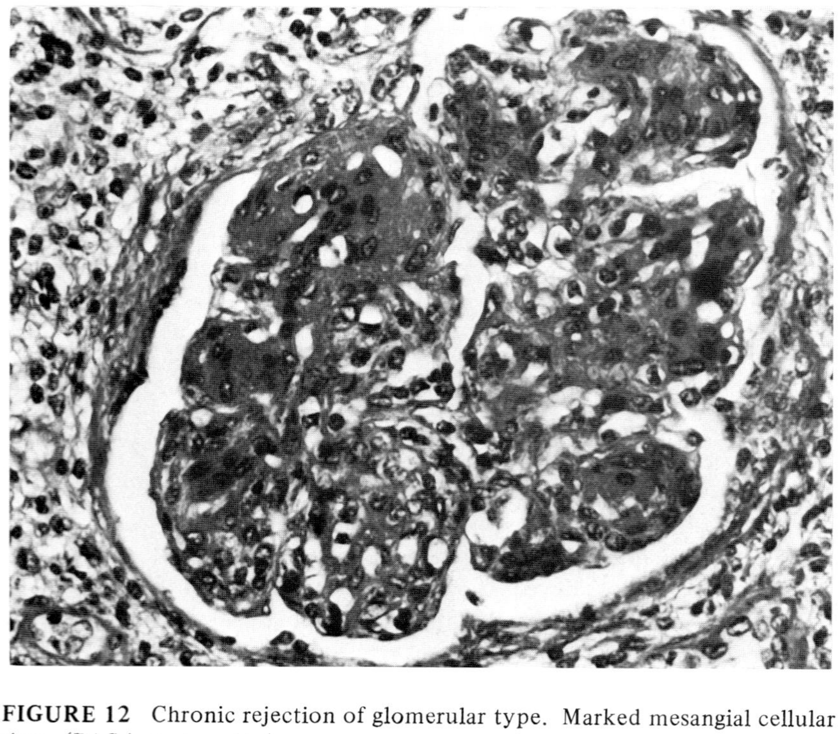

FIGURE 12 Chronic rejection of glomerular type. Marked mesangial cellular proliferation. (PAS-hematoxylin.)

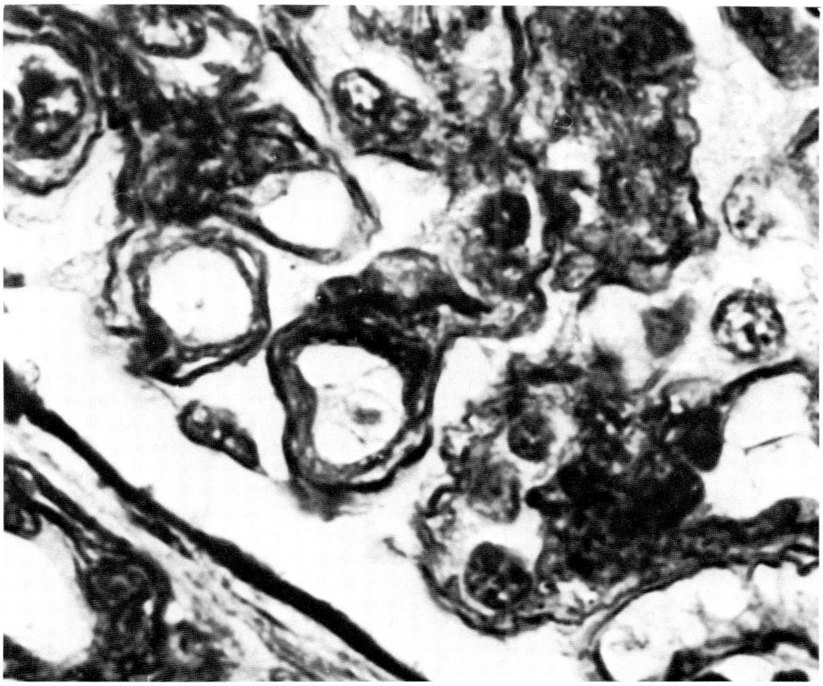

FIGURE 13 Chronic rejection of glomerular type. Peripheral mesangial interposition as in native membranoproliferative glomerulonephritis. (Silver-methenamine-hematoxylin.)

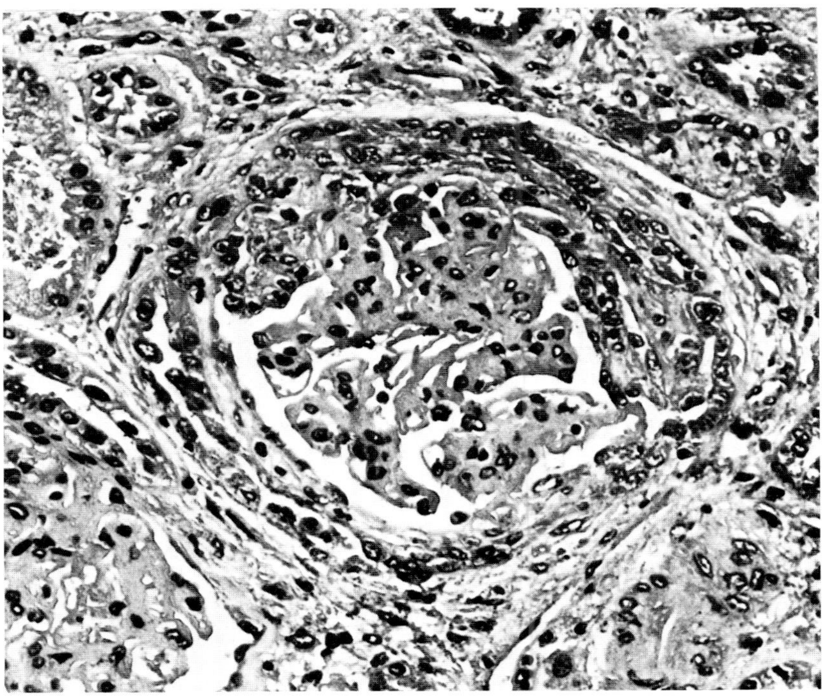

FIGURE 14 Chronic rejection of glomerular type. Epithelial crescent. (H&E.)

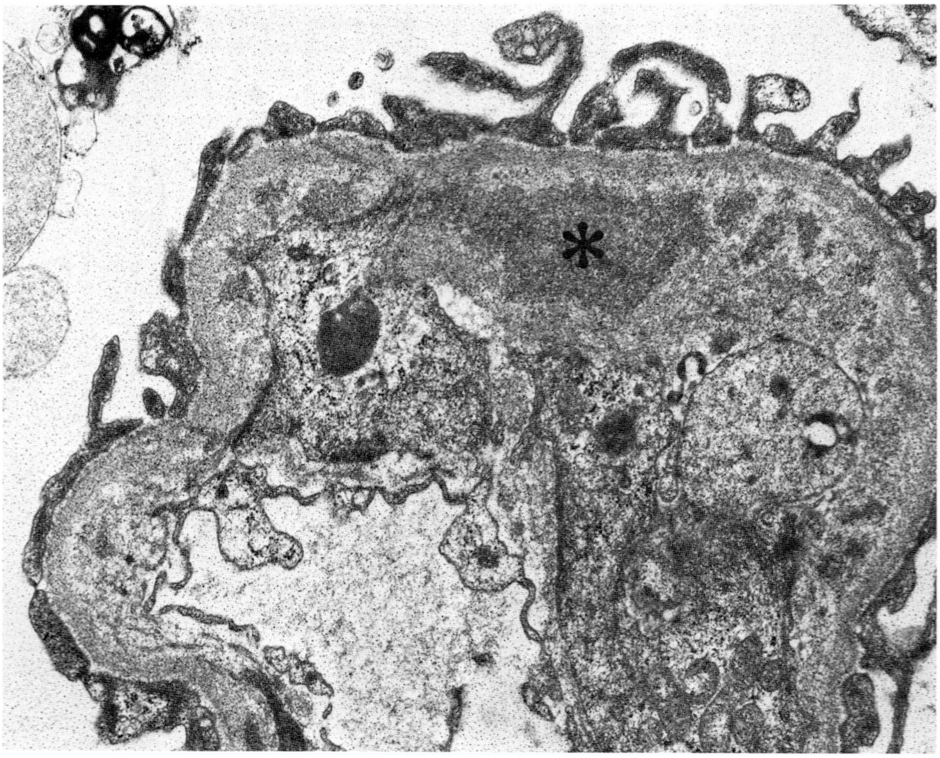

(A)

FIGURE 15 Chronic rejection. Types of abnormal basement membrane material. (Type 1 has been illustrated in Figure 8.) (A) Type 2 electron-dense material (asterisk) resembling that known from immune deposits in various forms of complex-mediated glomerulonephritis (X13,000). (B) Type 4 (arrows). Large vesicular particles and membranous profiles, type 5 (double arrows) (X23,000). (C) Small vesicular particles (type 3) (X60,000). (D) Type 5 profiles (X70,000). (For details of ultrastructure and occurrence of these structures, see Reference 24.)

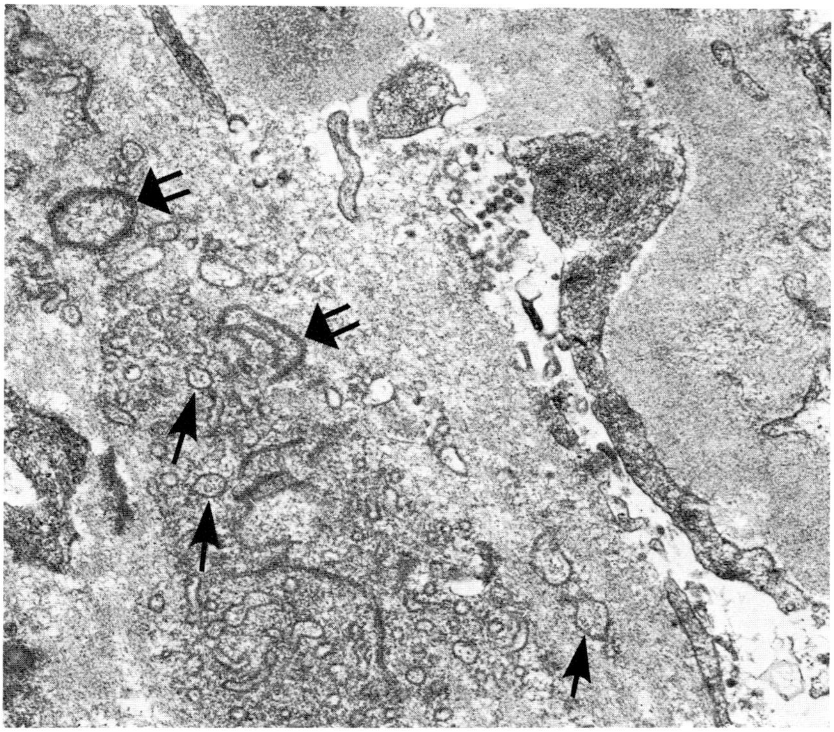

(B)

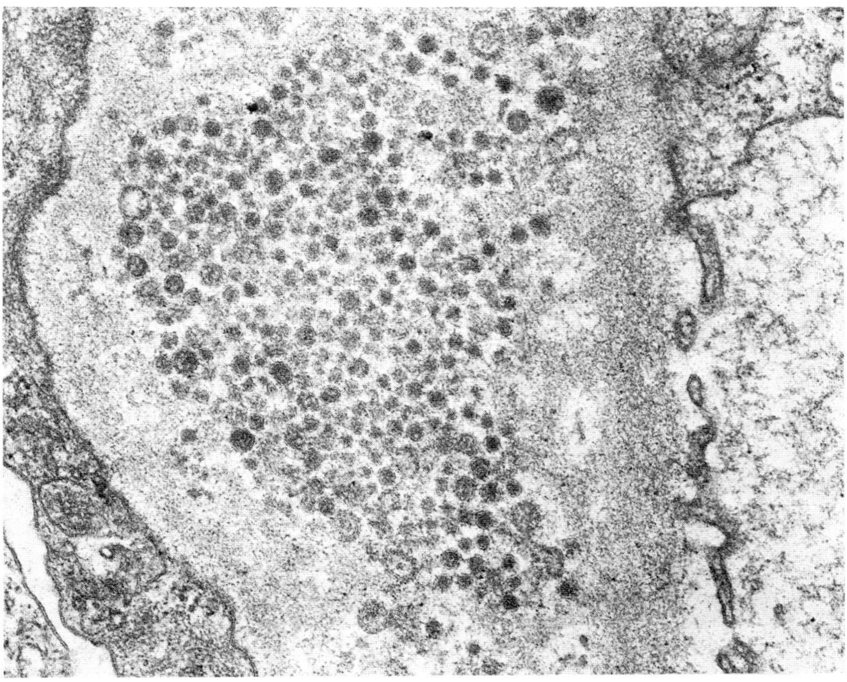

(C)

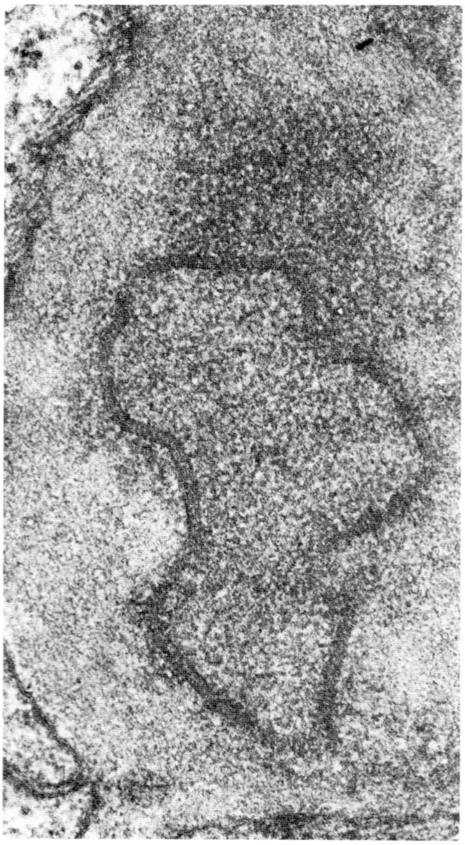

(D)
FIGURE 15 *(continued)*

On EM, five types of abnormal structures may be found in the thickened basement membrane in chronic rejection (Fig. 15) [24]. Type 1 is an electron-lucent flocculent material located in the widened region between the endothelial cells and the lamina densa of the glomerular basement membrane. This material looks like that commonly seen in early acute rejection. Type 2 is a finely granular, electron-dense material similar in appearance to deposits of immunocomplexes in native glomerulonephritis. This material may be subepithelial, intramembranous or subendothelial. Humplike structures (as in native post-streptococcal glomerulonephritis [15] or membranous lesions [24,29] may occasionally occur as part of the transplant glomerulopathy. Types 3 and 4 are small or large vesicular structures, formerly thought to be virus particles. A more probable interpretation is that they are membranes pinched-off from degenerating cells. Type 5 consists of large membranous profiles, probably material synthesized by the glomerular cells under pathologic conditions.

Arterial and glomerular changes may coexist, which is usually the case if the glomerular rejection appears with a loss of graft function, as well as in proteinuria. In rare cases, the morphologic picture may be almost pure, either arterial or glomerular. The difficult problem of delineating transplant glomerulopathy from other glomerular reactions in the graft will be discussed in the next section.

Ischemic glomerular alteration may also be present in chronic graft rejection. Thus, glomeruli may show wrinkling and collapse of the capillary basement membranes.

In addition to glomerular and vascular changes and their sequelae, there is always in the chronically rejecting graft some interstitial cell infiltration of the same type as described above in acute rejection.

THE PROBLEM OF GLOMERULONEPHRITIS IN THE ALLOGRAFT

The literature on this subject is complicated by imprecise and variable nomenclature and by the lack of definitions. Glomerular changes of glomerulonephritis may be expected to occur in the allograft in three main conditions.

1. Glomerulonephritis in the patient's native kidneys may recur in the graft due to persistence of the pathogenetic mechanism responsible for the original glomerular disease. This condition may be called *recurrent or transmitted glomerulonephritis.*
2. Glomerulonephritis may occur in the transplanted kidney due to an immune process induced by antigens present in the graft itself. The glomerular reaction in this situation is part of the rejection. Examples of such changes have been mentioned in sections on acute and chronic rejection. The term "acute or chronic *transplant glomerulopathy*" can be recommended for this condition.
3. Glomerulonephritis may occur in the allograft due to immune processes associated with an antigen neither responsible for a native glomerulonephritis nor present in the transplant. Deposition of immune complexes may thus be caused by bacterial or other infectious antigens or antigens introduced into the body for therapeutic purposes, such as antilymphocytic globulin. The term "*de novo* glomerulonephritis" has been applied to this situation. Since a transplant glomerulopathy could be designated as de novo with equal right, the more cumbersome (but also more precise) name "de novo glomerulonephritis, unrelated to histoincompatibility" might might be used to avoid confusion with transplant glomerulopathy.

It is not at all easy to determine the actual type of glomerulonephritis in a graft, and several reports in the literature of cases thought to represent one or another of the situations mentioned are supported by weak arguments. Ideally, the unequivocal determination of type can only be made if the antigen as well as the pathogenetic mechanism are known. In real life, this is unfortunately very seldom the case. For lack of such clear evidence, less reliable data have to be applied. The most used of these are identity or close resemblance of glomerular histopathology by LM and EM, as well as the glomerular immunoglobulin classes represented and their pattern as revealed by immunofluorescence microscopy. Due to the heterogeneity of the histologic picture of glomerular reaction in rejection, caution must be exercised in evaluating such data. Transplant glomerulopathy in chronic rejection may, therefore, take on a picture of diffuse membranoproliferative glomerulonephritis, and if this was also the patient's original disease, the case has sometimes been interpreted as transmission. This particular picture can, however, be present in a graft from a patient suffering from a nonglomerular native disease, as often documented [22,29], leaving only the possibilities 2 and 3. Other patterns of glomerular reaction can also be seen in chronic rejection. Membranous glomerulonephritis has been described in patients with this disease in the original kidneys as well as with nonglomerular native disease [24,29]. Focal proliferative and sclerosing lesions may also form part of the picture in chronic rejection.

Among the convincing examples of transmission are those that recur rather briefly after transplantation and with close recapitulation of the clinical picture, as well as identical LM and immunofluorescence pattern, as has been reported with rapidly progressive glomerulonephritis with crescents [28]. This has also been seen in the rare crescentic anti-glomerular basement membrane nephritis with linear fluorescent pattern (for literature and description of a case, see Reference 26). Another situation in which transmission has been based on firm evidence is in membranoproliferative glomerulonephritis type 2 (dense deposit disease) because of its unique electron microscopic characteristics [1,9]. For a discussion of other types of allegedly transmitted glomerulonephritis, see Reference 26.

A simple criterion, which seems to have convinced many authors about transmission, is the presence in the graft of marked glomerular changes by LM together with the presence of immunodeposits by EM as well as immunofluorescence microscopy. In our opinion, this criterion is not valid. We have studied renal transplant disease in 125 recipients surviving for more than 1-8 years after transplantation [24,29]. In this population, heavy proteinuria and/or declining graft function occurred in 22 patients. Glomerular transplant disease included a majority of 16 patients, constituting a rather homogeneous entity in terms of clinical course. Glomerular changes were severe and included endomesangial proliferation and focal crescent formation and thickening, as well as duplication of peripheral capillary walls. All cases revealed heavy glomerular immune deposits, most frequently IgG and IgM as well as complement, but IgA was also sometimes present. On EM, glomerular deposits were common. This type of glomerular allograft disease, which is present in the main part of chronically rejected grafts, occurred with equal incidence in patients with native glomerulonephritis and with nonglomerular disease. The development of the disease was clearly correlated with histoincompatibility. From these and other arguments, we concluded that this glomerulonephritis was a *de novo* disease probably due to the action of transplant antigens, not a transmission of the original glomerular disease.

The transmission of glomerulonephritis may obviously occur, but it is probably rare. In 400 consecutive renal allotransplantations from our series, there were 4 patients in whom transmission was considered likely. It is our conviction that most cases of glomerulonephritis in the graft occur as part of the rejection and should be termed "transplant glomerulopathy." The occurrence of a *de novo* glomerulonephritis caused by antigens other than those present in the graft is probably very rare.

CONCLUSION

A careful morphologic analysis of material from renal allografts may serve several important purposes. If the allograft has lost its function and has been surgically removed or if the patient has died, it is important to be able to disclose the cause. Was it a rejection, and if so, of what type? Was it due to causes other than rejection, and if so, what cause (infection, major vessel occlusion, possibly due to surgical complications, and others)? Reliable morphologic diagnoses are a prerequisite for the quality of rejection statistics and consequently for the evaluation of treatment strategies. Graft biopsies may aid this purpose by revealing the changes occurring during the course of the graft disease. Furthermore, biopsies are of great value for monitoring the treatment of the individual patient as well as for prognosis.

REFERENCES

1. Beaufils, H., Gubler, M. C., Karam, J., Gluckman, J. C., Legrain, M., and Küss, R. Dense deposit disease: Long term follow-up of three cases of recurrence after transplantation. *Clin. Nephrol.* 7:31-37, 1977.
2. Beschorner, W. E., Burdick, J. F., Williams, G. M., and Solez, K. The presence of Leu7 reactive lymphocytes in renal allografts undergoing acute rejection. *Transplant. Proc.* 17:618-622, 1985.
3. Brun, C., and Olsen, S. *Atlas of Renal Biopsy.* Munksgaard, Copenhagen, 1981.
4. Busch, G. J., Galvanek, E. G., and Reynolds, E. S. Human renal allografts. Analysis of lesions in long-term survivors. *Hum. Pathol.* 2:253-298, 1971.
5. Busch, G. J., Reynolds, E. S., Galvanek, E. G., Braun, W. E., and Dammin, G. J. Human renal allografts. The role of vascular injury in early graft failure. *Medicine (Baltimore)* 50:29-83, 1971.
6. Busch, G. J., Schamberg, J. F., Moretz, R. C., Stron, T. B., Tilney, N. L., and Carpenter, C. B. T and B cell patterns in irreversibly rejected human renal allografts: Correlation of morphology with surface markers and cytotoxic capacity of the isolated lymphoid infiltrates. *Lab. Invest.* 35:272-282, 1976.
7. Callard, P., Bedrossian, J., Idatte, J. M., Belair, M. F., Grossetete, J., Mandet, C., and Bariet, J. Les lésions arterielles au cours des phénomènes de rejet des allogreffes rénales. In *Actualités Nephrologiques de L'Hôpital Necker 1975.* Flammarian, Paris, 1975, pp. 165-185.
8. Curtis, J. J., Bhathena, D., Lucas, B. A., McRoberts, J. W., and Luke, R. G. "Hyperacute rejection" due to perfusion injury. *Clin. Nephrol.* 7:120-124, 1977.
9. Droz, D., Nabarra, B., Noel, L.-H., Leibowitch, J., and Crosnier, J. Recurrence of dense deposits in transplanted kidneys. I. Sequential survey of the lesions. *Kidney Int.* 15:386-395, 1979.
10. Farnsworth, A., Hall, B. M., Ng, A. B. P., Duggin, G. G., Horvath, J. S., Sheil, A. B. R., and Tiller, D. J. Renal biopsy morphology in renal transplantation. *Am. J. Surg. Pathol.* 8:243-252, 1984.
11. Finkelstein, F. O., Siegel, N. J., Bastl, C., Forrest, J. N., Jr., and Kashgarian, M. Kidney transplant biopsies in the diagnosis and management of acute rejection reactions. *Kidney Int.* 10:171-178, 1976.
12. Hamburger, J., Crosnier, J., and Dormont, J. Experience with 45 renal homotransplantations in man. *Lancet* 1:985, 1965.
13. Herbertson, B. M., Evans, D. B., Calne, R. Y., and Banerjee, A. K. Percutaneous needle biopsies of renal allografts: The relationship between morphological changes present in biopsies and subsequent allograft function. *Histopathology* 1:161-178, 1977.
14. Hus, A. C., Arbus, G. S., Noriega, E., and Huber, J. Renal allograft biopsy: A satisfactory adjunct for predicting renal function after graft rejection. *Clin. Nephrol.* 5: 260, 1976.
15. Hulme, B., Andres, G. A., Porter, K. A., and Ogden, D. A. Human renal transplants. IV. Glomerular ultrastructure, macromolecular permeability and hemodynamics. *Lab. Invest.* 26:2-10, 1972.
16. Jones, D. B. Scanning and transmission electron microscopy of tubular changes in acute renal failure. In *Acute Renal Failure: Correlation Between Morphology and Function.* K. Solez and A. Whelton, eds. Marcel Dekker, New York, 1983, pp. 71-96.

17. Kincaid-Smith, P. Histological diagnosis of rejection of renal homografts in man. *Lancet* 2:849-852, 1967.
18. Kissmeyer-Nielsen, F., Olsen, S., Petersen, V. P., and Fjeldborg, O. Hyperacute rejection of kidney allografts, associated with pre-existing humoral antibodies against donor cells. *Lancet* 2:662-665, 1966.
19. Kiaer, H., Hansen, H. E., and Olsen, S. The predictive value of percutaneous biopsies from human renal allografts with early impaired function. *Clin. Nephrol.* 13:58-63, 1980.
20. Lindquist, R. R., Guttmann, R. D., Merrill, J. P., and Dammin, G. J. Human renal allografts. Interpretation of morphologic and immunohistochemical observations. *Am. J. Pathol.* 53:851-881, 1968.
21. Lund, B., and Myhre Jensen, O. Renal transplantation in rabbits. II. Morphological alterations in autografts. *Acta Pathol. Microbiol. Scand.* [*A*] 78:701-712, 1970.
22. Mathew, T. H., Mathews, D. C., Hobbs, J. B., and Kincaid-Smith, P. Glomerular lesions after renal transplantation. *Am. J. Med.* 59:177-190, 1975.
23. Nabarra, B., and Descamps, B. Ultrastructure of cells infiltrating human kidney allografts. *Clin. Exp. Immunol.* 24:300-309, 1976.
24. Olsen, S., Bohman, S.-O., and Petersen, V. Ultrastructure of the glomerular basement membrane in long term renal allografts with transplant glomerular disease. *Lab. Invest.* 30:176-189, 1974.
25. Olsen, S., and Bohman, S.-O. Renal allograft rejection. In *Electron Microscopy in Human Medicine,* J. Vincents Johannesen, ed. McGraw Hill, New York, 1979, pp. 128-142.
26. Olsen, S. Pathology of the renal allograft rejection. In *Kidney Disease—Present Status,* IAP Monograph no. 20, Williams & Wilkins, Baltimore, 1979, pp. 327-355.
27. Olsen, T. S., Hansen, H. E., and Olsen. H. S. Tubular ultrastructure in acute renal failure: Alterations of cellular surfaces (branch-border and basolateral infoldings). *Virch. Archiv. A406*:91-104, 1985.
28. Petersen, V. P., Olsen, S., Kissmeyer-Nielsen, F., and Fjeldborg, O. Transmission of glomerulonephritis from host to human-kidney allotransplant. *N. Engl. J. Med.* 275: 1259-1273, 1966.
29. Petersen, V. P., Olsen, T. S., Kissmeyer-Nielsen, F., Bohman, S.-O., Hansen, H. E., Hansen, E. S., Skov, P. E., and Sølling, K. Late failure of human renal transplants. An analysis of transplant disease and graft failure among 125 recipients surviving for one to eight years. *Medicine* (*Baltimore*) 54:45-71, 1975.
30. Porter, K. A., Thomson, W. B., Owen, K., Kenyon, J. R., Mowbray, J. F., and Peart, W. S. Obliterative vascular changes in four human kidney homotransplants. *Br. Med. J.* 2:639-645, 1963.
31. Porter, K. A., Marchioro, T. L., and Starzl, T. E. Pathological changes in 37 human renal homotransplants treated with immunosuppressive drugs. *Br. J. Urol.* 37:250-273, 1965.
32. Porter, K. A., Rendall, J. M., Stolinski, C., Terasaki, P. I., Marchioro, T. L., and Starzl, T. E. Light and electron microscopic study of biopsies from 33 human renal allografts and an isograft 1¾-2½ years after transplantation. *Ann. N.Y. Acad. Sci.* 129:615, 1966.
33. Porter, K. A., Dossetor, J. B., Marchioro, T. L., Peart, W. S., Rendall, J. M., Starzl, T. E., and Terasaki, P. I. Human renal transplants. I. Glomerular changes. *Lab. Invest.* 16:153-181, 1967.
34. Richardson, W. P., Colvin, R. B., Cheeseman, S. H., Tolkoff-Rubin, N. E., Herrin, J. T., Cosimi, B., Collins, A. B., Hirsch, M. S., McCluskey, R. T., Russell, P. S., and Rubin, R. H. Glomerulopathy associated with cytomegalovirus viremia in renal allografts. *N. Engl. J. Med.* 305:57-63, 1981.

35. Starzl, T. E., Lerner, R. A., Dixon, F. J., Groth, C. G., Brettschneider, L., and Terasaki, P. I. Shwartzman reaction of human renal homotransplantation. *N. Engl. J. Med.* *278*:642-648, 1968.
36. Solez, K., McGraw, D. J., Beschorner, W. E., Kone, B. C., Racusen, L. C., Whelton, A., and Burdick, J. K. Reflections on use of the renal biopsy as the "gold standard" in distinguishing transplant rejection from cyclosporine nephrotoxicity. *Trans. Proc. 17* (Suppl. 1):123-133, 1985.
37. Williams, G. M., Hume, D. M., Hudson, R. P., Morris, P. J., Kano, K., and Milgrom, F. "Hyperacute" renal-homograft rejection in man. *N. Engl. J. Med.* 279:611-618, 1968.
38. Zollinger, H. U., Miharsch, M. J., Gudat, F., Thiel, G., Brunner, F., and Enderlin, F. Etiologic and prognostic significance of isolated acute renal hypoxic change (so-called tubular necrosis or shock kidney) in kidney transplants. *Clin. Nephrol.* 6:485-487, 1976.
39. Zollinger, H. U., and Mihatsch, M. J. *Renal Pathology in Biopsy.* Springer-Verlag, Berlin, 1978.

9

HYPERACUTE REJECTION AND PERFUSION INJURY

Kim Solez and G. Melville Williams
The Johns Hopkins University School of Medicine, Baltimore, Maryland

The greatest obstacle to the success of kidney transplantation as a therapy for end-stage renal disease is rejection. Rejection may be one of three types: hyperacute rejection, occurring within minutes after attaching the donor and recipient vessels, or acute or chronic rejection, occurring, respectively, weeks or months after the time of transplantation. The preceding chapter described acute and chronic rejection in some detail. In the present chapter we will consider hyperacute rejection [20] and a condition that may mimic hyperacute rejection–perfusion injury [6,15]. These two entities are the most common causes of the "soft blue kidney" syndrome in the immediate posttransplant period.

The appearance of the kidney during the first few minutes after release of the vascular clamps is very important to the transplant surgeon. If all has gone well, the initially flaccid kidney gradually pinks up and becomes firm. Brief compression of the venous anastomosis leads to swelling of the kidney due to the high arterial inflow. Under normal circumstances, the firm, orange-pink appearance of the kidney is maintained. However, if hyperacute rejection or perfusion injury is present, the kidney gradually turns a dusky bluish color and becomes soft. A biopsy with frozen section may be useful in distinguishing hyperacute rejection from perfusion injury or from thrombosis of the arterial anastomosis (Table 1).

HYPERACUTE REJECTION

Hyperacute rejection is due to preformed antibody in a recipient who has been previously sensitized to donor antigens present in the transplanted kidney. Hyperacute rejection cannot be treated with conventional immunosuppressive regimens and almost invariably results in loss of the transplanted kidney. Some investigators have advocated treating hyperacute rejection with large dosages of heparin and steroids. Although this treatment may restore some degree of function on occasion, severe systemic toxicity and consumption coagulopathy may develop [18]. Therefore, most surgeons favor the removal of grafts as soon as the diagnosis of hyperacute rejection is established. In its classic form, hyperacute rejection is extremely rare when modern cross-matching techniques are employed. More subtle forms of hyperacute rejection occasionally still occur. In these

TABLE 1 Intraoperative Assessment of the Soft Blue Kidney

Causes	Findings		
	Hilar pulsation	Effect of venous compression	Frozen section appearance
Diminished arterial inflow	Weak	No swelling	Normal
Perfusion injury	Strong, no thrill	No swelling	Glomerular capillary "plugs"
Hyperacute rejection	Strong, no thrill	No swelling	Polymorphonuclear leukocytes in peritubular capillaries

cases the graft may appear normal and even produce urine initially. A high fever and anuria occur 2-3 days later. If these signs are accompanied by a fall in the peripheral platelet count, which seems a more sensitive marker than a decline in fibrinogen or the appearance of fibrin split products, the diagnosis is almost certainly that of hyperacute rejection.

PERFUSION INJURY

Perfusion injury is due to mechanical damage to the endothelium of small blood vessels and capillaries. The mechanical damage in perfusion injury is thought to be due to inappropriate composition or pressure of the perfusion solutions used to preserve kidneys on a pulsatile perfusion machine in the interval between harvesting of the kidney and placement in the recipient [2,3,6,15]. Often, however, the origin of the damage is obscure, and occasional transplanted kidneys sustain injury similar to perfusion injury even though they are never placed on a perfusion machine. Perfusion injury tends to be self-limiting. In biopsies obtained immediately after transplantation, it may mimic the changes of hyperacute rejection, but whereas hyperacute rejection leads to death of the kidney, perfusion injury is frequently compatible with considerable return of kidney function.

Damage to the main renal artery induced by the perfusion cannula can lead to thrombosis or to later renal artery stenosis [10,17]. Indirect perfusion via an aortic cannula avoids this problem.

PATHOLOGIC FEATURES

In both hyperacute rejection and perfusion injury there is plugging of glomerular capillaries in the kidney with aggregates of fibrin, platelets, and red blood cells (Figure 1). Polymorphonuclear leukocytes accumulate in peritubular and glomerular capillaries (Figure 2). In both conditions the kidney is observed by the surgeon to turn blue after a short initial period when it has a normal pink color. This color change reflects the congestion and inadequate blood flow that results when many capillaries are plugged. The two conditions may often be differentiated in early (1 hr) biopsies (Table 1) because in hyperacute rejection the accumulation of polymorphs in peritubular capillaries tends to precede the capillary plugging [20], whereas in perfusion injury the sequence is the other way around [15]. In an early biopsy only capillary plugging may be seen in perfusion in-

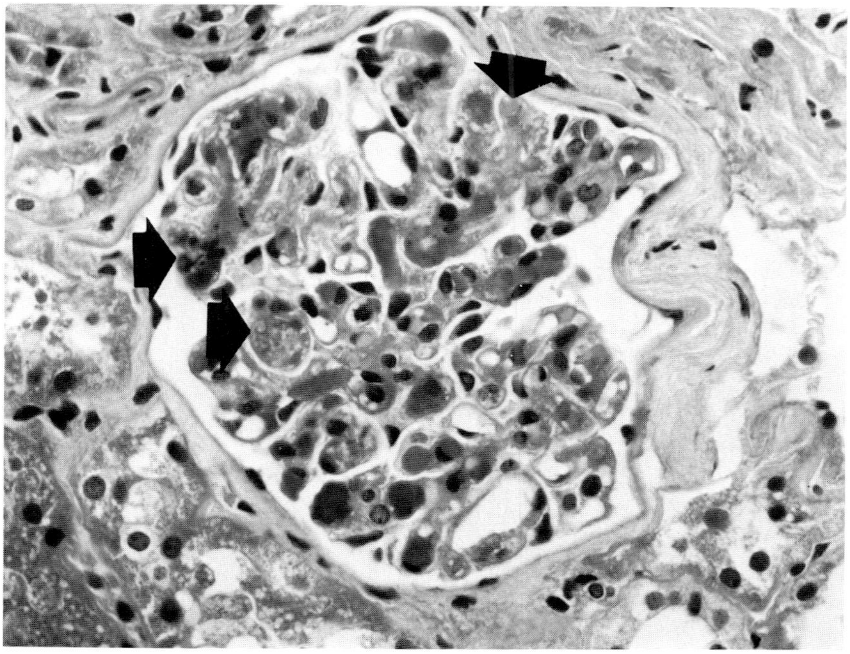

FIGURE 1 Perfusion injury as seen in a renal transplant biopsy obtained 1 hr after attaching the donor and recipient vessels. There is considerable plugging of glomerular capillaries by fibrin-platelet-red cell aggregates (arrows), and many capillaries have lost their endothelial lining cells. (H&E, X415)

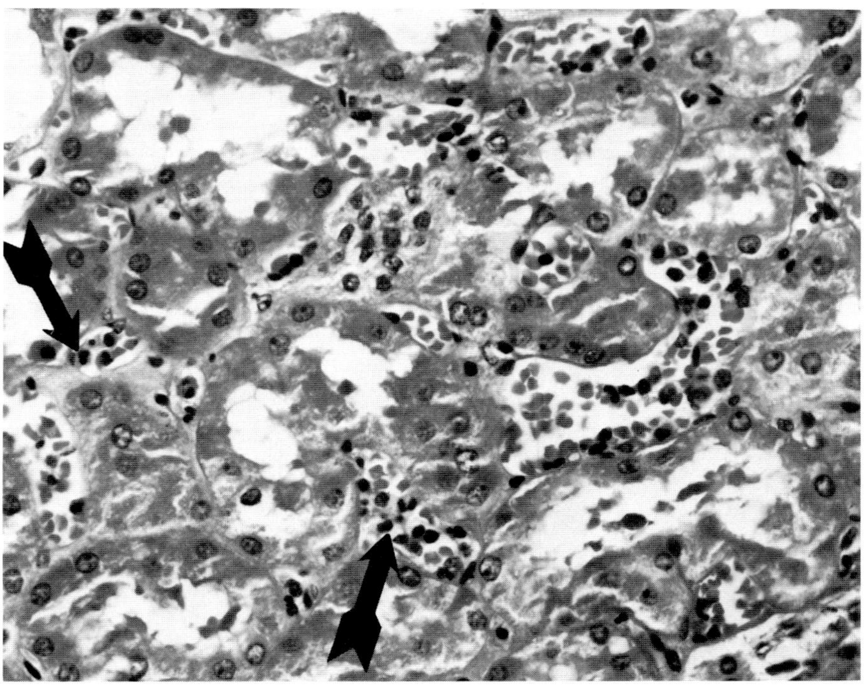

FIGURE 2 Accumulations of polymorphonuclear leukocytes (arrows) in peritubular capillaries in a case of hyperacute rejection. (H&E, X370)

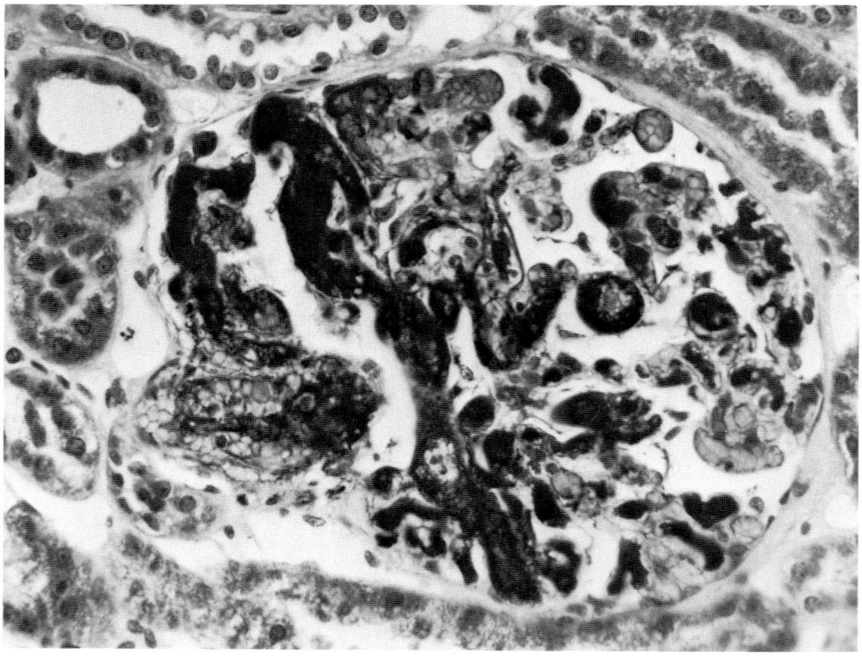

FIGURE 3 Extensive fibrin thrombi in glomerular capillaries due to perfusion injury in a biopsy obtained 1 hr posttransplant. This kidney had two renal arteries, only one of which was identified at the time of harvesting. A portion of the kidney was machine perfused through the single renal artery and after transplantation had the appearance seen here. (PTAH stain for fibrin, X370)

jury, as there may not have been enough time for the polymorphonuclear leukocyte reaction to be stimulated. On rare occasions, only a portion of kidney may manifest perfusion injury if there are two renal arteries, but only one is used during perfusion (Figures 3 and 4).

OTHER CONDITIONS SIMULATING PERFUSION INJURY

Perfusion injury has seemed sometimes to be a regional problem—some transplant centers believing that they have never seen a clear-cut case [4]—and in the 1980s it has become a rare problem nationwide, probably because of improvements in perfusion techniques, machines, and solutions. A number of other conditions can produce morphologic and/or clinical features similar to perfusion injury.

Cornstarch Emboli

Cornstarch particles used as a glove lubricant can find their way into the perfusion fluid and become lodged in glomerular capillaries [6,7]. These particles are refractile and highly periodic acid-Schiff (PAS) positive. In our experience and that of Hill et al. [6], the presence of these particles does not seem to be associated with transplant dysfunction.

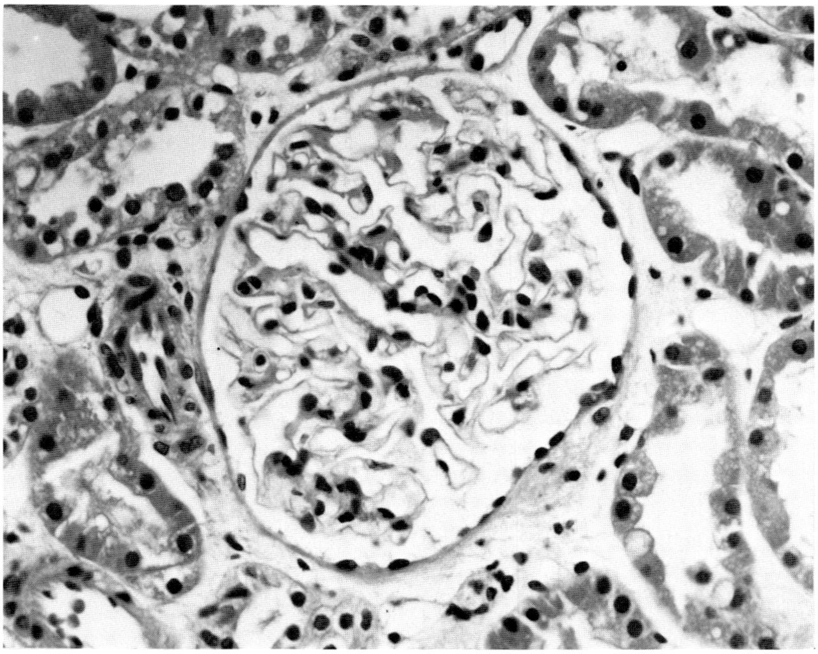

FIGURE 4 Normal renal morphology except for degenerative tubular changes in the nonperfused portion of same kidney as in Figure 3. This portion of the kidney remained pink after opening the anastomoses, while the perfused portion rapidly turned blue. (H&E, X370)

Cold-Reactive Antibody Injury

Lobo et al. [8] and Sturgill et al. [19] have recently alleged that cold-reacting IgM antibodies are a common cause of immediate transplant failure when the cold kidney is not rewarmed prior to releasing the vascular changes. The pathology described in their cases, many of which had machine preservation, is similar to that of perfusion injury. To determine whether it is possible that we had confused cold-reactive IgM injury with perfusion injury we retrospectively analyzed serum obtained around the time of transplantation from six patients diagnosed as having perfusion injury and six controls for cold IgM antibody reactive against a panel of lymphocytes. The only patient with clearly demonstrable cold-reactive IgM antibody came from the control group. Thus, we concluded that perfusion injury is not mediated through the mechanism of cold-reactive IgM antibody. This does not exclude the possibility that such antibodies can on occasion lead to early transplant failure.

Schweizer et al. [12] have described five patients in whom cold red blood cell autoagglutinins appeared to be responsible for immediate transplant nonfunction with thrombosis. These authors considered antibodies reactive at 22°C to be more significant in causing transplant failure than those reactive at 4°C and stated that the titer and thermal amplitude of such antibodies should always be determined before organ transplantation. The test for cold red blood cell autoagglutinins can be readily performed by most blood banks. It seems reasonable to suggest that kidneys transplanted into individuals with cold agglutinins be warmed by brief flushing prior to opening the anastomoses.

Pigmentation Abnormalities

Disease entities that may cause persistently blue or discolored kidneys include hemosiderosis, lipofuscin deposition, melanoma, or genetic abnormalities, such as the Hermansky-Pudlak syndrome [16]. Except for melanoma, these conditions in the donor probably have no adverse effect on transplant kidney function in the recipient.

Subclinical Glomerulonephritis

We recently encountered a donor with enlarged (400-g) kidneys that had scattered petechiae on their surface. Donor renal function and urinalysis were normal. A biopsy showed occasional superficial tubules containing red blood cells, corresponding to the petechiae seen grossly. One glomerulus contained a crescent with fibrin deposition in the capsular space (Figure 5). The remaining glomeruli, numbering more than 50, all appeared normal. Fibrin deposition was seen in occasional arterioles. This case probably represented subclinical microembolization or subclinical glomerulonephritis. The kidneys were not used for transplantation, but it is not certain that they would have led to problems in a potential recipient.

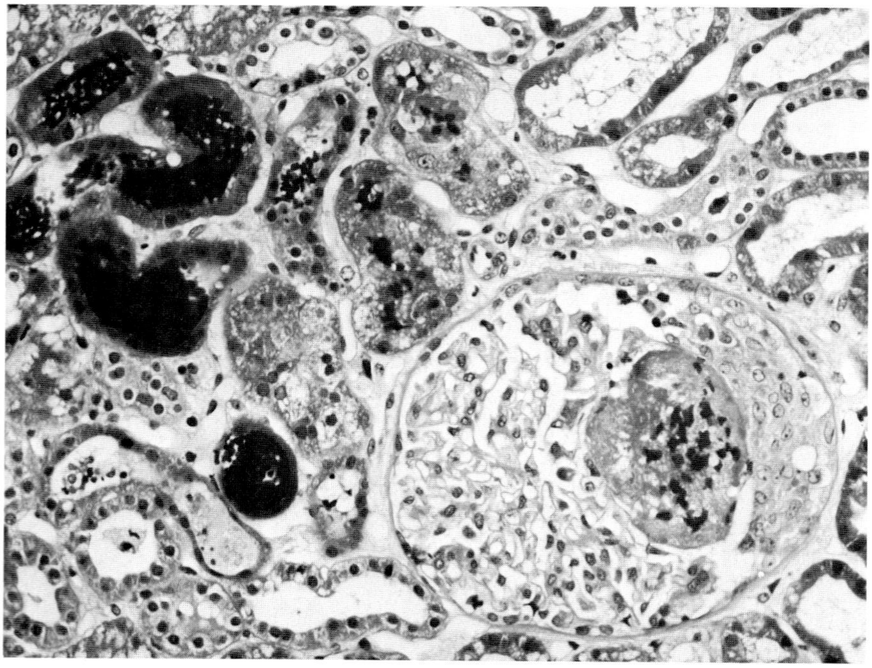

FIGURE 5 Thrombus material and epithelial crescent in a glomerulus from a donor kidney with surface petechiae. Red blood cells can be seen in nearby tubular cross sections. (H&E, X270)

The question of whether kidneys with subclinical glomerulonephritis should be transplanted comes up in another context. If one does immunofluorescence studies routinely on biopsies obtained 1 hr after transplantation, a certain number will contain mesangial deposits of IgA. This is not surprising since IgA nephropathy is a common condition and patients with liver disease often have asymptomatic mesangial deposits of IgA [1]. There is no evidence that such incidentally discovered IgA deposits cause glomerular disease in the recipient [11,13], although in one report [11] the incidence of rejection was high in kidneys exhibiting this feature.

Thrombotic Phenomena Associated with Cyclosporine Therapy

We have observed an apparent increased incidence of glomerular capillary thrombosis in 1-hr biopsies in transplanting patients pretreated with cyclosporine. Several of these patients have eventually had adequate transplant function, suggesting a self-limiting process. The kidneys had not been perfused, and no cold-reactive antibodies were detected. There are several reports of later intrarenal thrombotic phenomena associated with cyclosporine therapy [5,9,13]. It is possible that on occasion cyclosporine's effect on endothelium is evident as early as 1 hr posttransplant.

REFERENCES

1. Berger, J., Yaneva, H., and Nabarra, B. Glomerular changes in patients with cirrhosis of the liver. *Adv. Nephrol.* 7:3-14, 1978.
2. Cerra, F. B., Raza, S., Andres, G. A., and Segel, J. H. The endothelial damage of pulsatile renal preservation and its relationship to perfusion pressure and colloid osmotic pressure. *Surgery* 81:534, 1977.
3. Evan, A. P., Gattone, V. H., II, Filo, R. S., Leapman, S. B., Smith, E. J., and Luft, F. C. Glomerular endothelial injury related to renal perfusion. A scanning electron microscopic study. *Transplantation* 35:436-441, 1983.
4. Goldzer, R. C., Strom, T. B., and Tilney, N. L. Acute renal failure associated with renal transplantation. In *Acute Renal Failure,* B. M. Brenner and J. M. Lazarus, eds. W. B. Saunders, Philadelphia, 1983, pp. 555-566.
5. Green, L., Verani, R., Schoenberg, L., and Kahan, B. Comparative pathological review of 72 renal transplant nephrectomies of patients treated with cyclosporine or azathioprine (abstract). *Kidney Int.* 27:341, 1985.
6. Hill, G. S., Light, J. A., and Perloff, L. J. Perfusion-related injury in renal transplantation. *Surgery* 79:440-447, 1976.
7. Limas, C., Spector, D., and Wright, J. R. Histologic changes in preserved cadaveric renal transplants. *Am. J. Pathol.* 88:403-420, 1977.
8. Lobo, P. I., Sturgill, B. C., and Bolton, W. K. Cold-reactive alloantibodies and allograft malfunction occurring immediately posttransplant. *Transplantation* 37:76-81, 1984.
9. Neild, G., Reuben, R., Hartley, B., and Cameron, J. S. Glomerular thrombi in renal allografts associated with cyclosporin therapy. *Kidney Int.* 27:345, 1985.
10. Oakes, D. D., Spees, E. K., McAllister, H. A., and Saddler, W. Arterial injury during perfusion preservation: A possible cause of posttransplantation renal artery stenosis. *Surgery* 89:210-215, 1981.
11. Sanfilippo, F., Croker, B. P., and Bollinger, R. R. Fate of four cadaveric donor renal allografts with mesangial IgA deposits. *Transplantation* 33:370-376, 1982.
12. Schweizer, R. T., Bartus, S. A., Perkins, H. A., and Belzer, F. O. Renal allograft failure and cold red blood cell autoagglutinins. *Transplantation* 33:77-79, 1982.

13. Shulman, H., Striker, G., Deeg, H. J., Kennedy, M., Storb, R., and Thomas, E. D. Nephrotoxicity of cyclosporin A after allogeneic marrow transplantation. *N. Engl. J. Med.* 305:1392-1395, 1981.
14. Silva, F. G., Chander, P., Pirani, C. L., and Hardy, M. A. Disappearance of glomerular mesangial IgA deposits after renal allograft transplantation (letter to editor). *Transplantation* 33:214-216, 1982.
15. Spector, D., Limas, C., Frost, J. L., Zachary, J. B., Sterioff, S., Williams, G. M., Rolley, R. T., and Sadler, J. H. Perfusion nephropathy in human transplants. *N. Engl. J. Med.* 295:1217, 1976.
16. Spees, E. K., Lempert, N., Olson, J. L., Williams, G. M., Phillips, M. G., Mendez-Picon, G., and Rohr, M. Blue cadaver donor kidneys for transplantation (abstract). *J. Urol.* 131:338A, 1984.
17. Spees, E. K., Oakes, D. D., Hill, G. S., Light, J. A., Williams, G. M., and Ernst, C. B. Why some preserved kidneys do not function: A review of preservation-related endothelial injuries. *Transplant. Proc.* 14:80-85, 1982.
18. Starzl, T. E., Boehmig, H. J., Amemiya, H., Wilson, C. B., Dixon, F. J., Giles, G. R., Simpson, K. M., and Halgrimson, C. G. Clotting changes, including disseminated intravascular coagulation, during rapid renal-homograft rejection. *N. Engl. J. Med.* 283:383-390, 1970.
19. Sturgill, B. C., Lobo, P. I., and Bolton, W. K. Cold-reacting IgM antibody-induced renal allograft failure. Similarity to hyperacute rejection. *Nephron* 36:125-127, 1984.
20. Williams, G. M., Hume, D. M., Hudson, R. P., Morris, P. J., Kano, K., and Milgrom, F. Hyperacute renal-homograft rejection in man. *N. Engl. J. Med.* 279:611, 1968.

10

PATHOLOGY OF "ACUTE TUBULAR NECROSIS" AND ACUTE REJECTION

Observations on Early Systematic Renal Transplant Biopsies

Kim Solez, Daniel J. McGraw, William E. Beschorner, and James F. Burdick
The Johns Hopkins University School of Medicine, Baltimore, Maryland

BACKGROUND: THE RENAL BIOPSY AS THE "GOLD STANDARD" IN THE DIAGNOSIS OF REJECTION

The common causes of acute renal failure (ARF) in transplanted kidneys are postischemic ARF ("acute tubular necrosis"), cyclosporine nephrotoxicity, and acute rejection. Acute rejection occurs in a majority of renal transplant recipients and remains the greatest single obstacle to the success of kidney transplantation as a therapy for patients with end-stage renal disease. Acute rejection may be difficult to distinguish on clinical grounds from postischemic ARF or cyclosporine-induced ARF. Therefore, many centers routinely do a biopsy of the transplant at the time of suspected rejection to help guide therapeutic decision making. Renal biopsies performed at the time of renal dysfunction have been regarded as the "gold standard" definitely establishing the presence or absence of acute rejection [25,25a,66]. Heavy emphasis has been placed on the finding of an inflammatory infiltrate in the interpretation of such biopsies since it is known that an interstitial infiltrate of mononuclear cells is a prominent feature of experimental graft rejection [46,48]. Biopsies have rarely been performed in the first month posttransplant in patients with normal function or obvious acute tubular necrosis. It has often been assumed that the morphology of acute tubular necrosis was the same in transplanted and native kidneys and that normally functioning allografts had normal morphology. However, we have found that transplanted kidneys in patients with normal renal function or typical acute tubular necrosis often have a prominent interstitial inflammatory infiltrate and may even have such severe changes as focal infarction and interstitial hemorrhage. As will be described later, we have found these same changes in experimental rat isografts and similar changes have been described by others in experimental autografts and isografts [4,34,35,43]. Matas et al. [45] described 12 transplant patients who had an interstitial infiltrate on biopsy despite good function and the absence of any clinical signs of rejection. They were unable to relate the observed infiltrates to later episodes of rejection.

The presence of a prominent interstitial infiltrate in transplants without clinical rejection probably explains the seemingly curious fact that series of biopsies obtained at the time of suspected rejection have often been described as consisting of biopsies showing mild, moderate, and severe rejection, as if almost almost every patient with suspected re-

rejection indeed had rejection [5,22,32,37]. It is probable that many of the patients with nonrejection states were categorized as having mild or moderate rejection because of the prominence of the inflammatory infiltrate or other "rejection changes" observed on biopsy. In these studies patients with "mild cellular rejection" have almost always had a very favorable outcome regardless of the therapy employed. The probable overdiagnosis of acute rejection in these biopsy studies is an important issue. The bolus steroid therapy commonly used to treat rejection can cause considerable morbidity and should not be used in transplant patients who do not actually have rejection. Also, the efficacy of new anti-rejection therapies (such as cyclosporine or monoclonal antibodies) is difficult to evaluate if some of the treated patients *do not* actually have rejection. The new technique of fine-needle aspiration cytology of the transplant kidney, widely used in Europe to monitor renal transplant rejection, has been validated by comparison with standard needle biopsies [6,17,20,21,77]. Thus, if rejection is overdiagnosed in needle biopsies, it will also be overdiagnosed by aspiration cytology.

A recent editorial [67] states that "renal biopsies used to rule out rejection are far more important than ascertainment of drug levels in the management of suspected cyclosporine nephrotoxicity." However, the interpretation of biopsies performed to distinguish cyclosporine toxicity from rejection [39,60] is also made difficult by the lack of knowledge of the morphologic changes present when a transplant is not rejecting. Interstitial inflammation has been described as a prominent part of cyclosporine toxicity in transplanted human kidneys [60]. On the other hand, Farnsworth et al. [24] could find no difference in the inflammatory infiltrate in biopsies performed because of prolonged post-transplant renal failure in cyclosporine-treated and conventionally treated patients. Others have suggested that the infiltrate seen in cyclosporine-treated patients may be due to concomitant rejection [75]. Homan et al. have reported that cyclosporine can prevent rejection in rat renal allografts while still allowing cellular infiltration of the graft [33]. In animal models of cyclosporine nephrotoxicity in native kidneys, interstitial inflammation is an inconstant feature and is mild when it occurs [12,70,81,82]. It is important to know whether the pathology of "pure" cyclosporine toxicity really is different in transplanted and native kidneys, or whether, as our preliminary studies suggest, the inflammatory infiltrate seen in cyclosporine-treated renal transplant patients is unrelated to cyclosporine therapy.

An interstitial inflammatory infiltrate is often present in ischemic ARF (acute tubular necrosis) but generally is not ascribed a role in production of the renal failure [62-64, 74]. The interstitial infiltrate in acute rejection, on the other hand, is believed to be actively damaging the renal parenchyma and to be one of the main factors causing renal failure. It is logical to assume that the cell types making up these two inflammatory infiltrates ought to be different, but this remains to be demonstrated. Several studies [32,73] have described differences between cell types in inflammatory infiltrates in various types of rejection but have not presented data on nonrejection states. Platt et al. [54] found a difference in the cellular character of inflammatory infiltrates in renal allografts with "acute interstitial rejection" and "interstitial nephritis without rejection," but did not state the clinical criteria for distinguishing the two. In a subsequent study by the same group [53], inflammatory infiltrates in kidneys of transplant recipients with acute rejection were compared with infiltrates from kidneys of patients with cyclosporine toxicity. Differences in OKT4/OKT8 ratios were found, but the authors were uncertain whether the infiltrate in patients with cyclosporine nephrotoxicity was directly related to the cyclosporin treatment or was a nonspecific phenomenon. Other authors [57,72] have described differences in cellular composition and clinical significance of infiltrates in perivascular versus interstitial areas of the kidney. Clearly, there is a need to determine differences in cellular composition and location of renal allograft infiltrates seen in clinically well-defined states of acute rejection, ischemic ARF, cyclosporine toxicity, and normal function.

SYSTEMATIC EARLY TRANSPLANT BIOPSIES IN CLINICAL TRANSPLANTATION

To determine the histologic changes present in the transplant that is doing well, and thus to determine more clearly the features that truly correspond to active acute rejection, we have performed a series of routine allograft biopsies on patients early after renal transplantation, at a time when "acute tubular necrosis" (ATN) or normal function, but no apparent rejection or nephrotoxicity, was present. These were then compared to biopsies obtained during episodes of clinical rejection. We have found that an interstitial infiltrate of mononuclear cells is almost universally present, regardless of the clinical situation, and that a novel lymphocyte subset, appearing to express both T4 and T8 antigens, is found in many of these early biopsies. The presence of an intimal arteritis was found to be specific for acute rejection.

Our studies of these systematic biopsies are only about half completed, so that this chapter represents only a preliminary report based on biopsies from patients on steroid-azathioprine immunosuppression. We are in the process of obtaining an equal number of biopsies from patients on cyclosporine-steroid immunosuppression and will then be able to compare the two immunosuppressive regimens.

The allograft specimens studied were all from adult recipients of cadaver donor transplants treated routinely with prednisone and azathioprine immunosuppression. Horse anti-thymocyte globulin (ATGAM) was added for severe rejection. Under a protocol approved by the Johns Hopkins Joint Committee on Clinical Investigation and after obtaining informed consent, allograft biopsies were obtained systematically at 1 and 4 weeks after renal transplantation. The upper pole of the kidney was biopsied percutaneously at the bedside, using local anesthesia and a Tru-Cut needle. Aside from occasional transient hematuria, there was no morbidity. Specimens obtained at the time of clinically apparent rejection, incidentally during re-exploration of the transplant, or at transplant nephrectomy were also examined. An intraoperative wedge biopsy, taken at approximately 1 hr after restoring kidney blood flow at the time of transplantation, was available in each case. Also included in some comparisons were native kidney biopsies from patients with ATN, which have previously been described in detail [63].

Clinical status of the transplant patients was determined on the basis of renal function, presence or absence of signs of inflammation, including fever, and isotopic renal scan. In a blinded fashion, without knowledge of the histology results, the clinical status of each transplant recipient at the time of biopsy was assigned to one of four categories: normal function, ATN, acute rejection, or incipient acute rejection with a clinical rejection episode occurring within 4-5 days of the biopsy. In two cases, clinically apparent rejection developed within 48 hr after the biopsy, and these two patients were included in the rejection category.

Quantitation of the Interstitial Infiltrate

A total of 18 of the protocol specimens and 9 native kidney ATN biopsies at 1-4 weeks after onset were assessed for degree of interstitial inflammatory infiltrate in hematoxylin and eosin-stained sections. The infiltrate was quantitated using morphometry. A representative section was completely photographed using a Zeiss photomicroscope and high-resolution color transparency film at a magnification of 100. Projected images (×360, final magnification) were traced on white drawing paper, indicating the edges of the biopsy and the location of interstitial inflammatory cells, vessels, glomeruli, and areas of infarction or hemorrhage. These large drawings of each biopsy were then completely photocopied in numbered segments. For each segment the cells were counted and the excess paper trimmed off, leaving only the representation of the biopsy. This trimmed paper was weighed and the total actual area of the biopsy segment calculated from the magnification employed. This allowed calculation of the total number of cells per square millimeter in the entire biopsy.

Phenotypic Analysis of the Infiltrate

Specimens were prepared at 6-μm frozen sections. After inactivating endogenous peroxidase with methanol and hydrogen peroxide, and endogenous biotin and avidin receptors with avidin D and biotin (Vector Labs, Burlingame, CA), the sections were stained with OKT series (Ortho Pharmaceuticals, NJ) or Leu series (Becton-Dickinson, CA) monoclonal antibodies against monocyte subset antigens. The sections were washed and developed with the avidin-biotin immunoperoxidase technique, using diaminobenzidine and copper sulfate [13], and the percentage of staining cells enumerated by light microscopy. In order to avoid sampling error, a representative longitudinal section of each biopsy was counted in its entirety. To determine the approximate fraction of cells that stained with both OKT4 (or Leu 3) and OKT8 (or Leu 2), the monoclonals were added together on the same slide, and the subsequent steps performed similarly; the percentages of stained cells on these slides were then compared with the sum of the percentages obtained when the antibodies were employed separately. This allowed calculation of a "coexpression ratio," defined as

$$\frac{\text{Sum of \% cells stained with each antibody separately}}{\text{\% Cells stained with both antibodies used together}}$$

Interstitial Infiltrate in Different Clinical States and Specificity of Intimal Arteritis

In all but one case an infiltrate was apparent. This consisted of an often impressive interstitial accumulation of mononuclear cells, as illustrated in Figure 1 [(Color Plate 1) Color Plate section follows page 252]. In addition, an intimal arteritis was found in some specimens, an example of which is shown in Figure 2a (Color Plate 1). The results of morphometric enumeration of the total infiltrates in the entire biopsies are shown in Table 1. It is clear that the inflammatory infiltrate was considerable even in cases of ATN or normal function, although there was a statistically significantly greater overall infiltrate in the biopsies from patients with clinically apparent rejection ($p < 0.01$). The more important correlate with clinically apparent rejection in this series was the presence of vasculitis, as shown in Table 1.

Of the patients with infiltrates during quiescence, one subsequently died months later of cytomegalovirus infection, and one kidney never functioned, apparently due to a combination of severe ATN and later rejection. The remaining seven patients, who had

TABLE 1 Inflammatory Infiltrate and Intimal Arteritis in the Various Biopsy Groups

		No. of interstitial cells (cells/mm ± SEM)		
Patient status	N	Overall	Segment with greatest density	Intimal arteritis[a]
ATN in native kidney	9	451 ± 101[bc]	810 ± 229[b]	0/9
Transplant–normal function	4	1290 ± 179[b]	3276 ± 413	0/4
Transplant–normal function, but rejection 4-5 days later	2	807	1796	1/2
Transplant–ATN	7	1335 ± 182[b]	2800 ± 623	0/7
Rejection	5	2269 ± 215[c]	4690 ± 830	4/5[c]

[a]The number of small arteries present in the transplant biopsies ranged from 0 (in one normal function biopsy) to 7, with a mean of 2.4.
[b]Indicates significantly different from rejection group ($p < 0.01$).
[c]Indicates significantly different from transplant ATN group ($p < 0.01$).
Source: From Reference 14. Reprinted with permission.

nine biopsies containing a median of 1198 cells mm^{-2}, are all doing well with good transplant function.

Lymphocyte Phenotypes in Different Clinical States

Table 2 shows the fraction of cells staining for different lymphocyte subset antigens. There was noticeable inhomogeneity, with adjacent clusters of cells often differing in the predominant phenotype. Since all cells were counted on each section, this potential for sampling error was avoided insofar as possible. It may be seen that, both as regards total T lymphocytes present and the helper/suppressor ("4/8") ratio, there were no major differences that would allow discrimination of biopsies from patients with clinically apparent rejection from other settings.

Discussion

Since the demonstration by Medawar [46] that rabbit skin allograft rejection is immunologically mediated and involves an inflammatory infiltrate, the finding of such an infiltrate in any human renal allograft has been considered to represent evidence that rejection was present [32,38,60]. However, previous series describing human renal allograft histology have considered only biopsies performed at the time of suspected renal dysfunction, unlike our protocol, in which the routine biopsies were taken during a stable period. Our observations confirm that an interstitial infiltrate is an accompaniment of human renal allograft rejection (Table 1) in that the cells were, on the average, more numerous in specimens from patients with clinically apparent rejection than during stable quiescence. However, that nearly every biopsy showed an inflammatory infiltrate, even when the patient was without clinical evidence of rejection, indicates that the mere presence of an infiltrate is not necessarily a sign of rejection. This is further strengthened by the observation that subsequent follow-up of the patients with infiltrates revealed good graft survival, for the

TABLE 2 T-Cell Phenotypes in the Allograft Biopsies

Clinical status	% Staining			4:8 Ratio (mean ± SD)	% Staining		Leu3/leu2 ratio
	OKT11	OKT4	OKT8		Leu 3a	Leu 2b	
Acute rejection (n = 4)	39 ± 12	37 ± 18	28 ± 5	1.40 ± 0.69	40 ± 16	35 ± 21	1.60 ± 1.00
Normal/ATN (n = 23)	50 ± 25	32 ± 16	35 ± 21	1.05 ± 0.58	30 ± 17	33 ± 20	1.08 ± 0.70

Source: From Reference 14. Reprinted with permission.

2-year follow-up period we have completed thus far. Therefore, the infiltrates observed in these patients with steroids-azathioprine immunosuppression, did not represent a threat of ensuing renal damage in the next few months following the biopsies. On the other hand, the infiltrates in the allografts probably did represent a response to the allogeneic tissue, since they were much more extensive than those observed in native kidney ATN ($p < 0.01$; Table 1).

Although it has previously been noted that a mononuclear infiltrate on biopsy can exist during periods of continued good allograft function [44,58], ours is the first detailed report in which the situation in quiescence may be compared to that in rejection. The finding of infiltrates during quiescence has precedent in the observation by Balch et al. [4] that renal isografts in rats exhibited an interstitial infiltrate containing T cells. Acute tubular necrosis regularly produces a moderate infiltrate at the corticomedullary junction [63,64]. Therefore, it is not surprising that infiltrates were generally present in this study. In view of the good graft survival during the short follow-up available thus far, the cells observed in the allografts, if not totally impotent, must represent a very attenuated rejection process, perhaps only threatening the survival of the graft in the very long term. Alternatively, a process of resignation of the host to the transplant required for long-term graft survival may occur in mononuclear cells that have migrated into the graft; possible mechanisms for such adaptation include induction of suppressor cells [69], antibody-mediated enhancement [71] or induction of a suppressive effect due to anti-idiotype antibody [68].

The presence of a vasculitis, with intimal thickening and invasion by inflammatory cells, sometimes called vascular rejection, has been noted as a feature of rejection in the past [52]. Our data provide strong support for this as a very convincing histologic sign of rejection (Table 2). Clinical rejection was also definitely present in the absence of intimal arteritis in some biopsies, but the sampling error inherent in this assessment is a limiting factor.

Differentiation between cyclosporine nephrotoxicity and renal allograft rejection has proven to be difficult [27]. It has previously been suggested that an interstitial infiltrate in kidneys not undergoing rejection represented cyclosporine toxicity [60]. Although our data do not disprove this, that the infiltrate was observed in our stable patients, none of whom received cyclosporine, strongly suggests that the infiltrate described in previous studies was coincidental, not related to the use of cyclosporine.

There have been several studies of the phenotype of the infiltrating cells in biopsies from rejecting or rejected allografts; these generally have suggested that the percentage of T cells, or the helper-inducer/cytotoxic-suppressor (4:8), ratio is informative in determining the presence or progress of rejection. In particular, Platt et al. [53] and Hancock et al. [32] found a high fraction of OKT8$^+$ cells in biopsies during rejection and suggested that this is a particularly important population of lymphocytes in rejection. It was clear,

TABLE 3 Coexpression Ratio in Renal Allograft Biopsies[a]

	Coexpression ratio (mean ± SD)	
Clinical status	OKT4 and OKT8	Leu 3a and Leu 2b
Acute rejection (n = 4)	1.30 ± 0.40	1.31 ± 0.10
ATN/normal (n = 16)	1.32 ± 0.25	1.11 ± 0.35

[a]Coexpression ratio = sum of % cells stained with each Ab separately divided by % cells stained with both ABs used together.
Source: From Reference 14. Reprinted with permission.

as shown in Table 2, that a major proportion of the cells were T lymphocytes even in the absence of rejection. The predominance of OKT8$^+$ cells seen in studies of later, more established rejection was not seen commonly in our specimens. In our biopsies, the 4:8 ratio was not useful in diagnosing rejection. Because of the systematic nature of our biopsy protocol, our biopsies were performed on average much earlier than in other reports, which have generally dealt with nephrectomy specimens or biopsies taken longer after the onset of rejection. This may be one explanation for the differences in our observations as compared with previous reports. Also, the peroxidase technique for monoclonal antibody labeling that we used may allow more exact quantitation of the cell types than the fluorescein labeling technique used in some earlier studies.

The apparent coexpression of T4 and T8 antigen on a significant fraction of the same cells, as demonstrated by double-labeling studies (Table 3), was a very interesting result. Quantitative artefacts related to differences in intensity of staining of the two cell types or to sampling error could theoretically have produced a misleading appearance of coexpression. Therefore, direct double-labeling observations, using two different chromogens on the same slide, will be required to determine with certainty whether cells expressing both T4 and T8 do, in fact, exist in these biopsies. Such studies are currently under way. It was suggested some time ago by Dennert et al. [19] that the strict segregation of cells into different functional phenotypes may not be correct and that coexpression of functions may occur during the induction of an immune response. The joint expression of T4 and T8 may also relate to the recent concept that T4-bearing cells react to class II antigens to produce both a helper effect and cytotoxicity, and, correspondingly, T8-positive cells react to class I antigens to produce both help and cytotoxicity [11]. A previous report of 4^+8^+ cells in the peripheral blood of patients with myasthenia gravis suggested that these represented immature cells [7]. However, stimulated cloned cell lines have been found to express both T4 and T8 in some cases [3,79]. It has been shown that antigens may exist in undetectable form on the cell surface, becoming expressed when the membrane is perturbed [49]. Chatenoud et al. [16] have reported that coexpression of T4 and T8 may be seen in the peripheral blood in some transplant patients; these cells do not express T6, the immature thymocyte marker, which should be present if they were cells released from the thymus prematurely [10]. As was previously pointed out [16], the presence of these cells complicates the interpretation of the 4:8 ratio, in biopsies or in peripheral blood.

Similar coexpression of T4 and T8 has been found in peripheral blood lymphocytes stimulated in vitro with interleukin-2-containing supernate from Con-A treated mouse splenocytes [65] or in mixed lymphocyte culture [14].

Routine biopsies of heart allografts have been facilitated by the Biotome. The necessity for a percutaneous needle biopsy or intraoperative open biopsy of renal allografts, coupled with the impression that a "normal" biopsy would be expected in the absence of clinical rejection or nephrotoxicity, has prevented the routine use of renal allograft biopsies. It is not at present clear to what extent fine needle renal allograft aspirates, which may be performed repeatedly with minimal risk to the patient [77], may replace the standard percutaneous needle biopsy in diagnosing rejection. That there was no morbidity in this series, and that unexpected infiltrates and cell phenotypes were detected in these patients, both suggest that there may be a role for routine renal allograft biopsies in the clinical management of kidney transplant patients.

LEU 7$^+$ LYMPHOCYTES IN CLINICAL ACUTE REJECTION

Most monoclonal antibodies can only be used for cell characterizations in frozen sections. In the course of the analysis of the systematic transplant biopsies described above, we found that the Leu 7 antibody (Becton-Dickinson, Mountain View, CA) works equally well in standard paraffin sections. This allowed us to perform a large retrospective study of Leu 7 staining of infiltrates in transplanted and native kidneys.

Monoclonal antibodies have been used to characterize changes in peripheral blood and renal allograft lymphocyte subpopulations in renal allograft rejection [9,18,23,61]. Tissue studies to date have generally shown a low OKT4/OKT8 (helper/inducer to cytotoxic/suppressor) ratio in interstitial infiltrates in acute rejection in contrast to ratios observed in peripheral blood [30,32]. Some recent studies, however, have noted high 4:8 ratios in rejection [30,76]. Furthermore, the meaning of the OKT4/OKT8 ratio has been unclear since both cytotoxic and suppressor cells may have the OKT8 (and Leu 2a, Leu 2b) phenotype [56], and since some clones of class II antigen reactive cytotoxic cells have the OKT4, Leu 3a, Leu 3b phenotype [47,50].

As we will describe, we have found that the identification of Leu 7-positive intraepithelial lymphocytes (IEL) within tubules appears to be quite helpful in the recognition of early acute renal allograft rejection. The Leu 7 monoclonal antibody reacts with a small percentage of peripheral blood leukocytes, including some large granular lymphocytes (natural killer–NK–and K cells) and some Leu 2a (cytotoxic/suppressor T lymphocyte)-positive cells [1,2,40,41]. We have examined the profile of Leu 7-positive lymphocytes in paraffin sections of renal allograft needle biopsies and nephrectomies. Analysis of paraffin sections offers several advantages over frozen sections. A large retrospective analysis is possible, more tissue is available, and morphology is better.

Methods

The transplant specimens for this study included 41 needle biopsies and 16 nephrectomy specimens from 46 renal allograft recipients. For comparison we studied 8 needle biopsies and 7 nephrectomy specimens from nontransplanted patients with interstitial nephritis. These included 12 specimens representing chronic pyelonephritis, 1 fenoprofen-associated interstitial nephritis, 1 systemic lupus erythematosus-associated interstitial nephritis, and 1 focal glomerulosclerosis and idiopathic interstitial nephritis.

The transplant patients were adult recipients of cadaver donor renal allografts, most of whom were treated routinely with prednisone and azathioprine immunosuppression, with horse anti-thymocyte globulin (ATGAM) added for some rejection episodes. After obtaining informed consent, routine percutaneous transplant needle (Tru-Cut) biopsies were obtained using a protocol approved by the Johns Hopkins Joint Committee on Clinical Investigation. These were performed at approximately 1 and 4 weeks after transplantation, at which time acute tubular necrosis or normal function was generally present, without clinically apparent rejection. In addition, biopsies were studied that were obtained at the time of clinically suspected rejection, or in one case intraoperatively during transplant re-exploration.

The determination of which patients had acute rejection was made by one of us (JFB) on the basis of clinical criteria, independently of morphologic findings. There were 13 specimens obtained during episodes of early acute rejection, characterized by fever, recently altered renal function (present for a mean of 3.3 days; range, 1-11 days), and deteriorating radionucleotide scans. The 13 specimens, all nephrectomies, were designated as having end-stage rejection, since they were removed due to loss of function after longstanding rejection unresponsive to immunosuppressive therapy. These nephrectomies were performed on an average of 2.6 months (range, 1-6 months) after the onset of acute rejection. For 7 specimens, it was unclear clinically whether the patient had acute rejection within 24 hr of the time of the biopsy. These specimens were evaluated for Leu 7-positive lymphocytes but omitted from the statistical calculations. A total of 24 transplant biopsies were obtained during periods of normal function or acute tubular necrosis (stable or improving renal function).

The specimens were initially fixed in neutral-buffered formalin and embedded in paraffin by routine methods. For staining with the Leu 7 antibody, 6-μm sections were deparaffinized with xylene and alcohol and washed briefly with phosphate-buffered saline containing 0.2% bovine serum albumin (PBS). Endogenous peroxidase was inactivated with methanol and hydrogen peroxide and endogenous avidin and biotin receptors blocked with avidin D and biotin (Vector Labs, Burlingame, CA) [83]. The sections were incubated with the Leu 7 antibody (Becton-Dickenson, Mountain View, CA), washed with phosphate-buffered saline, and developed with the avidin-biotin complex immunoperoxidase procedure with diaminobenzidine and copper sulfate [78,83]. The slides were counterstained with Terry's methylene blue, dehydrated, and coverslipped.

Most of the monoclonal antibody-associated antigens are inactivated by one or more of the solvents or treatments used in paraffin embedding. The Leu 7 antigen, however, appears to be quite resistant to these procedures. With the Leu 7 antibody, the same relative number and distribution of Leu 7-positive lymphocytes were observed in paraffin sections and frozen sections of 8 lymph nodes and tonsils (staining scattered cells in the germinal centers), 4 B-cell lymphomas, and 12 renal biopsies in the present study.

The slides were examined (by WEB) for Leu 7-positive lymphocytes without knowledge of the clinical or histologic diagnoses. The overall relative number of Leu 7-positive lymphocytes was recorded, as well as the number of interstitial, intratubular (interepithelial), glomerular, and intra-arterial Leu 7-positive cells on a scale from 0 to 4^+, corresponding to 0 (absent), 1^+ (rare), 2^+ (common), 3^+ (many), 4^+ (numerous). For the overall grading, a 1^+ designation corresponded to 1-3 cells per section, 2^+ to 0.5-3 cells per high power field (HPF), 3^+ to 3-10 cells/HPF, and 4^+ to greater than 10 cells/HPF. Statistical analyses were carried out using the Mann-Whitney U test. The 24 slides with identifiable intratubular (interepithelial) Leu 7^+ lymphocytes (IEL) were ranked in order of relative number of Leu 7^+ IEL, and the remaining 48 slides without such cells were considered tied for the lowest rank [13].

TABLE 4 Biopsy and Nephrectomy Specimens with Leu 7⁺ Lymphocytes[a]

Group	Setting	n	Overall (% ≥ 2)	Intraepithelial (% ≥ 2)	Interstitial (2 ≥ 2)	Glomeruli (% ≥ 1)	Arteries (% ≥ 1)
I	Early acute rejection	13	69	69	54	31	23
II	End stage acute rejection	13	38	23	15	15	15
III	Stable function or acute tubular necrosis	24	33	0	33	29	4
IV	Interstitial nephritis	15	20	0	13	6	0

[a] $p = 0.05$ for group I versus group IV. $p < 0.001$ for group I versus group III and group I versus group IV. $p < 0.05$ for group I versus group II.
Source: From Reference 8. Reprinted with permission.

Results

Table 4 shows the extent of Leu 7-positive lymphocytes in different locations in the kidney in different transplant settings. For the overall assessment of tubular intraepithelial lymphocytes and interstitial lymphocytes, a division was made between cases with a 0-1 rating (fewer than 3 cells per specimen) and those with a 2-4⁺ rating (generally more than 1 cell per 2 HPF).

Although interstitial Leu 7-positive lymphocytes were more readily found in the patients with early acute renal allograft rejection, the fraction of specimens with such cells was not significantly different in the various transplant groups. Indeed, numerous Leu 7⁺ interstitial lymphocytes were observed in some nontransplant specimens. Leu 7-positive lymphocytes were seen only occasionally in glomeruli or as a component of the inflammatory cells within artery walls in a rejection arteritis.

In contrast, Leu 7⁺ intraepithelial lymphocytes were readily identified only in patients with acute renal allograft rejection and tended to be more prevalent in those with early acute rejection than those with end-stage rejection. Independent evaluation (by KS) of the Leu 7⁺ IEL in 37 specimens showed good interobserver agreement, both in grading (0-4+) of Leu 7⁺ IEL ($r = 0.87$; $p < 0.001$) and in distinguishing cases with 0-1⁺ Leu 7⁺ IEL and 2-4⁺ IEL (36 of 37 cases; $p < 0.0001$). The specimens were ranked on the basis of relative numbers of Leu 7-positive IEL per unit area [13]. The nontransplant specimens and recipients who had stable function or had acute tubular necrosis rarely had any such cells. Recipients with early acute rejection had significantly more Leu 7-positive IEL than other groups, including those with end-stage rejection ($p < 0.01$). By routine histology, intraepithelial lymphocytes were frequently evident in specimens with interstitial nephritis, but they were Leu 7 negative.

Figure 3 (Color Plate 2) demonstrates these interepithelial lymphocytes insinuated between tubular epithelial cells in a nephrectomy specimen from a patient with fulminant acute rejection. The Leu 7⁺ cells show sharp membranous brown staining, often with a rim of cytoplasmic sparing between the cell membrane and the nucleus, and are slightly larger than small resting lymphocytes. They are usually seen adjacent to the basement membrane between the tubular epithelial cells. It is clear that there is considerable enrichment of the Leu 7⁺ population within the tubules, accounting for the majority of the IEL in early acute rejection but less than 20% of the interstitial infiltrate. In the specimens with Leu 7⁺ IEL, the proximal tubules appeared injured, with considerable variability in cell size, focal absence of tubular cells, and patchy discontinuity of basement membranes.

In addition to lymphocytes, the Leu 7 antibody stained the cytoplasm or brush border of the tubular epithelium in several cases (including both transplant and nontransplant specimens) and occasionally stained the media of large arteries. This staining was distinct from the membranous staining of the lymphocytes and did not interfere with the recognition of Leu 7-positive lymphocytes. The cytoplasmic staining of tubular cells and arteries did not correlate with any particular pathologic processes or clinical states in this study.

Of the 57 renal transplant specimens, 7 were from patients with an atypical presentation and uncertain rejection status. Of these 7 problematic specimens, which were omitted from the above analyses, 3 had histologic evidence of acute rejection. Of these 3, 2 had prominent Leu 7^+ IEL. Two additional specimens had neither histologic evidence of rejection nor Leu 7^+ IEL. Finally, 2 specimens with equivocal histologic features of rejection lacked Leu 7^+ IEL.

Discussion

Leu 7-positive lymphocytes situated between tubular epithelial cells are frequently observed in moderate to large numbers in the early phase of acute renal allograft rejection. They are seen occasionally and in fewer numbers in end-stage rejection and only rarely in the absence of acute rejection or in nontransplant specimens. As a specific indicator of early acute rejection, the presence of intraepithelial Leu 7^+ cells complements other clinical and histologic indicators of acute rejection. If Leu 7^+ IEL are readily identified, acute rejection is probable. If they are not present, however, acute rejection cannot be totally excluded.

Although Leu 7 was initially developed as an antibody directed against NK cells, our observations do not prove that NK cells mediate renal injury in acute rejection. More recent studies have found that Leu 7 reacts with other lymphocyte populations not having NK activity, including Leu $2a^+$ T lymphocytes [41]. Preliminary studies in our laboratory indicate that many of the Leu 7-positive IEL may be cytotoxic T cells [8]. Hancock and Atkins [31] have recently commented on the frequent finding of Leu 7-positive cells in the interstitium in early acute rejection. They have assumed that these cells are natural killer cells.

For the purpose of this study, the presence or absence of rejection was determined solely on the basis of clinical findings. Thus, the observed relationship between Leu 7-positive interepithelial lymphocytes and rejection is not just a reflection of an association between two histologic features. In patients with acute rejection, Leu 7^+ IEL do not correlate with cytomegalovirus, renal tubular acidosis, or the outcome of the graft. Most of the patients in this study did not receive cyclosporin. Several specimens from patients receiving cyclosporin had neither Leu 7^+ IEL nor clinically evident acute rejection.

As a diagnostic aid, the Leu 7^+ antibody has advantages over other monoclonal antibodies against lymphocyte subsets in its ability to react with formalin-fixed, paraffin-embedded tissue. As a practical matter, generally only a small portion of a percutaneous renal biopsy is frozen for immunofluorescence and immunoperoxidase studies. Thus, antibodies that work in paraffin sections can be applied to larger pieces of tissue and sampling error is therefore less of a problem. In addition, paraffin-embedded tissue provides much better morphologic detail than frozen tissue.

In looking at the histology of these specimens, Leu 7^+ IEL appear to be quite independent of other important histologic features of acute rejection. As reported elsewhere, intimal arteritis, with subendothelial inflammatory cells, is frequently observed in acute rejection [15,55,62]. Most of these cells, however, are Leu 7 negative, and the intimal arteritis is evident in end-stage acute rejection as well as the early stages of rejection. Numerous lymphocytes and lymphoblasts staining with methyl green pyronine (MGP; reflecting RNA) have been reported in acute rejection [55]. Although such cells were seen in the patients in this study, they were more prevalent in long-term end-stage rejection (K. Solez, personal observation). Thus, histologic features, such as intimal arteritis, when present, are valuable in the detection of acute rejection during any phase. Methyl green pyronine-positive lymphoblasts are found in the later phases of acute rejection; Leu 7$^+$ IEL are particularly prominent in the early phases of acute rejection.

EXPERIMENTAL RENAL TRANSPLANTATION IN RATS

In these studies, which are still in progress, we are using the DA rat to Lewis rat renal allograft model described by Homan et al. and Lewis-Lewis isografts. There is a major histocompatibility barrier between the DA and Lewis rat strains, but rejection is prevented by daily cyclosporin A (CsA) in a dose of 10 mg/kg.

Surgical Procedure and Animal Groups

Primarily vascularized renal transplantation operations are performed (by DJM) using the technique described by Fisher and Lee [26] employing modifications described by Lee [42], White et al. [80], and Gutman et al. [29]. Under sodium pentabarbital anesthesia, a length of recipient aorta and vena cava is prepared to receive the allograft anastomoses. The donor artery, vein, and contiguous great vessels are dissected free. The left ureter is then freed and removed in continuity with a portion of bladder wall. The donor aorta and vena cava are then tied proximally and the aorta injected with a cold solution of heparinized physiologic saline to perfuse the kidney. Next, the left kidney, renal artery, and renal vein are removed from the donor en bloc with a portion of aorta and vena cava. The aorta and vena cava are trimmed appropriately, leaving a patch of each for anastamosis. The recipient great vessels are occluded proximally and distally and an arterotomy and venotomy made. The vessel anastomoses are performed in a running fashion under magnification (Zeiss OPMI microscope) using 8-0 sutures. The donor bladder patch with ureter attached will be anastomosed with 8-0 suture to a defect created in the recipient bladder. In our hands this transplant operation can now be reproducibly performed with a warm ischemia time of 30-40 min and good kidney function and animal survival. In allografts maintained for 28 days, we remove one native kidney at time of transplantation and the other at 1 week, at which time a biopsy of the transplant is obtained. At the present time, we have performed over 60 rat transplants. The preliminary results discussed here will be presented in greater detail elsewhere (McGraw et al., in preparation).

Unmodified Acute Rejection of DA-Lewis Allografts

The morphologic changes observed closely parallel those described previously by Guttman et al. [29] and Porter [55]. At 3 days, there was extensive margination of mononuclear cells in venules, peritubular capillaries, and the medullary vasa recta. Some lymphocytes appeared to be adherent to the endothelium of interlobular arteries. At 5 days, there was severe interstitial infiltration by mononuclear cells with an active intima arteritis in interlobular arteries. By 7 days, there was thrombosis of interlobular arteries with extensive tubular necrosis and interstitial infiltration. Periods longer than 7 days were not studied.

DA-Lewis Allografts Treated with Cyclosporine and Thrombotic Phenomena

At 3-5 days, there was a patchy, mild interstitial infiltrate of mononuclear cells mainly around arcuate veins in the allografts of rats treated with parenteral cyclosporine 10 mg/kg per day IP. By light microscopy this infiltrate was not significantly different from that seen in Lewis-Lewis isografts (see below). At 7 days, in addition to the mild inflammatory infiltrate, some rats showed a prominence of the endothelial cells in interlobular arteries but not definite lymphocytic infiltration of the vessels. Focal mild tubular vacuolization was seen both in allografts and in the native kidneys at 7 days. At 28 days, striking eosinophilic cytoplasmic inclusions were seen in proximal tubules. There was a patchy mild-to-moderate interstitial infiltrate of mononuclear cells with focal accumulations of mononuclear cells in cortical peritubular capillaries in some animals. There was patchy interstitial fibrosis and tubular atrophy in the outer cortex. These rats had good allograft function at 28 days (serum creatinine, 0.6 mg/dl).

Rats treated with a higher dose of cyclosporine, 50 mg/kg per day IP, usually did not survive beyond 6 days. At 5 days, the allografts from these rats showed extensive tubular vacuolization and a mild-to-moderate interstitial infiltrate of mononuclear cells. It is presumed that the deaths in the high-dose group were due to the central nervous system and liver toxicity of cyclosporine.

Of the 22 cyclosporine-treated rats, 5 showed evidence of venous or arterial thrombosis, a figure not different from the incidence of 4 of 14 in Lewis-Lewis isografts. The thrombosis and infarcts in Lewis-Lewis isografts could be attributed to technical complications, but there was a suggestion in the cyclosporine-treated DA-Lewis allografts that some of the thrombotic phenomena may be related to cyclosporine vascular injury [28, 51,59] or to a combination of cyclosporine vascular injury and subclinical rejection. At 28 days, 1 cyclosporine-treated DA-Lewis allograft showed recent nonocclusive thrombosis of an arcuate artery with extensive interstitial fibrosis and tubular loss in the region of cortex served by this artery. This graft had good function and did not otherwise appear to show signs of rejection.

Lewis-Lewis Isografts and Conclusions from Rat Transplant Data

All the Lewis-Lewis isografts had at least a mild interstitial infiltrate of mononuclear cells, usually around the arcuate veins. In animals with longer warm ischemic times, there was a somewhat more extensive interstitial infiltrate, including some just beneath the renal capsule. In the only rat with a warm ischemic time longer than 1 hr there was, in addition, papillary necrosis and patchy interstitial hemorrhage, with regenerative tubular changes in the cortex.

These preliminary rat transplant results tend to support the conclusions from the systematic renal biopsy study described earlier in this chapter. Nonrejecting grafts had an inflammatory infiltrate, although it was not as severe as that seen in rejecting grafts. An intimal arteritis was seen only in rejection.

REFERENCES

1. Abo, T., and Balch, C. M. A differentiation antigen of human NK and K cells identified by a monoclonal antibody (HNK-1). *J. Immunol.* 127:1024-1029, 1981.
2. Abo, T., Cooper, M. D., and Balch, C. M. Characterization of HNK-1+ (Leu-7) human

lymphocytes. I. Two distinct phenotypes of human NK cells with different cytotoxic capability. *J. Immunol.* 129:1752-1757, 1982.
3. Andrus, L., Granelli, Piperno, A., and Reich, E. Cytotoxic T cells both produce and respond to interleukin 2. *J. Exp. Med.* 159:647-652, 1983.
4. Balch, C. M., Wilson, C. B., Lee, S., and Feldman, J. D. Thymus-dependent lymphocytes in tissue sections of rejecting rat renal allografts. *J. Exp. Med.* 138:1584-1590, 1973.
5. Banfi, G., Imbasciati, E., Tarantino, A., and Ponticelli, C. Prognostic value of renal biopsy in acute rejection of kidney transplantation. *Nephron* 28:222-226, 1981.
6. Belitsky, P., Gupta, R., and Campbell, J. Diagnosis of acute cellular rejection in kidney allografts by fine needle aspiration cytology. *Transplant. Proc.* 16:1076-1079, 1984.
7. Berrih, S., Gaud, C., Bach, M.-A., Le Brigand, H., Binet, J. P., and Bach, J. F. Evaluation of T cell subsets to myasthenia gravis using anti-T cell monoclonal antibodies. *Clin. Exp. Immunol.* 45:1-8, 1981.
8. Beschorner, W. E., Burdick, J. F., Williams, G. M., and Solez, K. The presence of Leu 7 reactive lymphocytes in renal allografts undergoing acute rejection. *Transplant. Proc.* 17:618-622, 1985.
9. Bhan, A. K., Mihm, M. C., and Dvorak, H. F. T-cell subsets in allograft rejection. In situ characterization of T-cell subsets in human skin allografts by the use of monoclonal antibodies. *J. Immunol.* 129:1578-1583, 1982.
10. Bhan, A. K., Reinherz, E. L., Poppema, S., McCluckey, R. T., and Schlossman, S. F. Location of T cell and major histocompatibility complex antigens in the human thymus. *J. Exp. Med.* 152:771-782, 1980.
11. Biddison, W. E., Rao, P. E., Talle, M. A., Goldstein, G., and Shaw, S. Possible involvement of the OKT4 molecule in T cell recognition of class II HLA antigens: Evidence from studies of cytotoxic T lymphocytes specific for SB antigens. *J. Exp. Med.* 156: 1065-1076, 1982.
12. Blair, J. T., Thompson, A. W., Whiting, P. H., Davidson, R. J., and Simpson, J. G. Toxicity of the immune suppressant cyclosporin A in the rat. *J. Pathol.* 138:163-178, 1982.
13. Boitnott, J. K., and Solez, K. The use of ranking in the statistical assessment of morphologic data. In *Acute Renal Failure: Correlations Between Morphology and Function,* K. Solez and A. Whelton, eds. Marcel Dekker, New York, 1984, pp. 13-16.
14. Burdick, J. F., Beschorner, W. E., Smith, W. J., McGraw, D. J., Bender, W. L., Williams, G. M., and Solez, K. Characteristics of early routine renal allograft biopsies. *Transplantation* 38:679-684, 1984.
15. Busch, G. J., Reynolds, E. S., Galvanek, E. G., Braun, W. E., and Dammin G. J. Human renal allografts: The role of vascular injury in early graft failure. *Medicine (Baltimore)* 50:29-83, 1971.
16. Chatenoud, L., Chkoff, N., Kreis, H., and Bach, J. F. Interest in and limitations of monoclonal anti-T cell antibodies for the follow-up of renal transplant patients. *Transplantation* 36:45-50, 1983.
17. Cooksey, G., Reeve, R. S., Wenham, P. W., Botton, R. E., and Blamey, R. W. Comparison of fine needle aspiration cytology with histology in the diagnosis or renal allograft rejection. In *Renal Transplant Cytology,* H. Kreis and D. Droz, eds. Wichtig editore SRL, Milan, 1984, p. 73.
18. Cosimi, A. B., Colvin, R. B., Burton, R. C., Rubin, R. H., Goldstein, G., Kung, P. C., Hansen, W. P., Delmonico, F. L., and Russell, P. S. Use of monoclonal antibodies to T-cell subsets for immunologic monitoring and treatment in recipients of renal allografts. *N. Engl. J. Med.* 305:308-314, 1981.
19. Dennert, G., Weiss, S., and Warner, J. F. T cells may express multiple activities: Spe-

cific allohelp, cytolysis, and delayed-type hypersensitivity are expressed by a cloned T cell line. *Proc. Natl. Acad. Sci. USA* 78:4540-4543, 1981.

20. Devecchi, A., Egridi, F., Banfi, G., Imbasciati, E., Tarantino, A., and Ponticelli, C. Comparison of fine needle aspiration biopsy and needle biopsy in renal transplantation. In *Renal Transplant Cytology,* H. Kreis and D. Droz, eds. Wichtig Editore SRL, Milan, 1984, p. 67.
21. Droz, D., Campos, H., Noel, L. H., Adafer, E., and Kreis, H. Renal transplant fine-needle aspiration cytology (FNAC): Correlations to renal histology. *Abstracts of the IXth International Congress of Nephrology,* June 11-16, 1984, Los Angeles, p. 471A.
22. Durand, D., Segonds, A., Orfila, C., Deproc, F., Bories, P., Giraud, P., and Suc, J. M. Transplant biopsies and short-term outcome of cadaveric renal allografts. In *Advances in Nephrology,* J. Hamburger, ed., Vol. 12. Year Book Publishers, Chicago, 1983, pp. 309-330.
23. Ellis, T. M., Lee, H. M., and Mohanakumar, T. Alterations in human regulatory T lymphocyte subpopulations after renal allografting. *J. Immunol.* 127:2199-2203, 1981.
24. Farnsworth, A., Hall, B. M., Ng, A. B., Duggin, G. G., Horvath, J. S., Sheil, A. G. R., and Tiller, D. J. Renal biopsy morphology in renal transplantation. A comparative study of the light microscopic appearances of biopsies from patients treated with cyclosporin A or azathioprine-prednisone and antilymphocyte globulin. *Am. J. Surg. Pathol.* 8:243-252, 1984.
25. Feduska, N. J., Hricak, H., Terrier, F., and Vincenti, F. Magnetic resonance imaging (MRI) following renal transplantation. *Kidney Int.* 27:340, 1985.

25a. Ferguson, R. M., Rynasiewica, J. J., Sutherland, D. E. R., Simmons, R. L., and Najarian, J. S. Cyclosporin A in renal transplantation: A prospective randomized trial (discussion). *Surgery* 92:175-182, 1982.

26. Fisher, B., and Lee, S. Microvascular surgical techniques in research, with special reference to renal transplantation in the rat. *Surgery* 58:904, 1965.
27. French, M. E., Thompson, J. F., Hunnisett, A. G. W., Wood, R. F. M., and Morris, P. J. Impaired function of renal allografts during treatment with Cyclosporin-A: Nephrotoxicity or rejection? *Transplant. Proc.* 15:485-488, 1983.
28. Green, L., Verani, R., Schoenberg, L., and Kahan, B. Comparative pathological review of 72 renal transplant nephrectomies of patients treated with cyclosporine or azathioprine (abstract). *Kidney Int.* 27:141, 1985.
29. Guttman, R. D., Lindquist, R. R., Parker, R. M., Carpenter, C. B., and Merrill, J. P. Transplantation in the inbred rat. I. Morphologic, immunologic, and functional alterations during acute rejection. *Transplantation* 5:668-681, 1967.
30. Hall, B. M., Bishop, G. A., Farnsworth, A., Duggin, G. G., Horwath, J. S., Sheil, A. G. R., and Tiller, D. J. Identification of the cellular subpopulations infiltrating rejecting cadaver renal allografts. Preponderance of the T_4 subset of T cells. *Transplantation* 37:564-570, 1984.
31. Hancock, W. W., and Atkins, R. C. Immunohistological analysis of sequential renal biopsies from patients with acute rejection (abstract). *Kidney Int.* (in press, 1985).
32. Hancock, W. W., Thomson, N. M., and Atkins, R. C. Composition of interstitial cellular infiltrate identified by monoclonal antibodies in renal biopsies of rejecting human renal allografts. *Transplantation* 35:458-463, 1983.
33. Homan, W. P., Fabre, J. W., Williams, K. A., Millard, P. R., and Morris, P. J. Studies on the immunosuppressive properties of cyclosporin A in rats receiving renal allografts. *Transplantation* 29:361-366, 1980.
34. Howden, B., Jablonski, P., Rigol, G., Birrell, C., Rae, D., Marshall, V. C., and Tange, J. Studies in renal preservation using a rat kidney transplant model. II. The effect of reflushing with citrate. *Transplantation* 37:52-54, 1984.
35. Howden, B., Rae, D., Jablonski, P., Marshall, V. C., and Tange, J. Studies of renal

preservation using a rat kidney transplant model. I. Evaluation of citrate flushing. *Transplantation* 35:311-314, 1983.
36. Hsu, S.-M., Raine, L., and Fanger, H. Use of avidin-biotin-peroxidase complex (ABC) in immunoperoxidase techniques: A comparison between ABC and unlabeled antibody (PAP) procedures. *J. Histochem. Cytochem.* 29:577-580, 1981.
37. Kiaer, H., Hansen, H. E., and Olsen, S. The predictive value of percutaneous biopsies from human renal allografts with early impaired function. *Clin. Nephrol.* 13:58-63, 1980.
38. Kincaid-Smith, P., McKenzie, I. F. C., Morris, P. J., and Marshall, V. C. Biopsy features of early acute rejection in cadaveric renal grafts. *Transplant. Proc.* 1:287-289, 1969.
39. Klintmalm, G., Bergstrand, A., Ringden, O., Wasserman, J., Collste, H., Lundgren, G., Wilczek, H., and Groth, C. G. Graft biopsy for the differentiation between nephrotoxicity and rejection in cyclosporin A-treated renal transplant recipients. *Transplant. Proc.* 15:493-496, 1983.
40. Lanier, L. L., Le, A. M., Phillips, J. H., Warner, N. L., and Babcock, G. F. Subpopulations of human natural killer cells defined by expression of the Leu-7 (HNK-1) and Leu-11 (NK-15) antigens. *J. Immunol.* 131:1789-1796, 1983.
41. Lanier, L. L., and Loken, M. R. Human lymphocyte subpopulations identified by using three-color immunofluorescence and flow cytometry analysis: Correlation of Leu-2, Leu-3, Leu-7, Leu-8, and Leu-11 cell surface antigen expression. *J. Immunol.* 132:151-156, 1984.
42. Lee, S. An improved technique of renal transplantation in the rat. *Surgery* 61:771, 1967.
43. Lund, B., and Jensen, O. M. Renal transplantation in rabbits. II. Morphological alterations in autografts. *Acta Pathol. Microbiol. Scand.* [*A*] 78:701-712, 1970.
44. Matas, A. J., Sibley, R., Mauer, S. M., Kim, Y., Sutherland, D. E. R., Simmons, R. L. and Najarian, J. S. Pre-discharge, post-transplant kidney biopsy does not predict rejection. *J. Surg. Res.* 32:269-274, 1982.
45. Matas, A. J., Sibley, R., Mauer, M., Sutherland, D. E., Simmons, R. L., and Najarian, J. S. The value of needle renal allograft biopsy. I. A retrospective study of biopsies performed during putative rejection episodes. *Ann. Surg.* 197:226-237, 1983.
46. Medawar, P. B. The behaviour and fate of skin autografts and skin homografts in rabbits. *J. Anat.* 78:176-199, 1944.
47. Meuer, S. C., Schlossman, S. F., and Reinherz, E. L. Clonal analysis of human cytotoxic T lymphocytes: T4+ and T8+ effector T cells recognize products of different major histocompatibility regions. *Proc. Natl. Acad. Sci. USA* 79:4395-4399, 1982.
48. Mitchison, N. A., and Dube, O. L. Studies on immunological response to foreign tumor transplants in mouse. II. Relation between hemagglutinating antibody and graft resistance in normal mouse and mice pretreated with tissue preparations. *J. Exp. Med.* 102:179-197, 1955.
49. Mittler, R. S., Rao, P. E., Talle, M. A., Look, R., and Goldstein, G. Cell membrane perturbation of resting T cells and thymocytes causes display of activation antigens. *J. Exp. Med.* 158:99-111, 1983.
50. Moretta, L., Mingari, M. C., Sekaly, P. R., Moretta, A., Chapuis, B., and Cerottini, J.-C. Surface markers of cloned human T cells with various cytolytic activities. *J. Exp. Med.* 154:569-574, 1981.
51. Neild, G., Reuben, R., Hartley, B., and Cameron, J. S. Glomerular thrombi in renal allografts associated with cyclosporin therapy. *Kidney Int.* 27:145, 1985.
52. Olsen, S. Pathology of renal allograft rejection. In *Kidney Disease: Present Status,* J. Chung, B. H. Spargo, and F. K. Mostofi, eds. Williams & Wilkins, Baltimore, 1979, pp. 327-355.

53. Platt, J. L., Ferguson, R. M., Sibley, R. K., Gajl-Peczalska, K. J., and Michael, A. F. Renal interstitial cell populations in cyclosporine nephrotoxicity. Identification using monoclonal antibodies. *Transplantation* 35:343-346, 1983.
54. Platt, J. L., LeBien, T. W., and Michael, A. F. Interstitial mononuclear cell populations in renal graft rejection. Identification by monoclonal antibodies in tissue sections. *J. Exp. Med.* 155:17-30, 1982.
55. Porter, K. A. Renal transplantation. In *Pathology of the Kidney,* R. H. Heptinstall, ed. Little, Brown, Boston, 1983, pp. 1455-1547.
56. Reinherz, E. L., Kung, P. C., Goldstein, G., and Schlossman, S. F. A monoclonal antibody reactive with the human cytotoxic/suppressor T-cell subset, previously defined by a heteroantiserum termed TH-2. *J. Immunol.* 124:1301-1307, 1980.
57. Reitamo, S., Konttinen, Y. T., Ranki, A., and Hayry, P. The relation of different inflammatory cell types to the various parenchymal components of rejecting kidney allografts. *Histopathology* 4:517-532, 1980.
58. Russell, P. S., and Monaco, A. P. *The Biology of Tissue Transplantation.* Little, Brown, Boston, 1967.
59. Shulman, H., Striker, G., Deeg, H. J., Kennedy, M., Storb, R., and Thomas, E. D. Nephrotoxicity of cyclosporin A after allogeneic marrow transplantation. *N. Engl. J. Med.* 305:1392-1395, 1981.
60. Sibley, R. K., Rynasiewicz, J. J., Ferguson, R. M., Fryd, D., Sutherland, D. E. R., Simmons, R. L., and Najarian, J. S. Morphology of cyclosporine nephrotoxicity and acute rejection in patients immunosuppressed with cyclosporine and prednisone. *Surgery* 94:225-234, 1983.
61. Smith, W. J., Burdick, J. F., and Williams, G. M. Immunologic monitoring of renal transplant recipients. *Transplant. Proc.* 15: 182-1183, 1983.
62. Solez, K., McGraw, D., Bender, W. L., and Burdick, J. F. The morphology of clinically typical "acute tubular necrosis" (ATN), normal function, and acute rejection in transplanted human kidneys (abstract). *Kidney Int.* 25:226, 1984.
63. Solez, K., Morel-Maroger, L., and Sraer, J.-D. Morphology of "acute tubular necrosis" in man: Analysis of 57 renal biopsies and comparison with the glycerol model. *Medicine (Baltimore)* 58:362-376, 1979.
64. Solez, K., and Whelton, A. *Acute Renal Failure: Correlations Between Morphology and Function.* Marcel Dekker, New York, 1984.
65. Spiess, P. J., and Rosenberg, S. A. A simplified method for the production of murine T-cell growth factor free of lectin. *J. Immunol. Methods* 42:213-222, 1981.
66. Strom, T. B. Immunosuppressive agents in renal transplantation. *Kidney Int.* 26: 353-365, 1984.
67. Strom, T. B., and Loertscher, R. Cyclosporine-induced nephrotoxicity. Inevitable and intractable? *N. Engl. J. Med.* 311:728-729, 1984.
68. Suciu-Foca, N., Rohowsky, C., Kung, P., Lewison, A., Nicholson, R., Reemtsma, K., and King. D. W. MHC-specific idiotypes on alloactivated human T cells: In vivo and in vitro studies. *Transplant. Proc.* 15:784-789, 1983.
69. Thomas, J. M., Carver, F. M., Haisch, C. E., Fahrenbruch, G., Deepe, R. M., and Thomas, F. T. Suppressor cells in Rhesus monkeys treated with antithymocyte globulin. *Transplantation* 34:83-89, 1982.
70. Thomson, A. W., Whiting, P. H., Blair, J. T., Davidson, R. J. L., and Simpson, J. G. Pathologic changes developing in the rat during a three-week course of high dosage cyclosporin A and their reversal following drug withdrawal. *Transplantation* 32:271-277, 1981.
71. Tilney, N. L., and Bell, P. R. F. Studies on enhancement of cardiac and renal allografts in the rat. *Transplantation* 18:31-37, 1974.
72. van Es, A., Meyer, C. J. L. M., Oljans, P. J., Tanke, H. J., and van Es, L. A. Mononu-

clear cells in renal allografts. Correlation with peripheral blood T lymphocyte subpopulations and graft prognosis. *Transplantation* 37:134-139, 1984.
73. Vangelista, A., Frasca, G. M., Stefoni, S., and Bonomini, V. Graft biopsy in renal transplantation: Correlation with clinical, immunological, and virological investigations. *Kidney Int.* 14:541-545, 1983.
74. Venkatachalam, M. A. Pathology of acute renal failure. In *Acute Renal Failure,* B. M. Brenner and J. H. Stein, eds. Churchill Livingstone, New York, 1980, pp. 79-107.
75. Verani, R., Flechner, S., and Kahan, B. Acute cellular rejection (ACR) or cyclosporine A nephrotoxicity (CsANT)? A review of transplant renal biopsies. *Abstracts of the IXth International Congress of Nephrology,* Los Angeles, June, 1984, p. 496A.
76. von Willebrand, E. OKT4/8 ratio in the blood and in the graft during episodes of human renal allograft rejection. *Cell Immunol.* 77:196-201, 1983.
77. von Willebrand, E., Taskinen, E., Ahonen, J., and Hayry, P. Recent modifications in the fine needle aspiration biopsy of human renal allografts. *Transplant. Proc.* 15: 1195-1197, 1983.
78. Warnke, R., and Levy, R. Detection of T and B cell antigens with hybridoma monoclonal antibodies: A biotin-avidin-horseradish peroxidase method. *J. Histochem. Cytochem.* 28:771-776, 1980.
79. Wee, S.-L., Chen, L.-K., Strassmann, G., and Bach, F. H. Helper cell-independent cytotoxic clones in man. *J. Exp. Med.* 156:1854-1859, 1982.
80. White, E., Hildemann, W. H., and Mullen, Y. Chronic kidney allograft reactions in rats. *Transplantation* 8:602-617, 1969.
81. Whiting, P. H., Thomson, A. W., Blari, J. T., and Simpson, J. G. Experimental cyclosporin A nephrotoxicity. *Br. J. Exp. Pathol.* 63:88-94, 1982.
82. Whiting, P. H., Simpson, J. G., Davidson, R. J. L., and Thomson, A. W. Pathological changes in rats receiving cyclosporin A at immunotherapeutic dosage for 7 weeks. *Br. J. Exp. Pathol.* 64:437-444, 1983.
83. Wood, G. S., and Warnke, R. Suppression of endogenous avidin-binding activity in tissues and its relevance to biotin-avidin detection systems. *J. Histochem. Cytochem.* 29:1196-1204, 1981.

11

LOCALIZATION OF THE CELLULAR COMPONENTS OF ACUTE REJECTION

William E. Beschorner
The Johns Hopkins University School of Medicine, Baltimore, Maryland

To fully understand and monitor renal allograft rejection it is essential to understand the cellular participants within the graft itself. Intercepting the peripheral blood lymphocytes will provide insight into the messages sent between the lymphoid system and the graft. Catching the urinary lymphocytes could potentially tell us the end result of some components of rejection. But only by studying the graft itself can we tell what the actual effector cells are and what type of damage they are inflicting. Only the graft can tell us where the important antigens are, whether the rejection is directed against the vasculature or the tubules, whether the rejection is a direct cytolytic reaction against the antigen-bearing cells, an indirect injury through a delayed-type hypersensitivity reaction, or innocent bystander effect, considerations that may be important in designing specific antirejection therapies.

A few years ago our immunopathologic tools for answering these questions were rather limited. We could identify the type of necrosis, the relative number and location of lymphocytes, plasma cells, and macrophages, and whether there were detectable immune deposits present. Then the immunologists, working with lymphocyte suspensions, characterized in detail multiple types of effector cells and mechanisms and multiple types of regulatory cells to control these mechanisms. They then provided us with highly specific monoclonal antibodies for each lymphocyte subtype. Finally, they gave us immunohistochemical methods to identify individual cells. Needless to say, some of us pathologists felt like Willie Sutton strutting down Wall Street, and expectations for significant new findings were high.

This direct approach to eliciting the pathogenesis of rejection has, in fact, had mixed results. Some questions have been answered; some new questions have been posed. But there have also been multiple reports with conflicting data, and the limitations of the procedures have become quite apparent. Meanwhile, the clinical ante has been raised. Immunologists are taking a surgical approach to immune suppression, using monoclonal antibodies against the specific lymphocyte subtypes or relatively immune-specific drugs, such as cyclosporin A (CsA), in an attempt to remove or make ineffective the cells damaging the graft. We are now challenged to decide whether a particular type of rejection will respond to one specific approach or another.

This review will center on the identified target cells and the profile of mononuclear cells within the renal allograft. To limit the controversy, the discussion will be limited to acute rejection; hyperacute and chronic rejection will not be covered. Since most phenotype studies are of episodes of the cellular form of acute rejection, we will not discuss the humoral form. The role of antibodies in rejection is detailed in Chapter 3.

There are several possible reasons that many of the original goals and aims in this area have not been met. They include, along with others, three assumptions which proved to be premature.

First was the initial assumption that a highly specific monoclonal antibody would define a single functional genotype. We now realize that occasionally a very small epitope recognized by a monoclonal antibody can be expressed on widely divergent cell types. OKT6 and Leu 6 recognize cortical thymocytes and epidermal Langerhans cells [61,76]. OKT8 and Leu 2 are expressed on both cytotoxic and suppressor T cells and some natural killer cells [67,74]. Antibodies to OKT4 and Leu 3 were initially developed against helper and inducer T lymphocytes but later found to react with monocytes, macrophages, and select clones with cytotoxic activity (generally to class II antigen-bearing cells) [28,47,75]. Even one of the original pan-T markers, Leu 1, is now routinely detected on B-cell chronic lymphocytic leukemia [18].

Second, there is an underlying assumption that the relative number of lymphocytes counted in a specimen is proportional to their importance in the pathogenetic mechanism. Limiting dilution studies find that, with acute rejection, the number of antigen-specific effector cells in sponge allografts rise to only 1 in 200 lymphocytes [3]. Renal pathologists looking at cutaneous graft-versus-host disease (GVHD) in an irradiation chimera for the first time are usually surprised at the paucity of infiltrate. Often there is only a "one-on-one" relationship between effector cells and injured keratinocytes [86]. It is quite possible, then, that much of the heavy infiltrate observed in renal biopsies is irrelevant to the immune reaction.

Third, there has been the presumption that acute rejection is the only process; that is, if you understand the renal infiltrate in patients with rejection, you understand rejection. As detailed elsewhere in this volume, renal allografts without rejection and without impending rejection can have very significant interstitial mononuclear infiltrates [15]. It is probable that the grafts with rejection have these inflammatory processes in addition to their rejection.

RENAL ALLOGRAFT REJECTION COMPARED WITH ACUTE REJECTION OF OTHER TYPES OF GRAFTS

The acute rejection episodes of graft-versus-host disease, cardiac allograft rejection, and hepatic allograft rejection can provide some insight into kidney allograft rejection. These settings have a number of differences from and some similarities with kidney allograft rejection. By recognizing these differences and similarities, the other settings can lend support or help refute various hypotheses concerning the cellular mechanisms of rejection.

Bone marrow transplants in humans are usually performed between HLA-identical siblings. Thus, the reaction is primarily against minor histocompatibility antigens. The infiltrates are observed principally within the epithelium, including the epidermis, the hepatic bile ducts, bronchial mucosa, and intestinal crypts. Vascular infiltrates are quite rare, and involvement of the kidneys is most unusual. Solid organ allografts usually represent a small antigen load in a sea of hostile lymphocytes, but the bone marrow recipient presents a large antigen load to relatively few lymphocytes.

Bone marrow transplants are performed in human recipients after total-body irradiation or aggressive immunosuppression [83]. Here there are few host lymphocytes remaining for nonspecific recruitment. The remaining radioresistant host histiocytes and dendritic cells can serve as targets or antigenic stimulation.

Graft-versus-host disease has been induced in animals both by injecting incompatible marrow and spleen into an irradiated host simulating the human transplants and by the semiallogeneic model. Billingham described three requisites for acute GVHD:

1. The graft must be immunoreactive.
2. The graft must recognize antigens on the host.
3. The host must not be able to reject the graft; that is, the graft must have security of tenure [11].

The initial rodent models satisfied the third requisite by injecting inbred parental marrow and spleen into the F_1 hybrid of that parental strain and an unrelated parental strain. In contrast to the irradiation model, the host is not immune depleted. But although the host immunocytes are available for nonspecific recruitment, there are also many more cells available for antigenic stimulation.

The skin has been extensively studied in GVHD, both in humans and in animal models [6,81]. Compared with other rejection settings the lymphoid infiltrate is relatively sparse relative to the observed injury, present in the superficial dermis and extending into the epidermis. There is usually an intimate relation between lymphocytes ("satellite" lymphocytes) and injured epidermal cells. Cutaneous infiltrates in these patients are rare (occasional perivascular allergic reactions; leukemic infiltrates), so there is little interference in evaluating the process.

Acute GVHD therefore offers potential clues concerning reactions against minor histocompatibility antigens and reactions against epithelium. The infiltrates are sparse and more likely to be directly related to the rejection reaction. Obviously, nonspecific infiltrates and repair following surgery are not of any concern. Syngeneic and autologous transplants rarely show infiltrates resembling GVHD.

Although helpful, important differences prevent extrapolation to the renal allograft. Bone marrow recipients are much more immunosuppressed at the time of GVHD compared even with aggressively treated renal allograft recipients. They not only receive total-body irradiation and/or high-dose chemotherapy, but additional immunosuppression for GVHD. Graft-versus-host disease itself leads to immunosuppression through destruction of the thymic epithelium [84]. Secondly, because of their immune deficiency, they are at high risk for secondary infections. Finally, it remains enigmatic why the kidneys are almost never involved in GVHD, neither the vasculature nor the tubular epithelium.

The cardiac allograft rejection is almost the complete antithesis to GVHD. Donors are usually HLA mismatched and unrelated to the host, providing both major and minor antigen disparities [4]. The heart is a vascular organ, and the infiltrates are perivascular and subendothelial. Like the renal allografts, there is an extensive capillary bed as well as larger arteries and veins. The allograft represents a limited antigen load to a host with near-normal immunocompetence.

Like the renal allograft, the cardiac allograft may have infiltrates related to surgery. In the animal models, syngeneic grafts and autografts frequently have lymphocytic infiltrates that resolve by the first week posttransplant [40]. Aside from this, however, there are relatively few inflammatory processes to interfere with the rejection process (except in some of those transplanted for myocarditis).

Cardiac allograft rejection, therefore, can provide potential clues for understanding the vascular component of rejection and provides a system for studying the reaction against class I and class II major histocompatibility antigens.

Hepatic allograft rejection, like the renal allograft, falls between these two extremes. The graft is usually incompatible for HLA antigens and often for ABO antigens [42,69,90]. Like the renal allograft, it contains epithelium (bile ducts), various types of endothelium (capillaries, portal veins, hepatic arteries, and veins) and dendritic cells (Kupffer cells). Infiltrates have been described associated with both the bile ducts and hepatic veins [25]. Although the grafts are usually HLA incompatible, severe rejection episodes appear to be less frequent than with renal allografts. Like the kidney, the liver is subject to various infiltrates and drug toxicities that can interfere with the diagnosis of rejection.

Orthotopic liver transplants into miniature swine provide an animal model closely simulating the human setting [79].

Liver allograft rejection complements the study of renal allograft rejection as another solid allograft with many features in common. The hepatic epithelial component, however, is separate from the vascular components and dendritic cells, allowing some segregation of the rejection components.

CELLULAR TARGETS OF ACUTE REJECTION

To understand the graft rejection reaction at the tissue level, knowledge of the antigens involved and their distribution are a necessary starting point.

The major histocompatibility complex (MHC) antigens are well known to be important in acute rejection. Disparity in the MHC leads to a greater incidence of rejection, and immunoadsorption studies have established the presence of MHC antigens in kidneys [102]. Three areas of investigation, however, indicate that antigen expression is more complicated than simply a reservoir of stimulator cells and a target for effector cells. The type of cellular response and therefore the type of rejection may well depend on the antigen mismatch. Class I (HLA-A, B, and C) and class II (HLA-D and Dr) antigens stimulate the differentiation of different phenotypes of effector cells, as discussed later. Second, the expression of antigens is no longer believed to be a static situation but is seen to vary under different conditions. Third, kidney allografts that perform well demonstrate a different distribution of antigen expression than those that undergo repeated rejection [37].

In the normal kidney, class I antigens as defined by monoclonal antibodies to HLA-A, B, and C are expressed on the endothelium of the capillaries, arteries, and veins as well the glomeruli [33,104]. Expression on renal proximal tubular cells appears to be restricted to the cytoplasm. This apparent sparing of the tubular cell membrane has been confirmed by fine needle aspiration studies. The parietal cells of Bowman's capsule also appear to be stained with these antibodies.

The class II histocompatibility antigens appear more restricted in distribution. Immunohistochemistry has identified the HLA-D and HLA-DR antigens on most endothelial cells, including the glomeruli. No staining, however, was observed in the endothelium of the interlobular arteries and arterioles or in the proximal tubules.

From these findings, the expected pattern of rejection would be a vascular infiltrate, glomerulonephritis, and negligible if any tubulitis. In fact, a subendothelial lymphocytic infiltrate is a prominent component of rejection, as discussed elsewhere in this book. However, the glomeruli are rarely involved early in acute rejection, and there is frequently a lymphocytic tubulitis. Clearly, antigen expression in the normal kidney does not provide the entire explanation.

One proposed explanation for this discrepancy is that other class II antigens, such as SB, MB, and DC, may show a different distribution than the DR antigen [27,37]. The MB antigen has been found to be expressed primarily in the intertubular capillaries and veins. Antibodies, such as NFK1, which recognize not only the DR antigen but also the SB and DC antigens, detect strong presence in epithelial cells, including normal renal proximal tubules [24].

Second, the tissue expression of histocompatibility antigens may be variable. Different individuals demonstrate variable tissue patterns for the common determinant epitopes of the class II antigens. An individual demonstrates variability in tissue distribution at different times.

Major differences in class II antigen expression on various endothelial cells has been observed between different tissues for one species and between different species for a particular tissue [38,51]. Major arteries and veins in human kidneys and hearts stained for these antigens, whereas normal rat kidneys and hearts did not. On the other hand, normal rat liver demonstrated expression in the major vascular endothelium but human liver specimens did not demonstrate expression. In another study, HLA-DR was weak or absent in the major vascular endothelium of human kidneys. We have looked at the distribution of HLA-DR in donor heart atria prior to transplant. Although generally the larger vessels do not stain for this antigen, occasional donors are strongly positive for HLA-DR. The factors controlling expression are unknown.

Tissue expression of histocompatibility antigens appears related to graft survival. Renal tubular HLA-DR was observed in 25 of 25 biopsies with acute rejection but only 4 of 14 without rejection [29]. Of these 4 patients, 2 were recently treated for acute rejection, the other 2 later lost their grafts to chronic rejection. Another study of fine needle aspirates from repeatedly rejecting kidneys and "well-to-do" allografts found both HLA-ABC and HLA-DR on the endothelial cells with rejection but absent in the well-to-do patients and normal kidneys. In these studies, it is unclear whether the antigen expression was present in the graft prior to transplant, although the absence of endothelial antigens in normal kidneys in the latter study would infer that they were induced after transplant. If these antigens are induced, are they induced prior to the onset of rejection, and therefore in part responsible for rejection, or are they induced following the onset of rejection?

The induction of class II antigens has been well documented in other organs. The Ia antigen is evident in the duct epithelium of lactating but not resting breasts. It is also seen in the skin epithelium with mycosis fungoides. In human and rat marrow transplant recipients, Ia is evident in the skin epidermis, intestinal mucosa and bile duct epithelium with acute GVHD but is absent without acute GVHD [48,55]. In rats with acute GVHD, the hepatic veins also expressed class II antigens (OX-6), but the control groups did not [94]. Interestingly, the portal veins did not show induction of class II antigens. With human liver allograft rejection, the bile duct epithelium expresses HLA-DR [95].

With induction of class II antigens in the very target cells of acute rejection, the temptation is overwhelming to speculate that this induction is causally related to the rejection. We have made two observations, however, that indicate that such conclusions may be premature.

We have analyzed 65 sequential endocardial biopsies from 15 cardiac allograft recipients who experienced at least one episode of acute rejection. Prior to rejection, the major arteries and veins in these patients did not have detectable Ia antigen (OKIa1 with avidin-biotin complex immunoperoxidase). In the biopsies with moderate or quiescent rejection, however, strong staining was observed. Significantly, the "predictor" biopsies, those that preceded the first biopsy with histologically evident rejection, had Ia^- endothelium in the major vessels.

In addition, we have looked at the sequential skin biopsies of human marrow recipients undergoing acute GVHD. Consistent with the findings of Lampert et al. [48], we observed strong Ia staining of the basal cells and keratinocytes with well-established GVHD but not in syngeneic or autologous recipients or allogeneic recipients with GVHD. However, the initial diagnostic biopsies, taken within 24 hr of the onset of rash, showed only weak Ia staining in 7 of 25 biopsies, even though these biopsies had good evidence of GVHD with epidermal infiltrates and keratinocyte injury. The Ia staining was most intense and always evident in those specimens with active GVHD for more than 3 weeks.

In these two settings, the expression of Ia appears to follow the onset of rejection and cannot therefore be considered a requisite for rejection. Whether the induction of Ia prolongs or exacerbates the rejection episode is still open to speculation. The continued presence in patients with quiescent cardiac allograft rejection does not necessarily mean that it is irrelevant, since these patients may have developed tolerance or loss of reactive immunocytes. It is also possible that other class II antigens may precede the onset of rejection.

Finally, the discrepancy between the morphology of rejection and the distribution of MHC may be in part due to antigens outside the MHC. At least two antibodies against tubular basement membrane are known to be expressed in select strains of rats, but the antigens map outside the MHC as tested with MHC congenic strains [64]. Additional sera from transplanted rats reacted with Bowman's capsule but not the tubular basement membranes.

Male specific (H-Y) antigens have been associated with rapid renal allograft rejection in one female recipient of an HLA-identical graft from her brother [68]. Cell-mediated lysis (CML) could be elicited from her lymphocytes, but only after stimulation in a mixed lymphocyte culture. Screening these cells against a panel of lymphocytes resulted in CML only in haplotype-identical male donors but not haplotype-identical female donors.

Minor histocompatibility antigens may be expressed on either the epithelium or endothelium. Skin grafts placed on MHC-identical, multiple minor antigen-incompatible recipients have been reported to be rejected within 15 days [56]. Primarily vascularized heart grafts placed in congenic mice with only minor antigen mismatches are rejected as quickly as some strain combinations with class I and/or class II mismatches [17]. Both of these rejection reactions are vascular, with perivascular and subendothelial infiltrates, and the end point of rejection is thrombosis.

Acute GVHD is primarily a reaction against epithelium. Human bone marrow transplant donors are usually HLA-identical siblings and the mixed lymphocyte culture negative. Thus, acute GVHD in this setting is a reaction against minor histocompatibility antigens. Even with this extent of matching, the reaction is histologically detectable in 80% of the engrafted recipients and can contribute to the patient's death in 25% of those with GVHD. The injury consists of an intimate contact of lymphocytes with epidermal cells, bile duct epithelium, bronchial mucosa, and intestinal crypts [80]. Vascular and subendothelial infiltrates are rare. Rat and mouse radiation chimeras in minor antigen-incompatible hosts can demonstrate either acute or chronic GVHD [10,43,73]. Although the tissue manifestations of chronic GVHD are different with mixed cellular infiltrates and more fibrosis, vascular injury is still rare.

Some murine histocompatibility antigens mapping outside the MHC have been localized specifically in the epidermis and in fibroblasts [96]. Circulating CTL specific to these antigens have been identified with GVHD, and clones of CTL specific to one of these antigens, Epa-1, have been produced. When these clones are labeled and injected into susceptible strains of mice, they localize and are associated with cell injury in the epidermis [97,98]. These studies conclusively demonstrate the potential for minor antigens to stimulate a cytotoxic reaction against organ-specific alloantigens.

Thus far I have emphasized the distribution and induction of alloantigens on epithelium and endothelium to the exclusion of dendritic macrophages. In theory, they, too, could be potent stimulators of acute rejection. They are ubiquitous in tissues, including the renal interstitium and glomerular mesangium. Their membranes are rich in class II antigens and can stimulate a mixed lymphocyte reaction [3a,41,91]. In rats, renal allografts depleted of passenger leukocytes can be rendered more immunogenic by infusing dendritic cells [52].

In human recipients, however, the participation of dendritic cells has not been conclusively demonstrated. Glomerulonephritis with involvement of the mesangial cells is not a recognized component of early acute rejection. In the interstitium, the dendritic cells cannot be differentiated from the infiltrating cells, which include many (presumably host) macrophages.

Outside of renal allograft rejection, there are other indications that dendritic cells might not be important target cells. The relative number of dendritic cells is much greater in the liver than in the kidney. Yet, rejection may be less severe and less frequent in the liver [38]. In acute GVHD and in liver allograft rejection, the primary injury is seen in and around the bile ducts, not in the lobule, where there are numerous Kupffer cells [9, 82,88]. Host lung alveolar macrophages and Kupffer cells in bone marrow recipients are rapidly replaced with donor-type cells shortly after engraftment. This illustrates the mobility of these cells and may explain why these antigen-rich cells do not stimulate significant rejection.

In the skin, Langerhans cells have been hypothesized to be the target cells of GVHD. These cells can be easily monitored by their cytoplasmic ATPase activity and by the membranous OKT6 antigen, an antigen identified only on cortical thymocytes and Langerhans cells. Using these methods, the Langerhans cells have been noted to be depleted with acute GVHD [48]. However, in another study, the Langerhans cells were depleted in all recipients, including those who never developed GVHD [66]. In sex-mismatched patients, Langerhans cells were later found to be of donor phenotype after reconstitution [65]. Because these cells are so readily depleted and replaced with cells of the responder genotype, they are unlikely targets for GVHD.

METHODS FOR CHARACTERIZATION OF INTRAGRAFT INFLAMMATORY CELLS

What is the optimal method for monitoring the inflammatory reaction of acute renal allograft rejection? The most frequently used probe is the quantitation of cell phenotypes in the peripheral blood lymphocytes (PBL). The cells are easily obtained, and analysis can be performed as frequently as daily if necessary to detect a change in status. The flow cytometer provides a quantitative assessment of the relative number of each phenotype and can potentially analyze the PBL by relative size (actually light scatter), and fluorescence intensity (e.g., antigen molecules per cell). More specific subclassification of the phenotypes is now possible using antibodies with different fluorochromes to measure coexpression of multiple antigens [49].

The major limitation for this source is that it only samples the lymphocyte traffic between the graft and lymphoreticular system. In rat experiments with radiolabeled leukocytes, a considerable influx and outflux of cells takes place in the first 4 days post-transplant [62]. After that the traffic declines sharply, 3 days before the graft is rejected. The white cells in the graft, however, continue to proliferate and differentiate. With the sponge allograft model, precursor cytotoxic cells were shown to migrate from the host to the graft during the first 5 days [2,3]. Thereafter, the cells proliferated and differentiated in the graft and rejection was no longer dependent on the host lymphoreticular system.

There are currently two basic methods of monitoring human renal allografts commonly utilized today, and a third method was recently introduced. Most frequently, fresh needle core biopsies obtained for histologic purposes are also stained with antibodies to the lymphocyte phenotypes and analyzed by immunofluorescence or immunoperoxidase techniques. The profile of graft lymphocytes is readily determined, either by semiquantitative estimates or by counting. Of greater import, however, the relationship between the infiltrate and the tissue components is evident. Follicular B lymphocytes can be analyzed separately from the interstitial infiltrates. Lymphocyte phenotypes can be separately analyzed for perivascular regions, subendothelial areas, glomerular capillaries, proximal tubules, and so on.

The two major limitations to this technique are the difficulty in obtaining tissue on a regular basis and the technical difficulties of analyzing the infiltrates. Most of the membrane antigens are sensitive to the usual fixatives, necessitating the use of frozen tissue or tissue fixed in special cryopreservatives. This in turn compromises the overall morphology. Immunoperoxidase is subject to background staining from cells with endogenous peroxidase, Fc receptors, and endogenous avidin receptors [105], although most of this can be blocked. Immunofluorescence is generally less sensitive than immunoperoxidase for lymphocyte membrane antigens, requiring lower dilutions of antibodies and revealing fewer cells. With immunofluorescence, it is usually more difficult to relate the lymphocytes to the overall tissue organization. With intact tissue, interstitial antigens can interfere with the counting of intact lymphocytes. For example, interstitial immunoglobulins can interfere with the surface immunoglobulin of B cells. A major drawback to analyzing the cells *in situ* is that the functional genotype of the lymphocytes cannot be confirmed.

Fine needle aspirations offers a relatively risk-free method for analyzing the graft, allowing analysis as frequently as hourly if necessary [13,22,39]. The separated lymphocytes can be stained and readily quantitated after layering them on slides with the cytocentrifuge. The only limitations are the uncertainty brought about by the adjustment for contaminating peripheral blood and the lack of ability to relate cells to tissue structure. This technique is discussed at length elsewhere in this volume.

Recently, lymphocytes from needle core biopsies of human renal allografts have been cultured and expanded for analysis [58]. Small fragments of the biopsy are cultured in the presence of interleukin-2 (IL-2) until sufficient numbers are obtained. Not only can one quantitate the phenotypes of the graft lymphocytes with flow cytometry, but the cells can be functionally tested as well, including proliferation in mixed lymphocyte cultures, specific and nonspecific cytotoxicity, and natural killer activity. By doing limiting dilution studies, one could potentially quantitate the number of antigen-reactive cells. The limitation of this procedure is that it may select for cells sensitive to IL-2. More than 96% of the cultured cells were T lymphocytes; while most studies find 30-60% T cells and 30-60%

monocytes and B cells in the graft infiltrates. It was unclear whether the expansion in IL-2 effected the Th/Ts ratio.

INTERSTITIAL INFILTRATES

In a sequential series of biopsies and a nephrectomy specimen, Hancock suggests that the location and type of inflammatory cells depends on the duration of acute rejection [32,36]. Within the first 3-4 days, the specimens had prominent perivascular and periglomerular infiltrates with a mixture of T lymphocytes (40-60%) and macrophages (40-50%). The interstitial area had fewer inflammatory cells containing more than 80% macrophages. B lymphocytes were unusual (1-5%) at this time. Less than 1% of the T cells were activated, as monitored with the Tac-1 antibody against the IL-2 receptor [99]. The T lymphocytes also express class II antigens, another indication of activation [101]. By day 10, the interstitial infiltrate was more prominent and the number of activated T cells had risen to 15%. In the 30-day specimen, the overall T-cell component had dropped to 30% and macrophages accounted for 50-60% of the infiltrate. B cells and plasma cells now represented 10% of the infiltrate and were more evident in the perivascular regions.

As discussed earlier, the PBL lymphocyte profile should resemble the allograft profile about as much as an expressway should resemble a used car lot: in general, there is little resemblance between the two profiles. Most series of PBL analysis have concentrated on the ratio of helper T cells (OKT4, Leu 3a) to cytotoxic/suppressor T cells (OKT8, Leu 2a), referred hereafter as the Th/Ts ratio. Most recipients posttransplant have a low ratio, reflecting a chronic immune deficiency and paucity of helper cells. A rising Th/Ts ratio, however, was usually predictive of rejection [19,20,23,59,93]. In contrast, most interstitial infiltrates of acutely rejecting grafts tend to show a predominance of cytotoxic/suppressor cells and a Th/Ts ratio usually less than 0.5 [31,35,71]. The apparent disparity between PBL and graft cells was confirmed in direct comparisons for the same patients. Platt et al. found the Th/Ts ratio was higher in PBL in five of six patients [71]. The graft infiltrates in the perivascular regions and interstitial areas were separately estimated for relative T-cell subtypes by van Es et al. [100]. The perivascular infiltrates showed a significant correlation with the PBL lymphocytes ($r = 0.72$); the interstitial cells did not correlate as well. Two comparisons between fine needle aspirates and PBL failed to show significant correlation.

Ideally, these two analyses should complement each other, the PBL reflecting day-to-day changes in T-cell regulation, the graft reflecting the result of differentiated effector cells. However, these two distinct methodologies should be compared only with caution. Relative fluorescence in the flow cytometer is proportional to the number of molecules in a single drop, that is, the antigen number per cell. Under the microscope, the relative intensity of fluorescence or perioxidase staining is proportional to the antigens per membrane area unit. Therefore, small cells will appear to stain more intensely under the microscope; large cells, such as lymphoblasts, appear more intense in flow cytometry. For example, stains for the surface immunoglobulin of chronic lymphocytic leukemia appear "dim" on the flow cytometer but intense by immunoperoxidase. Large-cell lymphomas routinely display the converse pattern. Therefore, microscopy will tend to emphasize the smaller lymphocytes and some blasts normally detected by flow cytometry will stain below the detection threshold.

The antibodies to OKT4 and Leu 3 are now known to weakly stain not only helper T cells but also many monocytes and macrophages [28]. With greater sensitivity, the flow cytometer is more likely to count these OKT4$^+$, Leu 3$^+$ monocytes and give a higher Th/Ts ratio. Comparing fluorescent microscopy with flow cytometry, the number of Leu 3$^+$ cells, in fact, correlated poorly, particularly in immunosuppressed (such as those treated with anti-thymocyte globulin), but the cells stained with antibodies to Leu 2 and to Leu 4 (pan-T cell) correlated well with the two methods [28].

In contrast to the initial publications demonstrating a low Th/Ts ratio with acute rejection in tissue, several investigators have now reported acute rejection with high Th/Ts ratios. Analysis of 25 fine needle aspirates with acute rejection showed a low Th/Ts ratio in 19 [103]. In each of these 19 patients, however, rejection was reversible, but 4 of the 6 with high ratios lost their grafts. Another series found that 12 of 15 patients with vascular rejection had a Th/Ts ratio greater than 1, significantly greater than was evident with quiescent rejection or diffuse rejection [22]. In 28 of 31 biopsies with acute renal allograft rejection, the predominant interstitial lymphocyte was OKT4$^+$ [30]. In our own series at the Johns Hopkins Hospital, a prospective study of needle biopsies taken from all recipients at 7 and 28 days showed no significant difference between those with clinically evident acute rejection (Th/Ts ratio = 1.10 ± 0.63) or with stable or improving renal function (Th/Ts ratio = 1.08 ± 0.62) [16].

I cannot easily explain the discrepancy between these series. It does not appear to be related to posttransplant therapy since both groups included patients treated conventionally, with ATG and with CsA. Although each study used a different staining technique, this is an unlikely explanation since both included a sensitive immunoperoxidase procedure and demonstrated crisp membranous staining. The troublesome antibodies to OKT4 and Leu 3 could well be the source of some variation in results. Because of their weak affinity, those with low ratios should demonstrate that the use of fluorescence or cryopreservatives do not interfere with the detection of some helper T cells. On the other side, those using frozen sections and sensitive immunoperoxidase procedures must exclude or correct for any cross-reactivity of these antibodies with monocytes and macrophages.

The Th/Ts ratio was found by one group to be lower in specimens with diffuse cortical infiltrates compared with perivascular or cortical aggregate infiltrates [46]. This appears consistent with the above-mentioned correlation of vascular rejection and a high Th/Ts ratio. However, the studies with low Th/Ts ratios included patients with vascular rejections.

Until these differences are resolved, with more specific antibodies, more standardized staining procedures, or better quantitation, the Th/Ts ratio in renal allograft biopsies is of limited diagnostic use. If, in fact, there are helper-dominant rejection episodes and cytotoxic-dominant rejection episodes, then the Th/Ts ratio in tissue could potentially predict the response to different forms of therapy.

Such a precedent actually exists in cutaneous GVHD. This tissue is somewhat easier to analyze because the infiltrates are less dense than renal biopsies and the epidermal and vascular "compartments" are more readily distinguished. With acute GVHD, the infiltrate is principally along the basal cell layer of the epidermis and is predominantly OKT8$^+$, Leu 2$^+$, OKT11$^+$, consistent with cytotoxic T lymphocytes, with fewer numbers of monocytes and only rare T-helper cells [8,44,48,87]. Chronic GVHD (not equivalent to chronic renal rejection) consists of dermal and perivascular round cell infiltrates dominated by OKT4$^+$, Leu 3$^+$, OKT11$^+$ lymphocytes and monocytes and macrophages. Cytotoxic cells and epidermal lymphocytes are less frequently seen. These two reactions have different clinical outcomes. Acute GVHD is more likely to lead to breakdown of the epidermis. It responds better to therapy such as steroids or increased intravenous CsA. Chronic GVHD is more likely to progress to dermal fibrosis resembling scleroderma. It responds better to a combination of steroids and azathioprine.

With rejection of cardiac allografts, representing primarily a vascular rejection, the current limited experience suggests that the profile of perivascular and vascular infiltrates depends on the immune suppression. One study included 35 endocardial biopsies, 17 from patients receiving conventional therapy (azathioprine, corticosteroids, and ATG) and 18 from patients treated with CsA [78]. The conventionally treated patients had low Th/Ts ratios (mean, 0.4; 0.2-0.6). The CsA-treated patients had a greater infiltrate and widely variable Th/Ts ratios (mean, 1.4; 0.4-2.8). A second study of conventionally treated cardiac allograft recipients also demonstrated a low Th/Ts ratio. At the Johns Hopkins Hospital, all our recipients receive CsA posttransplant. In 65 endocardial biopsies from 15 patients experiencing at least one rejection episode, we found considerable variability in the Th/Ts ratio, although the OKT4/OKT8 ratio correlated well with the Leu 3/ Leu 2 ratio. The Th/Ts ratio did not predict outcome of the rejection or response to therapy.

Initial investigations in liver allografts with acute rejection resemble more the profile with cutaneous GVHD than with heart or kidney allografts. With acute rejection, the predominant lymphocytes in the periportal areas are $OKT8^+$ lymphocytes [85].

Within the thymic cortex, immature thymocytes express both OTK4 and OKT8 antigens simultaneously [76]. As they mature and differentiate into helper, cytotoxic, or suppressor T lymphocytes, the T lymphocytes lose one or the other of these antigens. In peripheral blood and lymph nodes of normal individuals, the expression of OKT4 and OKT8 was initially thought to be mutually exclusive.

In the renal transplant recipient, however, simultaneous coexpression of the OKT4 and OKT8 antigens is frequently observed. This was initially noted as a frequent problem in the determination of Th/Ts ratios in peripheral blood, where the $OKT4^+$ plus $OKT8^+$ cell subpopulations often exceeded the total T cells as determined with OKT3 [20]. Although they did not address the issue specifically, others had similar experiences, as evident in the accompanying tables. Coexpression has also been seen in rat kidney allograft recipients as measured by the W3/25 and OX8 antibodies [21].

We have routinely seen coexpression of the OKT4 and OKT8 antigens as well as the Leu 3a and Leu 2a antigens in the renal allograft biopsies. Because OKT4 and Leu 3a have been noted to stain some monocytes and because T lymphocytes could lose some pan-T markers, we repeated these analyses, comparing the Th cells plus Ts cells to the cells labeled when both antibodies were applied simultaneously. The biopsies showed from 10 to 85% of the defined "T" cells expressed both markers [15,16]. The coexpression is independent of the cell density and independent of the relative number of monocytes or macrophages. There is good agreement between the coexpression as determined with OKT4 and OKT8 antibodies and the coexpression measured with the Leu 3 and Leu 2 antibodies. The simultaneous expression of both markers on the same lymphocytes have been observed using double-label immunofluorescence [89].

The pathogenetic implications are not yet evident. The coexpression did not appear to be a function of acute rejection or of posttransplant therapy. Most of the evidence suggests that it is a nonspecific phenomenon related to T-cell activation. Smith has induced 30-100% coexpression in peripheral blood lymphocytes in a mixed lymphocyte culture with either normal lymphocytes or peripheral blood lymphocytes from transplant recipients. Similar results followed the stimulation of lymphocytes with interleukin-2 but no antigen [15]. Coexpression of T4 and T8 has also been induced in

PBL with the mitogen concanavalin A [12]. The coexpression in grafts does not seem to be due to dedifferentiation, since these cells do not express OKT6, usually observed in all cortical thymocytes. T-cell clones have also been isolated that coexpress OKT4 and OKT8 but have differentiated into functional helper cells [60].

Monocytes and macrophages compose a major portion of the overall renal allograft infiltrate, particularly in the later stages of rejection. In fact, in severe episodes, they can exceed the number of T lymphocytes [35]. They have been observed both in the interstitial regions and localized perivascularly [36,45]. The simple presence of monocytes and macrophages is not specific for rejection and does not necessarily indicate impending allograft injury. We have observed them in high numbers (detected with anti-OKM1) in prospectively performed renal biopsies at 7 and 28 days from patients with stable or improving renal function.

Their effector role in rejection is not clear [53]. It has been hypothesized that as a secretor of plasminogen activator, some of these macrophages may be responsible for fibrin deposition in the later stages of rejection. When the macrophages were identified as "activated" or "resting" with a monoclonal antibody, HTF-1, a direct correlation was observed between the relative number of "active" macrophages and fibrin deposition [36]. Additional studies stratifying the types, activation, and differentiation of monocytes and macrophages could help elucidate their specific action in allograft rejection.

The participation of natural killer (NK) and killer (K) cells in allograft rejection has been postulated but as yet not clearly established. In rat renal allografts, NK and K cells are the first cellular components to enter the graft and proliferate. These were identified by their appearance (large granular lymphocytes; LGL) and ability to lyse an NK target (the YAC-1 cell line) [63]. However, at day 4 they rapidly decline in number, long before the actual rejection occurs. An antigen presentation or regulatory role for these cells has not been proposed. In human allografts Leu 7^+ (HNK-1) lymphocytes are seen with increased frequency with acute rejection, particularly during the early phase of rejection. They are prominent in the peritubular capillaries. However, Leu 7 is no longer thought to be expressed solely on NK and K cells and in fact is present only on a subpopulation of LGL containing weak NK activity [49]. We have been unable to identify NK cells using anti-Leu 11 (NK-15), thought to be specific for NK cells and staining most NK cells. However, this antibody stained the tubular epithelial cytoplasm in some specimens, interfering with analysis of some biopsies. We have not observed any Leu 11^+ mononuclear cells in either skin with acute GVHD or endocardial biopsies with acute cardiac allograft rejection. We have observed moderate numbers of Leu 11^+ lymphocytes in some large-cell lymphomas and within the cortical sinuses of lymph nodes.

B lymphocytes and plasma cells generally comprise a minor component of the renal allograft infiltrate with acute rejection [30,31,35]. Most of the rejection episodes in these series would be considered the cellular form rather than the humoral form of acute rejection as discussed by Porter [72]. With acute cardiac allograft rejection and acute GVHD, we have rarely seen infiltrates containing more than 5% B lymphocytes as detected with the anti-B1 antibody. B lymphocytes are also rare in liver allografts undergoing acute rejection [85]. The role of antibodies in renal allograft rejection is discussed in more detail in Chapter 3.

INTRAVASCULAR INFILTRATES

Vascular involvement with acute rejection is clearly established as an indicator of poor prognosis [26,54,57]. Indeed, in the absence of an intimal arteritis, it is questionable whether an allograft infiltrate represents the actual acute rejection or a nonspecific inflammatory response to surgery, warm ischemia, or some other transient insult [15].

The infiltrate with acute rejection consists of subendothelial mononuclear cells, occasional neutrophils, and associated intimal edema. This picture is quite distinct from the usual vasculitis seen with immune complex disease, a transmural infiltrate of neutrophils. With acute rejection, these lesions contain only focal deposits of IgM and no C3, also suggesting a cellular reaction rather than a humoral or immune complex reaction [57].

In spite of the prognostic significance of these subendothelial infiltrates, they have not been well characterized. Considering the emphasis given to endothelial antigens and how these antigens might affect the cellular immune response, this is rather surprising. The reason is probably technical. The best infiltrates are seen with early rejection, before secondary effects following thrombosis. This limits the evaluable material to needle core biopsies. Second, most monoclonal antibodies require the use of frozen tissue, usually the smaller portion of a biopsy. The arteritis is often patchy in distribution, and often the biopsies have relatively few evaluable arteries which may not be present in the portion frozen for immunoperoxidase stains.

We have been able to stain and evaluate with monoclonal antibodies and immunoperoxidase four needle core biopsies with recent onset acute rejection. In each of these specimens, the *subendothelial* infiltrate consisted of $OKT8^+$ T lymphocytes with occasional $OKM1^+$ cells. In two of these cases, the *interstitial* infiltrate had a low Th/Ts ratio (0.2; 0.6). In the other two, the ratio was increased (1.5; 3.2). If these few cases are representative, the intimal infiltrate is not simply a reflection of the interstitial or perivascular infiltrates. The profile of the intimal cells is consistent with a CTL response to the class I or minor histocompatibility antigens expressed on the endothelium.

Using the anti-Tac-1 antibody, many of the lymphocytes in close approximation to the endothelial cells were found to express the IL-2 receptor [36].

INTRAEPITHELIAL INFILTRATES

Is acute renal allograft rejection principally a vascular rejection, as with heart allografts, or is there also a significant rejection of the epithelium, as with liver allograft rejection and acute GVHD? A comparison of the perivascular infiltrates to the interstitial infiltrates is not adequate to resolve this question. Because of the rich network of peritubular capillaries, a count of the "interstitial" cells could include many cells within capillaries. The interstitial and peritubular capillary populations can be particularly difficult to distinguish when the immunohistochemical analysis is done with frozen tissue.

Initial phenotype analysis used punctate α-naphthyl acetate esterase (ANAE) staining for marking T cells and diffuse cytoplasmic ANAE of lysozyme for macrophages. In cases of irreversible acute rejection, the larger blood vessels were surrounded by T lymphocytes but the infiltrates around the tubules and within the peritubular capillaries were predominantly macrophages [45,77].

Using monoclonal antibodies, including OKM1 and FMC32 [14], Hancock noted that monocytes and macrophages accounted for 40-50% of the interstitial infiltrate with mild to moderate rejection. With severe rejection, the monocytes and macrophages amounted to 60% of the infiltrate and were observed immediately adjacent to the proximal tubular cells [35,36].

A predominantly histiocytic infiltrate often indicates a secondary reaction to another insult or a delayed-type hypersensitivity reaction. In fact, a sequential study of renal allograft rejection indicates that the influx of monocytes and macrophages occurs in the later stages of acute rejection.

Recently we observed that the intraepithelial lymphocytes in the proximal tubules of biopsies with clinically evident acute rejection carry the Leu 7 (HNK-1) antigen [7]. [See Fig. 3 (Color Plate 2) in center of book]. Unlike most membrane antigens, the Leu 7 antigen is resistant to formalin and the tissue processing required for routine histology. Using this antibody and avidin-biotin complex immunoperoxidase on paraffin-embedded tissues, we determined the relative frequency and location of Leu 7^+ lymphocytes in 57 renal allograft specimens and 15 native kidney specimens.

Although tubulitis was seen in renal allograft biopsies without rejection and in some native kidneys with interstitial nephritis or pyelonephritis, the lymphocytes are Leu 7 negative. In 70% (9 of 13) of the specimens with recent onset acute rejection, however, most of the intraepithelial lymphocytes are Leu 7^+. With end-stage rejection, having an average duration of 2 months, 38% (5 of 13) have Leu 7^+ intraepithelial lymphocytes, although not as many as the recent onset cases. We have not observed any renal allograft specimens with acute tubular necrosis or stable function having more than a rare Leu 7^+ intraepithelial lymphocytes. These cells correlated with acute rejection regardless of whether the patient received conventional therapy (prednisone, azathioprine, or optional horse anti-thymocyte globulin) or CsA. Graft biopsies from patients with well-documented CMV infections but no rejection contained interstitial Leu 7^+ lymphocytes but no Leu 7^+ intraepithelial lymphocytes. Consistent with Hancock's recent findings, the interstitial infiltrate contained more Leu 7^+ lymphocytes during the earlier phase of acute rejection [32]. However, they were also evident in 8 of 24 specimens with stable or improving function and in 3 of 15 native kidney specimens. Glomerular and intravascular Leu 7^+ cells were rare and did not correlate with the graft status.

Paraffin sections allow for better morphology than usually seen with immunoperoxidase. The Leu 7^+ lymphocytes were just inside the tubular basement membrane, often elongated, and slightly larger than a resting lymphocyte [Figure 3 (Color Plate 2) in center of book]. The staining was clearly membranous, with cytoplasmic sparing. The invaded tubules showed signs of injury with desquamation of individual tubular cells and disorientation as well as patchy disruption of the tubular basement membrane.

The specificity of Leu 7^+ intraepithelial lymphocytes give them diagnostic importance. Their role in complementing other diagnostic features of rejection is discussed elsewhere in this volume. Here we will discuss some of the pathogenetic implications.

The intimate association of these intraepithelial lymphocytes with epithelial injury and their presence at the onset of rejection make them good candidates for the effector cells against epithelial cells. What are these Leu 7^+ cells? Leu 7 (HNK-1) was initially developed against the large granular lymphocytes (LGL) and thought to be specific for K and NK cells [1]. Peripheral blood lymphocytes contain only about 15% Leu 7^+ lymphocytes. Later studies, however, have shown that it is present only on a subpopulation of NK and K cells and is present on other cells as well. Leu 11 (NK-15) is now known to be more specific for NK cells with little if any cross-reaction with other cell populations. Separating the cells with flow cytometry and using separate fluorescent labels for these two antigens, the strongest NK activity was localized in the Leu 7^-, Leu 11^+ subpopulations [49]. Double-label flow cytometry showed that Leu 7 is present on 20-40% of the Leu $2a^+$ (cytotoxic/suppressor) cells [50]. They do not contain detectable NK activity.

In fact, we believe that the Leu 7^+ intraepithelial lymphocytes are probably not NK cells. For five biopsies with acute rejection and numerous Leu 7^+ intraepithelial lymphocytes, we stained frozen sections with B1, OKT11, Leu 1, Leu 3a, Leu 2a, OKT4, OKT8, OKM1, Leu 11, and Leu 7 antibodies and analyzed the intraepithelial lymphocytes [5]. The intraepithelial lymphocytes were predominantly T lymphocytes; a few were monocytes, but none were B lymphocytes. More than 85% of the intraepithelial lymphocytes were Leu 2^+, $OKT8^+$, but $OKT4^+$ or Leu 3^+ intraepithelial lymphocytes were only rarely observed. As with the paraffin sections, more than 90% of the intraepithelial lymphocytes stained with the anti-Leu 7 antibody. Anti-Leu 11 did not stain any intraepithelial lymphocytes in three of the cases. In the other two cases, anti-Leu 11 intensely stained the cytoplasm of the tubular epithelium, preventing analysis of the intraepithelial lymphocytes. The results suggest that this highly compartmentalized population of cells in a highly select group of patients is dominated by a single phenotype. The profile is more consistent with cytotoxic/suppressor T lymphocytes than with NK or K cells. With the early and intimate association with tubular injury, they are more likely cytotoxic T cells than suppressor T cells.

Are the Leu 7^+ intraepithelial lymphocytes a primary reaction to the epithelium or a secondary reaction to rejection-induced decreased renal blood flow? Subendothelial arteritis was also present in all specimens with moderate to numerous Leu 7^+ intraepithelial lymphocytes and evaluable arteries. These probably represent two independent components of rejection. The Leu 7^+ intraepithelial lymphocytes were most numerous at the onset or rejection, -1 to 4 days after deterioration of renal function. In these specimens, there was no evidence of thrombosis or hemorrhage. The peritubular capillaries were intact and patent, though they often contained mononuclear cells. In native kidneys with ischemic changes, Leu 7^+ intraepithelial lymphocytes were not seen.

In fact, the vascular and epithelial infiltrates may represent separate lymphocyte populations. In four specimens with acute rejection, moderate to numerous Leu 7^+ intraepithelial lymphocytes, and evaluable arteries on frozen sections, the subendothelial infiltrate consisted of $OKT8^+$, Leu 2^+ T cells that were Leu 7^-. When the factors responsible for Leu 7 expression on cytotoxic/suppressor T cells are clarified, the pathogenesis of these two components of rejection should be evident.

We cannot exclude at this point a complementary role for the intraepithelial lymphocytes following injury by a delayed-type hypersensitivity reaction, innocent bystander injury, or humoral reaction. The presence and relative number of Leu 7^+ intraepithelial lymphocytes was independent of the relative number of interstitial monocytes, B cells, plasma cells, and Th/Ts ratio. Since delayed-type hypersensitivity reactions usually consist of mixed infiltrates dominated by helper T cells and monocytes, rejection most likely does not require a predominantly delayed-type hypersensitivity reaction for Leu 7^+ intraepithelial lymphocyte-associated epithelial injury [70].

SUMMARY

At the moment, the characterization of graft cell infiltrates and cellular targets is at an awkward stage of development, similar to adolescence. Different approaches have been tried, and some show considerable promise. No approach is ideal, and we have detailed some of the limitations of each method. There is considerable room for improvement; not all of the potential advantages of looking at tissue have been developed. Yet, with an increasingly specific approach to therapy, the responsibilities and the need for characterizing the infiltrates will be considerably greater in the very near future.

The distribution of histocompatibility antigens in the normal kidney did not correlate with the distribution of the cellular injury of rejection. Several reasons for this discrepancy and the supporting evidence were explored, including a different distribution of recently discovered closely linked class II antigens, the induction of class II antigens, and the expression of minor histocompatibility antigens not linked to the MHC.

Acute cellular rejection begins with a perivascular infiltrate of T lymphocytes and later influx of monocytes and macrophages.

The T lymphocytes are activated lymphocytes bearing interleukin-2 receptors, class II antigens (Ia), and demonstrating coexpression of antigens usually found exclusively on helper *or* cytotoxic/suppressor cells. The cells are also seen in allografts without rejection, however, so "activation" alone is not sufficient. The relative numbers of helper and cytotoxic/suppressor T cells in the graft is still controversial, some reporting consistently cytotoxic/suppressor cell-dominated infiltrates, others seeing variable infiltrates in different patients. Most agree, however, that the graft infiltrate cannot be predicted from the peripheral blood profile, which routinely shows an increase in helper cells prior to rejection. The conflicting results from different groups may be due to technical factors or it may reflect differences in patient selection, therapy, or other factors. These controversies are becoming somewhat overshadowed by ensuing redefinition of the specificities of the monoclonal antibodies employed.

Monocytes and macrophages are a major participant in acute rejection, particularly in the later phases of rejection and in more severe cases. Evidence has been presented linking them to fibrin deposition.

The importance of natural killer cells, B lymphocytes, and plasma cells in acute cellular rejection is not known. These cells comprise only a minority of the overall infiltrate.

A chief advantage to analyzing tissue specimens is the ability to compartmentalize the infiltrates. Differences in cellular populations were seen between the perivascular and interstitial regions. The study of the intravascular and intraepithelial compartments allows for characterization of a very small fraction of the infiltrate that may well be specifically involved in the rejection. Initial reports suggest that the subendothelial infiltrate contains cytotoxic/suppressor T cells bearing IL-2 receptors. With most episodes of acute rejection, the intraepithelial lymphocytes between tubular epithelial cells consist of a second distinct population of cytotoxic/suppressor cells.

There is room for growth in this field at both the technical and theoretical levels.

High on the technical priority list is a toolbox containing more specific antibodies. This is critical for tissue analysis, in which the lymphocytes (particularly in select compartments) cannot readily be isolated and tested for function. The second generation of monoclonal antibodies offers some hope, as they are being developed not against cell populations but against epitopes of functional importance, such as the interleukin-2 receptor and T-cell receptor.

In the absence of more specific antibodies, the coexpression of multiple antigens on the same cells could define specific subpopulations. This potential has been realized with flow cytometry and has been used to a limited extent in tissue. However, the immunofluorescence techniques employed in tissue lack the sensitivity and specificity of other immunohistochemical techniques, and the significance of the apparent double-labeling is unclear.

The compartmentalization of infiltrates should be more extensively pursued. Most of the infiltrate with rejection may be irrelevant, and compartmentalization may select for the important participants and suggest their cellular mechanism. To best achieve this, however, it is necessary to obtain better morphology than is now realized with frozen tissue. Either antigens insensitive to fixation or better preservatives that do not destroy the antigens must be developed. It will also be necessary to be more quantitative than current estimates or cell counts. Computerized image analysis (CIA) could provide this and avoid errors of estimation, such as mistaking the relative intensity of membrane staining for the relative number.

At the theoretical and practical level, it is necessary to more precisely define the cellular profile specific for acute rejection. If there is more than one profile, what factors are responsible: antigen disparity, pretransplant immune status, warm ischemia, or others? Once rejection is better defined and understood, then the effects of different therapies, toxicities, and infections can be defined.

ACKNOWLEDGMENTS

I wish to gratefully acknowledge the technical assistance, persistence, and advice of Donna Suresch, Charlotte Shinn, and Sharyn Hedrick in the cited studies from our laboratory. This work was supported in part by grants CA15396 and CA28701 from the National Cancer Institute and AI20173 from the National Institute of Allergy and Infectious Diseases, National Institutes of Health.

REFERENCES

1. Abo, T., and Balch, C. M. A differentiation antigen of human NK and K cells identified by b monoclonal antibody (HNK-1). *J. Immunol.* 127:1024-1029, 1981.
2. Ascher, N. L., Chen, S., Hoffman, R., and Simmons, R. L. Maturation of cytotoxic effector cells at the site of allograft rejection. *Transplant. Proc.* 13:1105-1107, 1981.
3. Ascher, N. L., Hoffman, R., Hanto, D. W., and Simmons, R. L. Cellular events within the rejecting allograft. *Transplantation* 35:193-197, 1983.

3a. Austyn, J. M., Steinman, R. M., Weinstein, D. E., Granelli-Piperno, A., and Palladino, M. A. Dendritic cells initiate a two-stage mechanism for T lymphocyte proliferation. *J. Exp. Med.* 157:1101-1115, 1983.

4. Barnard, C. N., and Cooper, D. K. C. Clinical transplantation of the heart: A review of 13 years personal experience. *J. R. Soc. Med.* 74:670-674, 1981.
5. Beschorner, W. E., Burdick, J. F., Williams, G. M., and Solez, K. Phenotypic identification of intraepithelial lymphocytes (IEL) in acute renal allograft rejection. *Kidney Int.* 27:206, 1985.
6. Beschorner, W. E., Tutschka, P. J., and Santos, G. W. Sequential morphology of graft-versus-host disease in the rat radiation chimera. *Clin. Immunol. Immunopathol.* 22: 203-224, 1982.
7. Beschorner, W. E., Burdick, J. F., Williams, G. M., and Solez, K. The presence of Leu 7 reactive lymphocytes in renal allografts undergoing acute rejection. *Transplant. Proc.* 17:618-622, 1985.
8. Beschorner, W. E., Constantino, F. A., Tutschka, P. J., and Santos, G. W. Characterization of inflammatory cells of human skin with acute graft-versus-host disease (GVHD). *Exp. Hematol.* 10:6, 1982.
9. Beschorner, W. E., Pino, J., Boitnott, J. K., Tutschka, P. J., and Santos, G. W. Liver pathology of bone marrow transplantation: Effects of busulfan, carmustine, acute graft-versus-host disease and cytomegalovirus infection. *Am. J. Pathol.* 99:369-381, 1980.
10. Beschorner, W. E., Tutschka, P. J., and Santos, G. W. The sequential morphology of acute graft-versus-host disease in the rat radiation chimera. *Clin. Immunol. Immunopathol.* 22:203-228, 1982.

11. Billingham, R. E. The biology of graft-versus-host reactions. *Harvey Lect.* 62:21-78, 1966.
12. Blue, M.-L., Daley, J. F., Levine, H., and Schlossman, S. F. Coexpression of T4 and T8 on peripheral blood T cells demonstrated by two-color fluorescence flow cytometry. *J. Immunol.* 134:2281-2286, 1985.
13. Bolton, E. M., Thompson, J. F., Wood, R. F. M., and Morris, P. J. Immunoperoxidase staining of fine-needle aspiration biopsies and needle core biopsies from renal allografts. *Transplantation* 36:728-731, 1983.
14. Brooks, D. A., Zola, H., McNamara, P. J., Bradley, J., Bradstock, K. F., Hamcock, W. W., and Atkins, R. C. Membrane antigens of the monocyte macrophage lineage studied with monoclonal antibodies. *Pathology* 15:45-52, 1983.
15. Burdick, J. F., Beschorner, W. E., Smith, W. J., McGraw, D., Bender, W. L., Williams, G. M., and Solez, K. Characteristics of early routine renal allograft biopsies. *Transplantation* 38:679-684, 1984.
16. Burdick, J. F., Beschorner, W. E., Smith, W. J., McGraw, D., Bender, W., Williams, G. M., and Solez, K. Lymphocytes in early renal allograft Biopsies. *Transplant. Proc.* 17: 562-563, 1985.
17. Burdick, J. F., personal communication, 1985.
18. Burns, B. F., Warnke, R. A., Doggett, R. S., and Rouse, R. V. Expression of a T-cell antigen (Leu-1) by B-cell lymphomas. *Am. J. Pathol.* 113:165-171, 1983.
19. Burton, R. C., Cosimi, A. B., Colvin, R. B., Rubin, R. H., Delmonico, F. L., Goldstein, G., and Russell, P. S. Monoclonal antibodies to human T cell subsets: Use for immunological monitoring and immunosuppression in renal transplantation. *J. Clin. Immunol.* 2:142S-147S, 1982.
20. Chatenoud, L., Chkoff, N., Kreis, H., and Bach, J. F. Interest in and limitations of monoclonal anti-T-cell antibodies for the follow-up of renal transplant patients. *Transplantation* 36:45-50, 1983.
21. Claesson, K., Forsum, U., Klareskog, L., Larsson, E., Frodin, L., and Tufveson, G. T cell subsets and Ia-expressing cells in transplanted rat kidneys. *Transplant. Proc.* 17: 792-793, 1985.
22. Cooksey, G., Reeve, R. S., Paterson, A. D., Cotton, R. E., and Blamey, R. W. Lymphocyte subpopulations in cytologic aspirates from human renal allografts. *Transplant. Proc.* 17:630-632, 1985.
23. Cosimi, A. B., Colvin, R. B., Burton, R. C., Rubin, R. H., Goldstein, G., Kung, P. C., Hansen, W. P., Delmonico, F. L., and Russell, P. S. Use of monoclonal antibodies to T-cell subsets for immunologic monitoring and treatment in recipients of renal allografts. *N. Engl. J. Med.* 305:308-314, 1981.
24. Daar, A. S., Fuggle, S. V., Fabre, J. W., Ting, A., and Morris, P. J. The detailed distribution of MHC class II antigens in normal human organs. *Transplantation* 38:293-298, 1984.
25. Demetris, A. J., Lasky, S., Van Thiel, D. H., Starzl, T. E., and Dekker, A. Pathology of hepatic transplantation: A review of 62 adult allograft recipients immunosuppressed with a cyclosporine/steroid regimen. *Am. J. Pathol.* 118:151-161, 1985.
26. Finkelstein, F. O., Siegel, N. J., Bastl, C., Forrest, J. N., Jr., and Kashgarian, M. Kidney transplant biopsies in the diagnosis and management of acute rejection reactions. *Kidney Int.* 10:171-178, 1976.
27. Fuggle, S. V., Errasti, P., Daar, A. S., Fabre, J. W., Ting, A., and Morris, P. J. Localization of major histocompatibility complex (HLA-ABC and DR) antigens in 46 kidneys. *Transplantation* 35:385-390, 1983.
28. Ganghoff, O., Gross, U., Whitley, T. K., Roebuck, D., and Thomas, J. J. Factors in the accuracy and reproducibility of T cell and T cell subset measurements in transplant patients. *Transplant. Proc.* 17:640-641, 1985.

29. Hall, B. M., Bishop, G. A., Duggin, G. G., Horvath, J. S., Philips, J., and Tiller, D. J. Increased expression of HLA-DR antigens on renal tubular cells in renal transplants: Relevance to the rejection response. *Lancet* 2:247-251, 1984.
30. Hall, B. M., Bishop, G. A., Farnsworth, A., Duggin, G. G., Horvath, J. S., Sheil, A. G., and Tiller, D. F. Identification of the cellular subpopulations infiltrating rejecting cadaver renal allografts. Preponderance of the T4 subset of T cells. *Transplantation* 37:564-570, 1984.
31. Hammer, C., Land, W., Stadler, J., Koller, C., and Brendel, W. Lymphocyte subclasses in rejecting kidney grafts detected by monoclonal antibodies. *Transplant. Proc.* 15: 356-360, 1983.
32. Hancock, W. W., and Atkins, R. C. Immunohistological analysis of sequential renal biopsies from patients with acute renal rejection. *Kidney Int.* 27:341, 1985.
33. Hancock, W. W., Kraft, N., and Atkins, R. C. Demonstration of major histocompatibility antigens in the human kidney. *Pathology* 14:409-414, 1982.
35. Hancock, W. W., Thomson, N. M., and Atkins, R. C. Composition of interstitial cellular infiltrate identified by monoclonal antibodies in renal biopsies of rejecting human renal allografts. *Transplantation* 35:458-463, 1983.
36. Hancock, W. W. Analysis of intragraft effector mechanisms associated with human renal allograft rejection: Immunohistological studies with monoclonal antibodies. *Immunol. Rev.* 77:61-84, 1984.
37. Hayry, P., von Willebrand, E., Ahonen, J., and Eklund, B. Do well-to-do and repeatedly rejecting renal allografts express the transplantation antigens similarly on their surface? *Scand. J. Urol. Nephrol.* [*Suppl.*] 64:52-55, 1981.
38. Hayry, P., von Willebrand, E., Parthenais, E., Nemlander, A., Soots, A., Lautenschlager, I., Alfoldy, P., and Renkonen, R. The inflammatory mechanisms of allograft rejection. *Immunol. Rev.* 77:85-142, 1984.
39. Hayry, P., and von Willebrand, E. Transplant aspiration cytology. *Transplantation* 38: 7-12, 1984.
40. Herskowicz, A., Ueda, K., and Beschorner, W. E., submitted for publication.
41. Hofman, F. M., Danilovs, J. A., and Taylor, C. R. HLA-DR (Ia)-positive dendritic-like cells in human fetal nonlymphoid tissues. *Transplantation* 37:590-594, 1984.
42. Iwatsuki, S., Rabin, B. S., Shaw, B. W., Jr., and Starzl, T. E. Liver transplantation against T cell-positive warm crossmatches. *Transplant. Proc.* 16:1427-1429, 1984.
43. Jaffee, B. D., and Claman, H. N. Chronic graft-versus-host disease (GVHD) as a model for scleroderma. I. Description of model systems. *Cell Immunol.* 77:1-12, 1983.
44. Kaye, V. N., Neumann, P. M., Kersey, J., Goltz, R. W., Baldridge, B. D., Michael, A. F., and Platt, J. L. Identity of immune cells in graft-versus-host disease of the skin. Analysis using monoclonal antibodies by indirect immunofluorescence. *Am. J. Pathol.* 116: 436-440, 1984.
45. Klockers, M., Reitamo, S., and Collan, Y. Immunohistochemical identification of renal lysozyme during allograft rejection in man. *Histopathology* 3:433-443, 1979.
46. Kolbeck, P. C., Tatum, A. H., and Sanfilippo, F. Relationships among the histologic pattern, intensity, and phenotypes of T cells infiltrating renal allografts. *Transplantation* 38:709-713, 1984.
47. Krensky, A. M., Clayberger, C., Reiss, C. S., Strominger, J. L., and Burakoff, S. J. Specificity of OKT4+ cytotoxic T lymphocyte clones. *J. Immunol.* 129:2001-2003, 1982.
48. Lampert, I. A., Suitters, A. J., and Chisholm, P. M. Expression of Ia antigen on epidermal keratinocytes in graft-versus-host disease. *Nature* 293:149-150, 1981.
49. Lanier, L. L., Le, A. M., Phillips, J. H., Warner, N. L., and Babcock, G. F. Subpopulations of human natural killer cells defined by expression of the Leu-7 (HNK-1) and Leu-11 (NK-15) antigens. *J. Immunol.* 131:1789-1796, 1983.

50. Lanier, L. L., and Loken, M. R. Human lymphocyte subpopulations identified by using three-color immunofluorescence and flow cytometry analysis: Correlation of Leu-2, Leu-3, Leu-7, Leu-8, and Leu-11 cell surface antigen expression. *J. Immunol.* 132:151-156, 1984.
51. Lautenschlager, I., Nyman, N., Vaananen, H., Lehto, V. P., Virtanen, I., and Hayry, P. Antigenic and immunogenic components in rat liver. *Scand. J. Immunol.* 14:61-68, 1983.
52. Lechler, R. I., and Batchelor, J. R. Restoration of immunogenicity to passenger cell-depleted kidney allografts by the addition of donor strain dendritic cells. *J. Exp. Med.* 155:31-41, 1982.
53. MacPherson, G. G., and Christmas, S. E. The role of the macrophage in cardiac allograft rejection in the rat. *Immunol. Rev.* 77:143-166, 1984.
54. Magil, A., Rubin, J., Ladewig, L., Johnson, M., Goldstein, M. B., and Bear, R. A. Renal biopsy in acute allograft rejection. Significance of moderate vascular lesions in long-term graft survival. *Nephron* 26:180-183, 1980.
55. Mason, D. W., Dallman, M., and Barclay, A. N. GVHD induces expression of Ia antigen in rat epidermal cells and gut epithelia. *Nature* 293:150-151, 1981.
56. Mason, D. W., Dallman, M. J., Arthur, R. P., and Morris, P. J. Mechanisms of allograft rejection: The roles of cytotoxic T-cells and delayed-type hypersensitivity. *Immunol. Rev.* 77:167-184, 1984.
57. Matas, A. J., Scheinman, J. I., Rattazzi, L. C., Mozes, M. F., Simmons, R. L., and Najarian, J. S. Immunopathological studies of the ruptured human renal allograft. *Transplantation* 22:420-426, 1976.
58. Mayer, T. G., Lazarovitx, A. I., Boyle, L. A., Sullivan, E. R., Leary, C. P., Fuller, A. A., Fuller, T. C., Cosimi, A. B., Bhan, A. K., Colvin, R. B., Collins, A. B., and Kurnick, J. T. Functional allospecific T lymphocytes isolated from human renal allograft biopsies. *Transplant. Proc.* 17:816-818, 1985.
59. Mazaheri, R., Laupacis, A., Keown, P., Howson, W., Sinclair, N. R., and Stiller, C. R. Lymphocyte subsets in the allograft recipient: Correlation of helper to suppressor ratio with clinical events. *Transplant. Proc.* 14:676-678, 1982.
60. Mingari, M. C., Melioli, G., Moretta, A., Pantaleo, G., and Moretta, L. Surface markers of cloned human T cells with helper or suppressor activity on pokeweed mitogen-driven B cell differentiation. *Eur. J. Immunol.* 12:900-903, 1982.
61. Murphy, G. F. Monoclonal anti-T6 antibody and Langerhans cells. *Br. J. Dermatol.* 107:487-489, 1982.
62. Nemlander, A., Soots, A., von Willebrand, E., Husberg, B., and Hayry, P. Redistribution of renal allograft responding leukocytes during rejection. 2. Kinetics and specificity. *J. Exp. Med.* 156:1087-1100, 1982.
63. Nemlander, A., Saksela, E., and Hayry, P. Are "natural killer" cells involved in allograft rejection? *Eur. J. Immunol.* 13:348-350, 1983.
64. Paul, L. C., and Carpenter, C. B. Antigenic determinants of tubular basement membranes and Bowman's capsule in rats. *Kidney Int.* 21:800-807, 1982.
65. Pelletier, M., Perreault, C., Landry, D., David, M., and Montplaisir, S. Ontogeny of human epidermal Langerhans cells. *Transplantation* 38:544-546, 1984.
66. Perreault, C., Pelletier, M., Landry, D., and Gyger, M. Study of Langerhans cells after allogeneic bone marrow transplantation. *Blood* 63:807-811, 1984.
67. Perussia, B., Fanning, V., and Trinchieri, G. A human NK and K cell subset shares with cytotoxic T cell expression of the antigen recognized by antibody OKT8. *J. Immunol.* 131:223-231, 1983.
68. Pfeffer, P. F., and Thorsby, E. HLA-restricted cytotoxicity against male-specific (H-Y) antigen after acute rejection of an HLA-identical sibling kidney: Clonal distribution of the cytotoxic cells. *Transplantation* 33:52-56, 1982.

69. Pichlmayr, R., Brolsch, C., Wonigeit, K., Neuhaus, P., Siegismund, S., Schmidt, F. W., and Burdelski, M. Experiences with liver transplantation in Hannover. *Hepatology* 4(Suppl.):56S-60S, 1984.
70. Platt, J. L., Grant, B. W., Eddy, A. A., and Michael, A. F. Immune cell populations in cutaneous delayed-type hypersensitivity. *J. Exp. Med.* 158:1227-1242, 1983.
71. Platt, J. L., LeBien, T. W., and Michael, A. F. Interstitial mononuclear cell populations in renal graft rejection. Identification by monoclonal antibodies in tissue sections. *J. Exp. Med.* 155:17-30, 1982.
72. Porter, K. A. Renal transplantation. In *Pathology of the Kidney,* R. H. Heptinstall, ed. Little, Brown, Boston, 1983, pp. 1455-1546.
73. Rappaport, H., Khalil, A., Halle-Pannenko, O., Pritchard, L., Dantchev, D., and Mathe, G. Histopathologic sequence of events in adult mice undergoing lethal graft-versus-host reaction developed across H-2 and/or non-H-2 histocompatibility barriers. *Am. J. Pathol.* 96:121-142, 1979.
74. Reinherz, E. L., Kung, P. C., Goldstein, G., and Schlossman, S. F. A monoclonal antibody reactive with the human cytotoxic suppressor T cell subset previously defined by a heteroantiserum termed TH2. *J. Immunol.* 124:1301-1307, 1980.
75. Reinherz, E. L., Kung, P. C., Goldstein, G., and Schlossman, S. F. Further characterization of the human inducer T cell subset defined by monoclonal antibody. *J. Immunol.* 123:2894-2896, 1979.
76. Reinherz, E. L., and Schlossman, S. F. The differentiation and function of human T lymphocytes: A review. *Cell* 19:821-827, 1980.
77. Reitamo, S., Konttinen, Y. T., Ranki, A., and Hayry, P. The relation of different inflammatory cell types to the various parenchymal components of rejecting kidney allografts. *Histopathology* 4:517-532, 1980.
78. Rose, M. L., Gracie, J. A., Fraser, A., Chisholm, P. M., and Yacoub, M. H. Use of monoclonal antibodies to quantitate T lymphocyte subpopulations in human cardiac allografts. *Transplantation* 38:230-234, 1984.
79. Sachs, D. H., Leight, G. S., and Cone, J. Transplantation in miniature swine. I. Fixation of the major histocompatibility complex. *Transplantation* 22:559-567, 1976.
80. Sale, G. E. Pathology and recent pathogenetic studies in human graft-versus-host disease. *Surv. Synth. Pathol. Res.* 3:235-253, 1984.
81. Sale, G. E., Lerner, K. G., Barker, E. A., Shulman, H. M., and Thomas, E. D. The skin biopsy in the diagnosis of acute graft-versus-host disease in man. *Am. J. Pathol.* 89: 621-636, 1977.
82. Sale, G. E., Storb, R., and Kolb, H. Histopathology of hepatic acute graft-versus-host disease in the dog: A double blind study confirms the specificity of small bile duct lesions. *Transplantation* 26:103-106, 1978.
83. Santos, G. W. History of bone marrow transplantation. *Clin. Haematol.* 12:611-639, 1983.
84. Seemayer, T. A., Lapp, W. S., and Bolande, R. P. Thymic epithelial injury in graft-versus-host reactions following adrenalectomy. *Am. J. Pathol.* 93:325-338, 1978.
85. Si, L., Whiteside, T. L., Van Thiel, D. H., and Rabin, B. S. Lymphocyte subpopulations at the site of "piecemeal" necrosis in end stage chronic liver diseases and rejecting liver allografts in cyclosporine-treated patients. *Lab. Invest.* 50:341-347, 1984.
86. Slavin, R. E., and Santos, G. W. The graft-versus-host reaction in man following bone marrow transplantation: Pathology, pathogenesis, clinical features and implications. *Clin. Immunol. Immunopathol.* 1:472-498, 1973.
87. Sloane, J. P., Thomas, J. A., Imrie, S. F., Easton, D. F., and Powles, R. L. Morphological and immunohistological changes in the skin in allogeneic bone marrow recipients. *J. Clin. Pathol.* 37:919-930, 1984.

88. Snover, D. C., Weisdorf, S. A., Ramsay, N. K., McGlave, P., and Kersey, J. H. Hepatic graft versus host disease: A study of the predictive value of liver biopsy in diagnosis. *Hepatology* 4:123-130, 1984.
89. Solez, K. Unpublished observation, 1985.
90. Starzl, T. E., Iwatsuki, S., Van Thiel, D. H., Gartner, J. C., Zitelli, B. J., Malatack, J. J., Schade, R. R., Shaw, B. W., Jr., Hakala, T. R., Rosenthal, J. T., and Porter, K. A. Evolution of liver transplantation. *Hepatology* 2:614-636, 1982.
91. Steiniger, B., Klempnauer, J., and Wonigeit, K. Phenotype and histological distribution of interstitial dendritic cells in the rat pancreas, liver, heart, and kidney. *Transplantation* 38:169-175, 1984.
93. Stelzer, G. T., McLeish, K. R., Lorden, R. E., and Watson, S. L. Alterations in T lymphocyte subpopulations associated with renal allograft rejection. *Transplantation* 37:261-264, 1984.
94. Suitters, A. J., and Lampert, I. A. Class II antigen induction in the liver of rats with graft-versus-host disease. *Transplantation* 38:194-196, 1984.
95. Takacs, L., Szende, B., Monostori, E., et al. Expression of HLA-DR antigens on bile duct cells of rejected liver transplants. *Lancet* 2:1500, 1983.
96. Tyler, J. D., Burlingham, W. J., David, C. S., and Steinmuller, D. Cell-mediated cytotoxicity to non-MHC alloantigens on mouse epidermal cells. VI. Influence of the MHC on the tissue specificity of cytotoxic T-lymphocyte responses. *Immunogenetics* 16:23-36, 1982.
97. Tyler, J. D., Galli, S. J., Snider, M. E., Dvorak, A. M., and Steinmuller, D. Cloned LYT-2+ cytolytic T lymphocytes destroy allogeneic tissue in vivo. *J. Exp. Med.* 159: 234-243, 1984.
98. Tyler, J. D., and Steinmuller, D. Establishment of cytolytic T lymphocyte clones to epidermal alloantigen Epa-1. *Transplantation* 34:140-143, 1982.
99. Uchiyama, T., Broder, S., and Waldmann, T. A. A monoclonal antibody (anti-Tac) reactive with activated and functionally mature human T-cells. *J. Immunol.* 126: 1393-1397, 1981.
100. van Es, A., Meyer, C. J., Oljans, P. J., Tanke, H. J., and van Es, L. A. Mononuclear cells in renal allografts. Correlation with peripheral blood T lymphocyte subpopulations and graft prognosis. *Transplantation* 37:134-139, 1984.
101. van Es, A., Baldwin, W. M., Oljans, P. J., Tanke, H. J., Ploem, J. S., and van Es, L. A. Expression of HLA-DR on T lymphocytes following renal transplantation, and association with graft-rejection episodes and cytomegalovirus infection. *Transplantation* 37:65-69, 1984.
102. van Rood, J. J., De Vries, R. R. P., and Bradley, B. A. Genetics and biology of the HLA system. In *The Role of the Major Histocompatibility Complex in Immunobiology,* M. E. Dorf, ed. Garland STPM Press, New York, 1984, pp. 59-114.
103. von Willebrand, E. OKT4/8 ratio in the blood and in the graft during episodes of human renal allograft rejection. *Cell Immunol.* 77:196-201, 1983.
104. Williams, K. A., Hart, D. N. J., Fabre, J. W., and Morris, P. J. Distribution and quantitation of HLA-A, B, C and DR(Ia) antigen on human kidney and other tissues. *Transplantation* 29:274-279, 1980.
105. Wood, G. S., and Warnke, R. Suppression of endogenous avidin-binding activity in tissues and its relevance to biotin-avidin detection systems. *J. Histochem. Cytochem.* 29:1196-1204, 1981.

12

ASPIRATION CYTOLOGY IN MONITORING HUMAN ALLOGRAFTS

Pekka J. Häyry and Eeva von Willebrand
University of Helsinki, Helsinki, Finland

Renal transplantation poses several differential diagnostic problems, most of which focus on the graft. A number of attempts have been made to evaluate intragraft events from, for example, blood specimens, but few of these methods of "immunologic monitoring" have proven entirely satisfactory or are at present in general use. Therefore, needle biopsy has remained the only reliable method to assess the graft itself.

Needless to say, the needle biopsy is especially with the recently developed applications to immunohistochemistry, the most useful method to assess the graft. On the other hand, it carries a significant risk of complications and is therefore seldom applied repeatedly. With this difficulty in mind we have developed an alternative approach, which is based on aspiration cytology. In contrast to the needle biopsy, fine needle aspiration biopsies can be performed in, for example, human renal allografts repeatedly, daily if necessary, without any risk to the graft or the graft recipient. Compared with the needle biopsy, the information derived from the fine needle aspiration biopsy is, however, somewhat more limited. The purpose of this overview is to discuss the virtues, vices, and limitations of this new diagnostic method.

TECHNICAL ASPECTS

The approach is not new. Around the year 1000 A.D., the famed Arab physician Abul Casim Chalaf Ben Abbas el-Zahravi, physician-in-ordinary to the great Calif el-Hakim III of Cordoba, performed needle biopsies of the thyroid gland (cited by Merke, Reference 22). In the early 1960s, the Swedish physician Franzen [6] developed fine needle aspiration biopsy to be used as a practical diagnostic tool in urogenital malignancies. The first aspiration biopsies of human renal transplants were performed in 1970 by Pasternack in Helsinki [24]. At that time the cytology of allograft rejection was virtually unknown, and our subsequent studies with Pasternack [8,25] met with significant difficulties in the interpretation of the cytologic specimens. Therefore, a great many basic experiments had to be performed, first with sponge matrix allografts in mice [27] and later with rat and human renal allografts [16,33,36,37], before the cytologic sequence of events in renal allograft rejection became comprehensible. Our present method [10,31] is based on these investigations which have been recently reviewed [7,15,17,23] and will not be described in detail here.

The obtaining and processing of the aspiration biopsy specimen has been described elsewhere [9] and will be summarized here only briefly. The biopsy is performed under aseptic conditions at the bedside without local anesthesia. A 23 or 26 gauge needle (spinal needle, Becton Dickinson, East Rutherford, NJ) is inserted percutaneously into the kidney graft using ultrasound guidance, if necessary. On most occasions the graft is easily located. It is important that the needle samples the kidney cortical region; aspirations performed in the medullary region are nonrepresentative. The stylet is removed, and if no blood appears, a specimen of approximately 10-50 μl in volume is drawn by suction in a syringe with RPMI-1640 tissue culture medium containing 5 ml of 20% human serum albumin, 25,000 U heparin, and 1 ml 1 M Hepes-buffer per liter of medium. A "pistol" fitting a 10-ml or, preferably, a 20-ml syringe (Camecon AB, Täby, Sweden) with approximately 5 ml of medium in it, greatly facilitates the drawing of the specimen. Because of a variable blood contamination rate of the aspiration biopsy specimens, a blood sample of similar size is concomitantly drawn into another syringe from the fingertip. Both the inflammatory and renal parenchymal cells survive in this milieu at refrigerator temperature for at least 40 hr; hence specimens obtained during the weekend, for example, can be processed and analyzed (retrospectively) on Monday and the treatment of a patient corrected if the clinical diagnosis has been wrong.

When obtaining the biopsy, it is important for the needle is to be moved back and forth in its original direction over a distance of 1-1.5 cm. This ascertains that the needle tip hits several inflammatory foci and an "average" picture of inflammation (and other concurrent changes in the graft) is obtained.

Both specimens are processed for cytologic evaluation with a cytocentrifuge (e.g., Shandon-Elliott Cytospin, Camberley, Surrey, U.K.). This method gives an even distribution of the different cell types on the microscope slide. Several slides are made. We usually stain one to three slides with May-Grünwald-Giemsa; alternatively, air-dried specimens may be fixed and evaluated further by applying mono- or polyclonal antibodies and the indirect immunoperoxidase technique. On most occasions the May-Grünwald-Giemsa specimen is informative enough to provide the cytologic diagnosis.

Further information on the specimen may be obtained by using immunocytologic methods. We use mainly the indirect immunoperoxidase assay, as this method makes it possible to simultaneously evaluate the specimen morphologically. Use of antibodies directed to cyclosporin A (CsA) reveals deposits of this drug (or its immunologically cross-reactive by-products) in the renal parenchymal cells [34]. The structure of inflammation may be dissected further by using marker antibodies to the inflammatory cell subsets [32,39]. The origin of inflammatory blast cells, whether of donor or recipient, may be traced both by anti-class I alloantibodies directed to the donor or to the recipient and the *Staphylococcus aureus* Cowan I rosette assay [11]. The expression of the class I and II major histocompatibility (MHC) antigens on the graft vascular endothelial cells, for example, may be analyzed by the same method by using antibodies directed to the backbone or allelic determinants of the respective molecule [12]. Again, the technical details have been dealt with in the original communications and will not be repeated here.

INTERPRETATION OF CYTOLOGY SPECIMENS

In contrast to the needle biopsy, the fine needle aspiration biopsy specimen consists of single cells. Although occasionally the proximal tubular cells may appear in clumps and even whole glomeruli may be seen, the interpretation of the specimen is based on cytologic, not on histologic criteria.

Graft Parenchymal Components

The following types of graft parenchymal cells are seen in the cytologic specimens: whole glomeruli or parts of glomeruli, proximal tubular cells, distal tubular cells, and vascular endothelial cells [Figure 1, (see Color Plate 3) Color Plate section begins following page 252]. In case of doubt in regard to cytologic merphology, the following markers are useful in the identification of the cell types: anti-brush-border antibody for the proximal tubular cells, anti-Tamm-Horsfall antigen antibody for the distal tubular cells [4,5], and antibody to Factor VIII-related antigen(s) for the vascular endothelial cells [18].

Necrotic changes in the graft are reflected by deteriorating graft parenchymal cell morphology, until only necrotic cells are seen in the specimens.

In acute tubular necrosis (ATN), frequently complicating the immediate post-transplantation course, the tubular cells appear swollen and often vacuolized. These changes disappear and the morphology normalizes concomitantly with improving graft function.

Similar but more severe changes are seen in cyclosporin A toxicity. The tubular and vascular endothelial cells are greatly swollen, they often contain amorphic material, and even erythroautophagocytosis is seen. Deposits of CsA are concomitantly observed in the graft tubular cell cytoplasm (see below). Typical cytologic changes of renal allograft parenchymal cells in CsA toxicity are depicted in Figure 2 (see Color Plate 4).

Inflammation

All aspiration biopsies are contaminated with variable amounts of blood. This makes the evaluation of inflammation difficult, especially the quantitation of the inflammatory event. At present we use the following method [Fig. 3 (see Color Plates 4 and 5)] : white cell differential counts are performed separately for the graft and for the peripheral blood specimen. The number of parenchymal cells (per 100 inflammatory white cells) in the fine needle aspiration biopsy specimen is also recorded but with a separate cell counter. After the blood differential is deducted from the aspirate differential, those white cell types present in the graft but absent (or present in lower numbers) from the blood appear as positive values in the remaining "increment"; those present in the blood but absent from the graft appear negative. The following observations indicate that this method, as artificial as it may be, is probably the best available to quantitate the inflammatory events at present: the degree of inflammation in the fine needle aspiration biopsy and the concomitantly obtained needle biopsy are closely correlated [13]. Aspiration biopsies performed at the operation table right before extirpation of a failing allograft bear a close correlation to the cytologic composition of inflammation after enzymatic digestion and staining [13]. Only the relative frequency of macrophages is somewhat reduced in the aspiration specimens compared with the enzymatic dispersates. Finally, in 96 double-aspiration biopsies performed concomitantly to the same allograft, a high degree of correlation (correlation coefficient, 0.956) existed, provided that *both* specimens were representative, that is, contained at least 7 parenchymal cells per 100 inflammatory white cells [35]. Needless to say, the rules for the quantitation of inflammation are not yet final and the calculation of red cell number with electronic methods in the two specimens,

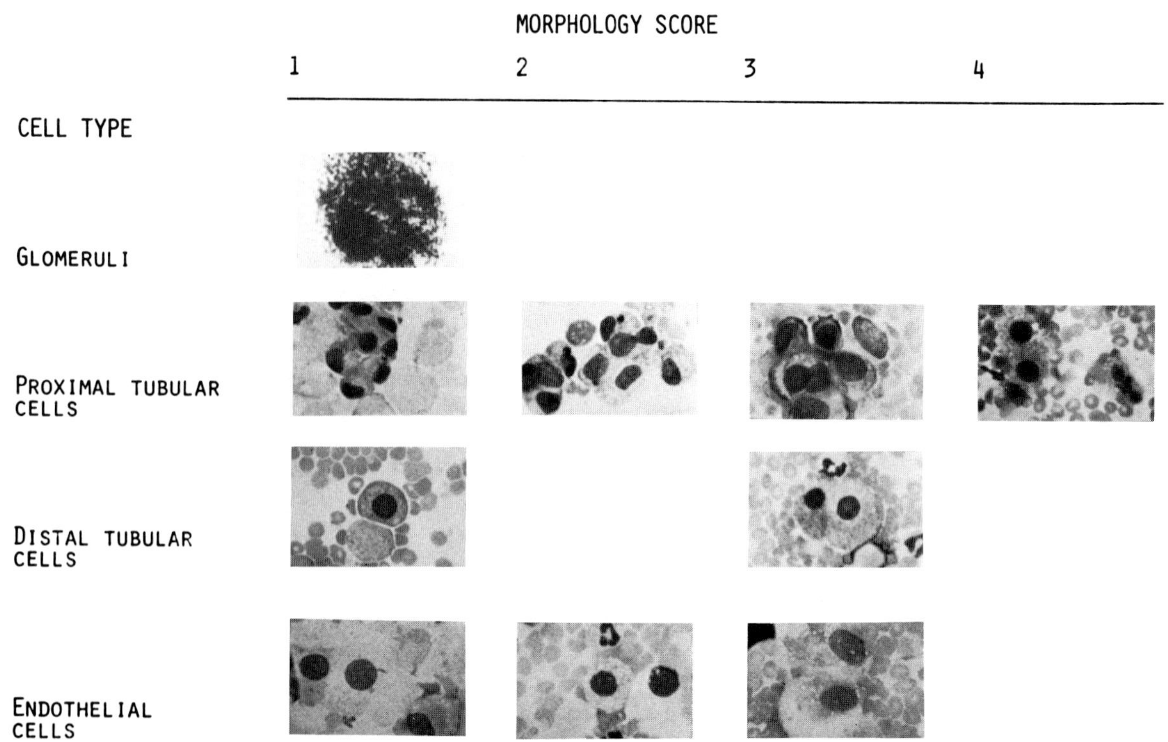

FIGURE 1 Renal parenchymal cells in the aspiration biopsy specimens. The following types of parenchymal cells can be identified: whole glomeruli, proximal tubular cells (displaying in indirect immunofluorescence with anti-brush-border antigen, not shown), distal tubular cells (displaying the Tamm-Horsfall antigen, not shown), and vascular endothelial cells (displaying the Factor VIII-associated antigens, not shown). Typical examples of parenchymal cells with pathologic morphology are also shown. Morphology score from 1 (normal) through 4 (necrotic cells) is indicated in the top. See also Color Plate 3.

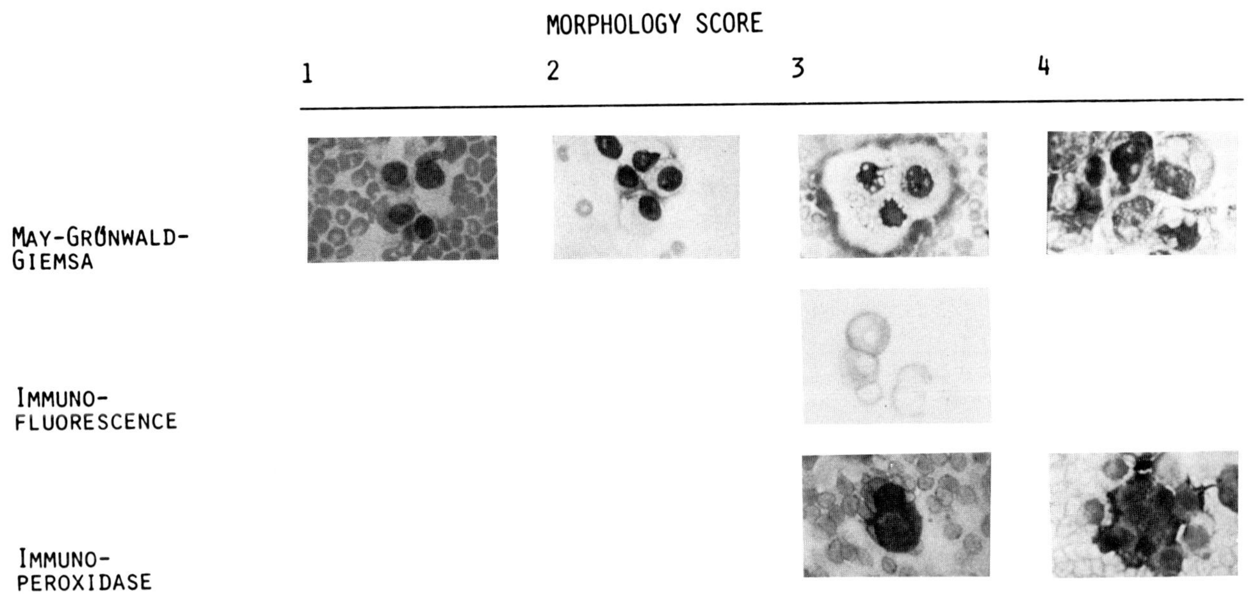

FIGURE 2 Morphologic alterations in renal parenchymal cells in cyclosporine nephrotoxicity. These changes are best identified by May-Grünwald-Giemsa staining (top). Cyclosporine deposits may be demonstrated by immunofluorescence and immunoperoxidase methods. Morphology score from 1 through 4 on the top. See also Color Plate 4.

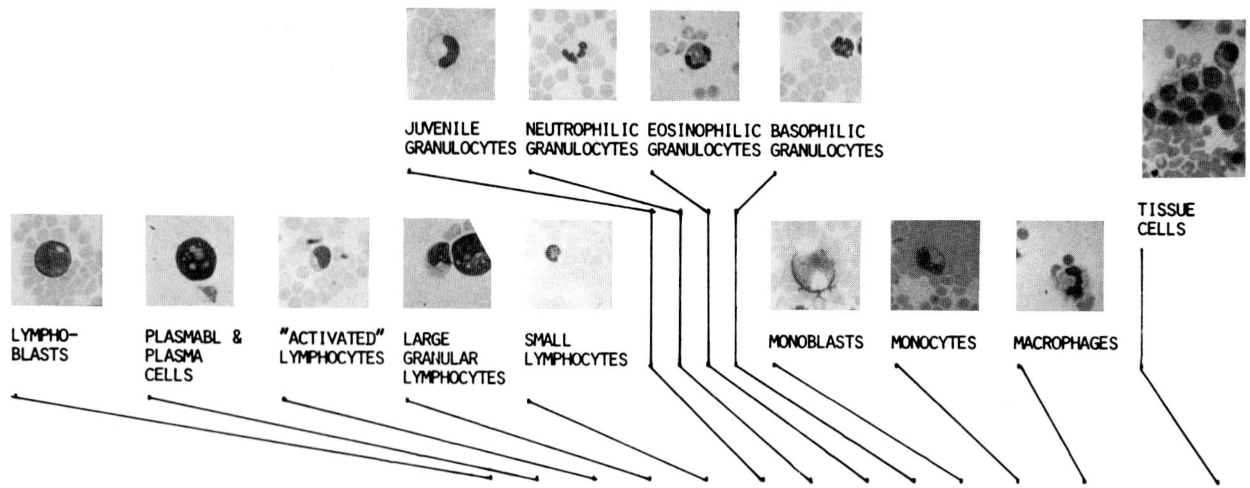

		LB	PB &PC	ALY	LGL	sLY	Juv	Neu	Eos	Bas	MBL	Mo	MP	TCI	TC
	FNAB DIFFERENTIAL (%)	4	8	4	4	31	1	20	20	1	1	15	1		15
(MINUS)	BLOOD DIFFERENTIAL (%)	0	1	1	1	5	2	68	9	2	0	10	0		
(IS)	"INCREMENT"	4	7	3	3	26	-1	-48	-1	-1	1	5	1		
(TIMES)	"CORRECTION FACTOR"	(1)	(1)	(.5)	(.2)	(.1)					(1)	(.2)	(1)		
(IS)	"CORRECTED INCREMENT"	4	7	1.5	0.6	2.6					1	1	1	<u>18.7</u>	

REPRESENTATIVITY: TC $\gtrsim$ 7
INFLAMMATION TCI $\gtrsim$ 2.5

FIGURE 3 Quantitation of inflammation. Currently the following types of inflammatory (white) cells may be recorded in May-Grünwald-Giemsa–stained specimens: lymphoblasts, plasmablasts and plasma cells, "activated" lymphocytes, large granular lymphocytes, and small lymphocytes; juvenile, neutrophilic, eosinophilic, and basophilic granulocytes; and monoblasts, monocytes, and tissue macrophages. See also Color Plates 4 and 5.

for example, as suggested by Hammer [20], may provide a better approach for the evaluation of the blood contamination rate in the future.

The following inflammatory cell types may be recorded in May-Grünwald-Giemsa-stained specimens: lymphoblasts (representing primarily T-blast cells), plasmablasts (representing primarily B-blast cells), plasma cells at different levels of maturation, "activated" lymphocytes, large granular lymphocytes (LGL), which include the natural killer (NK) cell population [28], small lymphocytes, different types of granulocytes, early monoblasts, monocytes, and tissue macrophages in different stages of morphologic maturation (Figure 3).

The functions of different inflammatory cell types in graft rejection, in combination with antibodies, is still incompletely understood. When comparing experimental rat renal allografts to autografts, the cell types most characteristic to the allograft inflammatory infiltrate are the different types of blast cells and mature tissue macrophages [17]. Therefore, in calculating the corrected increment (see above), different impact values have been assigned to these cell types according to their participation in experimental allograft rejection: lymphoblasts, plasmablasts, monoblasts, and mature macrophages have a full impact value of 1.0. The number of activated lymphocytes, LGL, and monocytes is multiplied by 0.2, that of lymphocytes by 0.1. Polymorphonuclear phagocytes are not an important component of inflammation before necrotic changes appear in the graft; hence their impact value is also 0.1. The sum of the "corrected" increment values represents "total corrected increment," that is, the degree of inflammation (Figure 3). Again, the system applied at present is probably not the best possible or only method to quantitate inflammation. However, this method makes it possible to compare the results from different laboratories more readily than a simple verbal description of the findings.

All transplants display a certain amount of inflammation in the cytologic specimens. This inflammation consists primarily of lymphocytes and monocytes with a notable absence of any blastogenic component or mature macrophages. In azathioprine and methylprednisolone immunosuppressed recipients, this inflammation subsides within days or weeks, unless signs of rejection appear. In CsA-immunosuppressed recipients the degree of inflammation is usually higher and persists longer, even for months after transplantation.

In approximately 80% of cases, acute rejection follows a distinct, relatively reproducible cytologic pattern: the number of monocytes and lymphocytes increases in the graft and a distinct blastogenic response, consisting of lymphoblasts (a minority), plasmablasts (a majority), and plasma cells, is observed in situ [10]. On most occasions the inflammation subsides and blast cells disappear from the graft, concomitantly with intensified anti-inflammatory therapy with steroids. In some cases, however, the number of blast cells increases, still more lymphocytes are seen in the fine needle aspiration biopsy, and a rapid maturation of blood-borne monocytes into tissue macrophages is the most prominent hallmark of prolonged and irreversible rejection.

In individual patients the inflammatory event(s) may, however, follow many different patterns, or "profiles" (Figure 4). On some occasions, only one short peak of inflammation is observed with minimal clinical signs. On other occasions, the inflammation may mount slowly and precede the appearance of clinical signs by 1 or 2 days. In still other cases, the inflammation may persist for several days or even weeks with frequent exacerbations and remissions and (usually) with a distinct reflection to the clinical behavior [11].

Reviewing the more than 5000 aspiration biopsies performed in our transplant recipients up to the present time, it has become obvious that qualitatively different patterns of inflammation also exist. In CsA-immunosuppressed patients, the early inflammatory

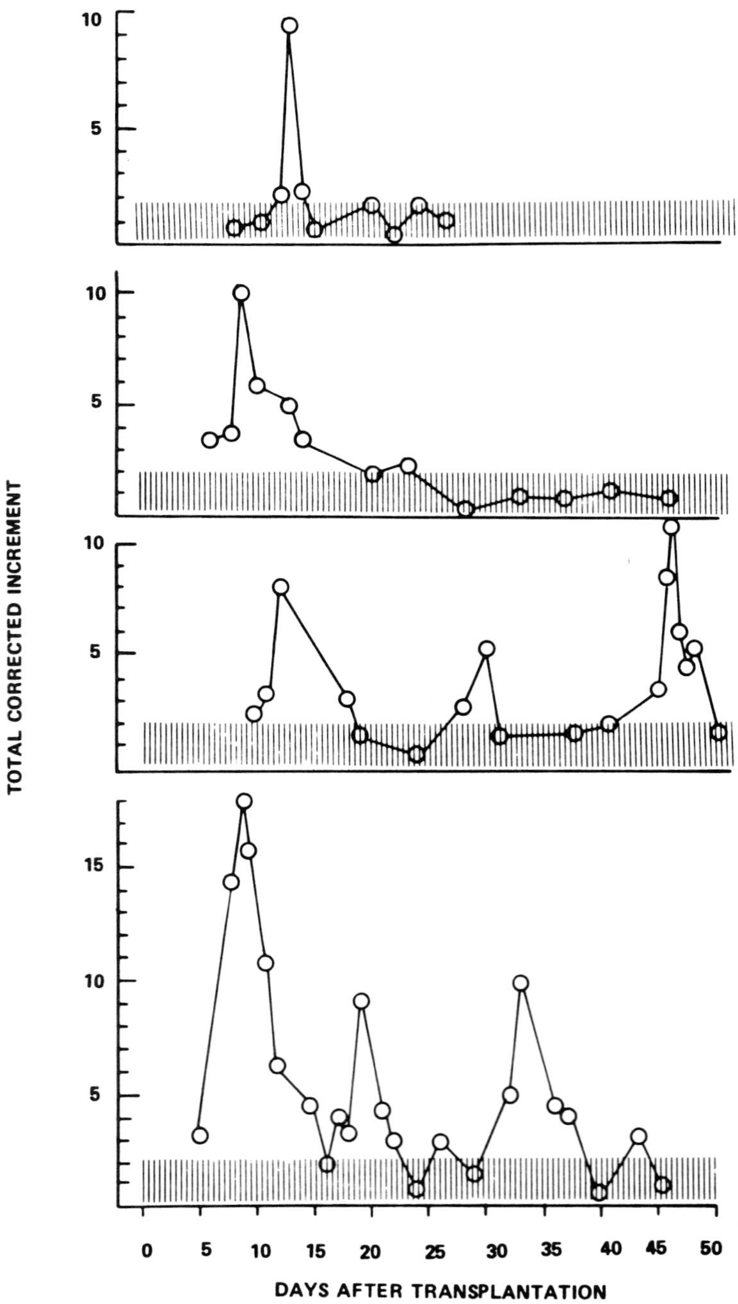

FIGURE 4 Different profiles of inflammation. The course of four different patients are represented. Shaded areas represent the background inflammation seen in clinically well-to-do grafts (±SD). (Reprinted through the courtesy of Excerpta Medica, Amsterdam-Oxford-Princeton: *Transplantation and Clinical Immunology,* Vol. 15.)

events may be dominated by a high frequency of early monoblasts, whereas in aspirates observed 1-6 months after transplantation or later, the blast cell component may be very small or even absent, with a cytologic pattern dominated by lymphocytes and mononuclear phagocytes.

Correlations with Histology

Histologic analysis of needle biopsies has demonstrated two major types of rejection, cellular rejection and vascular rejection. Cellular rejection is characterized by the appearance of inflammatory white cells, first around the blood vessels and later throughout the graft. The most prominent hallmark of vascular rejection is intimal proliferation and gradual "onion skinning" and obliteration of the graft arteries. Needless to say, most rejection episodes are combinations of these two types, perhaps with dominance of one or the other.

There is good evidence indicating that acute blastogenic inflammation corresponds to cellular rejection [19,30]. When fine needle aspiration biopsy are concomitantly performed on the same allograft, the inflammatory pattern with an infiltrate dominated by blast cells is compatible with cellular infiltrates of variable intensity in the allograft. There is also some experience, deriving primarily from Nottingham [3], that late inflammatory patterns dominated by lymphocytes and mononuclear phagocytes without any clear blastogenic component are more compatible with the vascular pattern of rejection. However, it should be stressed that at present only cellular rejections can be detected by the fine needle aspiration biopsy; the vascular pattern of rejection is much more difficult to evaluate and, needless to say, it is impossible to evaluate the degree of vascular damage from the fine needle specimen only. This always requires needle biopsy and histologic confirmation.

Immunocytologic Analysis of the FNAB Specimens

Further information on the intragraft events may be obtained by applying immunocytologic methods to the specimens. We have usually employed the indirect peroxidase-antiperoxidase technique, which gives good cytologic morphology, thus facilitating the evaluation of the specimen far better than immunofluorescence methods.

In cases of CsA nephrotoxicity, deposits of CsA (or immunologically cross-reactive by-products) may be demonstrated in the graft tubular cells by sheep anti-CsA antiserum (the standard antiserum for the Sandoz RIA kit). The degree of these deposits roughly correlates to the degree of morphologic changes in the May-Grunwald-Giemsa-stained specimens (Figure 2). Reduced administration of CsA, or transfer of the patient to azathioprine, is invariably followed by disappearance of these deposits from the allograft. The morphologic changes take a longer time to normalize [34].

If the cytologic specimen is treated with monoclonal anti-class I or II antibody before cytocentrifugation, washed, and *S. aureus* Cowan I bacteria are added, bacterial particles (due to their high contents of protein A) make rosettes with the antibody-binding cells [14]. After May-Grünwald-Giemsa staining, the rosette-forming cell type(s) may be evaluated on a morphologic basis. Human renal vascular endothelial cells, in particular the endothelial cells of glomeruli and the intertubular capillaries, usually display a high content of class II antigens in such cytologic specimens [14,26]. This is in striking contrast to rat renal vascular endothelial cells, for example, which are practically devoid of these antigens [36]. According to our fairly limited experience [12], the class

TABLE 1 Tracing the Origin of Inflammatory Cells by anti-HLA (AB) Alloantibody and Staphylococci

Biopsy no.	Inflammation (TCI)[a]	Antibody	Reactivity of inflammatory blast cells (%)[b] LB	PB	LY
1337	7.9	Anti-donor	5	50	40
		Anti-recipient	40	0	30
		Irrelevant	0	0	0
336	3.8	Anti-donor	70	70	70
		Irrelevant	0	0	0

[a]Total corrected increment units.
[b]Percentage of cells of a given type reactive with indicated antisera in *S. aureus* Cowan I rosette assay.
Source: Reprinted through the courtesy of Excerpta Medica, Amsterdam-Oxford-Princeton, *Transplantation and Clinical Immunology,* Vol. 15.

II antigens cannot be detected with this method in "well-to-do" (well-functioning) renal allografts, whereas most failing allografts with variable amounts of inflammation display the class II antigens on the endothelial cell surface. Postoperative administration of steroids is a likely candidate for the down-regulation of class II expression. It would be tempting to speculate that re-expression of class II antigens has induced rejection; however, the possibility that class II antigens have been exposed or induced as a consequence of inflammation is equally likely [21,29].

The structure of inflammation may also be analyzed further by using the aforementioned immunologic assays. The origin of inflammatory blast cells, whether of donor or recipient, may be investigated by using the *Staphylococcus* assay and alloantibodies directed to the class I antigens. In most rejections, all or the majority of the allograft-infiltrating inflammatory blast cells in the graft derive from the graft recipient (Table 1). Exceptions, however, exist: on some occasions a fair number of blast cells carry the HLA phenotype of the graft donor, or most of the blast cells are donor derived. These occasions resemble a bidirectional mixed lymphocyte culture (MLC) and apparently represent a local graft-versus-host (GVH) reaction in situ. In the absence of a systematic analysis of the fine needle aspiration biopsies in this respect, we have no idea how frequent is this inflammatory pattern of local GVH reaction.

The inflammatory event may be dissected further by using monoclonal marker antibodies directed toward the different inflammatory cell subtypes in the graft [2,32]. This approach, in combination with the peroxidase-antiperoxidase technique, enables the differentiation of T cells, B cells, the major subsets of T cells, and cells of the mononuclear phagocyte lineage in different stages of maturation. In most acute blastogenic rejections, the lymphoid cell compartment of the inflammatory population is heavily dominated by lymphoid T cells, the majority of which represent the T-suppressor/killer phenotype. However, on other occasions the T-helper subset may dominate [38]. According to our experience, the latter pattern of inflammation has a worse prognosis; however, this is not a final conclusion and must be confirmed with a larger series of patients.

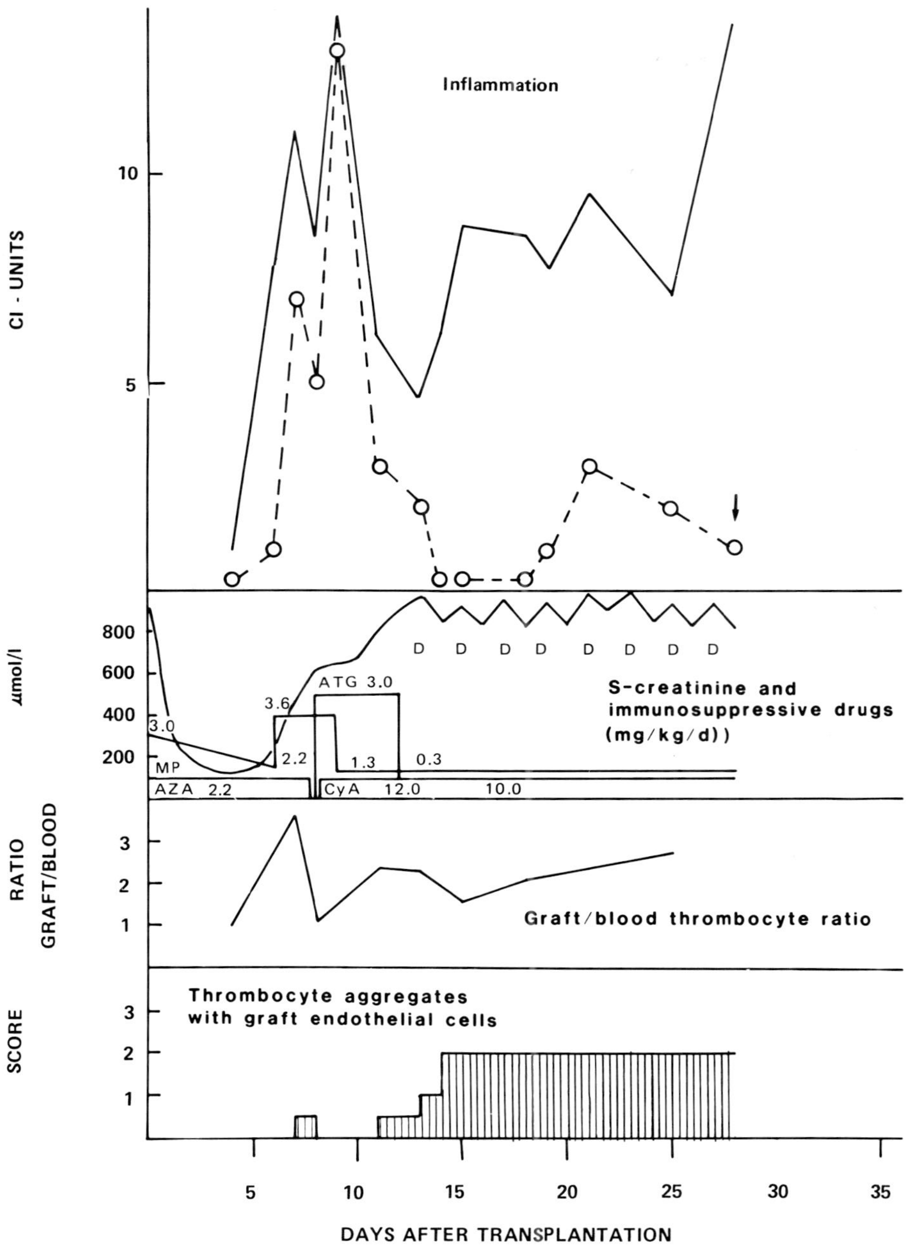

FIGURE 5 Entrapment of thrombocytes in a rejecting allograft during irreversible rejection. Top: inflammation in corrected increment units. Solid line, total inflammation; open circles and dashed line, blast cells. Second section: serum creatinine, postoperative dialysis treatment (D), and medication (mg/kg per day). Third section: graft/blood thrombocyte ratio analyzed by the FMC27 monoclonal antibody. Bottom: aggregates of thrombocytes with graft endothelial cells, scored from 1 through 3. (Reprinted through the courtesy of The Williams & Wilkins Co., Baltimore; *Transplantation 1984.*)

The final bone marrow-derived cell population intimately involved in allograft rejection is the platelet or thrombocyte. Thrombocytes are difficult to visualize in ordinary May-Grünwald-Giemsa-stained smears; they can be properly identified by combining monoclonal anti-thrombocyte antibody and the immunoperoxidase assay [38]. According to our recent experience (unpublished), "loose" thrombocyte aggregates, often in combination with granulocytes, are nearly invariably seen in renal allografts with acute rejection. The cytologic appearance of thrombocytes in the fine needle aspiration biopsy entirely overlaps with the entrapment of indium-111-labeled thrombocytes into the graft in the γ-camera assay (Figure 5). When the rejection is successfully treated, thrombocytes disappear from the transplant. In prolonged and irreversible rejection, increasing numbers of thrombocytes are observed in close association with and/or agglutinated on the graft endothelial cells. We now believe that the entrapment of thrombocytes in a rejecting allograft is a two-stage phenomenon where the second stage—thrombocyte-endothelial cell aggregate—indicates a prolonged course of rejection and an unfavorable outcome [38].

Monitoring Individual Patients with the Fine Needle Aspiration Biopsy

The great power of the technique is that it can be performed daily and, if necessary, even more often. This gives the investigator a chance to visualize the dynamic picture of rejection. Concomitant monitoring of the onset, size, type, and duration of the inflammatory episodes and morphologic changes in the graft tubular cells makes it possible to diagnose the onset, intensity, and duration of inflammation and—what is most important—the impact of immunosuppressive and anti-inflammatory therapy on the inflammatory events and on the graft. If the inflammatory cells disappear from the aspirates during intensified anti-inflammatory therapy, the therapy is obviously successful. If inflammation proceeds or increases in intensity and, in particular, if a concomitant gradual deterioration of the graft parenchymal cell morphology is observed, a diagnosis of prolonged and irreversible rejection is justified. Therefore, a change in the immunosuppressive regimen is warranted [1].

Aspiration Cytology as a Differential Diagnostic Tool

On most occasions acute rejection is easily diagnosed, provided that the renal allograft has a good initial function. If, however, the immediate postoperative course is complicated by prolonged acute tubular necrosis, the diagnosis of rejection may be more difficult to establish. In these cases, frequent aspiration biopsies make it possible to evaluate the onset of inflammation and to treat impending rejection guided only by the cytological specimens.

Cyclosporin A nephrotoxicity may further complicate the postoperative course. The differential diagnosis of CsA toxicity, rejection, ATN, or any of the combinations thereof, is possible to make with the fine needle aspiration biopsy (Table 2). If distinct parenchymal cell changes are present in the graft (and the graft does not function), the likely diagnosis is ATN. If inflammation is superimposed, rejection has occurred. If marked parenchymal cell changes appear in combination with CsA deposits in the graft, a plausible diagnosis is CsA nephrotoxicity. If inflammation is present in the graft together with concomitant CsA deposits and parenchymal cell changes, the therapeutic

TABLE 2 Differential Diagnosis Between Cyclosporine Nephrotoxicity and Other Reasons for Renal Transplant Failure by Fine Needle Aspiration Biopsy

	Fine needle aspiration biopsy			
S-Creatinine	Inflammation	Tubular cell changes	CsA deposits in graft	Explanation
Normal	–	+	±	Well-to-do graft
Elevated	–	++	–	ATN
Elevated	–[a]	+++	+++	CsA toxicity
Elevated	+++	+	–	Rejection
Elevated	+++	+++	+++	Rejection and CsA toxicity

[a]The possibility that CsA deposits occasionally induce some inflammation, is not entirely excluded.
Source: Reprinted through the courtesy of *Transplantation Proceedings,* Stony Brook, New York, 1983.

margin of this therapeutic regimen is obviously too small and a change in the immunosuppressive regimen is warranted [11].

CONCLUDING REMARKS

The great power of aspiration cytology lies in the ability to perform frequent biopsies of a single allograft. Currently, we biopsy all of our patients routinely every second day. This makes it possible to construct the picture of rejection as a dynamic process, with the onset and decline of inflammation and concomitant changes in the graft parenchymal component, and to analyze the impact of immunosuppressive and anti-inflammatory treatment on these components of rejection. The main drawback of the method is that information deriving from the fine needle aspiration biopsy specimen is limited: acute cell-mediated rejection may be diagnosed with certainty, vascular rejection is far more difficult to visualize, and it is impossible to evaluate the degree of vascular damage in the graft without a needle biopsy. Therefore, these two approaches are not mutually exclusive but should be applied concomitantly. As Hammer states, the needle biopsy gives a comprehensive and complete picture of rejection at the moment when it is performed; the fine needle aspiration biopsy makes it possible to evaluate whether the bicycle rider is moving forward or backward.

At the level of the individual patient, the fine needle approach is most useful in the evaluation of transplants with initial ATN and nonfunction. In such cases, we determine our immunosuppressive and anti-inflammatory treatment solely on the basis of the cytologic specimens.

The major difficulty of the cytologic approach is that even experienced pathologists are not often familiar with the inflammatory cell cytology of renal aspirates. We have found it useful for centers desiring to adopt this method to be trained in an experienced center already familiar with this approach. At present, several "experienced" transplant centers exist. They include, in addition to our own laboratory, the Department of Pathology, Hôpital Necker, Paris (Dr. Dominique Droz), Division of Nephrology, Ospedale Maggiore, Milan (Dr. Francesca Egidi), and Department of Experimental Surgery, Ludwig-

Maximilian University, Munich (Dr. Claus Hammer), to mention a few. Usually a 1-week training course has been sufficient for an experienced pathologist to establish this method.

Another obvious difficulty is that the method is not complete but requires still further modifications. Currently, the amount of information on the mechanics of graft rejection is rapidly growing and the inflammatory events occurring inside the allograft during rejection become easier to interpret. This necessitates continuous re-evaluation and remodification of the fine needle aspiration biopsy approach. It is also obligatory to have frequent contacts between the participating centers, and workshops on this method are now being organized every second year. Furthermore, it is mandatory to establish that all different centers using this method use the same cytologic criteria. This means international quality control analysis among the participating centers. One such analysis, with 32 different centers from Europe, Canada, Africa, and Australia participating, is currently underway.

ACKNOWLEDGMENTS

The authors wish to thank the personnel of the Department IV of Surgery and the Transplantation Laboratory, University of Helsinki, for their effort in the designing of this method. The secretarial help of Ms. Leena Saraste is gratefully acknowledged. The original work where this review is based upon has been financed by grants from the Sigrid Juselius Foundation, Finnish Academy of Sciences, the Association of Finnish Life Insurance Companies, Helsinki, Finland, and by grants 26882-01 through -06 and 31730-01 through -03 from the National Institutes of Health, Bethesda, Maryland.

REFERENCES

1. Ahonen, J. Clinical use of FNAB in renal transplantation. In *Renal Transplant Cytology* (Proc. 2nd Intern. Workshop), H. Kreis and D. Droz, eds. Wichtig Editore, Milan, 1984, pp. 31-38.
2. Bolton, E. M., Thompson, J. F., Wood, R. F. M., and Morris, P. J. Lymphocyte subpopulations in fine needle aspiration biopsies determined by immunoperoxidase staining. In *Renal Transplant Cytology* (Proc. 2nd Intern. Workshop), H. Kreis and D. Droz, eds. Wichtig Editore, Milan, 1984, pp. 207-210.
3. Cooksey, G., Reeve, R. S., Wenham, P. W., Cotton, R. E., and Blamey, R. W. Comparison of fine needle aspiration cytology with histology in the diagnosis of renal allograft rejection. In *Renal Transplant Cytology* (Proc. 2nd Intern. Workshop), H. Kreis and D. Droz, eds. Wichtig Editore, Milan, 1984, pp. 73-80.
4. Ekblom, P., Miettinen, A., and Saxen, L. Induction of brush border antigens of the proximal tubule of the developing kidney. *Dev. Biol.* 74:263-274, 1980.
5. Ekblom, P., Miettinen, A., Virtanen, I., Wahlström, T., Dawnay, A., and Saxen, L. In vitro segregation of the metanephric nephron. *Dev. Biol.* 84:88-95, 1981.
6. Franzén, S., Giertz, G., and Zaijcek, J. Cytological diagnosis of prostatic tumours by transrectal aspiration biopsy. *Br. J. Urol.* 32:193, 1960.
7. Häyry, P. Intra-graft events in allograft destruction. *Transplantation* 38:1, 1984.
8. Häyry, P., Lindström, B. L., Birolainen, M., Pasternack, A., and Lindfors, O. Immunobiological diagnosis of rejection in dogs with renal allografts. *Surgery* 71:494, 1972.
9. Häyry, P., and von Willebrand, E. Practical guidelines for fine needle aspiration biopsy of human renal allografts. *Ann. Clin. Res.* 13:288, 1981.

10. Häyry, P., and von Willebrand, E. Monitoring of human renal allograft rejection with fine needle aspiration cytology. *Scand. J. Immunol.* 13:87, 1981.
11. Häyry, P., and von Willebrand, E. Transplant aspiration cytology in the evaluation of a renal allograft. Proc. 15th International Course on Transplantation and Clinical Immunology. Excerpta Medica, Amsterdam, 1984.
12. Häyry, P., von Willebrand, E., Ahonen, J., and Eklund, B. Do well-to-do and repeatedly rejecting renal allografts express the transplantation antigens similarly on their surface? *Scand. J. Urol. Nephrol.* (*Suppl.*) 64:52, 1981.
13. Häyry, P., von Willebrand, E., Ahonen, J., Eklund, B., and Lautenschlager, I. Monitoring of organ allograft rejection by transplant aspiration cytology. *Ann. Clin. Res.* 13: 264, 1981.
14. Häyry, P., von Willebrand, E., and Andersson, L. C. Expression of HLA-ABC and DR locus antigens on human kidney endothelial, tubular and glomerular cells. *Scand. J. Immunol.* 11:303, 1980.
15. Häyry, P., von Willebrand, E., Parthenais, E., Nemlander, A., Soots, A., Lautenschlager, I., Alfödly, P., and Renkonen, R. The inflammatory mechanisms of allograft rejection. *Immunol. Rev.* 77:85-142, 1984.
16. Häyry, P., von Willebrand, E., and Soots, A. In situ effector mechanisms in rat kidney allograft rejection. III. Kinetics of the inflammatory response and generation of donor-directed killer cells. *Scand. J. Immunol.* 10:95, 1979.
17. Häyry, P., von Willebrand, E., Parthenais, E., Nemlander, A., Soots, A., Lautenschlager, I., Alföldy, P., and Renkonen, R. The inflammatory mechanisms of allograft rejection. *Immunol. Rev.* 77:85, 1984.
18. Jaffe, E. A. Endothelial cells and the biology of Factor VIII. *N. Engl. J. Med.* 296: 377-383, 1977.
19. Koller, C., Hammer, C., Gokel, J. M., Land, W., Hillebrand, D., Castro, L. A., Stadler, J., and Weber, B. Correlation between core biopsy and aspiration cytology. *Transplant. Proc.* xvi:1298, 1984.
20. Koller, C., Stadler, J., Hammer, C., Schneider, B., Land, W., and Brendel, W. Evaluation of FNAB and TAC by coulter counting. In *Renal Transplant Cytology* (Proc. 2nd Intern. Workshop), H. Kreis and D. Droz, eds. Wichtig Editore, Milan, 1984, pp. 39-44.
21. Krombach, F., Gebhard, F., Scholz, S., Danko, I., and Hammer, C. Expression of major histocompatibility antigens in kidney xenografts under cyclosporin A treatment. In *RenalTransplant Cytology* (Proc. 2nd Intern. Workshop), H. Kreis and D. Droz, eds. Wichtig Editore, Milan, 1984, pp. 181-188.
22. Merke, F. Geschichte und Ikonographie des Endemischen Kropfes und Kretinismus. Verlag Hans Huber, Bern, 1971, p. 109.
23. Möller, G. (ed.). Intragraft rejection mechanisms. *Immunol. Rev.* 77, 1984.
24. Pasternack, A. Fine-needle aspiration biopsy of human renal homografts. *Lancet* 2:82, 1968.
25. Pasternack, A., Virolainen, M., and Häyry, P. Fine needle aspiration biopsy in the diagnosis of human renal allograft rejection. *J. Urol.* 109:167, 1973.
26. Paul, L. C., van Es, L. A., and Baldwin, W. M., III. Antigens in human renal allografts. *Clin. Immunol. Immunopathol.* 19:206, 1981.
27. Roberts, P. J., and Häyry, P. Effector mechanisms in allograft rejection. I. Assembly of "sponge matrix" allografts. *Cell. Immunol.* 26:160, 1976.
28. Saksela, E., Timonen, T., Ranki, A., and Häyry, P. Morphological and functional characterization of isolated effector cells responsible for human natural killer activity to fetal fibroblasts and to cultured cell line targets. *Immunol. Rev.* 44:71, 1979.
29. de Wall, R. M. W., Bogman, M. J. J., Maass, C. N., Cornelissen, L. M. H., Tax, W. J. M., and Koene, R. A. P. Variable expression of Ia antigens on the vascular endothelium of mouse skin allografts. *Nature* 303:426, 1983.

30. De Vecchi, A., Egidi, F., Banfi, G., Imbasciati, E., Tarantino, A., and Ponticelli, G. Comparison of fine needle aspiration biopsy and needle biopsy in renal transplantation. In *Renal Transplant Cytology* (Proc. 2nd Intern. Workshop), H. Kreis and D. Droz, eds. Wichtig Editore, Milan, 1984, pp. 67-72.
31. von Willebrand, E. Fine needle aspiration cytology of human renal transplants. *Clin. Immunol. Immunopathol.* 17:309, 1980.
32. von Willebrand, E. OKT4/8 ratio in the blood and in the graft during episodes of human allograft rejection. *Cell.Immunol.* 77:196, 1983.
33. von Willebrand, E., and Häyry, P. Composition and in vitro cytotoxicity of cellular infiltrates in rejecting human kidney allografts. *Cell. Immunol.* 41:358, 1978.
34. von Willebrand, E., and Häyry, P. Cyclosporin A deposits in renal allografts. *Lancet* 2:189, 1983.
35. von Willebrand, E., and Häyry, P. Reproducibility of the fine needle aspiration biopsy. Analysis of 93 double biopsies. *Transplantation* 38:314, 1984.
36. von Willebrand, E., Parthenais, E., and Häyry, P. Expression of the major AgB histocompatibility complex antigens on different structural components of rat kidney and heart. *Cell. Immunol.* 52:313, 1980.
37. von Willebrand, E., Soots, A., and Häyry, P. In situ effector mechanisms in rat kidney allograft rejection. I. Characterization of host cellular infiltrate in rejecting allograft parenchyma. *Cell. Immunol.* 46:309, 1979.
38. von Willebrand, E., Zola, H., and Häyry, P. Thrombocyte aggregates in renal allografts. Analysis by the fine needle aspiration biopsy and monoclonal anti-thrombocyte antibodies. *Transplantation* 39:258, 1985.
39. Wood, R. F. M., Bolton, E. M., Thompson, J. F., and Morris, P. J. Monoclonal antibodies and fine needle aspiration cytology in detecting renal allograft rejection. *Lancet* 2:278, 1982.

13

MONITORING THE COMPONENTS OF THE IMMUNE SYSTEM

William J. Smith
The Johns Hopkins University School of Medicine, Baltimore, Maryland

Renal transplantation has been the focus of immunologic studies for more than 20 years, and yet questions remain about the mechanisms of graft rejection, optimal methods of immunosuppression, and differential diagnosis of renal failure episodes. Analysis of the immune components active in the allograft response holds the promise of providing the clinician with much of the necessary information on which to base clinical decisions in the management of transplant recipients. Unfortunately this promise has not as yet been fulfilled.

One of the most obvious impediments to our full understanding of the allograft response is the extreme complexity of the immune response networks. Definition of the interactions between lymphoid and nonlymphoid cells and their mutual interaction with humoral factors is still in the investigative stage. Our understanding of the nature and function of the T-cell receptor and the family of biologic response modifiers has only recently reached the formulative stage. Although blaming much of our lack of progress in transplant immunology on the immune networks, investigators in the field must share in the responsibility due to years of failing to establish uniform techniques and terminology and thereby leaving much data unsubstantiated. Fortunately, since 1979, many of these interlaboratory differences have been addressed through the convening of four international symposia on immunologic monitoring of the transplant recipient.

Many laboratories active in renal transplantation immunology are engaged in research involving the matching of donor and recipient, defining immunobiologic mechanisms active in the allograft recipient, assessing the efficacy of immunosuppressive therapy regimens, and profiling the immune status of the recipients. At first glance it would appear that no single laboratory is capable of following so many research directions, yet, although that may be true in some cases, all these goals are tied to one common denominator—understanding the role of the components of the immune response active in the regulation or effector functions of the allograft response. Efforts in these directions have generated volumes of data well beyond the scope of this review. Since other chapters in this volume discuss the cellular and humoral mechanisms of rejection and immune regulation, the clinical management of rejection and the use of biopsy and fine needle aspiration cytology for defining intragraft events, this chapter will focus on the application of peripheral blood analysis of cellular and humoral components that define the occurrence of active or impending rejection events and more specifically on those procedures that can be employed with sufficient frequency to provide a clinically useful adjunct to the management of renal allograft recipients.

METHODOLOGIES EMPLOYED IN IMMUNOLOGIC MONITORING

The assay systems employed in transplantation immunology are, for the most part, common to the general field of immunobiology. These systems can be broadly grouped into assays of humoral, blastogenic, cytotoxic, or suppressor functions or phenotypic analysis of cell surface determinants. Recent reviews have addressed many of the problems of the cellular functional assays [28,52,125] and phenotypic analysis [69,101]. In this chapter I will describe the techniques, terminology, and peculiarities that affect their use in transplantation immunology.

Blastogenic Assays

The mixed lymphocyte reaction (MLR), used principally in pretransplant studies, is frequently employed posttransplant to assess the development of anti-donor or broad-based cellular reactivity.

Several laboratories routinely monitor the ability of peripheral blood leukocytes (PBL) to evidence blastogenic reactivity in vitro following stimulation with mitogens or soluble antigens. The blastogenic activity is usually measured by the incorporation of radiolabeled DNA precursors or more recently by measurement of protein synthesis kinetics by uptake of radiolabeled amino acids. It is assumed that alteration of the blastic responses will accompany in vivo increases in cellular activity caused by allogeneic stimulation. In much the same vein, it has been known since the early 1970s that circulating lymphocytes from allograft recipients have increased blastic activities in the absence of in vitro stimulation [56]. This spontaneous blastogenesis (SB) is employed by several laboratories for routine monitoring.

Many of the blastogenic procedures have attained routine utilization in most immunology laboratories, but their application to transplantation involves a unique set of problems which must be addressed. First, the patients providing the cells for analysis are being treated with a variety of immunosuppressive drugs that, by their very nature, interfere with normal immunocyte function. Types and schedules of drugs taken must be included in the day-to-day evaluation of patient responses and can seriously interfere with analysis of a large group of patients. Second, most laboratories use simple well-defined procedures for the isolation of the assay cells without considering the nature of the isolates from immunosuppressed patients. Our laboratory and others have reported on the problem of nonlymphoid contamination of presumed lymphocyte preparations obtained through bouyant density centrifugation of peripheral blood of allograft recipients [18,112]. Changes in the standard procedures employed in normal subjects may be necessary when attempting to evaluate cellular immune functions in these patients.

Cytotoxic and Suppressor Assays

While providing more direct assessments of the functional capacities of the recipient's immune system, cytotoxic and suppressor assays are subject to technical difficulties and interpretive complexities that have given rise to confusion. Only those laboratories well established in these procedures have been able to approach even the most basic of correlations between in vitro tests and clinical events.

Whereas the blastogenic assays provide a means to demonstrate activation events of recipient cells, primarily lymphocytes, the functional assays can be used to evaluate either cellular or humoral capabilities. Cytotoxic antibodies are usually defined through the complement-dependent cytotoxicity assay using vital staining of the target cells to assess killing. Recent studies attempting to define the significance of anti-donor antibodies have shown that many of these antibodies react weakly and are often missed in the standard microcytotoxicity test. In these cases, it is best to use chromium-51 labeling of target cells for maximum sensitivity [26].

A second type of antibody test that may be of significance to the transplant immunologist is the assay for antibodies that mediate the destruction of donor tissue by killer (K) cells. This reactivity, known as antibody-dependent cellular cytotoxicity (ADCC), is a source of terminologic difficulty that may result in the misinterpretation of data. The antibody active in this system should be referred to as lymphocyte-dependent antibody (LDA), and the assay involves ^{51}Cr-labeled target cells bearing major histocompatibility (MHC) antigens of the donor incubated with sera containing the presumed LDA and exposed to peripheral blood leukocytes from normal control individuals. Measurement of LDA activity is determined by ^{51}Cr release. Use of the ADCC assay to measure K-cell activity will be discussed below.

Tests of humoral cytotoxicity are for the most part free of interfering substances that alter the results. Certainly, patient serum samples may contain substances, either contributed by the clinical condition of the patient or as by-product of the patient's therapy, that can be cytotoxic to target cells. Fortunately, since most of the incubations with patient sera are of short duration and controlled for within the assay, interpretation of this type of test is usually straightforward.

Assays of cellular function are technically more difficult, often lack interlaboratory (and even intralaboratory) reproducibility, and are subject to the use of inconsistent terminology in their publication. These problems are especially unfortunate since this group of assays might have the potential of providing the most complete information on mechanisms of cellular rejection, function of cellular components active in regulation of the immune response, and efficacy of immunosuppressive treatments.

The ability of patient lymphocytes to lyse donor or third-party target cells can be assessed either immediately after isolation of the effector cells from the circulation or following in vitro stimulation by allogeneic stimulator cells in mixed lymphocyte culture (MLC). Direct assessment of circulating cytotoxic T lymphocytes should be referred to as lymphocyte-mediated cytotoxicity (LMC) to distinguish it from the demonstration of MLC-generated cytotoxic T cells in the cell-mediated lympholysis (CML) assay [125]. This may appear as only a matter of semantics, but this confusion has contributed to misinterpretations in the past. The LMC assay is designed to demonstrate the presence of competent, or nearly competent, cytotoxic T cells in the circulation of graft recipients. The CML assay evaluates the ability of circulating cells to generate competent T-effector cells from the precursors in the peripheral circulation.

Further significant considerations are the duration of incubation of the cytotoxic phase of the assay and the nature of target cells employed. Almost all assays of this type use ^{51}Cr-labeled target cells, but whether these cells are freshly isolated or incubated in phytohemagglutinin (PHA) for 3 days may make a difference. The PHA exposure often is capable of bringing out expression of surface antigens only weakly expressed in fresh isolates. On the other hand, this treatment may elicit target cell antigens against which the effectors may react but that are irrelevant to the in vivo response. In a similar manner, effector and target incubations of 4-6 hr generally provide sufficient exposure to demonstrate cytotoxic T-cell activity. When this activity is present but weak, the short incubation may be insufficient and the assay may require an incubation of 16-18 hr. Some laboratories find, however, that the longer incubations increase spontaneous release to the point of making a statistical assessment of specific ^{51}Cr release impossible. It is necessary to invest considerable time and effort to establish and perfect these procedures if one hopes to develop informative data bases from cell-mediated immune tests.

As described in the humoral cytotoxicity section, ADCC assays can be used to demonstrate the presence of killer cells in patient peripheral circulation. Target cells (^{51}Cr-labeled) from any of several sources, RBC or nucleated cells, coated with appropriate antibody, are incubated in the presence of peripheral blood mononuclear cells from the study subject. If K-cell activity is present, lysis will be signaled by ^{51}Cr release. We will henceforth describe the test for antibody as LDA and the evaluation of K-cell activity as ADCC.

The final cytotoxic test to be discussed is the evaluation of natural killer (NK) cell activity. In general, this activity is measured by incubation of peripheral blood mononuclear cells, without antibody, with any of several ^{51}Cr-labeled susceptible target cells [55], most frequently K562, a human myelogenous leukemia cell line.

Determinations of suppressor cell function are plagued with many of the same difficulties as cytotoxic cell testing since the test systems employed generally involve addition of the suppressor population as second- or third-party reactants to antigen or mitogen blastogenic assays or to MLR or MLC-CML reactions. Further complicating the demonstration of suppressor activity is the requirement that the cell preparation lack cytotoxic activity against the reactant cell population. If such cytotoxicity exists, it could produce artefactual suppression of the test reaction.

Phenotypic Analysis

These assays have been well documented over the past few years and require minimal description. They include the demonstration of receptors on cells capable of binding sheep red blood cells (E-RFC), or RBC coated with antibody (EA), or antibody and complement components (EAC) [63,64,126]. Although the rosetting assays were the principal phenotypic characterization methods for peripheral blood lymphocytes for many years, they have been supplanted by monoclonal antibodies directed against cell surface determinants [69,101]. Methods for monoclonal antibody quantitation of cell types include complement cytotoxicity [67,132], immunoenzymatic procedures [91], and fluorescent techniques, either microscopic or flow cytometric [51,57].

The most significant technical problems encountered with these procedures are interfering effects of immunosuppressive therapy and aberrant antigenic expression. The ability of T cells to bind sheep RBC is altered by treatment of the patient with anti-thymocyte reagents (ATS or ATG), possibly due to steric hinderance from the ATG at the receptor site [124]. This problem is largely but not completely overcome by the use of pan-T-cell reactive monoclonal antibodies (OKT3, Anti-Leu 4). In using monoclonal antibodies, care should be exercised to eliminate the possibility of antigenic modulation [15,39], giving rise to false-negative results or the congenital occurrence of abnormal antigenic profiles [60,69] generating false interpretations of the data.

CLINICAL RELEVANCE OF MONITORING DATA

Humoral Immunity—Donor Specific

The ability to assess the formation of anti-donor antibodies in transplant recipients is hindered by the rapid absorption of these antibodies onto the donor tissue cells of the graft. Elution studies using rejected kidneys have shown a considerable variety of antibodies present in the graft without defining which of these may have been critical factors in graft destruction [85,100]. Even with the restrictions imposed by tissue absorption, several antibody types have been identified following transplantation when frequent serial samples of recipient sera have been collected. Among those that may be important are complement-fixing antibodies [26,68] and antibodies with specificity against DR antigens [87], endothelium-monocyte (EM) antigen [6,87], B-cell lines [74], or donor tissue [100]. Part of the problem in using assays for these antibodies is that long-range planning is required. Antibody detection systems are less complex than those for detection of cellular reactivities; the type of antibody testing required in the posttransplant period involves the isolation and storage of donor tissues, in particular B cells, vascular endothelium, and biopsy tissue sections prepared for use in immunoenzymatic and fluorescent antibody staining procedures.

If testing the above antibodies would provide us with a reliable indicator of donor immune status, much of the effort required would be readily undertaken. Unfortunately, the presence of these antibodies has been shown to be associated both with rejection events and with periods of quiescence [26,68,74,98].

These results raise questions as to the relevance of donor-specific antibody screening after transplantation, but individual laboratories have established firm associations between changes in circulating antibody activity and immune responses. Stiller et al. [115] have shown that the sequential analysis of patient sera can, when used in complement-mediated cytotoxicity with ^{51}Cr-labeled target cells, be associated with rejection. These results have been extended to include correlation between antibodies cytotoxic to a panel of unrelated target cells and rejection [26]. Anti-endothelial antibodies may be studied without the need for donor-specific tissue [6] and therefore may be extensively analyzed throughout the posttransplant period. Lastly, though antibody-dependent cellular cytotoxicity (ADCC) techniques may not be routine in many laboratories, some investigators have routinely employed this technique in monitoring recipients and find development of anti-donor tissue LDA to be significantly associated with rejection [48].

In conclusion, although antibody detection is generally considered an easier approach to monitoring than cellular assays, the routine use of complement-mediated cytotoxicity, ADCC, and other assays evaluating anti-donor reactivities is hampered by tissue availability and interpretive problems. Individual laboratories should continue to study antibody responses, especially if they have available tissue banks from donors, sera banks from recipients, and established protocols for these techniques.

Humoral Immunity—Nonspecific Factors

Numerous factors can be found in patient serum that relate to the degree of specific and nonspecific immune activity in the patient. As our knowledge of these factors continues to grow, we become aware of the extensive networks of soluble substances far beyond our earlier concerns with antibody molecules. From acute phase reactants, through enzymatic activities, to lymphokine and monokine activity, our knowledge of chemical intermediaries of the immune response continues to grow. It is a reasonable assumption that some of these factors may function as signals of immune activation that may assist the clinician in the diagnosis of rejection.

The first and most obvious humoral factor to be considered is circulating immunoglobulin level. If we assume that many immune events are activated in preparation for rejection episodes, then it is only logical that broad-based B-cell activation occurs with concomitant production of immunoglobulins of all types. Indeed, when circulating levels of IgG and IgM were studied, increases in both but principally IgM were noted at rejection [8]. On the other hand, this same report noted that posttransplantation levels of Ig were altered from controls, probably due to the immunosuppressive therapy. In fact, the patterns of increase observed were not consistent from patient to patient and were not useful in predicting rejection. Spontaneous plaque formation using protein A-coated erythrocytes is an assay that determines the overall level of B-cell activation. This system has been used successfully to detect an association between B-cell activation, probably through lymphokine production, and onset of rejection [106].

If antibodies are involved in rejection, then it would be safe to assume that complement levels should be altered through complement consumption. However, complement levels are for the most part stable through periods of rejection or quiescence [8]. Occasionally individual patients will show changes, but there has been no correlation established in these patients whether the consumption is due to antibody activity or the presence of antigen-antibody complexes.

Circulating immune complexes (CIC) themselves have been the target of a number of investigations and were shown [90] to increase in association with antibody-mediated vascular rejection. Unfortunately, several other studies have failed to confirm a diagnostic role for the presence of CIC [59].

In summary, nonspecific humoral factors directly related to the immune response, that is, immunoglobulins, complement, and antigen-antibody complexes, have failed to provide a reliable diagnostic indicator to the onset of rejection. Fortunately, serum contains many more factors than those just described and some of these may hold more promise as tools of immunologic monitoring.

Acute phase reactants, proteins found in response to inflammatory activity, have been extensively studied, and two, C-reactive protein (CRP) and β_2-microglobulin, have shown the most promise. White et al. [137] initially showed that C-reactive protein detected by radial immunodiffusion exhibited elevation prior to rejection episodes. More recently, rate immunonephelometry has been shown to be a faster and more precise technique for CRP determination [45]. Both reports establish a link between the inflammatory activity of rejection and CRP increase, and both also demonstrate the occurrence of CRP increases without apparent rejection.

Similar findings have been demonstrated for β_2-microglobulin. Elevations in β_2-microglobulin have been associated with rejection [7,8,42,43] and appear to be detectable before creatinine elevations. Similar elevations, however, can be seen during viral and bacterial infections and other inflammatory processes. Therefore, the diagnostic utility of β_2-microglobulin is limited. On the other hand, those laboratory groups that use this indicator in concert with creatinine determinations for the diagnosis of rejection are quite certain that the two markers provide the earliest possible diagnosis and set the stage for better graft prognosis.

A growing area of interest is in the detection of products of altered metabolism demonstrated in serum or urine due to rejection processes. Neopterin [78] and urine thromboxane

COLOR PLATES 1-7

PLATE 1
(Chapter 10)

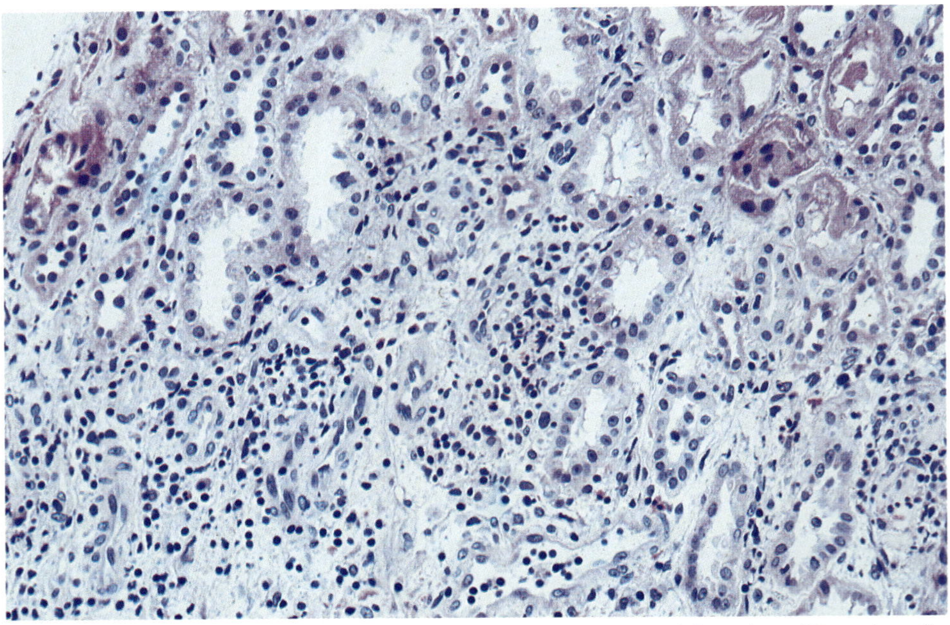

FIGURE 1 Interstitial infiltrate in a patient with stable renal function. (Hematoxylin and eosin stain, ×270.)

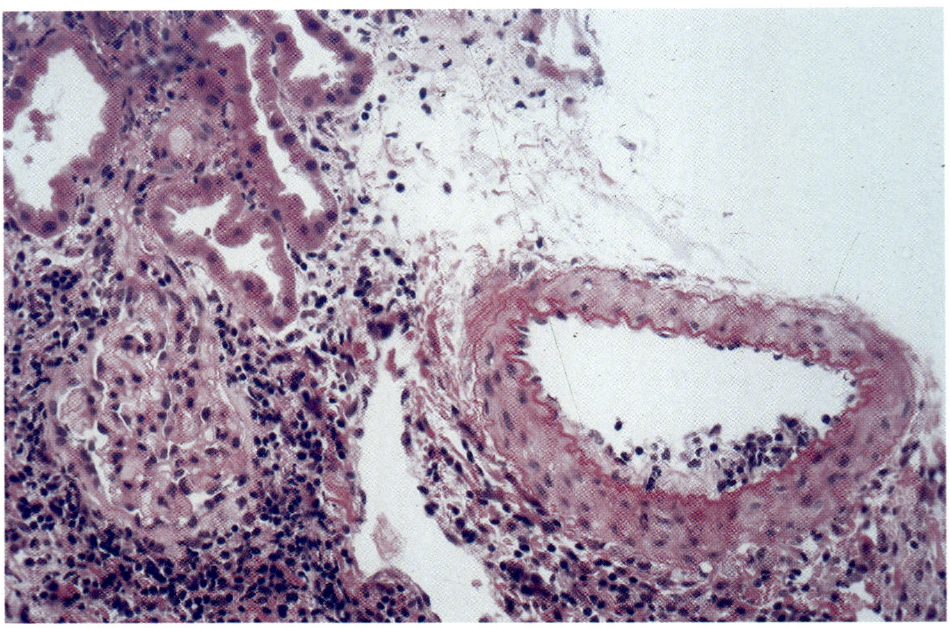

FIGURE 2a Typical intimal arteritis in a patient with rejection. (H & E stain, ×270.)

PLATE 2
(*Chapter 10*)

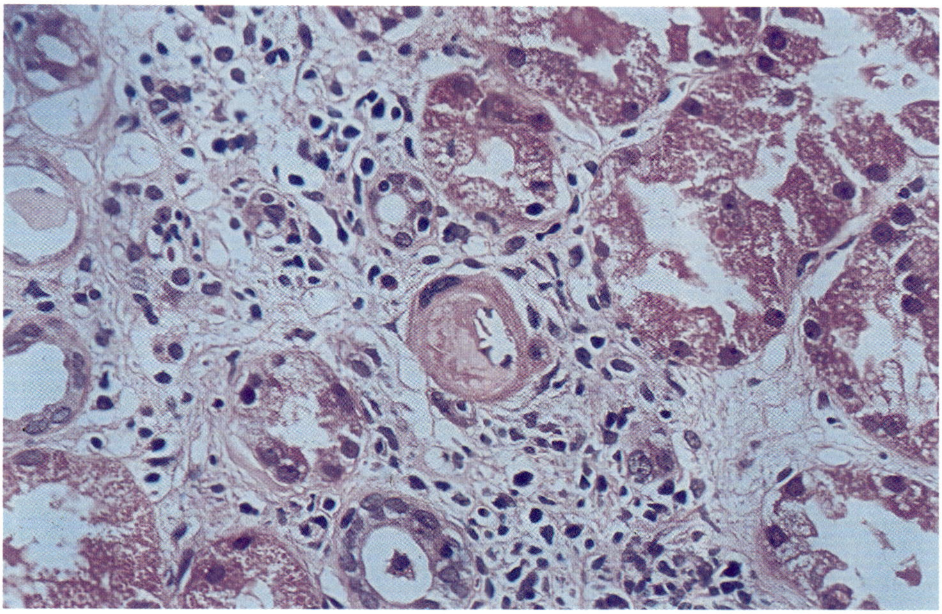

FIGURE 2b Cyclosporine arteriolopathy in a patient with cyclosporine nephrotoxicity. Note difference in size of vessel affected and character of the pathologic change. (H & E stain, ×270.)

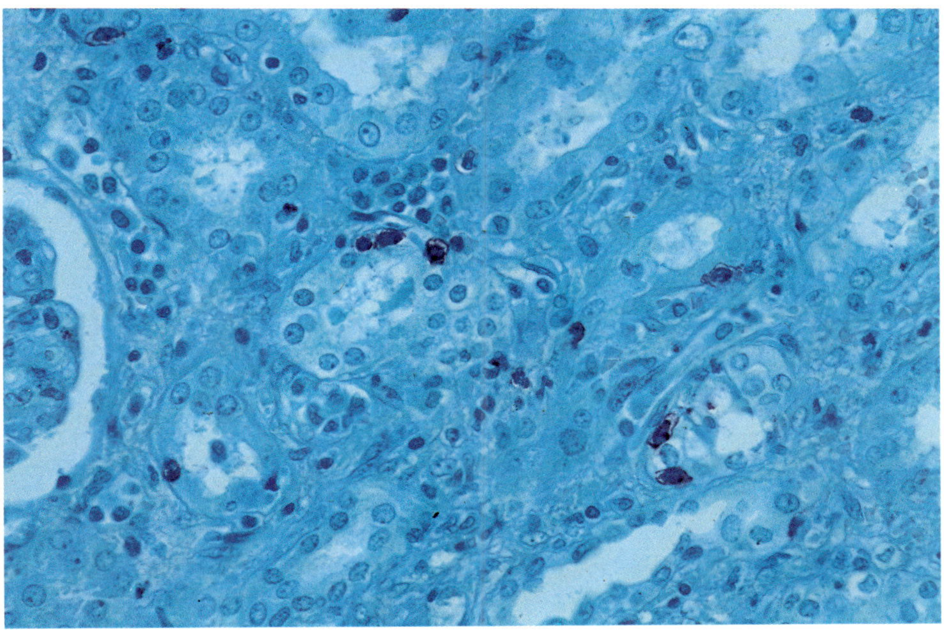

FIGURE 3 Acute renal allograft rejection with Leu 7 positive lymphocytes between tubular epithelial cells. The positively staining lymphocytes appear black. Note that the Leu 7 positive lymphocytes are adjacent to the tubular basement membrane. (Avidin-Biotin complex immunoperoxidase, methylene blue counter-stain, ×400.)

PLATE 3
(*Chapter 12*)

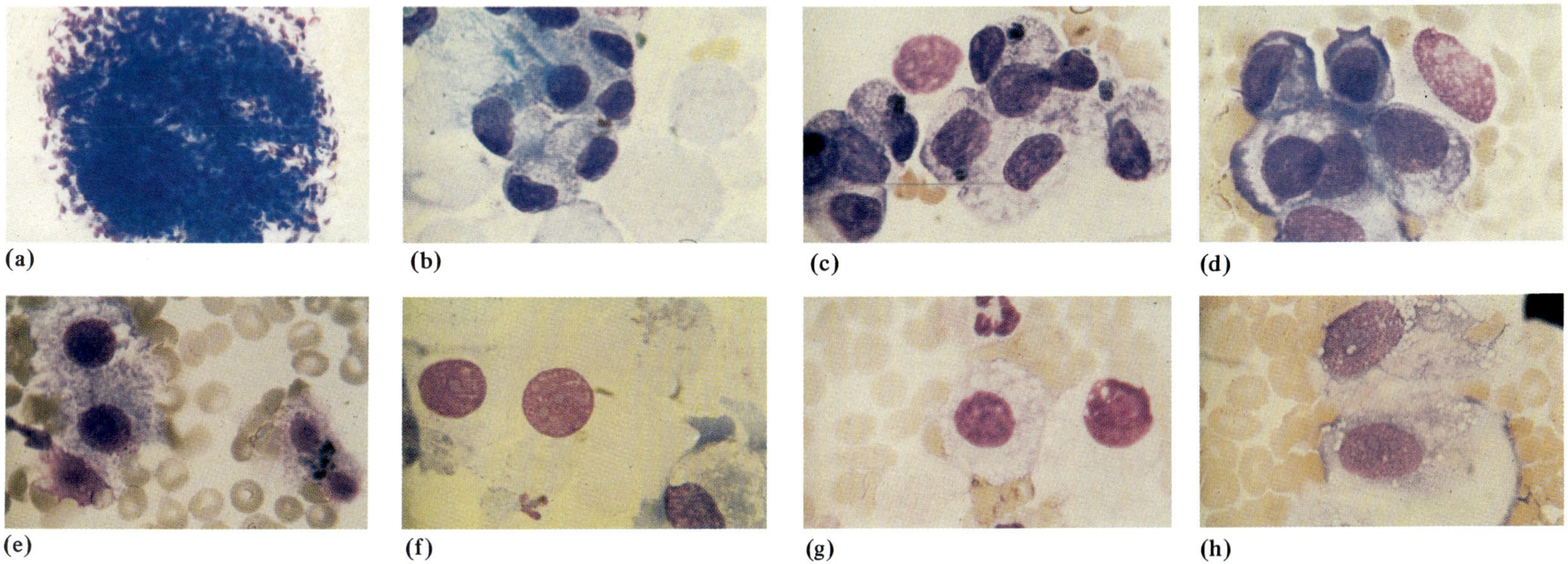

FIGURE 1 Parenchymal cell cytology with May-Grunwald-Giemsa staining of fine needle aspiration biopsy (FNAB) specimens. (a) Whole glomerulus in a FNAB specimen. Detailed glomerular structures are impossible to visualize in the May-Grunwald-Giemsa stained-specimen (×400). (b) Well preserved epithelial cells from proximal tubules. Note the compact cytoplasm with good morphologic integrity (×1000). (c) Proximal tubular cells with slight cytoplasmic changes, swelling and vacuolization, coinciding with clinical ATN. (d) As in (c) but the alterations are more severe. (e) Necrotic tubular cells in the fine needle specimen during advanced irreversible rejection. It is not possible to judge whether these cells are from proximal or distal tubules. (f) Vascular endothelial cells with good morphologic integrity. Note the distinct bluish nucleoli, transparent cytoplasm, and polygonal shape. (g) Endothelial cells with cytoplasmic swelling and vacuolization during advanced rejection. (h) Two endothelial cells with "bubbly" cytoplasmic vacuolization, often encountered in CyA nephrotoxicity. Note the large nucleoli in these cells, indicating increased metabolic activity.

PLATE 4
(*Chapter 12*)

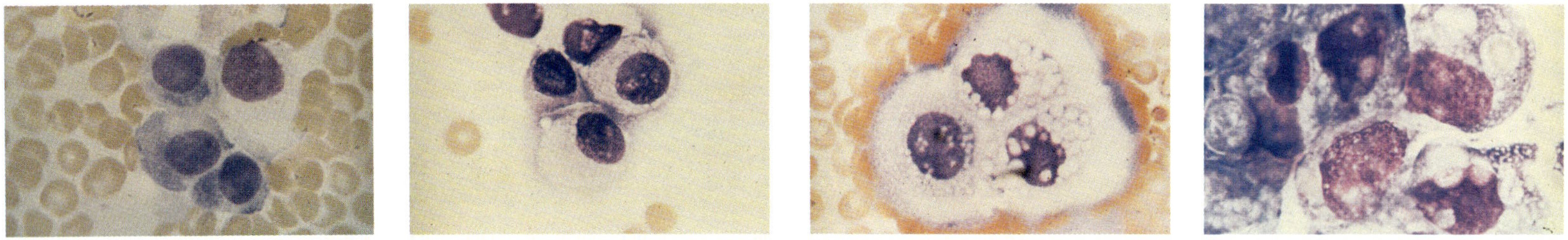

(a) (b) (c) (d)

FIGURE 2 Characteristic cytologic alterations in cyclosporine nephrotoxicity. (a) Proximal tubular cells with good morphological integrity with no evidence of CyA toxicity. (b) Proximal tubular cells with distinct swelling and "bubbly" cytoplasmic vacuolization. (c) Proximal (?) tubular cells with very distinct cytoplasmic vacuolization and swelling. (d) Proximal (?) tubular cells with extreme swelling, cytoplasmic vacuolization, inclusions, and erythrophagocytosis.

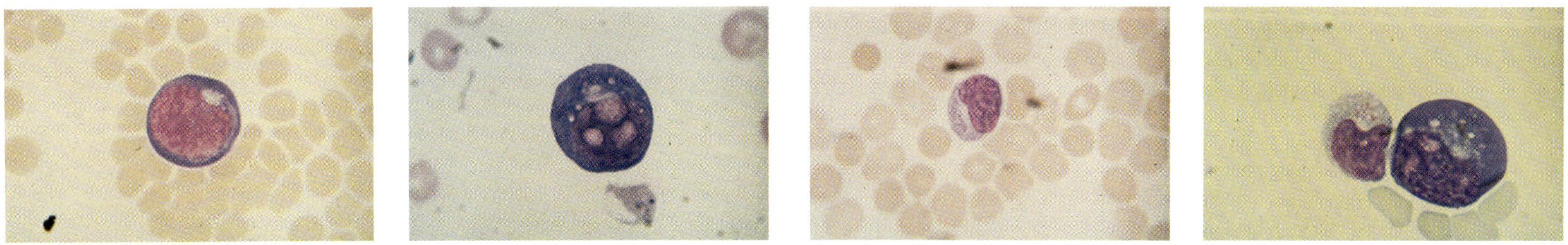

(a) (b) (c) (d)

FIGURE 3 Inflammatory cell cytology in May-Grunwald-Giemsa staining. (a) A blast cell with 1 to 2 distinct nucleoli, relatively scanty cytoplasm, and fine chromatin, of T-cell lineage, as identified by cell surface markers (not shown). (b) A blast cell with large amount of highly basophilic cytoplasm, several prominent nucleoli, and cytoplasmic vacuolization. This type of blast cells usually contain intracellular immunoglobulin, indicating that they are of B-cell lineage. (c) An "activated" lymphocyte. Note the large size and perinuclear halo. (d) A blast cell of B-cell lineage and a large granular lymphocyte (LGL) in the field. LGL can be distinguished by their large size and clear azurophilic granulation in the cytoplasm, corresponding to the site of Golgi apparatus.

PLATE 5
(*Chapter 12*)

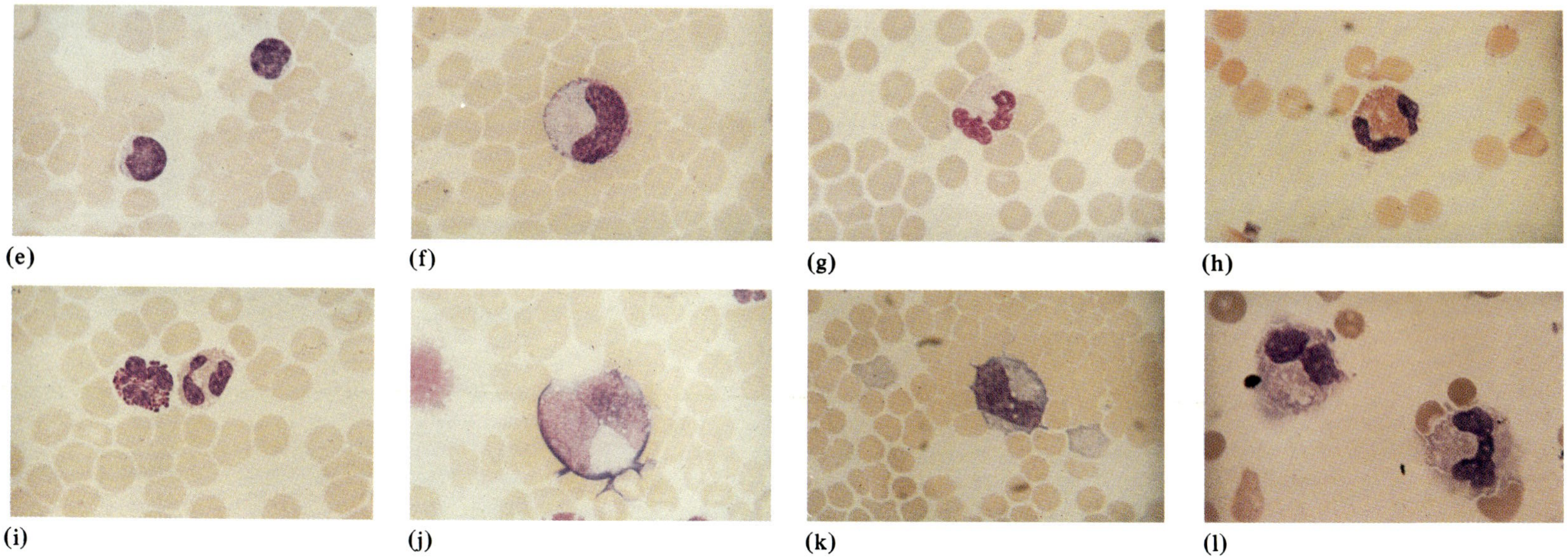

FIGURE 3 (continued) (e) Small lymphocytes. (f) A stab-formed granulocyte. (g) Neutrophil. (h) Eosinophil. (i) Basophil and an eosinophil. (j) A monoblast, frequently observed in the inflammatory infiltrate of cyclosporine-treated recipients. (k) A monocyte with beginning morphological transformation to a tissue macrophage. (1) Mature tissue macrophages.

PLATE 6
(*Chapter 18*)

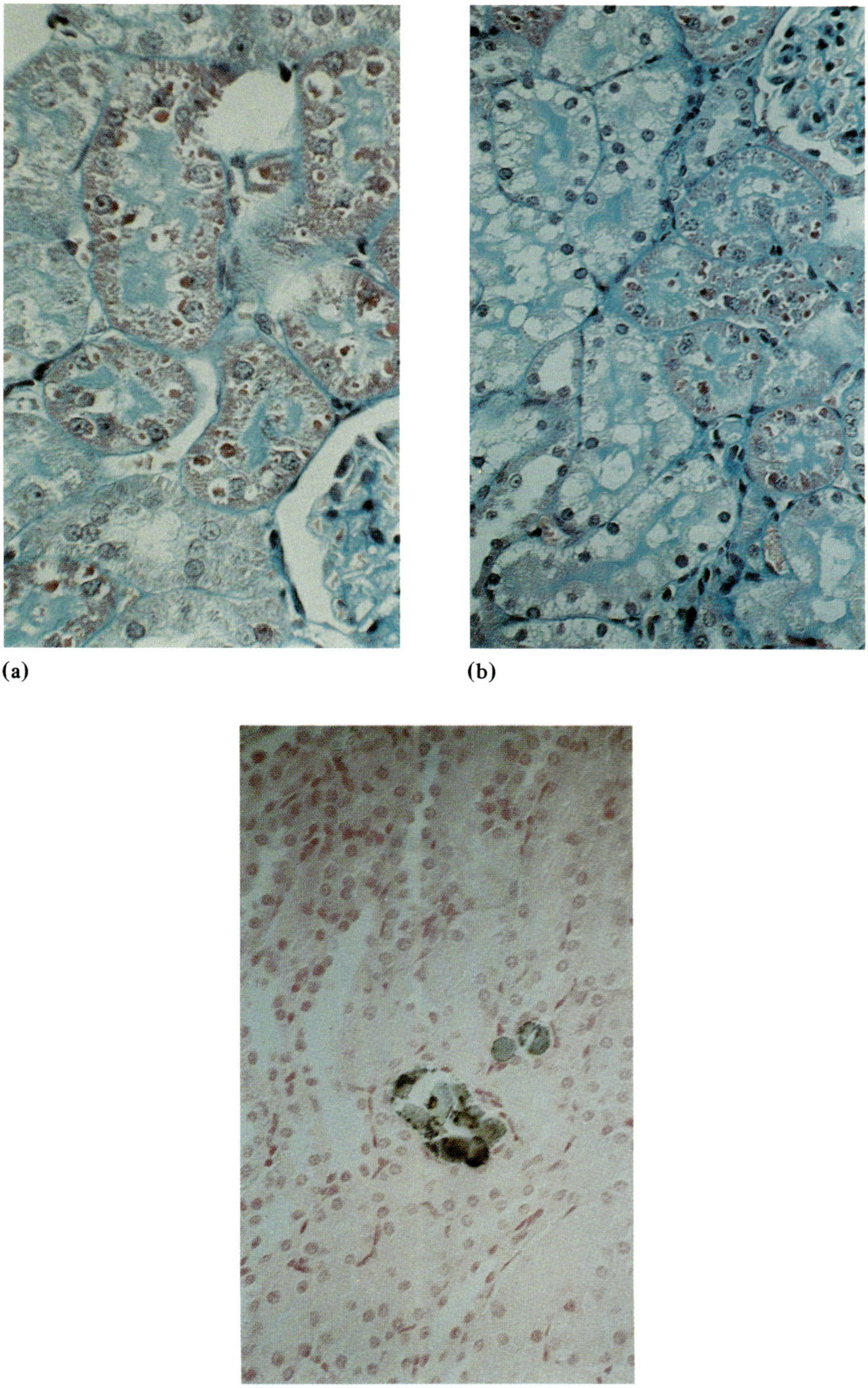

(a) (b) (c)

FIGURE 1 Renal tubular lesions in CsA-treated rats consisting of chromotrope aniline blue-positive inclusion bodies (a), vacuolization (b), and microcalcification (c).

PLATE 7
(*Chapter 18*)

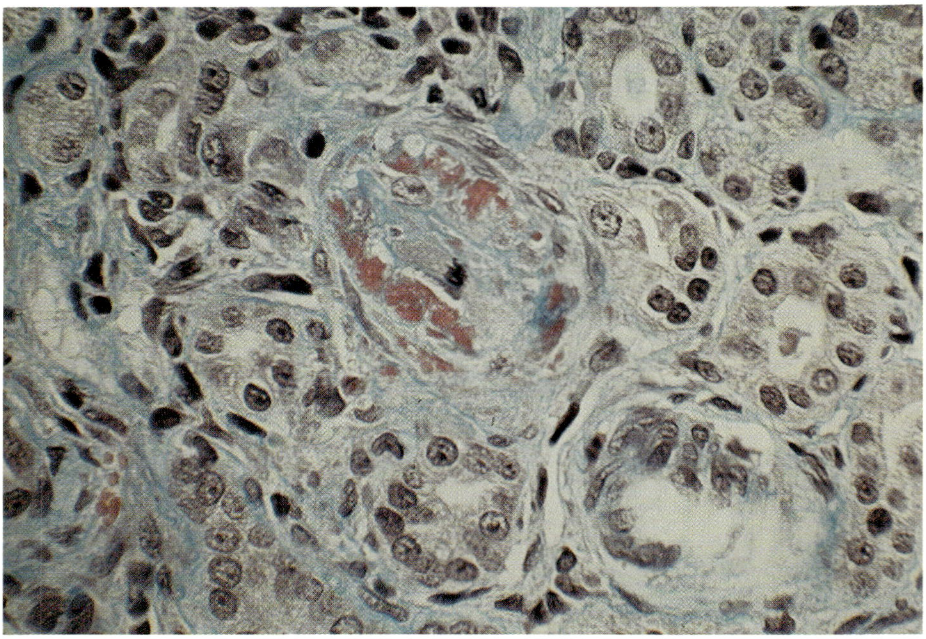

(a)

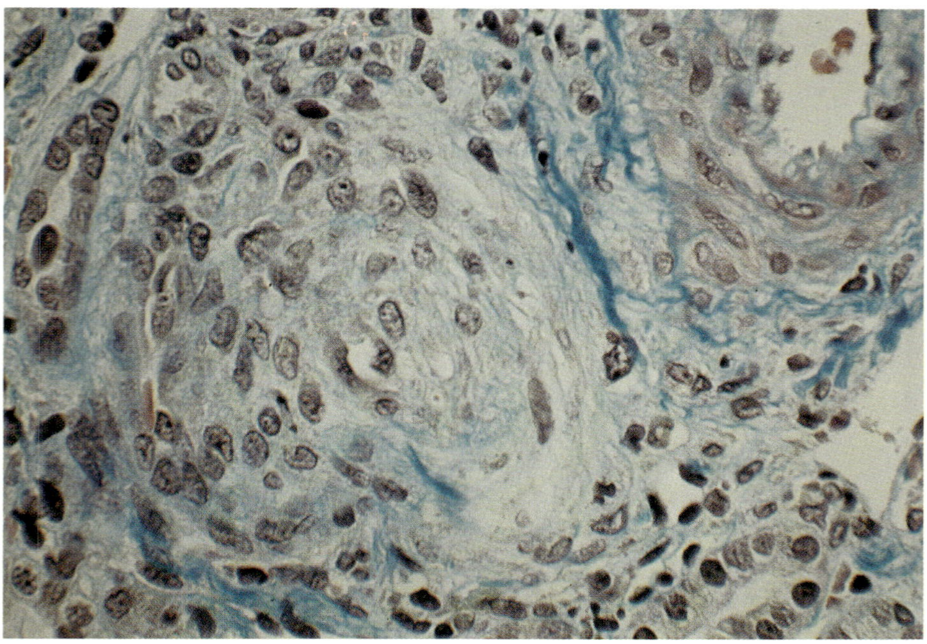

(b)

FIGURE 3 Arteriolar lesions in CsA-treated spontaneously hypertensive rats. Exudative type with media necrosis (a) and proliferative type (b) with obliteration of the vessel lumen. (Chromotrope aniline blue stain.)

[44] are examples. Continued studies in this area may prove fruitful in the future, but as of yet, these substances provide no better indicators of rejection than creatinine determinations.

Last among the humoral factors that will be discussed here are the chemical mediators of the immune response produced by lymphocytes or monocytes, the lymphokines and monokines. These substances are rapidly becoming a principal focus of many immunology laboratories. Elucidation of their central roles in cellular communication is leading to better understanding of immune relationships and pointing the way to future immunosuppressive regimens. An alteration in the ability of patient peripheral blood leukocytes to produce migration inhibitory factor in response to donor antigens has been reported to correlate with poor graft prognosis [76]. This altered production can be detected at a time immediately preceding the onset of rejection. The presence of a migration inhibiting factor in the serum of patients at rejection was recently shown [68]. Serum concentrations of interleukin-2 (IL-2) decrease following transplantation, probably due to drug treatments. However, increases in IL-2 levels can be detected at the time of rejection [117]. Research into interleukins, activation factors, and cytotoxic factors will undoubtedly provide more indicators of immune activation in the future.

Cellular Immunity–Donor Specific

Many laboratories have attempted to detect cell-mediated immunity (CMI) in allograft recipients against their donor tissue. Since CMI has historically been accepted as the principal mediator of acute rejection processes, it seems logical that demonstration of donor-specific cytotoxicity would be compelling evidence that rejection processes have been activated. Unfortunately, as we shall see, very few laboratories have produced cellular assays that are predictive of rejection. The reasons for this paucity of correlating data are not fully understood, but certain facts stand out as possibilities. First, as mentioned in defining the problems of donor-specific antibody analysis, most assays have used peripheral blood cells for the effector cell source. It is valid to argue that the donor-specific effector cells of the recipient will be present in the peripheral circulation for only a short period before taking up residence in the graft. There are data to support the notion that fully competent effector cells may never be found in the peripheral circulation because they undergo final differentiation in the graft itself [2]. Although intragraft events are critical to the rejection process, data also exist to support the idea that the peripheral circulation contains, at various times in the posttransplantation period, representative cells with effector and suppressor function that can be analyzed in vitro with at least some correlations to rejection.

Several reports indicate that cytotoxic effectors, as assessed in the LMC assay, can be detected using ^{51}Cr-labeled target cells and a 16-hr cytotoxicity test [68,115]. Using this technique, Stiller et al. [115] have been able to utilize the LMC assay as a predictor of rejection. On the other hand, several other laboratories have failed to establish the same correlations [28,48]. Even though correlated with poor graft outcome, LMC changes do not occur early enough to be helpful in the diagnosis of rejection [68]. Anti-viral cytotoxic T cells are readily demonstrated in the circulation [103], but it is possible that only precursors to allogeneic cytotoxic lymphocytes are found in the peripheral circulation and these require longer periods of incubation to develop into fully competent effector cells. Quantitation of precursor cytotoxic cells in vitro [10,11] and improved understanding of the target antigens recognized by alloreactive T cells [20,77,104] will lead to improved prognostic tests of transplant recipients.

Since patients have T cells active against donor antigens, it would seem likely that peripheral blood cells from recipients would have a high degree of reactivity against donor cells in mixed lymphocyte reactions. However, although a few laboratories have demonstrated increased MLR responsiveness prior to rejection, these results have not been reproducible [5,38,58,116]. Long-term allograft recipients have decreased allogeneic [96] and autologous MLR [38], suggesting the presence of suppressor cells. Phenotypic characterization of some cells with suppressor activity in tolerant recipients has been reported [14], but the phenotypic and functional characteristics of all such suppressor cells is an area of current study (see Chapter 7).

Development of cytotoxic T cells following in vitro stimulation in MLR is generally found when peripheral blood lymphocytes from normal individuals are used. When responder cells are drawn from recipients with long-term surviving grafts, however, they often fail to generate cytotoxic effector cells [49]. This lack of CML responsiveness might be due to deletion of alloreactive clones or allospecific suppressor cells. When followed chronologically, patients with CML nonresponsiveness to their donors developed donor-specific CML at the time of rejection [89]. The role of nonspecific [129] or specific suppressor cells [14,80] in this altered responsiveness has yet to be clarified.

Further progress in our understanding of suppressor cells and their action in graft recipients is central to the attainment of tolerance in all patients. The ability of recipients to generate donor-specific suppressor cells in vitro has been demonstrated [47]. Phenotypic characterizations of T-cell [14] and B-cell [19] suppressors have begun.

In summary, assays of donor-specific cellular responses are cumbersome and subject to factors that affect their reproducibility, both inter- and intralaboratory. When used in a consistent manner, they have shown that cytotoxic T cells can be detected in the peripheral circulation, and their occurrence is correlated with rejection events. Patients who fail to generate donor-specific cytotoxic T cells have a good graft prognosis. Future developments may determine whether the long-term acceptance of grafts is dependent on deletion of alloreactive T-cell clones or production of allospecific suppressor cells.

Cellular Immunity–Non-donor Specific

Considerable efforts have been expended on analysis of donor-specific humoral and cellular responses, but very few clinically relevant data have emerged. For the most part, non-donor-specific assays have been more productive in generating clinical associations [28,125]. In this section, we will discuss quantitation of T lymphocytes and their subsets, NK, ADCC, and monocyte responses.

Quantitation of T lymphocytes has proven of value in establishing whether individuals possessed sufficient effector cells to mount a rejection response [84,126]. Patients undergoing ATG therapy fail to properly demonstrate the E-RFC receptor and must have their T cells measured through the use of pan-T monoclonal antibodies [124]. These monoclonal anti-T-cell reagents have been shown to be effective means of monitoring immunotherapy [25].

With the introduction of monoclonal antibodies capable of reacting with differentiation antigens unique to subpopulations of T cells [69,101], studies were initiated to evaluate the significance of subset dynamics in disease. Subsets have proven useful in characterizing lymphoid neoplasms [66], demonstrating changes in autoimmunity [97], and suggesting immune mechanisms of other diseases [3,4]. Early studies in renal allograft recipients suggested a possible correlation between subset activity and clinical events [22,35] and pointed the way to potential use of these reagents in immunotherapy [22,23]. Unfortunately, the diagnostic promise of these reagents has not been attained.

Patients undergoing transplantation can be broadly grouped into two sets based on the peripheral blood ratios of helper to suppressor cells in the early posttransplant period. The majority of patients maintain near-normal ratios (>1.0), whereas only 10-20% have low ratios (<1.0). Several laboratories reported that the individuals with low ratios were apparently immunodeficient and had less chance of exhibiting rejection episodes [9,22, 110]. Other laboratories, including our own, have failed to confirm this association [13, 113].

The kinetics of T-subset changes have been extensively studied. Some reports suggested that helper/suppressor ratios were diminished during acute rejection [22,112]. A number of laboratories, however, have seen the opposite, a marked increase in ratio signaling impending rejection [17,24,34,35,84,86,114]. Subset ratios may fluctuate in individual patients, but when populations of patients are studied, ratio changes do not appear to be diagnostic [54,65,113,123,135]. Very low ratios may put the patient at risk of infection and may indicate that immunosuppressive therapy should be reduced [110]. Apparent rejection episodes occurring in the presence of very low ratios may, instead, be due to irreversible "transplant glomerulopathy" [21].

Considering individual subpopulation changes, Mohanakumar et al. [84] have found that increases in the helper ($OKT4^+$) subset signal the onset of rejection processes, provided there are sufficient numbers of cells to effect rejection. Our laboratory, using similar techniques and frequency of analysis, failed to establish a statistical correlation between $OKT4^+$ increases and rejection but did see a significant increase in suppressor/cytotoxic ($OKT8^+$) cells at the onset of rejection [113].

In summary, quantitation of T-cell subpopulations with monoclonal antibody reagents has yet to prove clinically useful in the broad screening programs. Changes are often detectable when clinical events occur, and individual laboratories have established statistical correlations and find these procedures to be useful in monitoring immunotherapy. With all the efforts expended to this point, it is discouraging that more usefulness has not been attained. Progress in this area will be dependent on the development of more specific reagents and better understanding of the factors that can influence T-cell populations.

Subset ratios can be altered by circadian cycles [83] and physical activity [33]. Immunosuppressive therapy can have pronounced effects [127]. Prednisolone treatment can result in a decrease in helper/suppressor ratios [46,121] but apparently not in all patients [18,50]. Azathioprine itself only produces weak alterations [18], but combined azathioprine and prednisolone with or without ATG results in decreased ratios [18,37,72]. Effects produced by ATG can be dependent on the animal of origin with horse ATG having little to no effect, but rabbit ATG able to produce a pronounced reduction in patient ratios [124]. Cyclosporine does not appear to have a pronounced effect [81], but immunologic monitoring of cyclosporine patients may be useful for differentiating nephrotoxicity from immune events [61] and as a means of assessing the immunosuppressive efficacy of therapy [40].

Infections in allograft recipients may affect levels of lymphocyte subpopulations. Several laboratories have reported a marked decrease in ratios as a consequence of cytomegalovirus or other viral infections [31,41,105]. This association has not been confirmed in our laboratory [113] or in cyclosporine-treated patients [99].

Monoclonal antibodies to other cell populations besides lymphocytes have been produced, and these cell types may have a role in rejection processes. Cytotoxic activity of

NK cells has been associated with the improved outcome of viral infections in renal transplant recipients [102], and many immunosuppressive drugs markedly reduce circulating NK cells [32,93,94]. Increased NK activity has been associated with rejection [73], but this association has not been confirmed [36,134]. Clarification of the role of NK cells in rejection may be dependent on better definition of their antigenic phenotype [17, 108] or requirements for in vitro demonstration [75].

Increased killer cell activity as measured in ADCC may reflect the onset of rejection [1]. The possible role of ADCC effector cells in rejection is supported by the observation that, although most patients exhibit steroid-sensitive ADCC [93,118,122], those with steroid-resistant in vitro ADCC have poor graft outcome [29] unless rescued by ATG [30]. On the other hand, K-cell activity failed to correlate with rejection in a recent study [36].

In contrast to the intense scrutiny of lymphocytes and related cell types, monocyte studies in renal allograft recipients are sparse. Histologic demonstration of monocytes as components of the inflammatory infiltrates of rejection within the graft is indicative of poor outcome [53,131]. One study that failed to demonstrate any correlation of T-subset changes and rejection did demonstrate increases in the levels of $OKM1^+$ cells prior to rejection [13]. This marker may reflect more than monocyte populations [79]; our laboratory has also presented preliminary data suggesting increases in circulating monocyte levels may precede rejection [113].

Non-donor-specific suppressor cell activity may reflect the efficacy of immunosuppression or provide insight into immune regulation in graft recipients. Following treatment with rabbit ATG, adherent, prostaglandin-dependent cells capable of depressing mitogen stimulation of patient lymphocytes have been demonstrated [129]. Failure to develop these cells signals a poor prognosis. Concanavalin-inducible suppressor cells increase in patients following blood transfusions [111] and have been phenotypically characterized as displaying T8 and Ia-like antigens. It is possible that they exhibit MHC products comparable to the I-J determinant of murine suppressor cells [71]. Differentiation of peripheral blood lymphocytes based on theophylline sensitivity has suggested that suppressor cells are theophylline sensitive and decrease at rejection [109]. Unfortunately, theophylline-sensitive and theophylline-resistant cells cannot be differentiated by monoclonal antibodies against T-cell antigens [120].

ACTIVATION MARKERS AND FUTURE DIRECTIONS

We have reviewed a large number of assay systems without conclusively establishing any as clinically useful adjuncts in the management of the renal allograft recipient. However, changes are detectable among immune components in the peripheral circulation of patients, which may indicate that the potential usefulness of immunologic monitoring is still waiting to be uncovered.

Among humoral components, acute phase reactants and biologic response modifiers may, when incorporated into a larger profile of patient symptoms, provide an easily monitored panel that would greatly improve our ability to interpret ongoing clinical events. Nonspecific activation of B-cell events and better understanding of the critical antibody specificities responsible for rejection episodes may provide more timely indicators of impending rejection crises.

Cellular events, such as LMC reactivity or failure to develop donor-specific CML reactivity, provide test systems to analyze the specific functions of cells responsible for graft destruction. Improvements in defining effector and target cell populations may allow these assays to produce results that are closely linked with in vivo events. The use of T-cell antigenic determinants has yet to prove relevant, but the numerous changes in subset levels, although they do not provide useful data for large populations of patients, may provide insight into activities occurring within individual patients. Certainly, individual laboratories have made substantial progress in studies in this area. It should be remembered that we have been using reagents that are first-generation and reactive against very broad groupings of cells. As the repertoire of reagents and the differentiation antigens they detect increases, so will the significance of the data they provide. We already have available monoclonal antibodies that detect surface determinants unique to activated cells, and these reagents may provide a signal for that most crucial immune event, cellular activation in response to allogeneic recognition.

Among the cells capable of reacting in the E-rosette test are those that have a high affinity for sheep RBC, the active E-RFC. Kerman et al. [64] demonstrated that recipients with high pretransplant levels of these active E-RFC cells had poor graft prognosis. Since fluctuations in the levels of these cells are seen coincident with rejection [62,63] and they express the T8 surface antigen [107]., it has been suggested that they are activated surveillance cells [64]. Supporting the concept that activated cells can be found in the peripheral circulation at the time of rejection are the observations that periopheral blood lymphocytes exhibit an increased level of spontaneous blastogenesis immediately prior to rejection [61,62,88,128]. The cells active in spontaneous blastogenesis have been shown to exhibit the T8 equivalent Leu 2 antigen. Besides the presence of activated T cells by E-rosette and spontaneous blastogenesis testing, increased levels of lymphocyte lactate dehydrogenase [136] suggests increased T-cell activity in the peripheral circulation coincident with rejection.

Whole families of activation antigens are being studied [119], and reports have shown that T cells in graft recipients are often large blast cells [51] bearing the T10 antigen [70,82] and Ia-like determinants [12,27,70,130]. Unique antigenic expression may also indicate activation events. The mutual exclusion of T4 and T8 antigens on cell surfaces that was once thought to exist appears to break down with in vitro cellular activation [12,113], and cells bearing both markers have been observed in renal transplant recipients [16,17,113] and during CMV infections [41].

As our knowledge of activation events progresses and reagents for detecting activated cells become available, our ability to more reliably and quickly recognize immune changes in the recipients will improve dramatically. Multiparameter analysis of cell cycles, DNA, and surface determinants by flow cytometric techniques [113,138] may become the required norm of immunologic monitoring laboratories of the future.

REFERENCES

1. Arnesen, E., and Bondevik, H. Donor-specific cellular and humoral immunity after clinical kidney transplantation. *Transplantation* 21:489-497, 1976.
2. Ascher, N. L., Hoffman, R., Hanto, D. W., and Simmons, R. L. Cellular events within the rejecting allograft. *Transplantation* 35:193-197, 1983.
3. Bach, M. A., and Bach, J. F. The use of monoclonal anti-T-cell antibodies to study T cell imbalances in human disease. *Clin. Exp. Immunol.* 45:449-456, 1981.
4. Bach, M. A., and Bach, J. F. Imbalances in T cell subsets in human diseases. *Int. J. Immunopharm.* 3:269-273, 1981.
5. Bakran, A., Taylor, G. M., Read, I., Johnson, R. W. G., and Harris, R. Cellular function

and T cell subsets in patients with long-surviving renal transplants. *Transplant. Proc.* 16:1558-1560, 1984.

6. Baldwin, W. M., Class, F. H., van Es, L. A., and van Rood, J. J. Distribution of endothelial-monocyte and HLA antigens on renal vascular endothelium. *Transplant. Proc.* 13:103-107, 1981.
7. Barnes, R. M., Alexander, L. C., and West, C. R. Beta-2-microglobulin and renal graft rejection: Relationship to plasma creatinine during stable transplant function and graft rejection. *Transplant. Proc.* 16:1613-1615, 1984.
8. Barnes, R. M., Hart, C. A., Alexander, L. C., and Steen, S. Immunological evaluation of renal transplant patients: Changes in levels of beta-2-microglobulin, immunoglobulins and complement components during graft rejection. *J. Clin. Lab. Immunol.* 12: 17-22, 1983.
9. Binkley, W. F., Valenzuela, R., Braun, W. E., Deodhar, S. D., Novick, A. C., and Steinmuller, D. R. Flow cytometry quantitation of peripheral blood (PB) T cell subsets in human renal allograft recipients. *Transplant. Proc.* 15:1163-1165, 1983.
10. Bonavida, B., Bradley, T. P., and Grimm, E. A. The single-cell assay in cell-mediated cytotoxicity. *Immunol. Today* 4:196-200, 1983.
11. Bryan, D. J., Pinto, C. E., and Fuller, T. C. Direct estimation of the frequency of human cytotoxic T lymphocytes and their precursors following in vitro allosensitization. *Hum. Immunol.* 6:31-44, 1983.
12. Burns, G. F., Battye, F. L., and Goldstein, G. Surface antigen changes occurring in short-term cultures of activated human T lymphocytes: Analysis by low cytometry. *Cell Immunol.* 71:12-26, 1982.
13. Carter, N. P., Cullen, P. R., Thompson, J. F., Bewick, A. L. T., Wood, R. F. M., and Morris, P. J. Monitoring lymphocyte subpopulations in renal allograft recipients. *Transplant. Proc.* 15:1157-1159, 1983.
14. Charpentier, B. M., Bach, M. A., Lang, P., and Fries, D. Expression of OKT8 antigen and FcG receptors by suppressor cells mediating specific unresponsiveness between recipient and donor in renal-allograft tolerant patients. *Transplantation* 36:495-501, 1983.
15. Chatenoud, L., Baudrihaye, M. F., Kreis, H., Goldstein, G., Schindler, J., and Bach, J. F. Human in vivo antigenic modulation induced by the anti-T cell OKT3 monoclonal antibody. *Eur. J. Immunol.* 12:979-982, 1982.
16. Chatenoud, L., Chkoff, N., Kreis, H., and Bach, J. F. Correlation between immunoregulatory T cell imbalances and renal allograft outcome. *Transplant. Proc.* 15:1184-1185, 1983.
17. Chatenoud, L., Chkoff, N., Kreis, H., and Bach, J. F. Interest in and limitations of monoclonal anti-T cell antibodies for the follow-up of renal transplant patients. *Transplantation* 36:45-50, 1983.
18. Chatenoud, L., Kreis, H., Jungers, P., and Bach, J. F. The effect of immunosuppressive agents on T cell subsets as evaluated by use of monoclonal anti-T cell antibodies. *Transplant. Proc.* 13:1651-1656, 1981.
19. Clement, L. T., Grossi, C. E., and Gartland, G. L. Morphologic and phenotypic features of the subpopulation of Leu-2+ cells that suppress B cell differentiation. *J. Immunol.* 133:2461-2468, 1984.
20. Collins, T., Krensky, A. M., Clayberger, C., Fiers, W., Gimbrone, M. A., Burakoff, S. J., and Pober, J. S. Human cytolytic T lymphocyte interactions with vascular endothelium and fibroblasts: Role of effector and target cell molecules. *J. Immunol.* 133: 1878-1884, 1984.
21. Colvin, R. B., Cosimi, A. B., Burton, R. C., Delmonico, F. L., Jaffers, G., Rubin, R. H., Tolkoff-Rubin, N. E., Giorgi, J. V., McCluskey, R. T., and Russell, P. S. Circulating T cell subsets in 72 human renal allograft recipients: The OKT4/OKT8 cell ratio corre-

lates with reversibility of graft injury and glomerulopathy. *Transplant. Proc.* 15: 1166-1169, 1983.
22. Cosimi, A. B., Colvin, R. B., Burton, R. C., Rubin, R. H., Goldstein, G., Kung, P. C., Hansen, W. P., Delmonico, F. L., and Russell, P. S. Use of monoclonal antibodies to T cell subsets for immunologic monitoring and treatment in recipients of renal allografts. *N. Engl. J. Med.* 305:308-314, 1981.
23. Cosimi, A. B., Colvin, R. B., Jaffers, G. J., Giorgi, J. V., Delmonico, F. L., Fuller, T. C., and Russell, P. S. Immunologic monitoring of monoclonal antibody therapy: Comparison of five antibodies as immunosuppressants of renal allograft rejection. *Transplant. Proc.* 16:1459-1461, 1984.
24. Daniel, V., Opelz, G., and Dreikorn, K. Lymphocyte subset monitoring in renal transplant recipients. *Transplant. Proc.* 16:1564-1565, 1984.
25. Delmonico, F. L., Nelson, P. W., Colvin, R. B., and Cosimi, A. B. Immunologic monitoring of antithymocyte globulin treatment for acute allograft rejection. *Transplant. Proc.* 16:1492-1493, 1984.
26. Descamps, B., Gagnon, R., van der Gaag, R., Feuillet, M. N., and Crosnier, J. Antibody dependent cell mediated cytotoxicity (ADCC) and complement dependent cytotoxicity (CDC) in 229 sera from human renal allograft recipients. *J. Clin. Lab. Immunol.* 2:303-309, 1979.
27. DiMario, U., and Guy, K. Evaluation of class II antigen positive T cells: A simple double staining method using monoclonal antibodies. *J. Clin. Lab. Immunol.* 13:203-204, 1984.
28. Dossetor, J. B., and Myburgh, J. A. Posttransplant immunologic monitoring: A summation. *Transplant. Proc.* 10:661-670, 1978.
29. Dumble, L. J., Clunie, G. J. A., Macdonald, I. M., Bowes, L. G., Dowling, J. P. G., and Kincaid-Smith, P. Diminished incidence of rejection in renal allograft recipients with ADCC sensitive to in vitro steroids. *Transplant. Proc.* 15:1954-1956, 1983.
30. Dumble, L. J., Clunie, G. J. A., Macdonald, I. M., Bowes, L. G., and Kincaid-Smith, P. Antithymocyte globulin-induced prolongation of human renal allograft survival in recipients with in vitro steroid-resistant ADCC. *Transplant. Proc.* 16:1503-1505, 1984.
31. Dummer, J. S., Ho, M., Rabin, B. P., Griffith, B. P., Hardesty, R. L., and Bahnson, H. T. The effect of cytomegalovirus and Epstein-Barr virus infection on T lymphocyte subsets in cardiac transplant patients on cyclosporine. *Transplantation* 38:433-435, 1984.
32. Dupont, E., Huygen, K., Schandene, L., Vandercruys, M., Palfliet, K., and Wybran, J. Depressed natural killer cell function in transplant recipients: An analysis. *Transplant. Proc.* 16:1506-1508, 1984.
33. Edwards, A. J., Bacon, T. H., Elms, C. A., Verardi, R., Felder, M., and Knight, S. C. Changes in the populations of lymphoid cells in human peripheral blood following physical exercise. *Clin. Exp. Immunol.* 58:420-427, 1984.
34. Ellis, T. M., Berry, C. R., Mendez-Picon, G., Goldman, M. N., Lower, R., Lee, H. M., and Mohanakumar, T. Immunologic monitoring of renal allograft recipients using monoclonal antibodies to human T lymphocyte subpopulations. *Transplantation* 33:317-319, 1982.
35. Ellis, T. M., Lee, H. M., Mohanakumar, T. Alterations in human regulatory T lymphocyte subpopulations after renal allografting. *J. Immunol.* 127:2199-2203, 1981.
36. Ellis, T. M., Mohanakumar, T., Mendez-Picon, G., Goldman, M. H., Lower, R., and Lee, H. M. Posttransplant monitoring of circulating K-cell, NK-cell, and total T-cell levels: Lack of association with renal allograft rejection. *Transplant. Proc.* 15: 1830-1831, 1983.
37. Ellis, T. M., Mohanakumar, T., Muakkassa, W., Lower, R., and Lee, H. M. Influence

of immunosuppressive therapy and blood transfusions on human T cell subpopulations. *Transplant. Proc.* 15:1173-1175, 1983.

38. Ellis, T. M., Reinitz, E. R., Mohanakumar, T., and Lee, H. M. Depressed proliferative responses in autologous mixed lymphocyte cultures and to soluble antigen by lymphocytes from long-term renal allograft recipients. *Transplant. Proc.* 16:1530-1531, 1984.
39. Estabrook, A., Mittler, R., LoGerfo, P., Hardy, M., Edelson, R. L., and Berger, C. L. Antigenic modulation of pan-T-cell and T-cell subset-specific markers. *Diagn. Immunol.* 1:199-204, 1983.
40. Ferguson, R. M., and Fidelus-Gort, R. The immunosuppressive action of cyclosporine in man. *Transplant. Proc.* 15:2350-2356, 1983.
41. Fiche, M., Soulillou, J. P., Bignon, J. D., Billaudel, S., and Guenel, J. T lymphocyte monitoring in kidney transplant recipients undergoing cytomegalovirus infection or rejection episodes. *Transplantation* 37:421-423, 1984.
42. Fields, B. L., Sollinger, H. W., Glass, N. R., Carlson, I. H., and Belzer, F. O. Beta-2-microglobulin versus creatinine as the sole indicator of rejection in renal transplants. *Transplant. Proc.* 16:1591-1593, 1984.
43. Finn, W. F., Huffman, K. A., Forman, D. T., and Mandel, S. R. Value of serum beta-2-microglobulin/serum creatinine ratio following renal transplantation. *Transplant. Proc.* 16:1609-1612, 1984.
44. Foegh, M. L., Alijani, M., Helfrich, G. B., Schreiner, G. E., and Ramwell, P. W. Urine thromboxane as an immunologic monitor in kidney transplant patients. *Transplant. Proc.* 16:1603-1605, 1984.
45. Freed, B., Walsh, A., Pietrocoia, D., MacDowell, R., Laffin, R., and Lempert, N. Early detection of renal allograft rejection by serum monitoring of serum C reactive protein. *Transplantation* 37:215-218, 1984.
46. Frey, B. M., Walker, C., Frey, F. J., and de Weck, A. L. Pharmacokinetics and pharmacodynamics of three different prednisolone prodrugs: Effects on circulating lymphocyte subsets and function. *J. Immunol.* 133:2479-2487, 1984.
47. Fuller, L., Kyriakides, G., Flaa, C., Esquenazi, V., and Miller, J. In vitro generation of human mixed lymphocyte culture suppressor cells. I. Cellular characterization and specificity. *Transplantation* 29:54-60, 1980.
48. Gailiunas, P., Suthanthiran, M., Person, A., Strom, T. B., Carpenter, C. B., and Garovoy, M. R. Posttransplant immunologic monitoring of the renal allograft recipient. *Transplant. Proc.* 10:609-611, 1978.
49. Goulmy, E., Perslin, G. G., Blokland, E., D'Amaro, J., and van Rood, J. J. Cell-mediated lympholysis studies in renal allograft recipients. *Transplantation* 31:210-217, 1981.
50. Green, W. F., Niblack, G. D., Richie, R. E., Johnson, H. K., MacDonell, R. C., and Tallent, M. B. High-dose versus low-dose steroid therapy in conjunction with rabbit anti-human lymphocyte serum: Flow cytometric monitoring of lymphocyte parameters. *Transplant. Proc.* 16:1517-1519, 1984.
51. Guttmann, R. D., and Poulsen, R. S. Fluorescent activated cell sorter analysis of lymphocyte subsets after renal transplantation. *Transplant. Proc.* 15:1160-1162, 1983.
52. Haynes, B. F., Katz, P., and Fauci, A. S. Immune responses of human lymphocytes in vitro. In *Progress in Clinical Immunology,* R. S. Schwartz, ed. Grune & Stratton, New York, 1982, vol. 4, pp. 23-62.
53. Hayry, P. Intragraft events in allograft destruction. *Transplantation* 38:1-6, 1984.
54. Helling, T. S., and Cross, D. E. Identification of renal allograft rejection using selected monoclonal antibodies to human lymphocyte subsets. *Transplant. Proc.* 16:1548-1549, 1984.
55. Herberman, R. B. Natural Killer (NK) cells. In *The Lymphocyte,* K. W. Sell and W. V. Miller, eds. Alan R. Liss, Inc., New York, 1981, pp. 33-43.
56. Hersh, E. M., Butler, W. T., Rossen, R. D., Morgan, R. D., and Suki, W. In vitro studies

of the human response to organ allografts: Appearance and detection of circulating activation lymphocytes. *J. Immunol.* 107:571-578, 1971.

57. Hoffman, R. A., Kung, P. C., Hansen, W. P., and Goldstein, G. Simple and rapid measurement of human T lymphocytes and their subclasses in peripheral blood. *Proc. Natl. Acad. Sci. USA* 77:4914-1917, 1980.
58. Jeffrey, J. R., Cheung, K., Masniuk, J., and Taylor, D. Mixed lymphocyte responses: Lack of correlation with cadaveric renal allograft survival and blood transfusions. *Transplantation* 38:42-45, 1984.
59. Junor, B. J. R., D'Apice, A. J. F., and Kincaid-Smith, P. Circulating immune complexes after renal transplantation. *Transplantation* 30:111-113, 1980.
60. Karol, R. A., Eng, J., Dennison, D. K., Faris, E., and Marcus, D. M. Hereditary abnormalities of the OKT4 human lymphocyte epitope in two families. *J. Clin. Immunol.* 4:71-74, 1984.
61. Kerman, R. H., Flechner, S. M., Van Buren, C. T., Payne, W., and Kahan, B. D. Immunologic monitoring of renal allograft recipients treated with cyclosporine. *Transplant. Proc.* 15:2302-2305, 1983.
62. Kerman, R. H., Floyd, M., Van Buren, C., McConnell, B. J., McConnell, R., and Kahan, B. D. Correlation of nonspecific immune monitoring with rejection or impaired function of renal allografts. *Transplantation* 32:16-23, 1981.
63. Kerman, R. H., and Geis, W. P. Total and active T cell dynamics in renal allograft recipients. *Surgery* 79:398-407, 1976.
64. Kerman, R. H., Ing, T. S., Hano, J. E., and Geis, W. P. Prognostic significance of the active thymus-derived rosette-forming cells in renal allograft survival: A preliminary report. *Surgery* 82:607-612, 1977.
65. Kerman, R. H., Van Buren, C. T., Payne, W., Flechner, S., and Kahan, B. D. Monitoring of T cell subsets and immune events in renal allograft recipients. *Transplant. Proc.* 15:1170-1172, 1983.
66. Knowles, D. M., Dodson, L. D., Raab, R., Mittler, R. S., Talle, M. A., and Goldstein, G. The application of monoclonal antibodies to the characterization and diagnosis of lymphoid neoplasms: A review of recent studies. *Diagn. Immunol.* 1:142-149, 1983.
67. Kovithavongs, T., and Dossetor, J. B. The real meaning of changing peripheral blood helper to cytotoxic/suppressor cell ratio during renal allograft rejection. *Transplant. Proc.* 16:1486-1489, 1984.
68. Kovithavongs, T., Schlaut, V., Pazderka, V., Lao, V., Razderka, F., Bettcher, K. B., and Dossetor, J. B. Posttransplant monitoring with special consideration of technique and interpretation of LMC. *Transplant. Proc.* 10:547-551, 1978.
69. Kung, P. C., Berger, C. L., Estabrook, A., and Edeslson, R. L. Monoclonal antibodies for clinical investigation of human T lymphocytes. *Int. J. Dermatol.* 22:67-74, 1983.
70. Kurnick, J. T., Warrens, A. R., Moscicki, R. A., and Leary, C. P. T-cell subsets in human lymphocytes maintained in IL-2 medium after PHA or mixed lymphocyte reaction activation. *Clin. Immunol. Immunopathol.* 27:444-451, 1983.
71. Lehner, T., Brines, R., Jones, T., and Avery, J. Detection of cross-reacting murine I-J like determinants on a human subset of $T8^+$ antigen binding, presenting and contrasuppressor cells. *Clin. Exp. Immunol.* 58:410-441, 1984.
72. Lewis, R. E., Kirchner, K., Preuss, T., Raju, S., Krueger, R., Cuchens, M., Bower, J. D., and Cruse, J. M. Serial monitoring of T cell subset ratios with monoclonal antibodies in steroid- and antithymocyte globulin-treated patients with renal allotransplants. *Clin. Immunol. Immunopathol.* 31:241-253, 1984.
73. Lipinski, M., Tursz, T., Finale, Y., and Amiel, J. L. Dissociation of natural killer cell activity and antibody-dependent-cell-mediated cytotoxicity in kidney allograft recipients receiving high-dose immunosuppressive therapy. *Transplant. Proc.* 29:214-218, 1980.

74. Lordon, R. E., Stelzer, G. T., Garrison, R. N., and Ferrone, S. Early determination of renal allograft survival: A correlation between cytotoxic antibodies in recipient sera, renal pathology, and response to antirejection therapy. *Transplant. Proc.* 16: 1588-1590, 1984.
75. Lotze, M. T., Marquis, D. M., Carey, A. S., Byer, B. J., Hoy, W. E., and May, A.G. Two new assays for the early detection of transplant rejection: IL-2 response and PHA-augmented NK activity. *Transplant. Proc.* 15:1796-1799, 1983.
76. MacSween, J. M., Cohen, A. D., and Rajaraman, K. Donor-specific cellular responses and preexisting nonspecific responsiveness as interrelated determinants of renal transplant survival. *Transplant. Proc.* 16:1410-1412, 1984.
77. Manca, F., Barocci, S., Kunkl, G., Guerreri, G., Constantini, M., and Celada, F. Recognition of donor fibroblast antigens by lymphocytes homing in the human grafted kidney. *Transplantation* 36:670-674, 1983.
78. Margreiter, R., Fuchs, D., Hausen, A., Huber, C., Reibnegger, G., Spielberger, M., and Wachter, H. Neopterin as a new biochemical marker for diagnosis of allograft rejection. *Transplantation* 36:650-653, 1983.
79. Marolda, R., Tilden, A. B., Abo, T., Dougherty, P. A., and Balch, C. M. Characterization of a subset of human natural killer cells that express OKM1 but lack HNK-1 (Leu-7) antigens. *Scand. J. Immunol.* 20:261-265, 1984.
80. Mathew, M., Kovithavongs, T., and Dossetor, J. B. Donor-specific suppressor cells and donor-specific loss of cell-mediated lympholysis in renal allograft recipients: A comparative study. *Transplant. Proc.* 16:1478-1480, 1984.
81. Mazaheri, R., Stiller, C. R., Keown, P., McKenzie, N., Howson, W., Farrow, K., McFarlane, D., and Sinclair, N. R. Temporal effect of cyclosporine immunosuppression on T lymphocyte subsets, Ia-reactive cells, and donor-specific immunity in cardiac allograft recipients. *Transplant. Proc.* 16:1537-1539 (1984).
82. Mittler, R. S., Lock, R., Sheffler, B., Talle, M. A., Rao, P. E., and Goldstein, G. Resting and activation antigens of T cells: Studies with OKT10 and OKT20 monoclonal antibodies. *Diagn. Immunol.* 1:120-128, 1983.
83. Miyawaki, T., Taga, K., Nagaoki, T., Seki, H., Suzuki, Y., and Taniguchi, N. Circadian changes of T lymphocyte subsets in human peripheral blood. *Clin. Exp. Immunol.* 55: 618-622, 1984.
84. Mohanakumar, T., Ellis, T. M., Reinitz, E. R., Page, S. D., Mendez-Picon, G., Goldman, M. H., Lower, R., and Lee, H. M. Daily monitoring of T cell subpopulations in renal allograft recipients: High-resolution measurement of T cell kinetics and their relevance to clinical course. *Transplant. Proc.* 16:1490-1491, 1984.
85. Mohanakumar, T., Waldrep, J. C., Phibbs, M., Mendez-Picon, G., Kaplan, A. M., and Lee, H. M. Serological characterization of antibodies eluted from chronically rejected human renal allografts. *Transplantation* 32:61-66, 1981.
86. Nanni-Costa, A., Vangelista, A., Frasca, G. M., Stefoni, S., and Bonomini, V. T cell subsets in renal allograft recipients. *Transplant. Proc.* 15:1176-1177, 1983.
87. Nunez, G., McPhaul, J., and Stastny, P. Characterization of B cell and monocyte antibodies in recipient sera and in eluates from rejected kidney allografts. *Transplant. Proc.* 13:111-113, 1981.
88. Oka, T., Yoshimura, N., Ohmori, Y., Aikawa, I., Matsumura, T., Usui, T., Arakawa, K., and Hashimoto, I. Analysis of lymphocytes concerned in spontaneous blastogenesis during acute rejection. *Transplant. Proc.* 15:2298-2301, 1983.
89. Ono, E., Dohi, K., Fukuda, Y., Asahara, T., Yahata, H., and Ezaki, H. Cell mediated lympholysis in kidney transplant recipients. *Transplant. Proc.* 16:1594-1597, 1984.
90. Ooi, Y. M., Ooi, B. S., Vallota, E. H., First, M. R., and Pollack, V. E. Circulating immune complexes after renal transplantation. Correlation of increased 125-I-C1q bind-

ing activity with acute rejection characterized by fibrin deposition in the kidney. *J. Clin. Invest.* 60:611-619, 1977.

91. Paradis, I. L., Merrall, E. J., Krell, J. M., Dauber, J. H., Rogers, R. M., and Rabin, B. S. Lymphocyte enumeration: A comparison between a modified avidin-biotin-immunoperoxidase system and flow cytometry. *J. Histochem. Cytochem.* 32:358-362, 1984.
92. Pfeffer, P. F., Thorsby, E., and Hirshberg, H. Cell-mediated cytotoxicity toward the donor in patients with well-functioning kidney grafts. *Transplantation* 35:546-551, 1983.
93. Prince, H. E., Ettenger, R. B., Dorey, F. J., Fine, R. N., and Fahey, J. L. Azathioprine suppression of natural killer activity and antibody-dependent cellular cytotoxicity in renal transplant recipients. *J. Immunol.* 4:312-318, 1984.
94. Ramsey, K. M., Djeu, J. Y., and Rook, A. H. Decreased circulating large granular lymphocytes associated with depressed natural killer cell activity in renal transplant recipients. *Transplantation* 38:351-356, 1984.
95. Raskova, J., Ghobrial, I., Shea, S. M., Eisinger, R. P., and Raska, K. Suppressor cells in end-stage renal disease: Functional assays and monoclonal antibody analysis. *Am. J. Med.* 76:847-853, 1984.
96. Redlich, P. N., Leapman, S. B., Marder, P., Schmidtke, J., Smith, E. J., Fineberg, N., and Filo, R. S. Evaluation of lymphocyte subsets and suppressor cell function in long-term renal transplant recipients. *Transplant. Proc.* 16:1555-1557, 1984.
97. Reinherz, E. L., Rubinstein, A., Geha, R. S., Strelkausas, A. J., Rosen, F. S., and Schlossman, S. F. Abnormalities of immunoregulatory T cells in disorders of immune function. *N. Engl. J. Med.* 301:1018-1022, 1979.
98. Rhodes, C. L., Goldman, M. H., Mendez-Picon, G., Lee, H. M., and Mohanakumar, T. Multiple specificities of B lymphocyte-reactive antibodies and their significance in renal allograft survival. *Transplant. Proc.* 16:1425-1426, 1984.
99. Rinaldo, C. R., Hamoudi, W. H., De Biasio, R. L., Rabin, B., Hakala, T. R., and Liebert, M. Cellular immune response and cytomegalovirus infection in renal transplant recipients receiving cyclosporine. *Transplant. Proc.* 15:2775-2778, 1983.
100. Rolley, R. T., Williams, G. M., Lerner, R. A., Hanscom, G., and Hume, D. M. Characterization of antibodies following human renal homograft rejection. *Transplant. Proc.* 1:275-278, 1696.
101. Romain, P. L., and Schlossman, S. F. Human T lymphocyte subsets: Functional heterogeneity and surface recognition structures. *J. Clin. Invest.* 74:1559-1565, 1984.
102. Rook, A. H., Frederick, W. R. J., Burns, W. H., Djeu, J. Y., Kirmani, N., Jackaon, L. B., Manischewitz, J. F., Saral, R., Santos, G. W., and Quinnan, G. V. Natural killer cell activity and interferon release predict survival from viral infection in bone marrow transplant recipients. *Transplant. Proc.* 15:1773-1776, 1983.
103. Rook, A. H., Smith, W. J., Burdick, J. F., Manischewitz, J. F., Frederick, W., Siegel, J. P., Williams, G. M., and Quinnan, G. V. Virus-specific cytotoxic lymphocyte responses are predictive of the outcome of cytomegalovirus infection of renal transplant recipients. *Transplant. Proc.* 16:1466-1469, 1984.
104. Roth, D., Kyriakides, G. K., Fuller, L., and Miller, J. Human peripheral blood and splenic T lymphocyte reactions versus kidney cortical cells. *Transplant. Proc.* 16:1532-1534, 1984.
105. Rubin, R. H., Carney, W. P., Schooley, R. B., Colvin, R. B., Burton, R. C., Hoffman, R. A., Hansen, W. P., Cosimi, A. B., Russell, P. S., and Hersch, M. S. The effect of infection on T lymphocyte subpopulations: A preliminary report. *Int. J. Immunopharm.* 3:307-312, 1981.

106. Satomi, S., Tanimura, S., Kunori, T., Taguchi, Y., and Kasai, M. Monitoring of B lymphocyte response with protein-A plaque assay in kidney transplant patients. *Transplantation* 35:324-328, 1983.
107. Schandene, L., Steen, F. V., Romasco, F., and Wybran, J. Active T rosettes, human autologous T rosettes, OKT8 and OKT4 cells, Con A-induced suppressive activity, and autoantibodies: Clinical correlations. *Clin. Immunol. Immunopathol.* 28:147-154, 1983.
108. Schlesinger, M., Lew, F., and Bekesi, J. G. Surface antigen determinants in subpopulations of peripheral blood NK and T cells separated by Percoll density fractionation. *J. Clin. Lab. Immunol.* 13:195-202, 1984.
109. Shapira, Z., Shohat, B., Boner, G., Levi, J., Joshua, H., and Servadio, C. Theophylline: A possible immunoregulator of T cells. *Transplant. Proc.* 14:113-115, 1983.
110. Shield, C. F., Blackmore, M., Lemon, J. A., and Cook, J. L. Posttransplant immune monitoring with monoclonal antibodies. *Transplant. Proc.* 16:1496-1498, 1984.
111. Smith, M. D., Williams, J. D., Coles, G. A., and Salaman, J. R. Blood transfusions, suppressor T cells, and renal transplant survival. *Transplantation* 36:647-650, 1983.
112. Smith, W. J., Burdick, J. F., and Williams, G. M. Immunologic monitoring of renal transplant recipients. *Transplant. Proc.* 15:1182-1183, 1983.
113. Smith, W. J., Burdick, J. F., and Williams, G. M. Fluorescent and light microscopic analysis of peripheral blood leukocytes from human renal allograft recipients. *Transplant. Proc.* 16:1546-1547, 1984.
114. Stelzer, G. T., McLeish, K. R., Lorden, R. E., and Watson, S. L. Alterations in T lymphocyte subpopulations associated with renal allograft rejection. *Transplantation* 37:261-264, 1984.
115. Stiller, C. R., Sinclair, N. R. S., Abrahams, S., McGirr, D., Singh, H., Howson, W. T., and Ulan, R. A. Anti-donor immune responses in prediction of transplant rejection. *N. Engl. J. Med.* 294:978-982, 1976.
116. Suciu-Foca, N., Woodward, K., Reed, E., Khan, R., Godfrey, M., Hardy, M., and Reemtsma, K. Posttransplant evaluation of T- and B-cell function. *Transplant. Proc.* 13:1584-1588, 1981.
117. Suthanthiran, M., Kaye, W. A., Rubin, A. L., and Stenzel, K. H. Interleukin-2 profiles in renal graft recipients. *Transplant. Proc.* 16:1473-1474, 1984.
118. Suthanthiran, M., Kaye, W. A., Vogel, R. M., Solomon, S. D., Rubin, A. L., Novogrodsky, A., and Stenzel, K. H. Immunosurveillance mechanisms operative in renal allograft recipients. *Transplant. Proc.* 15:1800-1801, 1983.
119. Talle, M. A., Allegar, N., Makowski, M., and Goldstein, G. Distinct classes of human T cell activation antigens. *Cell. Immunol.* 84:285-298, 1984.
120. Talpaz, M., and Mavligit, G. M. Characterization of the human effector and suppressor T cells by their activity in mixed lymphocyte reaction and by monoclonal antibody phenotyping. *J. Clin. Lab. Immunol.* 12:217-220, 1983.
121. TenBerge, R. J. M., Sauerwein, H. P., Yong, S. L., and Schellekens, P. T. A. Administration of prednisolone in vivo affects the ratio of OKT4/OKT8 and the LDH-isoenzyme pattern of human T lymphocytes. *Clin. Immunol. Immunopathol.* 30:91-103, 1984.
122. Ten Berge, R. J. M., Schellekens, P. T. A., Surachno, S., The, T. H., Ten Veen, J. H., and Wilmink, J. M. The influence of therapy with azathioprine and prednisone on the immune system of kidney transplant recipients. *Clin. Immunol. Immunopathol.* 21:20-32, 1981.
123. Thomas, F., Griesedieck, C., Thomas, J., Carver, M., Whitley, T., Watten, R., and Williams, D. Use of newer immunologic assays for individualized immunodulation after renal transplant. *Transplant. Proc.* 16:1520-1521, 1984.

124. Thomas, F. T., Griesedieck, C., Thomas, J., Carver, M., Whitley, T., Warren, R., and Williams, D. Differential effects of horse ATG and rabbit ATG on T cell and T cell subset levels measured by monoclonal antibodies. *Transplant. Proc.* 16:1561-1563, 1984.
125. Thomas, F. T., Lee, H. M., Lower, R. R., and Thomas, J. M. Immunologic monitoring as a guide to the management of transplant recipients. *Surg. Clin. North Am.* 59:253-281, 1979.
126. Thomas, F., Lee, H. M., Lower, R. R., and Thomas, J. M. Value of immunologic monitoring studies of human E, EA, and EAC rosetting lymphocyte subpopulations in renal and cardiac transplantation. *Transplant. Proc.* 13:1599-1603, 1981.
127. Thomas, F., Thomas, J., Mendez, G., Lower, R., and Lee, H. M. Differential effects of immunosuppressive drugs on human T, B, and K lymphocytes. *Transplantation* 24:435-441, 1977.
128. Thomas, J. H., Kinnaman, M. L., Pierce, G. E., Shaw, L. W., and Clancy, J. Spontaneous blastogenesis and protein synthesis as monitors of renal allograft rejection. *Transplant. Proc.* 16:1600-1602, 1984.
129. Thomas, J. M., Carver, F. M., Foil, M. B., and Thomas, F. T. Role of prostaglandin-dependent suppressor cells in the immunosuppressive action of rabbit antithymocyte globulin. *Transplant. Proc.* 15:1770-1772, 1983.
130. van Es, A., Baldwin, W. M., Oljans, P. J., Tanke, H. J., Ploem, J. S., and van Es, L. A. Expression of HLA-DR on T lymphocytes following renal transplantation, and association with graft rejection episodes and cytomegalovirus infection. *Transplantation* 37:65-69, 1981.
131. van Es, A., and Meyer, C. Mononuclear cells in renal allografts: Correlation with peripheral blood lymphocyte subpopulations and graft prognosis. *Transplantation* 37:134-138, 1984.
132. van Wauwe, J., and Goosens, J. Monoclonal anti-human T lymphocyte antibodies: Enumeration and characterization of T cell subsets. *Immunology* 42:157-164, 1981.
133. Walle, A., Suthanthiran, M., Taufield, P. A., Yankiver, B., Rubin, A. L., Stenzel, K. H., and Darzynkiewicz, Z. Multiparameter analysis of cell activation in renal allograft recipients. *Transplant. Proc.* 16:1586-1587, 1984.
134. Waltzer, W. C., Bachvaroff, R. J., Anaise, D., and Rappaport, F. T. Natural killer cell activity after renal transplantation. *Transplant. Proc.* 16:1527-1529, 1984.
135. Waltzer, W. C., Bachvaroff, R. J., Anaise, D., and Rappaport, F. T. Lymphocyte subpopulations in renal transplantation. *Transplant. Proc.* 16:1544-1545, 1984.
136. Wang, T., Abbasnezhad, M., Yasmineh, W., and Foker, J. E. Lymphocyte lactate dehydrogenase as a marker in predicting allograft rejection in organ transplantation patients. *Transplant. Proc.* 15:1827-1829, 1983.
137. White, J., Meyer, E., and Hardy, M. A. Prediction of onset and termination of renal allograft rejection by serum levels of C-reactive protein. *Transplant. Proc.* 13:682-685, 1981.
138. Williams, J. M., Christenson, L., Araujo, J. L., Carpenter, C. B., Milford, E. L., Shapiro, H. M., and Strom, T. D. A new approach to the monitoring of kidney transplant patients via flow cytometric analysis of T-cell subsets, activation antigens, and DNA content. *Transplant. Proc.* 15:1957-1961, 1983.

14

CYTOMEGALOVIRUS INFECTION IN RENAL TRANSPLANTATION

Clinical Importance and Control

Robert H. Rubin and Robert B. Colvin
Massachusetts General Hospital and Harvard Medical School, Boston, Massachusetts

The single most important infection that complicates the course of renal transplantation is that due to cytomegalovirus (CMV). Cytomegalovirus is ubiquitous among transplant patients, causes a broad range of clinical syndromes that play a significant role in determining both patient and allograft survival, and is modulated by the two major phenomena that underline the transplant experience—allograft rejection and immunosuppression [66, 71,74]. It is the purpose of this chapter to summarize the current status of CMV infection in renal transplantation, concentrating particularly on those factors and events that directly influence patient and allograft survival.

VIROLOGIC CHARACTERISTICS OF CMV

Cytomegalovirus, like the other members of the herpes virus group (which in humans includes Epstein-Barr virus, herpes simplex virus, and varicella zoster virus, as well as CMV), is a double-stranded DNA virus with an icosahedral capsid of 162 capsomeres. Perhaps the most important virologic properties of these viruses, in that they are major determinants of clinical events, are their ability to exhibit *latency,* a high degree of *cell association,* and *oncogenicity* [35].

With most viral infections, once clinical recovery has occurred and the virus can no longer be isolated from the host, the host is rendered immune and free of further risk of clinical disease from this agent. This is not true for CMV (or the other herpes viruses). Following primary infection, although a certain resistance to exogenous reinfection can be demonstrated, CMV remains dormant in a variety of cells throughout the body, capable of being reactivated if subjected to certain influences. The most notable of these influences are immunosuppression, allograft rejection, and the hormonal changes of pregnancy. When such events occur, although conventional virologic techniques have heretofore been unable to demonstrate the presence of the virus, CMV now emerges from its latent state, again capable of causing clinical disease. For all practical purposes, anyone who has had primary CMV infection in the past (and thus has circulating anti-CMV antibodies today), harbors latent virus that will be reactivated at any time when subjected to one of these influences. The sites of CMV latency have not been totally elucidated. In a murine CMV model, molecular biologic techniques of DNA hybridization have shown that splenic B lymphocytes, salivary gland tissue, the prostate, testes, and probably, macrophages harbor latent CMV DNA. Less complete information in humans suggests that peripheral blood leukocytes, the kidney, and some colonic tumors can harbor the virus in latent form. It is likely that CMV DNA will be found in other human tissues as well [35,66].

The second major characteristic of CMV that helps to determine its clinical effects is its high degree of cell association, with cell-to-cell spread of the virus characteristic. With direct contact between cells so important in the pathogenesis of the infection, neutralizing antibodies and complement are rendered relatively inefficient as host defenses, and an increased emphasis is placed upon cell-mediated immunity as the primary host defense against CMV. The corollary to this observation is that any clinical situation, such as transplantation, in which cell-mediated immunity is impaired, will be associated with an increased incidence and increased severity of CMV infection [35,66,74].

Finally, CMV must be regarded as a potentially oncogenic agent. Portions of the CMV genome are homologous to the *myc* oncogene [27,72,78], and both the intact virus and cloned CMV DNA fragments have been shown to transform (the in vitro correlate of oncogenesis) a variety of cell lines [51]. In other species, under special conditions, administration of the virus has been associated with the production of malignancy [35]. In humans, CMV has been closely associated with the pathogenesis of Kaposi's sarcoma (see below), and, to a lesser degree, with colonic cancer.

EPIDEMIOLOGY OF CMV INFECTION IN THE RENAL TRANSPLANT PATIENT

There are two major epidemiologic patterns of CMV infection observed in renal transplant patients [5,36]. The first is primary CMV disease in which a transplant recipient who has no detectable antibodies to CMV prior to transplant (the laboratory marker for the lack of significant past experience with the virus) receives latently infected cells from a seropositive donor and then reactivates dormant virus from such cells posttransplant. These cells are transmitted to the seronegative recipient in one of two ways. Some 80-90% of transplant patients who develop primary CMV infection posttransplant receive their infection via the renal allograft itself. That is, although no detectable virus can be isolated from the seropositive donor by conventional virologic techniques, the kidney derived from such a seropositive individual harbors latently infected cells capable of being reactivated posttransplant, thus causing primary infection in the seronegative recipient. The nature of the latently infected cells within the allograft is currently unknown, with an important question whether it is renal tissue per se or so-called passenger leukocytes within the graft that harbor the dormant virus. This question is of more than academic interest, since, if the passenger leukocytes within the graft are the major source of primary infection, pretreatment of the donor with cyclophosphamide, for example, to deplete the allograft of these leukocytes could be of use in preventing primary CMV infection [5,36,71].

In approximately 10-20% of cases of primary CMV infection, the source of such infections is posttransplant blood transfusions. Preliminary data would suggest that there is no difference in either the incidence of symptomatic disease (approximately 70% of patients with laboratory evidence of primary CMV posttransplant develop symptomatic disease) or the severity of these symptoms whether the source of primary infection is a latently infected allograft or blood transfusion [35,66,71,74]. Not all blood products carry an equal risk of transmitting primary CMV, as the latently infected cells in blood harboring the virus appear to lie within the leukocytic fraction. It is believed that the allogeneic reaction directed against transfused white blood cells is responsible for the reactivation of latent CMV posttransfusion. For this to occur, viable leukocytes must be present.

Whereas packed red blood cell preparations depleted of leukocytes carry essentially no risk of transmitting the virus, even to the most immunosuppressed recipient, leukocyte transfusions carry a high risk [35,40,41,66,81]. There are, then, two strategies available to protect the seronegative transplant recipient against posttransplant primary CMV infection: the use of units of blood only from seronegative donors, a strategy that works but that requires the elimination of 40-75% of donors, and the use of leukocyte-free units of blood for transfusion [1,7,81,85]. Perhaps the most efficient means of accomplishing this is by the use of frozen, deglycerolyzed red blood cells, which are essentially free of viable leukocytes, for posttransplant transfusion [7,81]. Thus, in one study we have noted that none of 21 seronegative adult patients seroconverted after receiving a total of 157 units of such blood [81]. Other investigators working with a variety of adult populations have noted similar findings [4,40]. Recently, Brady et al. [7], in a study of blood transfusions in neonates, an immunosuppressed population perhaps more akin to transplant recipients, reported that none of 106 infants transfused an average of 5.7 units each, 51.4% of which were from CMV seropositive donors, developed serologic or clinical evidence of posttransfusion CMV infection. Therefore, although there remains some controversy about whether frozen red blood cells pretransplant provide as much antirejection prophylaxis as regular units of blood, there seems to be little reason not to use the frozen red cell preparation posttransplant in CMV seronegative individuals.

The second, and more common, epidemiologic problem of CMV infection posttransplant is reactivation infection. In this form of CMV, patients with past experience with the virus (and thus seropositive prior to transplant) reactivate their own latent virus after transplantation. Present data would suggest that essentially every seropositive individual will manifest laboratory evidence (viral isolation and/or rise in serum antibody levels) posttransplant, with approximately 20% of these patients developing clinical disease on this basis [35,66,71,74].

An important unanswered question is whether CMV superinfection can occur; that is, is the clinical outcome of transplanting an allograft or transfusing a unit of blood from a seropositive donor into a seropositive recipient any different from the outcome when the donor is seronegative? In the laboratory, it can be shown that strains of human CMV isolated from different patients exhibit considerable genomic and antigenic heterogeneity; for example, if CMV antigen is prepared from two different strains of human CMV, very different antibody titers can be observed in the same serum specimens using the different antigen preparations [35]. The significance of these laboratory findings, however, is unclear. Detailed virologic studies of congenital CMV infection in infants has shown that superinfection can occur, but it is a rare event [37]. Fryd et al. [26] have reported that the transplantation of kidneys from seropositive donors into seropositive recipients indeed does have a worse clinical outcome than if kidneys from seronegative donors are used, suggesting that superinfection in clinical transplantation is indeed important. However, in a multicenter study (involving 50 different transplant centers in North America), we have been unable to confirm this finding, so the importance of reinfection remains an open issue [73]. As will be discussed subsequently, the answer to this question will have an impact on efforts to develop a monovalent vaccine against CMV, the proper deployment of antiviral strategies, and, possibly, even in the choice of donors for a given recipient.

It should be emphasized that a major factor influencing the effects of CMV infection in a transplant population is the level of CMV infection in the community served by a particular transplant center. In the community, there is a steady rate of acquisition of CMV seropositivity, with intimate mucosal content, especially venereal contact, the principal mode of spread after infancy. In general, in most of Western Europe and North America approximately 15% of individuals will be seropositive by age 2, 30% by age 25, and 50-60% after age 50 [35]. Significantly higher rates of CMV seropositivity are observed among male homosexuals, heterosexuals who are sexually promiscuous, and among lower socioeconomic groups [35]. Therefore, the incidence of CMV infection, the percentage of cases due to primary or reactivation disease, and the occurrence of clinical disease will vary from transplant center to center, depending upon the age, socioeconomic level, and sexual practices of both the donor and recipient population [71].

Notable by its absence from this discussion is person-to-person spread among dialysis and transplant patients and personnel. It does not appear to occur [4,81]. In contrast, there is the occasional transplant patient who is seronegative prior to transplant and remains free of CMV infection for the critical first 4-6 months posttransplant, only to develop community-acquired primary CMV infection thereafter. Such cases account for approximately 5% of cases of posttransplant primary CMV and, although lethal cases of this type have been reported, usually have a benign course—presumably due to the low level of immunosuppressive therapy administered at this point posttransplant [71]. Linnemann et al. [44] have reported a fascinating variation on this theme: a 53-year-old man who was seronegative prior to transplant, transiently seroconverted 6 weeks posttransplant, and then developed lethal disseminated CMV infection 16 months posttransplant. This unusual case presumably represents either an atypical case of late reactivation infection or superinfection acquired in the community in an individual with an impaired host response to his first experience with the virus.

FACTORS INFLUENCING THE COURSE OF CMV INFECTION IN THE RENAL TRANSPLANT PATIENT

The two experiences that differentiate the transplant patient from other patients, chronic immunosuppression and allograft rejection, are, at the same time, the most important modulators of the course of CMV infection posttransplant. In particular, both the form of immunosuppression and its intensity have been shown to profoundly influence the clinical consequences of CMV infection in these patients. A historical perspective underlines this observation. Prior to 1966, when corticosteroids alone were utilized for immunosuppression, CMV infection was virtually unknown. Following the introduction of azathioprine, cyclophosphamide, and antilymphocyte preparations, CMV became the important clinical problem that it is today [35]. Dowling et al. [22], in another population of patients being treated with immunosuppression, patients with rheumatologic disease, have documented this same phenomenon: CMV could not be isolated from 86 patients treated with steroids alone, whereas 5 of 9 patients treated with cyclophosphamide began to shed this virus.

Of all the immunosuppressive agents commonly used, antilymphocyte preparations, when given in addition to azathioprine and prednisone therapy (as is commonly done), appear to have the greatest potentiating effect on CMV infection [19,46,55]. In particular, in a carefully controlled study, Cheeseman et al. [19] reported a higher rate of viremia and symptomatic disease and an attenuation of the beneficial effects of a prophylactic course of α-interferon in patients treated with antithymocyte globulin (ATG). However, in a subsequent study, it was shown that not all the blame for virus-promoting effects should be directed at the ATG. In this second study, the ATG patients received 50% as much azathioprine and prednisone as the patients receiving just those two conventional agents. There was no difference in the two groups in terms of either viral isolation or clinical disease, suggesting that it is the net immunosuppressive effect or net cytotoxic (lymphocytotoxic ?) effect that is the determining factor, not just the immunosuppressive agent employed, in modulating the effect of CMV infection in the transplant patient [68].

Recent experience with cyclosporine suggests that regimens that include this drug plus low-dose steroids are associated with a lower rate of symptomatic CMV disease than regimens formerly employed [57,64]. However, it should be emphasized that such observations are still preliminary and may, in part, be influenced by the kind and intensity of immunosuppression previously utilized by a particular transplant center. Thus, a program that predominantly employed an intensive immunosuppressive program including an antilymphocyte preparation is far more likely to show less CMV infection with a cyclosporine regimen than a program that previously used lesser amounts of immunosuppression without an antilymphocyte preparation. Again, the concept of the net state of immunosuppression must be emphasized in evaluating the data.

Since the amount of allograft rejection is closely linked to the type and intensity of immunosuppression administered, there is little direct evidence to prove that allograft rejection influences the course of CMV infection. However, there are several lines of indirect evidence that are consistent with this hypothesis. Cytomegalovirus is both more common and more virulent in recipients of allografts from cadaveric donors as opposed to living related donors (with the former having considerably more rejection than the latter) [35,54,66]. In a murine model of chronically infected mice, the placement of skin grafts from histoincompatible donors significantly increased the titer of CMV in the spleen and kidneys of the graft recipients [84]. Finally, it is believed that the allogenic reaction (which is akin to allograft rejection) induced by donor leukocytes after blood transfusion is the factor responsible for reactivation of latent CMV posttransfusion [40, 42,81].

CLINICAL EFFECTS OF CMV IN THE RENAL TRANSPLANT PATIENT

Because of the chronicity of CMV infection, the inherent properties of this herpes group virus, and the chronic state of immunosuppression characteristic of the renal transplant patient, the clinical effects of this virus are much broader than those usually associated with most infectious agents. These effects may be grouped as follows [72]:

1. The production of a variety of infectious disease syndromes by the virus itself, ranging from prolonged fevers to chorioretinitis, from hepatitis to pneumonia.
2. The production of a state of immunosuppression by the virus in addition to that induced by the immunosuppressive drugs being administered. This contributes significantly to the patient's net level of immunosuppression and potentiates superinfection with a variety of opportunistic pathogens.
3. The production of a form of allograft injury induced or contributed to by the virus that is distinct from classic allograft rejection.
4. The production of malignant disease by a process in which CMV is at least an important cofactor.

Each of these clinical effects is of both practical and theoretical importance in the transplant patient.

Direct Infectious Disease Effects

More than 90% of patients who develop clinical manifestations of CMV infection, whether due to primary or reactivation infection, do so in the period 1-6 months posttransplant. Both because of the direct effects of the virus in producing infectious disease syndromes and because of its role in potentiating other infections, this time period is the most critical in terms of risks of life-threatening infection (Figure 1) [35,66,71,74]. The importance of CMV infection after renal transplantation is underlined by the observation that approximately 50% of all fevers posttransplant are due to this virus and that during the period 1-6 months posttransplant, at least two-thirds of febrile episodes are due to active CMV infection [46,58].

Although the incidence of clinically recognizable disease is two to three times more common in patients with primary rather than reactivation infection, in the individual patient the intensity of the clinical manifestations can be equally great in the two forms of CMV disease. In both instances, clinical manifestations usually begin insidiously with constitutional complaints of fever without rigors, anorexia, and malaise, sometimes accompanied by myalgias and arthralgias, dominating the clinical picture. In approximately one-third of symptomatic patients, no other manifestations of CMV develop, and the clinical picture is closely analogous to that seen in nonimmunosuppressed patients with CMV mononucleosis. In approximately one-third of transplant patients with fever due to CMV, a dry, nonproductive cough develops within a few days of the onset of constitutional symptoms. Initially, dyspnea and tachypnea are not seen, but over the course of several days progressive respiratory diseases can develop. This slowly progressive course bears emphasis, because acute respiratory deterioration over a few hours suggests superinfection with bacterial or fungal pathogens rather than CMV pneumonia by itself [35,58,66,69,71,74].

Of the common manifestations of CMV infection in the transplant patient, pneumonia is the one that separates serious illness from more benign disease. The most common form of CMV pneumonia observed in the transplant patient is a bilateral, symmetrical, peribronchovascular (interstitial) process that begins in the lung periphery and predominantly affects the lower lobes (Figure 2) [69]. Less commonly, a focal consolidation more suggestive of bacterial or fungal infection may be seen [69], and even a solitary pulmonary nodule has been reported as due to CMV along [62]. However, the important question for the clinician dealing with transplant patients 1-6 months posttransplant with pneumonia is not whether CMV is present but, rather, is anything else present? Superinfection is the usual cause of death in patients with CMV pneumonia–superinfection with *Pneumocystis carinii, Aspergillus fumigatus,* or Gram-negative bacilli being the major concerns. *Pneumocystis carinii* is the major concern, both because of its frequency in association with CMV and because its clinical manifestations are virtually identical to CMV pneumonia–insidious onset, peak incidence 1-6 months posttransplant, and identical x-ray manifestations [35, 66,69,71,74].

The two other organ systems commonly affected by CMV infection in the transplant patient are the hematologic and hepatic. A low-grade atypical lymphocytosis (5-10% of circulating leukocytes), leukopenia, and thrombocytopenia are quite common (at least 50% of patients with symptomatic CMV infection). A mild to moderate degree of hepatocellular dysfunction occurs in 25-35% of symptomatic patients [69]. Less clear is how

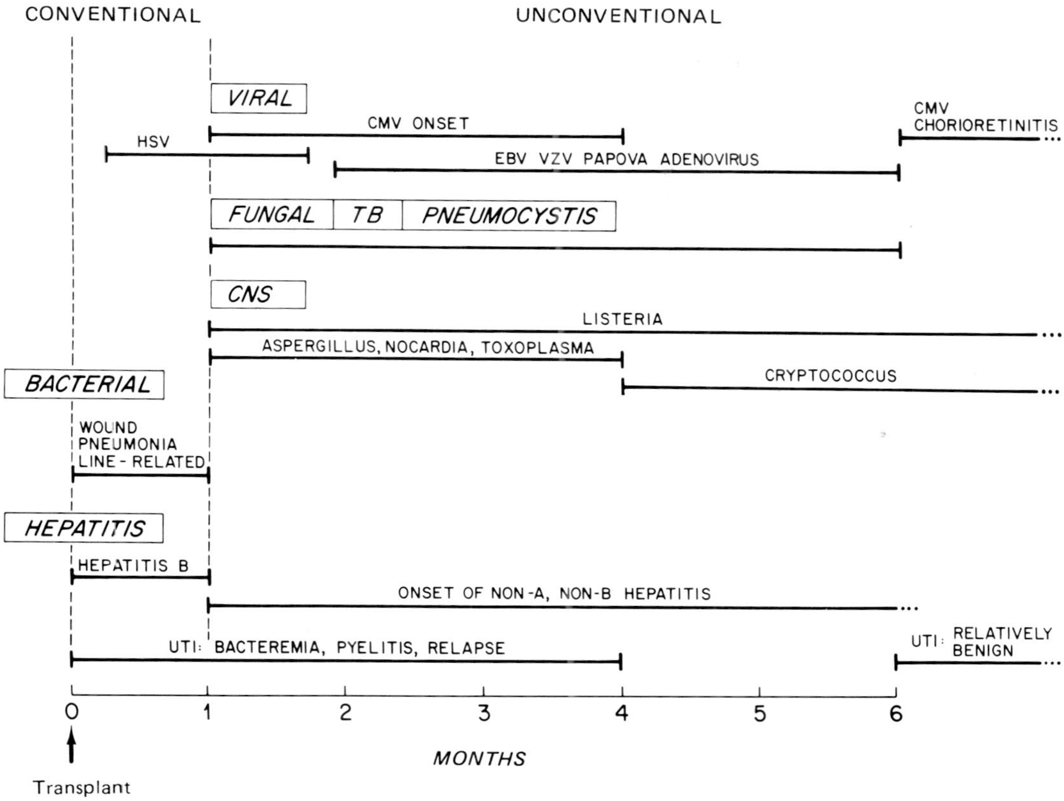

FIGURE 1 Timetable for the occurrence of infection in the renal transplant patient. Note that cytomegalovirus occupies a central position during the period 1-6 months posttransplant, the most critical period for the occurrence of infectious disease post transplant. Abbreviations used: CMV, cytomegalovirus; HSV, herpes simplex virus; EBV, Epstein-Barr virus; VZV, varicella zoster virus; CNS, central nervous system; UTI, urinary tract infection. (Modified from Rubin, et al. [74]. Reprinted by permission from the *American Journal of Medicine.*)

often CMV causes more severe forms of acute hepatitis or chronic liver disease now being attributed to so-called non-A, non-B hepatitis. It should be emphasized that the combination of fever, transient hepatocellular dysfunction, leukopenia, and/or thrombocytopenia 1-6 months posttransplant is virtually diagnostic of CMV infection [35,66,69,71,74].

Simmons and his colleagues at the University of Minnesota have described a group of patients with a "lethal CMV syndrome" [76,77], which, fortunately, is much rarer with current immunosuppressive protocols. Such patients present with fever and leukopenia and then rapidly develop severe pulmonary and hepatic dysfunction, encephalopathy, and gastrointestinal hemorrhage. Death results from either opportunistic superinfection or bowel hemorrhage. In patients with gastrointestinal hemorrhage, typical CMV inclusion bodies may be seen at the site of ulceration and the virus can be isolated. The right colon, especially the cecum, is the usual site of ulceration [3,77,80]. Similar lesions have been described in nontransplant patients with idiopathic ulcerative colitis, colonic adenocar-

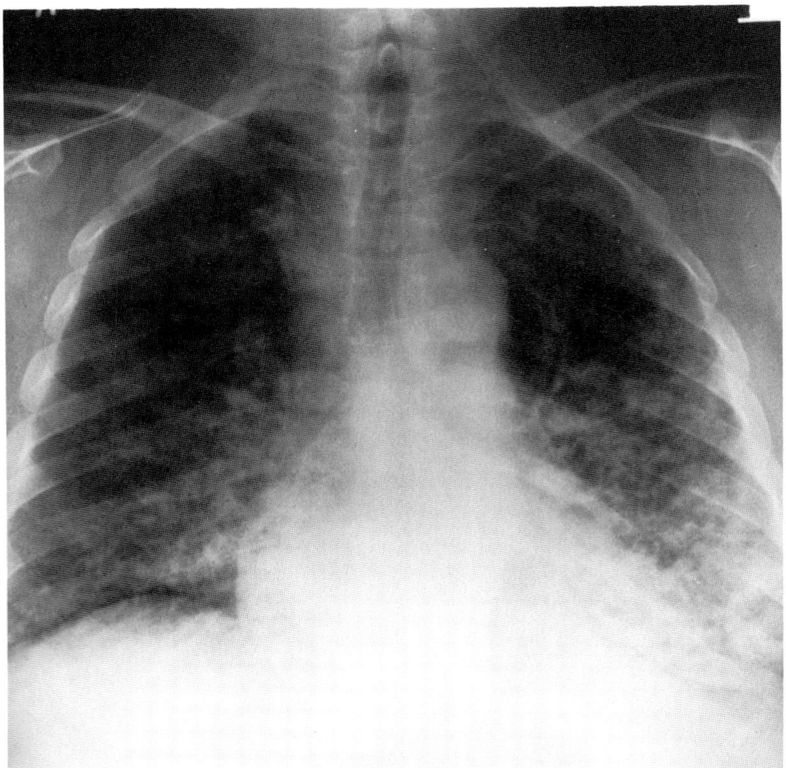

FIGURE 2 Biopsy-proven cytomegalovirus pneumonia in a recipient of a cadaver donor renal allograft. Chest x-ray and lung biopsy performed 8 weeks posttransplant.

cinoma, and other nonneoplastic forms of colonic disease. Indeed, several authors have proposed that the virus is responsible for the local ulceration, hemorrhage, and perforation that may be observed in such patients [35,66].

There is one manifestation of CMV infection that commonly begins more than 4 months posttransplant–progressive chorioretinitis, which is first discovered 4-8 months after transplantation. Although the eye disease may be unilateral at this time of presentation, it commonly progresses to involve both eyes. Typically, patients present with complaints of blurred vision, scotoma, and decreased visual acuity, although it is occasionally discovered at routine ophthalmologic evaluation of asymptomatic individuals. The initial retinal lesion appears as scattered white dots or granular particles when viewed with the ophthalmoscope. Irregular sheathing of adjacent retinal vessels is common. The funduscopic picture of hypopigmented (white) areas surrounding atrophic retina is due to the retinal pigment epithelium becoming so necrotic that its proliferative capacity is lost. Involved retinal arterioles have a white, cordlike appearance due to the sloughing of infected endothelial cells from the retinal vessels, which leads to subendothelial hemorrhage and the collection of serofibrinous material. Not uncommonly, retinal detachment or an anterior uveitis with secondary glaucoma may develop as the retinitis progresses, causing further loss of vision [9,15,47,50].

It is important to emphasize that the isolation of CMV from the urine or saliva of a transplant patient or the demonstration of a change in antibody titer do not prove that clinical disease is due to the virus—it only raises the possibility. Thus, occasional reports of encephalitis [21] and cutaneous vasculitis [49] due to CMV in transplant patients must be viewed with some caution, as the rate of asymptomatic CMV infection is quite high (reaching levels of 60-75% in patients with reactivation infection). Viremia, as opposed to peripheral excretion of the virus, is usually associated with clinically significant disease [8,19], but the absence of viremia does not rule out that possibility. A better laboratory marker of significant infection needs to be developed.

Not only will asymptomatic patients transiently excrete CMV in their urine and/or saliva, but more sustained asymptomatic viral excretion is common (in patients with previously symptomatic or asymptomatic infection). Approximately 50% of patients with acute CMV infection will continue to excrete the virus in their saliva and/or urine 2-5 years posttransplant, with approximately 20% continuing thereafter. The significance of such prolonged peripheral excretion of the virus is unclear. Of more interest, some 1-5% of patients will develop chronic viremia, which is associated with progressive chorioretinitis [20].

CMV Effects on Host Defenses and Their Significance

Cytomegalovirus infection is an important contributor to the net state of immunosuppression present in a given renal transplant patient. Indeed, it is probably fair to say that the most important "infectious disease" effect of this virus is not the array of clinical syndromes it produces by itself (see above), but rather the superinfection with a variety of opportunistic pathogens that is potentiated by the immunosuppressive effects of the virus [66,69,71,72,74].

The most important immunosuppressing effect of CMV appears to be on cell-mediated immunity. Patients with CMV infection have markedly impaired responses to skin testing to *Candida,* SKSD, mumps, and tuberculin antigens, and their in vitro lymphocyte responsiveness to these antigens and lectin stimulation is likewise depressed. It is equally interesting that individuals with demonstrable cell-mediated immunity to CMV prior to transplant lose this response in the first month posttransplant, with continuing hyporesponsiveness over the ensuing 4-6 months [35,66].

Cytomegalovirus infection is associated with suppressed monocyte function and monocyte-induced suppression of lymphocyte function [13]. A number of studies, in a variety of clinical situations, have suggested that cellular cytotoxic function, involving both natural killer cells and antibody-dependent cellular cytotoxicity, are important in the recovery from CMV infection and that defects in interleukin-2 (IL-2) production may be important pathogenetically [65]. Studies of T-lymphocyte subsets in normal individuals [14] and renal transplant patients [75] being treated with azathioprine and prednisone (+/- antithymocyte globulin) have demonstrated that CMV infection (and/or EBV infection) is associated with a marked decrease in circulating helper-T cells and an increase in the suppressor-cytotoxic T cells. If the normal ratio of helper-T cells to suppressor-cytotoxic T cells is approximately 1.5, patients with CMV infection have ratios of 0.1-0.5, so-called inverted ratios. Recently, Dummer et al. [24] have reported similar findings in cardiac transplant patients being treated with cyclosporine and prednisone, particularly in patients with clinical CMV disease, viremia, or dual infection with CMV and EBV. Patients with nonviremic, asymptomatic CMV infection (for example, renal transplant patients being treated with cyclosporine and with only peripheral excretion of the virus) may not change their T-cell subsets [64].

These T-cell subset alterations have been associated with important clinical correlations:

1. The great majority of opportunistic infections occur in the subset of renal transplant patients with inverted ratios. Therefore, serial measurement of T-cell subsets can be helpful in guiding immunosuppressive therapy—inverted ratios connoting viral infection, an increased risk of invasive superinfection, and a need for decreased immunosuppressive therapy [24,75].
2. The few instances of opportunistic infection that occur in the face of normal T-cell subsets are usually due to an excessive challenge with the invading pathogen. Thus, the few cases of invasive aspergillosis or Legionnaires' disease we have seen in patients with normal T-cell subsets occurred in the setting of a nosocomial epidemic and was an important clue to the presence of a major environmental hazard [71].

Another important marker of CMV-induced host defense depression is leukopenia. Severe leukopenia (white blood cell count less than $1500/mm^3$) in conjunction with symptomatic CMV disease of greater than 5 days' duration has been associated with a greater than 50% mortality due to superinfection of either the lung or bloodstream. In the lung, *P. carinii* and *A. fumigatus* have been the primary pathogens, and septicemia with *Listeria monocytogenes, Candida* species, and a variety of Gram-negative bacilli have been important problems [69].

The murine CMV model has provided useful information relevant to the consideration of host defense deficits induced by CMV in humans. In the murine model, CMV has been shown to suppress both primary and secondary humoral responses to sheep red blood cells, the degree of suppression being directly proportional to the size of the viral inoculum, to prolong skin graft survival across H-2 and H-Y histocompatibility barriers, to decrease responsiveness in vitro to T- and B-cell mitogens in mixed lymphocyte culture, and to impair development of cytotoxic T lymphocytes [35,66]. Probably most relevant to the clinical situation is the demonstration of a synergistic effect of CMV and *Pseudomonas aeruginosa, Staphylococcus aureus,* and *Candida albicans.* When sublethal infection with one of these organisms is added to sublethal CMV infection, mortality ensues—a direct analogy to what is believed to occur in humans [31].

Effect of CMV Infection on Renal Allograft Function

In 1970, Simmons et al. [77] first suggested that CMV infection could be associated with an increased risk of allograft dysfunction and loss. Since that publication, there has been much controversy in this area [35,66]. The major difficulties in settling this issue have been in two areas: the lack of an adequate laboratory marker for distinguishing clinically important from trivial CMV infection, and the inclusion in most studies of too few patients to allow consideration of all the variables that might be important in answering this question—type of donor, degree of histocompatibility match, form of immunosuppression employed, donor and recipient CMV status pretransplant, and others. Data that have been emerging from several sources in the past few years that attempt to avoid these two pitfalls enable us to answer a qualified "yes" to the question of whether infection can adversely influence renal allograft function.

CMV GLOMERULOPATHY

In 1981, Richardson et al. [63] described a distinctive pattern of glomerular injury in renal allografts that they associated with CMV viremia. Clinically, these patients had progressive azotemia a few weeks to months after transplantation. The salient pathologic features were diffuse endothelial hypertrophy and necrosis, accompanied by accumulation of fine fibrillar webs of periodic acid-Schiff (PAS)-positive material and mononuclear cells that resulted in the obliteration of the glomerular capillaries (Fig. 3). Fibrin and small amounts of IgM and C3 were found by immunofluorescence, and occasional subendothelial deposits were found by electron microscopy. Raji cell reactivity, presumed to be immune complexes, was present in the serum of the two patients studied. No viral particles were detectable by electron microscopy, nor were any viral antigens detected using polyclonal anti-CMV antibodies or two monoclonal antibodies to CMV early and late antigens [29] (Colvin et al., unpublished). One important feature was the minimal degree of inter-

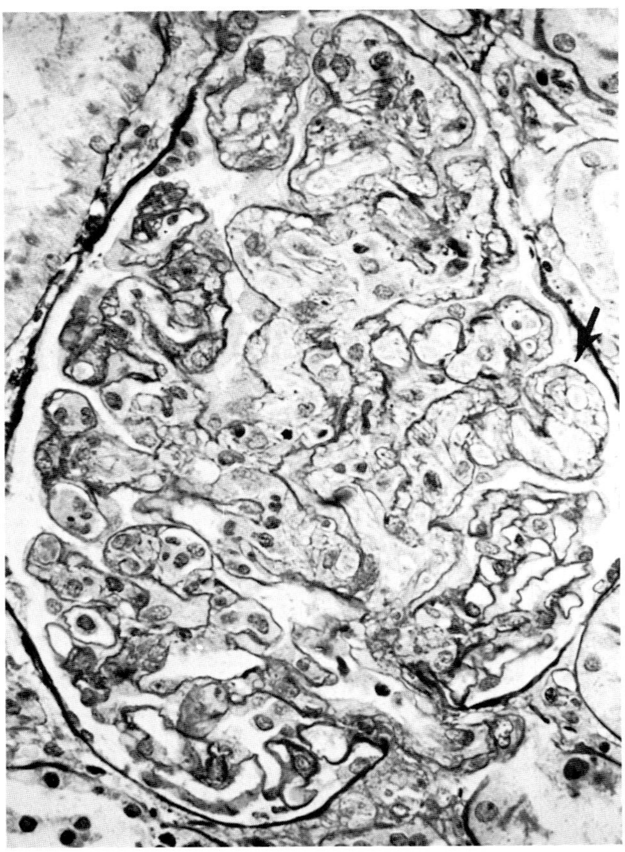

FIGURE 3 Glomerulopathy in a patient with CMV infection. Most of the capillary loops contain swollen endothelial cells and mononuclear leukocytes. The arrow points to a capillary with webs of material reactive with periodic acid-Schiff (PAS stain) (X400). (Reprinted from Reference 63 with the permission of the *New England Journal of Medicine.*)

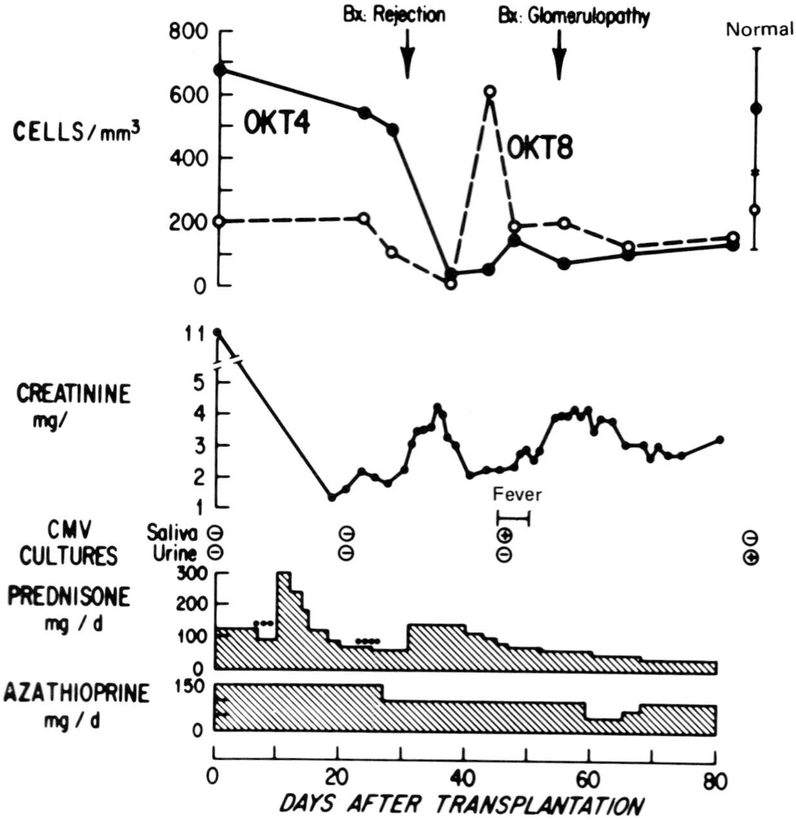

FIGURE 4 Clinical course of a patient who had sequential biopsies that showed interstitial rejection (1) and glomerulopathy (2), the latter associated with positive CMV cultures and a rise in the $T8^+$ cells in the blood [75]. (Diagram reprinted from Reference 59 with permission from the *N Engl J Med*.)

stitial mononuclear infiltrate that accompanied the glomerulopathy. Vascular injury was seen in one of the original cases and several subsequent ones [16].

Although the absence of interstitial rejection helped in the initial recognition of this injury, subsequent cases have been seen in association with typical interstitial infiltrates. One example is particularly instructive (Fig. 4). The initial biopsy showed a combination of interstitial rejection and the glomerulopathy. The patient was treated with OKT3 and initially responded, but renal function worsened after therapy was completed. A biopsy showed resolution of the interstitial process but a progression of the glomerulopathy, a strong argument that the two types of injury have a different pathogenesis. Repeat biopsies on other cases that have resolved clinically reveal that the endothelial reaction diminishes but the glomeruli are left with extensive basement membrane duplication.

How distinctive is the glomerulopathy? The glomerulus is normally relatively spared in acute cellular rejection. The accumulation of a few mononuclear cells in glomerular capillaries can sometimes be seen [2], but the number of lymphocytes is greater in the glomerulopathy (see below) and the endothelial reaction is more marked. In our experience, PAS-stained 2-μm sections are the best for demonstrating the characteristic features. Glomerular thrombosis and necrosis can accompany severe vascular rejection [11], but in the glomerulopathy global necrosis and thrombosis are not prominent. Others have confirmed the distinctiveness of the lesion [32,33] (Kincaid-Smith, personal communication), but there remains controversy about the importance of CMV. A prior episode of CMV allograft glomerulopathy can account for some of the cases of duplication of the glomerular basement membrane that is seen commonly in late biopsies of renal allografts, but at this stage the appearance is not diagnostic.

How strong is the evidence that the glomerulopathy is associated with CMV? Obviously, the frequency and sensitivity of the viral cultures will influence the number of CMV infections detected, particularly the buffy coat cultures. In our original series, five of eight patients with viremia had the glomerulopathy (67%), whereas none of seven without viremia had the lesion, results comparable to those from another transplant center, in which four of seven with the glomerulopathy had viremia [32]. Subsequent studies [16, 75] showed that the glomerulopathy could occur in the absence of demonstrable CMV viremia (seven patients with the glomerulopathy had negative buffy coat cultures within 4 days of the renal biopsy) [75]. Overall, in our experience CMV-infected recipients who are viremic have about twice the frequency of glomerulopathy of those who are nonviremic (58 versus 32%). Thus, viremia is a major risk factor but is neither necessary nor sufficient for the development of the glomerulopathy. In our experience, however, the glomerulopathy has not been found in patients in the absence of CMV. Since about 50% of the patients in our institution have an active CMV infection in the first 100 days after transplantation [75], there remains the possibility that the association is fortuitous. However, of the 36 biopsies taken for renal allograft dysfunction, the glomerulopathy was seen in 12 of 25 (48%) of those with CMV and 0 of 11 of those with negative CMV cultures and/or antibody titers within 3 weeks of the biopsy ($p < 0.005$) [75]. Thus, in this group of patients studied intensively for CMV, the glomerulopathy was observed only in those with demonstrable CMV infection. It should be noted, however, that at least one transplant unit does not detect an association of the glomerulopathy with CMV infections [32].

The other clinical abnormality associated with the glomerulopathy is an inverted T4/T8 ratio. In our series, 9 of 11 (82%) with the glomerulopathy have had T4/T8 ratios < 1.0, compared with 7 of 26 (27%) without the glomerulopathy ($p = 0.003$) [16]. A depression of the number of $T4^+$ cells and an increase in the number of $T8^+$ cells occurs in heavily immunosuppressed recipients of unrelated kidneys who develop CMV infection [75], as well as normal individuals with CMV mononucleosis [14].

The occurrence of the glomerulopathy is independent of the particular type of immunosuppressive therapy (although probably not the intensity), the histocompatibility match, and the patient's original disease. We have observed the glomerulopathy in patients treated with ATG, OKT3, cyclosporine, and azathioprine and steroids alone; in patients with transplants from HLA-identical siblings; and in patients whose original disease was nonglomerular (e.g., tuberculosis).

An essential component in the glomerulopathy, however, is the allograft itself. Patients without allografts who contract CMV infection do not develop this lesion, although a mild mesangial proliferative glomerulonephritis has been reported [52]. Furthermore, immunosuppressed patients with acquired immune deficiency syndrome (AIDS) and CMV infection do not have this glomerulopathy [53]. An interesting study [33] indicated that recipients of bone marrow transplants who had CMV infection did not have the glomerulopathy, an observation we can confirm (unpublished).

There is no animal model of the glomerulopathy known to us. Wehner and Smith [83] have described a mesangiopathic glomerulonephritis in mice, in which cells in the mesangium are infected with CMV, as indicated by their characteristic cytopathic changes by light microscopy and viral particles by electron microscopy. This is clearly different from the human CMV glomerulopathy, in which direct viral infection of the glomerular cells is not demonstrable. If the murine strain of CMV is capable of causing the glomerulopathy, CMV inoculation of a mouse carrying a renal transplant and the native kidney might provide key information about the requirement for alloantigens in the glomeruli.

The mechanism of the glomerular lesion remains unknown; viral antigens or viral particles are not detected in the glomeruli. Despite the presence of Raji-reactive material in the circulation, immune complex deposition in glomeruli is not prominent, ranging from trace to 1^+, as judged by immunofluorescence. Electron-dense deposits are found occasionally, but not uniformly. The most likely possibility, in our opinion, is that the virus alters the graft rejection process so that the glomerulus becomes the target. This might be due to humoral factors released in response to the virus or to direct cytotoxicity mediated by lymphocytes or macrophages. One such factor, α-interferon, produced by leukocytes in response to viral infection, can enhance the expression of H-2 antigens on spleen cells when given to mice [25]. Surface expression of HLA class I antigens and susceptibility to T-cell lysis by human cells are increased by α-interferon in vitro [39,43]. Systemic recombinant α-interferon has led to glomerular injury in three of eight patients with renal allografts, as judged by the development of nephrotic-range proteinuria [59]. The glomerular lesion in the one case studied showed "intracapillary proliferative glomerulonephritis" with extensive IgM, C3, and fibrin. Without illustrations it is hard to judge its similarity with the CMV glomerulopathy. A second antiviral agent, γ-interferon, is produced by T cells in response to antigenic stimuli. γ-Interferon activates macrophages and increases the expression of HLA class II antigens on vascular endothelial cells [82]. Thus either of these mediators has the potential, in principle at least, to increase alloantigen expression in the glomerulus. To determine whether cells were directly involved in the glomerulopathy and their nature, we have performed an immunoperoxidase analysis of the intraglomerular cells for surface makers [17]. We found a significant accumulation of $T3^+$ (anti-Leu 4) T cells, 12.0 ± 2.8 per glomerulus in the glomerulopathy, compared with 1.3 ± 0.5 per glomerulus in interstitial rejection. All these T cells could be accounted for by the $T8^+$ (OKT8) cells (12.9 ± 3.0 per glomerulus), which were selectively concentrated from the blood, in which 65% of the $T3^+$ cells were $T8^+$. T4 (anti-Leu 3a) was present on a minority of the cells (4.1 ± 1.1 per glomerulus), some of which had the appearance of macrophages. The intraglomerular mononuclear cells displayed activation markers, including HLA-DR, HLA-DC, and the IL-2 receptor. These data provide evidence that the glomerulopathy is mediated by a subset of T lymphocytes, namely $T8^+$ cells, that are activated within the glomerulus. This subset includes both suppressor effector cells and cytotoxic cells primarily reactive to HLA class I antigens and the subset whose absolute numbers increase in severe CMV infections [14].

We conclude from the available data that the acute glomerulopathy is a distinct form of allograft rejection, related to CMV and perhaps other initiators, in which the glomeruli become the primary target of $T8^+$ T cells, presumably to HLA class I antigens. Whatever the mechanism of injury, only 18% recovered renal function, compared with 85% without glomerulopathy. If both a low T4/T8 ratio and glomerulopathy are present, the recovery rate is even worse, only 9%. In contrast, if neither is present recovery is 95%. At this time the optimal therapy for the glomerulopathy in unknown. A few patients have recovered after decreased immunosuppression [63] and a few after ATG [16] (Cosimi et al., unpublished). We hope that improved recognition and understanding of its pathogenesis will lead to improved prevention and therapy.

ROLE OF CMV IN POSTTRANSPLANT MALIGNANCY

The major tumor linked with CMV infection is Kaposi's sarcoma, which accounts for approximately 3% of all malignancies occurring in renal transplant patients (five times the figure in the general population), with most of these tumors beginning approximately 3 years posttransplant [56]. Data supporting that CMV is involved in the pathogenesis of Kaposi's sarcoma is of two types: seroepidemiologic studies of populations with high-incidence figures for Kaposi's sarcoma, and molecular biologic or immunologic studies in which CMV antigen or DNA is sought in biopsied tumor tissue.

Seroepidemiologic studies among African patients with Kaposi's sarcoma and among acquired immune deficiency syndrome patients with this tumor reveal that virtually every individual in these high-risk groups are seropositive for CMV, as are 75-100% of the non-homosexual, non-drug addict European or American patients with sporadic Kaposi's sarcoma [71,72]. Now that the human T-cell leukemia virus type III (HTLV-III) has been widely recognized as the cause of AIDS, studies of AIDS patients are particularly revealing regarding the possible role of CMV in the pathogenesis of Kaposi's sarcoma. The two major clinical manifestations of AIDS are recurrent opportunistic infections and an aggressive form of Kaposi's sarcoma. Although all the AIDS high-risk groups (male homosexuals, hemophiliacs, Haitians, drug abusers, and, perhaps, recipients of multiple blood transfusions) have difficulties with opportunistic infection, there is a very different incidence of Kaposi's sarcoma in these different populations with AIDS—Kaposi's sarcoma is particularly common in homosexuals with AIDS, but less common in the other groups. Whereas active CMV infection is ubiquitous among the homosexuals with AIDS, it is much less common in other AIDS patients. On the other hand, studies in Zaire have shown that patients with Kaposi's sarcoma without other manifestations of AIDS are frequently seronegative for HTLV-III (while seropositive for CMV). In contrast, Zairian patients with AIDS are HTLV-III seropositive [6,30,67].

Such seroepidemiologic observations have led to the so-called two-step model to explain the occurrence of Kaposi's sarcoma [30,67]. The first step is the induction of a profound state of immunosuppression, leading to a markedly increased risk of opportunistic infection. The second step is the induction of the malignancy secondary to prolonged CMV infection in an immunodeficient host. In the case of renal transplant patients, the first step is the creation of an overimmunosuppressed state by the chronic immunosuppressive therapy administered; in the case of AIDS patients, the cause of the immunodeficiency state is primary infection with HTLV-III [6,30,64].

More direct evidence for a role for CMV in the pathogenesis of Kaposi's sarcoma comes from studies demonstrating that CMV DNA can be found within the nucleus of tumor cells and CMV antigen can be demonstrated on the surface of these cells, but not in surrounding tissues [35,69]. One of the more complete studies of this was performed by Drew et al. [23] on 10 homosexual men with Kaposi's sarcoma. In these patients, all 9 tested had IgG class anti-CMV antibody, and 7 of 9 had Ig M class antibody. The CMV could be isolated from body secretions or blood from 7 of these patients. Viral cultures of the tumor were negative in all patients, but CMV RNA was detected by in situ hybridization in tumor tissue from 2 of 3 patients tested and CMV antigens by immunofluorescence in 6 of 9 tumor samples tested. In contrast, biopsies of normal tissue from 3 of the positive patients failed to show any evidence of CMV.

Thus, there is a broad array of evidence consistent with the hypothesis that CMV plays an important role in the pathogenesis of Kaposi's sarcoma in such immunosuppressed patients as renal transplant recipients. Although it is our belief that CMV is indeed involved in the pathogenesis of Kaposi's sarcoma, we are not suggesting that this is proven. The question remains which comes first: does the virus play a causative role, or does the tumor develop first and then supply a suitable site for abortive viral growth? Definitive evidence to choose between these two possibilities is not yet available.

PREVENTION AND TREATMENT OF CMV INFECTION IN THE RENAL TRANSPLANT PATIENT

Given the profound effects of CMV on the transplant recipient, it is not surprising that a great deal of effort has gone into attempts to either prevent or treat CMV infection [70]. At the present time, preventive therapy has much more to offer than treatment after the development of clinical disease. There are three categories of preventive strategy currently available to limit the effects of CMV: decreasing the risk of virus acquisition and reactivation, specific immunologic manipulations, and antiviral chemotherapy [70,71].

The first of these strategies, limiting the risk of virus acquisition, primarily applies to patients who are seronegative for CMV prior to transplant. Such a strategy consists of two parts: a blood transfusion policy, in which either blood from CMV seronegative donors or frozen blood free of viable leukocytes are the only blood products utilized; and the protective matching of donor and recipient pairs so that an organ from a seropositive donor is not placed in a seronegative recipient. The first of these two could and probably should be implemented at the present time, as the use of such blood products carries no disadvantages for the patient [70,71].

The protective matching, however, is more problematic. Data generated from a multicenter study [73] strongly suggest that the advantages of an individual receiving a kidney from a living related donor far outweigh the disadvantages of possible CMV acquisition. In cadaveric donor transplants, however, particularly if the immunosuppressive program will include an antilymphocyte preparation, protective matching will show benefit in terms of patient and graft survival. It is clear, though, that the form of immunosuppression to be used is an important variable to be considered when contemplating the possibility of protective matching. If the initial data [57,64] suggesting that cyclosporine immunosuppression is associated with a lower rate of symptomatic CMV infection in renal transplant recipients holds up, then this would appear to be a more satisfactory approach to the seronegative patient than to limit that patient's pool of potential donors.

There are two specific anti-CMV immunologic manipulations that are currently under investigation [70]: active immunization prior to transplantation with the attenuated Towne strain live CMV vaccine, and passive immunization posttransplant with a hyperimmune anti-CMV globulin preparation. There are two concerns with the vaccine: efficacy and possible reversion to virulence (as can occur with attenuated murine CMV virus in vivo) [38], causing either acute disease or long-term adverse effects. These latter concerns have not been borne out, but there are still important questions regarding efficacy in the immunosuppressed patient. Preliminary studies have shown that when the Towne strain CMV vaccine is given to seronegative dialysis patients, an antibody response usually develops, there are no changes in T-lymphocyte subsets, and a significant minority of patients fail to develop in vitro evidence of anti-CMV cell-mediated immunity. Posttransplant, all recipients of the vaccine lose evidence of cell-mediated immunity against the vaccine. A further question that can be asked is whether such a monovalent vaccine is capable of giving broad enough protection against the genomic and antigenic heterogeneity of different CMV strains in nature. These questions are not meant to deny the desirability of an effective CMV vaccine; rather, they are raised to underline the difficulties of such an approach. On-going clinical trials should provide answers to these questions [12,28,61,79].

High-titered hyperimmune anti-CMV globulin or serum preparations, drawn from a large number of patients (and hence directed against many CMV strains), appear to offer promise when used prophylactically. Two studies on bone marrow transplant patients, in whom CMV is an even more challenging problem than it is in renal transplant recipients, suggest that this approach can be used quite effectively [18,48]. Studies now being carried out in renal transplant patients should assess the merits of this approach in this population as well.

At present, no effective antiviral drugs may be used as specific therapy against CMV. The nonspecific agent interferon, however, does have significant anti-CMV effects when utilized prophylactically. Hirsch et al. [34] have recently reported that a 14-week course of α-interferon (3×10^6 units thrice weekly for 6 weeks and twice weekly for 8 weeks, total dose 102×10^6 units) given to renal transplant patients at risk for reactivation CMV was quite effective in preventing clinical disease and may also decrease the incidence of both opportunistic superinfection and the CMV-associated glomerulopathy. Whether such a program is as effective for patients at risk for primary disease remains to be demonstrated.

Cytomegalovirus infection, like many infectious diseases, is better prevented than treated. At present, clinical management of overt CMV infections consists primarily of decreasing immunosuppression, with the cessation of any antilymphocyte therapy that might be on-going. Because of the close association between CMV and *P. carinii* infection, we have chosen to begin trimethoprim-sulfamethoxazole prophylaxis in patients with clinical CMV disease [66,71,74]. Specific antiviral therapy is not currently available. Initial attempts to use adenine arabinoside in renal transplant patients with serious CMV disease were associated with a catastrophic neurologic syndrome, possibly due to excess accumulation of the drug in patients with poor renal function [45]. Pollard et al. [60] have reported improvement in CMV chorioretinitis in patients treated with 20 mg/kg per day of adenine arabinoside, but with hematologic and gastrointestinal side effects serious enough to bar the use of this regimen for routine therapy. Acyclovir is without efficacy, and therapeutic interferon is unlikely to be effective. Anecdotal reports suggest that high-titered anti-CMV antibody preparations might have value therapeutically [10,60], but controlled testing has yet to be done. All in all, the reason for the emphasis on prevention is rather clear—specific therapy for CMV disease in the renal transplant patient is not yet available.

SUMMARY

Cytomegalovirus has been the most important single infectious agent marring the course of the renal transplant patient. The characteristics of the virus, particularly its capacity for latency and the modulation of its effects by the two major elements of transplantation—rejection and chronic immunosuppression—have led to a broad array of clinical effects. One of the more remarkable observations that has grown out of CMV research in transplant patients is that the "non-direct infectious disease effects" of this virus—its depressing effects on host defenses, its probable role in renal allograft injury, and its possible role in the development of Kaposi's sarcoma—are much more important to the patient than the infectious disease syndromes the virus causes by itself. Because of these effects, continuing effort is going into decreasing acquisition of the virus, and when this is not feasible, preventing clinical disease with specific immunotherapy and/or prophylaxis with interferon. True control of CMV, however, awaits the development of better antirejection strategies, of which cyclosporine may be a prime example, and specific, nontoxic, antiviral drugs that could be utilized either prophylactically or therapeutically. We have learned much about the effects of the virus; we have much more to learn about how to control it.

ACKNOWLEDGMENT

This work was supported in part by Grant No. HL 18646 from the United States Public Health Service.

REFERENCES

1. Adler, S. P., Chandrika, T., Lawrence, L. and Boggett, J. Cytomegalovirus infections in neonates acquired by blood transfusions. *Pediatr. Infect. Dis.* 2:114-118, 1983.
2. Atkins, R. C., Holdsworth, S. R., Hancock, W. W., et al. Cellular immune mechanisms in human glomerulonephritis: The role of mononuclear leukocytes. *Springer Semin. Immunopathol.* 5:269-296, 1982.
3. Ayulo, M., Aisner, S. C., Margois, K., et al. Cytomegalovirus-associated gastritis in a compromised host. *JAMA* 243:1364, 1980.
4. Betts, R. F., Cestero, R. U. M., Freeman, R. B., and Douglas, R. G., Jr. Epidemiology of cytomegalovirus infection in end stage renal disease. *J. Med. Virol.* 4:89-96, 1979.
5. Betts, R. F., Freeman, R. B., Doublas, R. H., Jr., et al. Transmission of cytomegalovirus infection with renal allograft. *Kidney Int.* 8:385-392, 1975.
6. Biggar, R. J., Melbye, M., Kestems, L., et al. Kaposi's sarcoma in Zaire is not associated with HTLV-III infection. *N. Engl. J. Med.* 311:1051-1052, 1984.
7. Brady, M. T., Milan, J. D., Anderson, D. C., et al. Use of deglycerolized red blood cells to prevent posttransfusion infection with cytomegalovirus in neonates. *J. Infect. Dis.* 150:334-339, 1984.
8. Braun, W. E., and Nankervis, G. Cytomegalovirus viremia and bacterimia in renal allograft recipients. *N. Engl. J. Med.* 299:1318-1319, 1978.
9. Broughton, W. L., Cupples, H. P., and Parver, L. M. Bilateral retinal detachment following cytomegalovirus retinitis. *Arch. Ophthalmol.* 96:618-619, 1978.
10. Brown, C. B., Nicholls, A. J., Edward, N., et al. Hyperimmune immunoglobulin therapy for cytomegalovirus infections in renal transplant patients. *Proc. Eur. Dial. Transplant Assoc.* 20:271-279, 1983.
11. Busch, G. J., Reynolds, E. S., Galvanek, E. G., Braun, W. E., and Dammin, G. J. Human renal allografts: The role of vascular injury in early graft failure. *Medicine (Baltimore)* 50:29-83, 1971.
12. Carney, W. P., Hirsch, M. S., Iacoviello, V. R., et al. T-lymphocyte subsets and proliferative responses following immunization with cytomegalovirus vaccine. *J. Infect. Dis.* 147:958, 1983.

13. Carney, W. P., and Hirsch, M. S. Mechanisms of immunosuppression in cytomegalovirus mononucleosis. II. Virus-monocyte interactions. *J. Infect. Dis.* 144:47-54, 1981.
14. Carney, W. P., Rubin, R. C., Hoffman, R. A., et al. Analysis of T lympnocyte subsets in cytomegalovirus mononucleosis. *J. Immunol.* 126:2114-2116, 1981.
15. Carson, S., and Chatterjee, S. N. Cytomegalovirus retinitis: Two cases occurring after renal transplantation. *Ann. Ophthalmol.* 10:275-279, 1978.
16. Colvin, R. B., Cosimi, A. B., Burton, R. C., et al. Circulating T-cell subsets in 72 human renal allograft recipients: The $OKT4^+/OKT8^+$ cell ratio correlates with reversibility of graft injury and glomerulopathy. *Transplant. Proc.* 15:1166-1169, 1983.
17. Colvin, R. B. Flow cytometric analysis of T cells: Diagnostic applications in transplantation. *Ann. N.Y. Acad. Sci.* 428:5-13, 1984.
18. Condie, R. M., and O'Reilly, R. J. Prophylaxis of CMV infection in bone marrow transplant recipients by hyperimmune CMV gamma-globulin. *Dev. Biol. Stand.* 52:501-513, 1982.
19. Cheeseman, S. H., Rubin, R. H., Stewart, J. A., et al. Controlled clinical trial of prophylactic human leukocyte interferon in renal transplantation. Effect on cytomegalovirus and herpes simplex virus infections. *N. Engl. J. Med.* 300:1345-1349, 1979.
20. Cheeseman, S. H., Stewart, J. A., Winkle, S., et al. Cytomegalovirus excretion 2-14 years after renal transplantation. *Transplant. Proc.* 11:71-74, 1979.
21. Dorfman, L. J. Cytomegalovirus encephalitis in adults. *Neurology (NY)* 23:316-344, 1973.
22. Dowling, J. N., Saslow, A. R., Armstrong, J. A., and Ho, M. Cytomegalovirus infection in patients receiving immunosuppressive therapy for rheumatologic disorders. *J. Infect. Dis.* 133:399-408, 1976.
23. Drew, W. L., Conant, M. A., Mines, R. C., et al. Cytomegalovirus and Kaposi's sarcoma in young homosexual men. *Lancet* 2:125-127, 1982.
24. Dummer, J. S., Ho, M., Rabin, B. P., Griffith, B. P., Hardesty, R. L., and Bahnson, B. T. The effect of cytomegalovirus and Epstein-Barr virus infection on T lymphocyte subsets in cardiac transplant patients on cyclosporine. *Transplantation* 38: 433-435, 1984.
25. Fellous, M., Kamoun, M., Gresser, I., et al. Enhanced expression of HLA antigens and 2-microglobulin on interferon-treated human lymphoid cells. *Eur. J. Immunol.* 9:446-449, 1984.
26. Fryd, D. S., Peterson, P. K., Ferguson, R. M., et al. Cytomegalovirus as a risk factor in renal transplantation. *Transplantation* 30:436-439, 1980.
27. Gelmann, E. P., Clanton, D. J., Jariwalla, R. J., and Rosenthal, L. J. Characterization and location of *myc* homologous sequences in human cytomegalovirus DNA. *Proc. Natl. Acad. Sci. USA* 80:5107-5111, 1983.
28. Glazer, J. P., Friedman, H. M., Grossman, R. A., et al. Live cytomegalovirus vaccination of renal transplant candidates; a preliminary trial. *Ann. Intern. Med.* 91:676-683, 1979.
29. Gleaves, C. A., Smith, T. F., Shuster, E. A., et al. Rapid detection of cytomegalovirus in MRC-5 cells inoculated with urine specimens by using low-speed centrifugation and monoclonal antibody to an early antigen. *J. Clin. Microbiol.* 19:917-919, 1984.
30. Gottlieb, M. S., Groopman, J. E., Weinstein, W. M., et al. The acquired immunodeficiency syndrome. *Ann. Intern. Med.* 99:208-220, 1983.
31. Hamilton, J. R., Overall, J. C., Jr., and Glasgow, L. A. Synergistic effect on mortality in mice with murine cytomegalovirus and *Pseudomonas aeruginosa, Staphylococcus aureus,* or *Candida albicans* infections. *Infect. Immun.* 14:982-989, 1976.

32. Harmon, J. B., Sibley, R. K., Peterson, P., et al. Cytomegalovirus viremia and renal allograft morphology: Are there distinct pathologic features? (abstract) *Lab. Invest.* 46:35A, 1982.
33. Harrera, G. A., Cooley, C. E., Alexander, R. W., et al. Cytomegalovirus glomerulopathy: Fact or fancy? (abstract) *Lab. Invest.* 50:25A, 1984.
34. Hirsch, M. S., Schooley, R. T., Cosimi, A. B., et al. Effects of interferon-alpha on cytomegalovirus reactivation in renal transplant recipients. *N. Engl. J. Med.* 308: 1489-1493, 1983.
35. Ho, M. *Cytomegalovirus: Biology and Infection.* Plenum Press, New York, 1982.
36. Ho, M., Suwansirikul, S., Dowling, J. N., et al. The transplanted kidney as a source of cytomegalovirus infection. *N. Engl. J. Med.* 293:1109-1112, 1975.
37. Huang, E. S., Alford, C. A., Reynolds, D. W., Stagno, S., and Pass, R. F. Molecular epidemiology of cytomegalovirus infection in women and their infants. *N. Engl. J. Med.* 303:958-962, 1980.
38. Jordan, M. C. Adverse effects of cytomegalovirus vaccination in mice. *J. Clin. Invest.* 65:798-803, 1980.
39. Kramer, P., ten-Kate, F. W., and Bijnen, A. B. Recombinant leucocyte interferon A induces steroid-resistant acute vascular rejection episodes in renal transplant recipients. *Lancet* 1:989-990, 1984.
40. Lang, D. J. Cytomegalovirus infections in organ transplantation and posttransfusion: An hypothesis. *Arch. Ges. Virusforsh.* 37:36-77, 1972.
41. Lang, D. J., Ebert, P. A., Rodgers, B. M., Boggess, H. P., and Rixse, R. S. Reduction of postperfusion cytomegalovirus infection following the use of leukocyte depleted blood. *Transfusion* 17:391-395, 1977.
42. Lang, D. J. Transfusion and perfusion-associated cytomegalovirus and Epstein-Barr virus infections: Current understanding and investigation. In *Transmissible Disease and Blood Transfusion,* T. J. Greenwalt and G. A. Jamieson, eds. Grune & Stratton, New York, 1975, pp. 153-173.
43. Lindahl, P., Gresser, I., Leary, P., et al. Interferon treatment of mice: Enhanced expression of histocompatibility antigens on lymphoid cells. *Proc. Natl. Acad. Sci. USA* 73:1284-1287, 1976.
44. Linnemann, C. C., Jr., Dunn, C. R., First, M. R., et al. Late onset of fatal cytomegalovirus infection after renal transplantation; primary or reactivation infection? *Arch. Intern. Med.* 138:1247-1250, 1978.
45. Marker, S. C., Howard, R. J., Groth, K. E., et al. A trial of vidarabine for cytomegalovirus in renal transplant patients. *Arch. Intern. Med.* 140:1441-1444, 1980.
46. Marker, S. C., Howard, R. J., Simmons, R. L., et al. Cytomegalovirus infection: A quantitative perspective study of 320 consecutive renal transplants. *Surgery* 89:660-671, 1981.
47. Merritt, J. C., and Callender, C. O. Adult cytomegalic inclusion retinitis. *Ann. Ophthalmol.* 10:1059-1063, 1978.
48. Meyers, J. D., Leszcynski, J., Zaia, J. A., et al. Prevention of cytomegalovirus infection by cytomegalovirus immune globulin after marrow transplantation. *Ann. Intern. Med.* 98:442-446, 1983.
49. Minars, N., Silverman, J. F., Escobar, M. R., and Martinez, A. J. Fatal cytomegalovirus inclusion disease; associated skin manifestation in a renal transplant patient. *Arch. Dermatol.* 113:1569-1571, 1977.
50. Murray, H. W., Knox, D. L., Green, W. R., and Susel, R. M. Cytomegalovirus retinitis in adults; a manifestation of disseminated viral infection. *Am. J. Med.* 63:574-584, 1977.
51. Nelson, J. A., Fleckenstein, B., Galloway, D. A., and McDougall, J. K. Transformation of NIH 3T3 cells with cloned fragments of human cytomegalovirus strain AD 169. *J. Virol.* 43:83-91, 1982.

52. Ozawa, T., and Stewart, J. A. Immune-complex glomerulonephritis associated with cytomegalovirus infection. *Am. J. Clin. Pathol.* 72:103-107, 1979.
53. Pardo, V., Aldana, M., Colton, R. M., et al. Glomerular lesions in the acquired immunodeficiency syndrome. *Ann. Intern. Med.* 101:429-434, 1984.
54. Pass, R. F., Long, W. K., Whitley, R. J., et al. Productive infection with cytomegalovirus and herpes simplex virus in renal transplant recipients: Role of source of kidney. *J. Infect. Dis.* 137:556-563, 1978.
55. Pass, R. F., Reynolds, D. W., Whelchel, J. D., Diethelm, A. G., and Alford, C. A. Impaired leukocyte transformation response to cytomegalovirus and phytohemagglutinin in recipients of renal transplants: Association with antithymocyte globulin. *J. Infect. Dis.* 143:259-265, 1981.
56. Penn, I. Kaposi's sarcoma in renal transplant recipients. *Transplantation* 27:8-11, 1979.
57. Peterson, P. K., Balfour, H. H., Fryd, D. S., et al. Risk factors in the development of cytomegalovirus-related pneumonia in renal transplant recipients. *J. Infect. Dis.* 148:1121, 1983.
58. Peterson, P. K., Balfour, H. H., Jr., Marker, S. C., et al. Cytomegalovirus disease in renal allograft recipients: A prospective study of the clinical features, risk factors and impact in renal transplantation. *Medicine (Baltimore)* 59:283-300, 1980.
59. Pober, J. S., Gimbonre, M. A., Jr., Cotran, R. S., et al. Ia expression by vascular enthothelium is inducible by activated T cells and by human α-interferon. *J. Exp. Med.* 157:1339-1353, 1983.
60. Pollard, R. B., Egbert, P. R., Gallagher, J. G., and Marigan, T. C. Cytomegalovirus retinitis in immunosuppressed hosts. I. Natural history and effects of treatment and adenine arabinoside. *Ann. Intern. Med.* 93:655-664, 1980.
61. Quinnan, G. V., Jr., Delery, M., Rook, A. H., et al. Comparative virulence and immunogenicity of the Towne strain and a nonattentuated strain of cytomegalovirus. *Ann. Intern. Med.* 101:478-483, 1984.
62. Ravin, C. E., Smith, G. W., Ahern, M. J., et al. Cytomegaloviral infection presenting as a solitary pulmonary nodule. *Chest* 71:220-222, 1977.
63. Richardson, W. P., Colvin, R. B., Cheeseman, S. H., et al. Glomerulopathy associated with cytomegalovirus in renal allografts. *N. Engl. J. Med.* 305:57-63, 1981.
64. Rinaldo, C. R., Hamoudi, W. H., DiBaiasio, R. L., Rabin, B., Hakala, T. R., and Liebert, M. Cellular immune response and cytomegalovirus infection in renal transplant patients receiving cyclosporine. *Transplant. Proc.* 15:2775-2779, 1983.
65. Rook, A. H., Masur, H., Lane, H. C., et al. Interleukin-2 enhances the depressed natural killer and cytomegalovirus-specific cytotoxic activities of lymphocytes from patients with the acquired immune deficiency syndrome. *J. Clin. Invest.* 72: 398-403, 1983.
66. Rubin, R. H. Infection in the renal transplant patient. In *Clinical Approach to Infection in the Compromised Host,* R. H. Rubin and L. S. Young, eds. Plenum Press, New York, 1981, pp. 553-605.
67. Rubin, R. H., Infection in the immunosuppressed host. In *Scientific American Textbook of Medicine,* E. Rubinstein and D. D. Federman, eds. Scientific American, New York, 1984, Section 7, Chapter X, pp. 1-28.
68. Rubin, R. H., Cosimi, A. B., Hirsch, M. S., et al. Effects of anti-thymocyte globulin in cytomegalovirus infection in renal transplant recipients. *Transplantation* 31:143-145, 1981.
69. Rubin, R. H., Cosimi, A. B., Tolkoff-Rubin, N. E., Russell, P. S., and Hirsch, M. S. Infectious disease syndromes attributable to cytomegalovirus and their significance among renal transplant recipients. *Transplantation* 24:458-464, 1977.
70. Rubin, R. H., Russell, P. S., Levin, M., and Cohen, C. Summary of a workshop of

cytomegalovirus infections during organ transplantation. *J. Infect. Dis.* 139:728-734, 1979.

71. Rubin, R. H., and Tolkoff-Rubin, N. E. The problem of cytomegalovirus infection in transplantation. In *Progress in Transplantation,* Volume 1, P. J. Morris and N. L. Tilney, eds. Churchill Livingstone, New York, 1984, pp. 89-114.
72. Rubin, R. H., and Tolkoff-Rubin, N. E. Viral infection in the renal transplant patient. *Proc. Eur. Dial. Transplant Assoc.* 19:513-528, 1982.
73. Rubin, R. H., Tolkoff-Rubin, N. E., Oliver, D., et al. Multicenter seroepidemiologic study of the impact of cytomegalovirus infection on renal transplantation. *Transplantation,* 40:243-249, 1985.
74. Rubin, R. H., Wolfson, J. S., Cosimi, A. B., and Tolkoff-Rubin, N. E. Infection in the renal transplant patient. *Am. J. Med.* 70:405-411, 1981.
75. Schooley, R. T., Hirsch, M. S., Colvin, R. B., et al. Association of herpes virus infection with T-lymphocyte subset alterations, glomerulopathy, and opportunistic infections after renal transplantation. *N. Engl. J. Med.* 308:307-313, 1983.
76. Simmons, R. L., Matas, A. J., Rattazzi, L. C., et al. Clinical observations of the lethal cytomegalovirus infection following renal transplantation. *Surgery* 82:537-546, 1977.
77. Simmons, R. L., Weil, R., Tallent, M. B., et al. Do mild infections trigger the rejection of renal allografts? *Transplant. Proc.* 2:419-423, 1970.
78. Spector, D. H., and Vacquier, J. P. Human cytomegalovirus (strain AD 169) contains sequences related to the avian retrovirus ocogene *v-myc. Proc. Natl. Acad. Sci. USA* 80:3889-3893, 1983.
79. Starr, S. E., Glazer, J. P., Friedman, H. M., Farqehar, J. D., and Plotkin, S. A. Specific cellular and humoral immunity after immunization with live Twone strain cytomegalovirus vaccine. *J. Infect. Dis.* 143:585-589, 1981.
80. Sutherland, D. E. R., Chan, F. Y., Foucar, E., et al. The bleeding cecal ulcer in transplant patients. *Surgery* 86:386-398, 1979.
81. Tolkoff-Rubin, N. E., Rubin, R. H., Keller, E. E., Baker, G. P., Stewart, J. A., and Hirsch, M. S. Cytomegalovirus infections in dialysis patients and personnel. *Am. Intern. Med.* 89:625-628, 1978.
82. Tuazon, T. V., Bhan, A. B., Schneeberger, E. E., et al. Intraglomerular T cell phenotype in cytomegalovirus (CMV)-associated allograft glomerulopathy (abstract). *Kidney Int.* 27:224, 1985.
83. Wehner, R. W., and Smith, R. D. Progressive cytomegalovirus glomerulonephritis: An experimental model. *Am. J. Pathol.* 112:313-325, 1983.
84. Wu, B. C., Dowling, J. N., Armstrong, J. A., and Ho, M. Enhancement of mouse cytomegalovirus infection during host versus graft reaction. *Science* 190:56-58, 1975.
85. Yeager, A. S., Grumet, F. C., Hafleigh, E. B., et al. Prevention of transfusion-acquired cytomegalovirus infections in newborn infants. *J. Pediatr.* 98:281-287, 1981.

NEW IMMUNOSUPPRESSIVE AGENTS

15

THE BIOLOGY OF IMMUNOSUPPRESSION MEDIATED BY ANTILYMPHOCYTE ANTIBODIES

James F. Burdick
The Johns Hopkins University School of Medicine, Baltimore, Maryland

The development of monoclonal antibodies has resulted in major advances in the characterization of cell surface antigens and other molecules involved in the immune response, as witnessed by the results described in other chapters in this book. Because of the success of polyclonal antilymphocyte sera (ALS) as immunosuppressive agents, it seemed likely that monoclonal antibodies could also be employed therapeutically. In this chapter I shall review progress to date in the experimental analysis of in vivo immunosuppressive effects of antilymphocyte antibodies, as background for the following chapter, by Cosimi and Delmonico, on the current clinical status of these agents. Excellent symposia and reviews on polyclonal antilymphocyte sera are available (e.g., References 73, 126, and 167), so they will be only briefly considered, and the emphasis of this chapter will be on monoclonal agents. The many functional and antigenic specificities potentially available with monoclonal reagents encompass a plethora of possible agents; since immunoglobulin class and the function served by the target antigen have greater implications for in vivo effects than for many in vitro uses, choosing a specific monoclonal agent most likely to be effective in vivo is a particularly complex enterprise. Therefore, the therapeutic promise of monoclonal antibodies may not be fully realized until a considerably greater understanding of the effect of these various factors has been achieved.

Several antibodies of different subclasses, directed against different lymphocyte surface antigens, have been evaluated clinically as immunosuppressive agents (see Chapter 16), and each produced different effects. It is not surprising that these rather different agents would differ in their therapeutic effectiveness; it further seems likely, given more extensive basic knowledge about the biology of the in vivo effects of different immunoglobulin subclasses and their interactions with different antigens, that choices of appropriate agents for clinical trials could be made quickly and inexpensively, rather than subjecting each possible agent to extensive clinical or nonhuman primate testing.

POLYCLONAL ANTILYMPHOCYTE SERA

Preparation and Active Components of ALS

A wide variety of sensitization regimens and preparative techniques have been successful in producing effective antilymphocyte sera. Thymic, lymph node, and spleen cells seem equally effective as sources of antigen. The unabsorbed sera have a variable amount of activity against different types of lymphoid cells, as well as against a variety of other antigens, including red blood cells, platelets, and, occasionally, kidney basement membrane. It has generally been found that the IgG fraction of ALS contains the immunosuppressive antibodies. Production techniques have generally involved extensive absorption with nonlymphoid cells and, often, fractionation to obtain the IgG portion of the serum. The degree of reproducibility for immunosuppressive potency has been somewhat unpredictable, even when comparing two lots that were raised and processed in as identical a fashion as possible.

Mechanism of Action of ALS

Early experiments with ALS revealed its capacity to kill lymphocytes in vitro. The in vivo administration of ALS was found to cause marked lymphopenia. When it was shown that graft rejection and other in vivo immunologic reactions could be inhibited by ALS [168], one mechanism for its immunosuppressive effect seemed likely to be classic complement-mediated lysis of lymphocytes. Clearance of lymphocytes due to reticuloendothelial system uptake of the cells opsonized by ALS also seemed to be a likely immunosuppressive mechanism, since it was found that ALS-coated thymocytes are sequestered in the reticuloendothelial system [89]. However, it became clear that the immunosuppressive effect of ALS considerably outlasted the treatment period, and that this long-lasting effect was not necessarily accompanied by lymphopenia. Therefore, other mechanisms of action have been considered. Loss of lymphocyte function due to "sterile activation" has been suggested, since it was found that many ALS preparations can cause lymphocyte proliferation. However, this possibility seems unlikely since the correlation between mitogenic potential and immunosuppressive potency is poor. Another explanation for prolonged immunosuppressive effect after resolution of the lymphopenia might lie in the finding, in certain experimental situations, that suppressor cells have become detectable in animals after successful treatment using ALS [86,102,134,149]. One preparation used clinically that does not have an experimental counterpart is the antilymphoblast globulin that binds T cells, which then, in part, remain in the circulation with masked antigens [104], which may result in blocking of lymphocyte function. Another likely contribution to a continued immunosuppressive effect, after severe lymphocyte depletion has resolved, is that the repopulation is initially by short-lived lymphocytes, and the restoration of the long-lived recirculating lymphocytes of particular importance for graft rejection requires a much longer time, during which interval the immunosuppressive effect persists (discussed in Reference 126).

One corollary to the inadequate understanding of the mechanism(s) of ALS action is the lack of an effective in vitro test for potency. Complement-dependent ALS-mediated lymphocyte killing and lymphocyte mitogenesis do not correlate well with immunosuppressive potency. Tests of the effectiveness of ALS for opsonization, such as its inhibition of various rosetting assays [2,36], are sometimes more useful. However, the effect in vivo on primate allograft survival seems to be the most reliable predictor of clinical effect [25].

Side Effects of ALS

Experimentally evident side effects, other than the major potential for dangerous overimmunosuppression, seem to hinge particularly upon two factors (reviewed in Reference 73). The first is the administration of a large amount of foreign protein, with resultant anti-ALS antibodies, which may cause acute allergic reactions, immune complex deposition, or amyloid deposits after long-term use. The second factor is the presence, even after proper absorption, of antibody with specificity for nonlymphocyte antigens, so that, for instance, anemia, pancytopenia, or venous sclerosis may be produced by ALS administration.

COMPARISONS BETWEEN MONOCLONAL AND POLYCLONAL SERA

The most important feature of monoclonal antibodies is their reproducible specificity for a certain haptene. This does not imply total specificity for a given complex antigen in the body, since different proteins might share a certain haptenic site regardless of their differences otherwise. Even so, in practice the specificity obtainable with monoclonal antibodies is extremely good.

The limits of clonal stability place a theoretical limit on the perpetual availability of any given monoclonal reagent. However for good clones, the frozen initial aliquots of early generation hybridoma will provide their originators with a degree of immortality, and the reproducibility of the reagent during the life of a given clone is essentially perfect, in marked contrast to the difficulties with reproducibility in the production of ALS. Furthermore, at least for many specificities, it may be reasonably easy to replace particularly useful clones that become exhausted, with nearly identical new monoclonal antibodies.

In spite of the theoretically spotless nature of monoclonal antibodies in comparison with ALS, it must be remembered that monoclonal antibodies are biologic products, and large-scale production at present usually involves purification from rodent ascites, so that possible residual impurities may remain. Monoclonal antibodies may also contain extraneous material even if derived from tissue culture fluid, since many clones are the result of fusions with "producer" myeloma lines and may secrete immunoglobulin light or heavy chains in addition to the desired antibody. Finally, the myeloma lines theoretically may contain oncogenic rodent viruses. It seems unlikely that oncogenic viral contamination, even if present, would be pathogenic for human cells, and furthermore, viruses should almost certainly be removed by the purification process. However, by contrast with ALG, where this is not as evident a consideration, oncogenic viral contamination remains a theoretical consideration in therapy with monoclonal antibodies.

Many techniques and antigen sources have been evaluated in the production of polyclonal ALS. However, the possible variations are minimal compared with the number of possible monoclonal reagents that might be employed to influence just one cell surface antigen. A partial list of the relevant variables includes epitope recognized on the antigen, function of the antigen, and immunoglobulin class of the antibody. Considering in addition the variety of different antigens that have been identified on lymphocytes and monocytes, it is clear that the possible number of different monoclonal reagents that might influence the immune system in vivo is very large. Polyclonal ALS contains an uncontrolled mixture of these ingredients, plus whatever antibody against nonlymphocyte antigens may have arisen. This distribution of antibodies in polyclonal sera presumably results in the presence of some antibodies of the desired characteristics in most ALS preparations; if the remaining majority of the immunoglobulin is irrelevant, or at least not too toxic, then the desired immunosuppressive effect will be achieved. A given monoclonal antibody, on the other hand, if it is of the wrong sort in any of the variables just noted, may be totally impotent as an immunosuppressive agent in vivo, regardless of its in vitro characteristics.

There are at least three ways that monoclonal antibodies do not represent any apparent improvement over ALS as an immunosuppressive agent. In the first place, monoclonal antibodies produced against T-lymphocyte differentiation antigens will still not distinguish T cells of a certain subset that are useful in defense against infection, from the cells in that subset that cause graft rejection. Thus there is still a risk, with monoclonal antibody treatment, of compromised defenses against infection. It is true that the risk may well be somewhat less, since ALS in some instances probably has activity against non-T-lymphocyte populations, such as natural killer (NK) cells, which would be spared by anti-T-cell monoclonal antibody, in which case the monoclonal agents should be safer. The second similarity is that immunoglobulin therapy with immunoglobulin of either sort must be parenteral, so that long-term treatment is impractical. Finally, the immune response of the recipient against these foreign proteins may be a limiting factor, as described for monoclonal agents under Induction of Anti-idiotype.

POSSIBLE MECHANISMS OF ACTION OF MONOCLONAL ANTIBODIES

Clearance of Cells

By analogy with ALS, a major goal of monoclonal antibody therapy might be to remove all T lymphocytes circulating in the bloodstream. The requirements for opsonizing antibody to produce clearance seem to include either complement-fixing capacity [35,57, 129] or capacity to interact with Fc receptors that will produce reticuloendothelial cell uptake [35,54]. Anti-Lyt 1 monoclonal antibodies can be shown to cause depletion of Lyt 1-positive cells from spleen and lymph nodes in mice [97,139,140]. Evaluation of peripheral blood clearance is more difficult in rodents but is of interest since it is the usual clinical approach. An example in mice of clearance from the peripheral blood of the appropriate cell type by administration of anti-Lyt 1 (clone TIB 104, from American Type Culture Collection, immunoglobulin prepared by Dr. K. Ishizaka) is shown in Figure 1. A parallel depletion of appropriate lymphocytes from the spleens of these mice was found, and Thy 1 (and Lyt 2)-positive cells also decreased, confirming that this disappearance of cells represented clearance, not masking of antigens on cells remaining in the circulation. Similar Lyt 2-positive cell clearance was produced by an antibody directed against this antigen (clone TIB 105). Although these are IgG_{2a} antibodies, they are interesting in that they do not fix complement well, indicating that complement fixation was not a critical factor for in vivo clearance.

The monoclonal antibody against human T cells, OKT3, is, to date, the most effective clinical in vivo application of monoclonal antibody immunosuppression. This antibody produces rapid and profound clearance of circulating cells in the human (Chapter 16). It has been very effective for the reversal of renal allograft rejection and fairly effective against graft-versus-host disease [43]. Other OKT series antibodies have been tested in primates, including OKT4/4A and OKT8 (recognizing helper/inducer and cytotoxic/suppressor subsets, respectively). Cynomolgus monkeys can be shown to undergo a partial decrement in circulating T4-bearing lymphocytes after treatment with OKT4

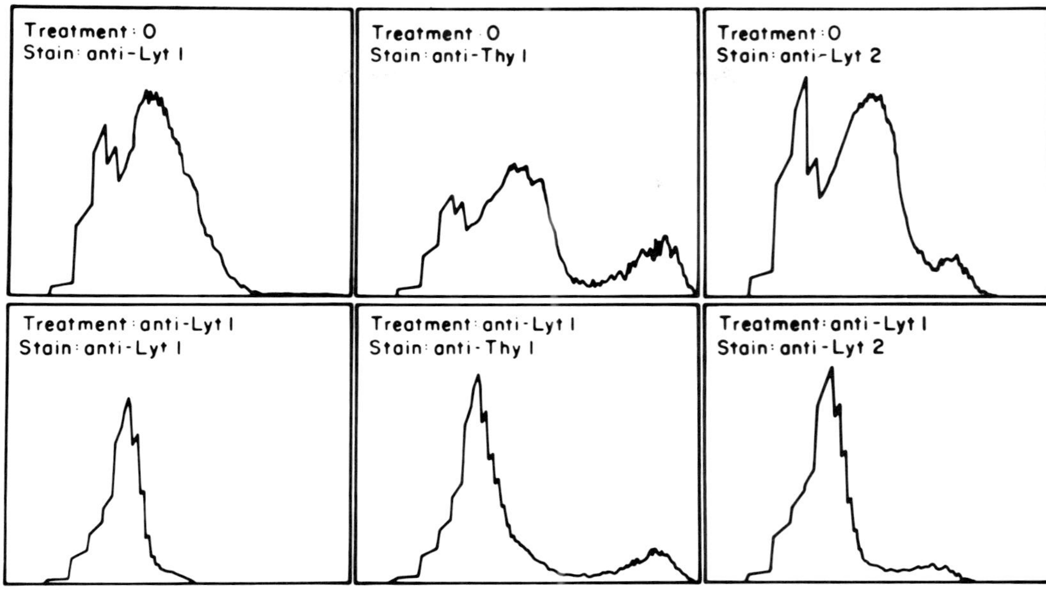

FIGURE 1 Clearance of lymphocytes from the peripheral blood of mice treated with anti-Lyt 1 monoclonal antibody. Antibody was given on day –1 and 0, and peripheral blood was then characterized for the specificities designated using the fluorescence-activated cell analyzer.

[23]. In one study it was found that neither OKT4 nor OKT4A individually would produce clearance from the peripheral blood of rhesus monkeys, but a combination of both antibodies administered simultaneously provided prompt clearance [61]. Similarly, a pool of monoclonal antibodies against cytotoxic T cells provided clearance of the cells in rhesus monkeys, whereas the antibodies employed singly were ineffective [62]. This might represent a complementary effect of different qualities of the Fc portions of the individual antibodies; alternatively, it might stem from a quantitative restriction on the degree to which antibody bound to one epitope can effect clearance, overcome by an additive effect of a second antibody to a different epitope.

The use of monoclonal antibodies in the treatment of leukemia and lymphoma is conceptually akin to using antilymphocyte antibodies to produce immunosuppression by clearance of normal lymphocytes from the blood, or from the inflammatory infiltrate in a graft during rejection. Treatment of T-cell leukemia with an anti-T-cell monoclonal antibody can result in marked clearance of the leukemic cells from the circulation, with uptake of the cells initially by the lungs [17,118] and later by the liver and spleen [98]. Addition of complement is required for maximum success in certain leukemia systems [6,11]. However, complement is more typically found not to be important in the effect of monoclonal antibodies against tumors [11,56].

A milestone in the therapeutic use of monoclonal antibodies was the demonstration that treatment with an anti-idiotype against the combining site of the surface immunoglobulin on a lymphoma, using large doses over a long period of time, was quite successful [99]. There is a general sense that IgG is more effective in tumor immunotherapy than IgM [3,7,58-60,65], although in one report, monoclonal antibody therapy of hepatomas was effective if the antibody was IgG_{2a} or IgM, but not IgG_1 [131]. Treatment of solid tumors with monoclonal antibodies against tumor-associated antigens has apparently also been effective in some other instances [32,131]. Monoclonal antitumor antibody used to treat nonlymphoid tumors is apparently usually effective only if it is of the IgG_{2a} subclass, perhaps because destruction by macrophages is mediated by IgG_{2a} antibody [51,136,137]. However, other factors are involved, since an IgG_{2a} antibody that was effective against one tumor in vivo actually potentiated tumor growth when it was used to treat another tumor [65].

The effectiveness of IgG_{2a} in clearance of cells from the circulation is not totally predictable. When IgG_2 antibodies were prepared similarly against the allotypic portions of Lyt 1 of different strains, one produced clearance of Lyt 1^+ cells when employed in vivo in the appropriate strain, whereas another, similar, antibody produced no clearance of cells in its appropriate strain [17]. An IgG_{2b} anti-Thy 1 monoclonal antibody was effective in clearing cells and treating experimental lupus in one mouse strain [166].

If lymphocyte depletion is to be the mechanism of action of a monoclonal antibody, then whether opsonization and clearance of lymphocytes from the circulation or removal from the graft is more important might determine which subclass is desirable. IgM stays within the circulation longer than IgG, and is more effective in opsonizing and clearing bacteria [36]. IgG, on the other hand, would be expected to enter the graft and produce its effect there more efficiently. However, in the situation noted above, IgM was as effective as an IgG_{2a} antibody in the inhibition of tumor growth [131], which presumably required the antibody to pass out into the tissue. By analogy, it might be that IgM can pass out of the bloodstream into other inflamed areas, such as allografts undergoing rejection. Lymphocytes in the thymus may be protected from the effect of antibody, which does not fix complement well, since there are no macrophages there to act with the antibody even if it can enter this area [145].

However, as with ALS, this sort of clearance may not be the required mechanism. Depletion of Lyt 1-positive cells from lymph nodes and spleen by anti-Lyt 1 monoclonal antibody was found to correlate with the immunosuppressive effect in mice [97,139, 140], but studies with the OKT series of anti-human lymphocyte antibodies in rhesus monkeys showed no correlation of clearance of the cells from the circulation with immunosuppressive effect [62]. Clinically, although anti-T12 produced very effective clearance of cells, the immunosuppressive effect of this antibody was not as reproducibly evident [66]. Different subsets of B lymphocytes are reconstituted at different rates after monoclonal anti-Ia antibody treatment [160], similar to the difference in reconstitution of short- and long-lived T cells after ALS treatment, and similar results are likely to be found with monoclonal anti-T-cell antibodies. Therefore, there may be marked differences in immunologic status after antibody treatment even when the overall lymphocyte levels seem normal.

Functional Receptor Blocking

A prime example of a powerful immunosuppressive effect without destruction of the lymphocytes involved is to be found in the experiments by McDevitt's group [125]. They employed F_1 mice that were heterozygous for immune response genes controlling responses to two different antigens. Treatment of the mice with monoclonal anti-Ia antibody against the Ia specificity of one strain abolished antibody formation against the antigen for which that strain was a responder. However, the response against the alternate antigen, facilitated by the other I region, remained intact unless the alternate anti-Ia antibody was employed. Since both Ia antigens are expressed on each cell, this means that the effect did not involve destruction of the lymphocytes. A likely mechanism would be interference with function of the Ia antigens due to steric hindrance by the bound antibody.

A concept that may separate the effect of monoclonal antibodies into two functional categories is the distinction between adhesion antigens and activation antigens on the T-cell surface. Adhesion antigens potentiate approximation between the surfaces of appropriate cells, and include T4 and its rodent equivalent, L3T4, which direct helper (or class II-reactive) cells [31,74,77,93,114,141,161], T8 or Lyt 2, which direct the adhesion of cytotoxic/suppressor (or class I-reactive) cells [55,77,113,157,165], perhaps T12 (whose function has not been identified), and lymphocyte function-associated antigen [52,135], which is thought to play a role in lymphocyte, monocyte, and polymorphonuclear adhesion (see Binding Sites and Affinity). Antibody against these antigens can inhibit specific functions in vitro, perhaps by blocking the adhesion necessary for interaction between cells in immunologic responses, and might produce a similar effect in vivo.

The other type of antigen is particularly involved in activation. The prototype for this is T3, which strongly stimulates T cells under appropriate conditions, as described under Pharmacologic Effect on Lymphocytes or Lymphokines. T3 is closely related to the Ti receptor molecules (Figure 2) [73,91,95,120,124] and theoretically is responsible for triggering the T cell to activate the interleukin-2 mechanism and to proliferate [124, 164]. In one study, blocking with anti-T4 or anti-T8 antibody did not inhibit proliferation, whereas blocking with anti-T3 inhibited proliferation as well as cytotoxicity [92]. It has recently been reported that T11, the sheep erythrocyte receptor, is also able to produce striking lymphocyte activation when treated with appropriate monoclonal antibodies and may represent a primitive intrathymic stimulatory mechanism [96].

Of course, all these antigens could serve merely as appropriate targets against which to direct antibody designed to kill or clear the lymphocytes bearing that antigen, but other effects on stimulation or on adhesion might play a significant role in ways not yet appreciated. As an example, anti-T3 will block cytotoxicity in vitro at appropriate concentrations [9,18,76,115,142], in addition to its capacity to activate T cells and its potential to opsonize for clearance of cells.

Monoclonal antibodies have been made against suppressor factor [85] and against interleukin-2 (IL-2) [107]. Interleukin-2 is centrally involved in T-cell activation (see Chapter 4) [95] and anti-interleukin-2 antibody blocks the generation of cytotoxic lymphocytes in vitro [42]. Monoclonal antibodies against rat [107] and human [82,

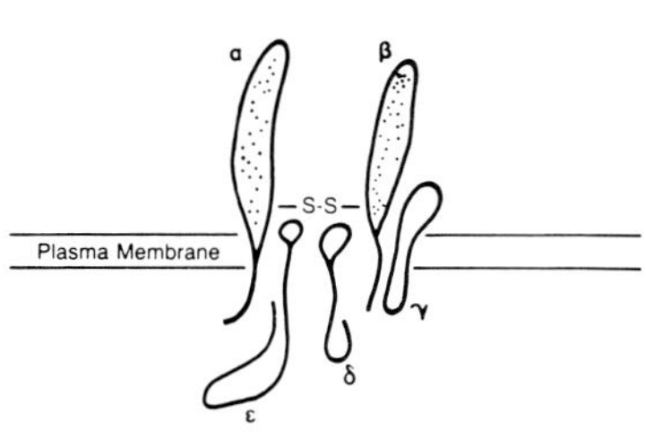

FIGURE 2 The T-cell receptor/T3 complex. The unstippled chains represent the T3 complex in this conceptualization. (From Weiss, A., Imboden, J., Hardy K., Manger, B., Terhorst, C., Stobo, J., The role of the T3/antigen receptor complex in T cell activation, *Ann. Rev. Immunol.* in press, 1986.)

146] interleukin-2 receptors have also been made, and these can inhibit T-cell function in vitro [87]. Antigens of the human D region (or murine IA region) are involved in the initiation of the IL-2 mechanism when T-cell activation occurs, and therefore an immunosuppressive effect of anti-Ia antisera might be due to an indirect inhibition of induction of interleukin-2 and its receptors [71,108,109], as well as by simple blocking of interactions by cells bearing Ia. Interference with the interleukin-2 mechanism is a particularly interesting possible application for monoclonal antibodies, since the result might resemble the excellent effectiveness of cyclosporine, for which a major mechanism of action seems to be interference with the interleukin-2 mechanism. Recently, it was demonstrated that interleukin-2 is important for B-cell as well as T-cell function [154], so that interference with this mechanism might not prove to be as specific for T-cell function as had been presumed. Another likely mechanism to exploit for immunosuppression might be blocking either γ-interferon or its receptor [117] by a monoclonal antibody, and the interleukin-1 mechanism (Chapter 4) might similarly be exploited.

Pharmacologic Effect on Lymphocytes or Lymphokines

Another explanation for the immunosuppressive effect of anti-Ia antibody described above could be modulation or shedding of the functionally necessary antigen from the cell surface. In order for this mechanism to contribute to immunosuppression, the molecule in question must be important for immunologic function of the cell. Modulation was found to have occurred in patients effectively treated with OKT3, as described in Chapter 16. Modulation of T3 in vitro is associated with activation of the cell; therefore, this effect was initially cited as a defect in the immunosuppressive potential of this agent. It has become clear that this is a complex phenomenon. The T3 molecule is an invariant structure that occurs in intimate association with the variable antigen-specific Ti portion of the T-cell receptor (Figure 2) [91,120]. Antibody to T3 alone or Ti alone in solution will not cause activation and, in fact, can block reactions in vitro [9,18,76,115,127]; however, when coupled to a surface these agents are powerful instigators of T-cell proliferation and interleukin-2 production [94]. This is a sudden event: within a minute of interaction with antibody a burst of oxidative metabolism occurs [30]. In more physiologic situations this mitogenesis requires the participation of monocytes [30,63,75,122,153,162], and the reason that Leu 4, unlike OKT3, is able to induce proliferation only in cells from certain individuals is apparently related to a failure of successful interaction with monocytes in the unstimulated cases [63,147,163]. The T3 molecule may function as a calcium channel "trigger" that normally is induced by perturbation of the adjacent antigen receptor molecules, resulting in activation [164]. Exceptions to the requirement for monocytes in the production of T-cell activation by monoclonal antibodies thus far reported are the stimulation produced in the absence of accessory cells by anti-Thy 1 [44] and anti-$T11_2$ plus anti-$T11_3$ together [96].

In view of its capacity to activate cells, why is OKT3 immunosuppressive rather than actually harmful for the treatment of rejection? This relates to the functional status of the cells in these patients that lack T3 due to modulation but express other usual T-lymphocyte antigens, such as T4 and T8: it is now known that T3 and Ti comodulate (reviewed in Reference 124). Therefore, it seems very likely that the circulating lymphocytes that lack expression of T3 antigen due to modulation also lack antigen receptors. Thus the choice of T3 as a target of immunosuppressive action may have been particularly serendipitous in that the gross clearance that may be required for effective action by monoclonal antibodies directed against other cell surface structures may be unnecessary for the action of OKT3. Furthermore, it might well be that a reagent against, for example, an invariant portion of one of the chains of Ti, might be equivalently effective in modulation of the antigen receptor, although this might also produce the initial stimulation caused by OKT3. This brief activation, which may be similar to that occurring naturally due to antigen stimulation [45] prior to establishment of a (theoretically) receptorless, nonfunctional, cell, apparently does not represent a problem for immunosuppression in view of the clinical effectiveness of OKT3 and the observation that lymphocytes taken from patients during a period of OKT3 treatment did not show evidence of activation [12]. Furthermore, activation could theoretically have a beneficial pharmacologic effect, as noted under Induction of Suppressor Cells.

Antigens vary in the degree to which they can be made to undergo modulation or shedding by antibody binding. In the mouse, Thy 1 can be seen to shed [159], and the anti-Lyt 1 and Lyt 2 antibodies used in Figure 1 will cause modulation or shedding of their target antigens in vitro (Ishizaka, personal communication). Abolition of some functionally active molecule other than the T3-T-cell receptor complex by such a mechanism might also be a particularly safe and reversible form of immunosuppression. This has not been directly investigated experimentally.

Another effect of a monoclonal antibody might be to alter the metabolism of the lymphocyte, if binding to the target antigen by the antibody caused a signal similar to the normal interaction of the cell with antigen or other cells [45,79,94]. Stimulation of some function might result, which could theoretically interfere with the desired inhibition of function. However, this does not necessarily follow, since the known capacity of OKT3 to induce lymphocyte proliferation under certain conditions in vitro does not render it ineffective for immunosuppression in vivo. Interestingly, as described below, activation of suppressor cells by stimulatory antibody is delayed for days beyond the immediate proliferation exhibited by helper cells, so that the final long-term result of activation of all T cells in this way could be a net suppressive effect of pan-T activation in this way.

Induction of Suppressor Cells

Direct attempts to induce active suppression of allograft rejection with monoclonal antibodies might include (1) "resetting" the regulatory level by allowing suppressor cell response to the antigen to develop while the generation of an effector mechanism is inhibited, as mentioned above; (2) stimulation of a suppressor cell response by antibody reacting against a functional cell surface antigen of the suppressor cell; and (3) induction of suppression through antiidiotype stimulation, which in clinical practice would be logistically difficult due to the large number of major and minor histocompatibility antigens on an allograft.

One intriguing example of alteration of function by monoclonal antibody interaction is represented by the discovery that suppressor T cells react in a special way to stimulation by antibody directed against Ti. Unlike the immediate stimulation produced in other T cells, suppressor cells become quiescent for about 72 hr, following which they become metabolically active and proliferate [5]. This mechanism presumably contributes to immune regulation. It might also be a useful effect to exploit for immunosuppression, and indeed, ATGAM or OKT3 therapy may in some instances have produced just this effect through interaction with the T3 molecule, conceivably resulting in the induction of suppressor cells that persist after treatment because their activation is delayed relative to the helper cells.

Prolonged treatment with anti-Ia monoclonal antibody may produce an effect that far outlasts the treatment, and this seems to be best explained by the generation of suppressor cells [112] during the time the antigen is present but a positive response is prevented by the antibody. Several other reports have implicated the generation of suppressor cells in the immunosuppressive effect of anti-Ia antibodies [13,72,80,130]. However, in vitro, anti-Ia antibody can interfere with immune response by blocking cell activities [71,80]; as with ALS it is apparent that different lymphocyte subpopulations become restored at widely different rates after monoclonal antibody treatment [160], and lymphocyte depletion followed by the slow return of cells capable of primary responses could be an alternative explanation for the long-term effects in other systems.

Donor Tissue Treatment

The use of antibodies to remove allogeneic passenger leukocytes, which may be responsible for stimulation of rejection, is appealing. In considering the use of monoclonal anti-Ia sera for this [169], the antigenic complexity of the glycoproteins and glycolipids now known to comprise this varied group of antigens (see under Antigen Recognized) must be taken into account, since each individual monoclonal antibody will not necessarily recognize the functionally important form of Ia. It may be that monoclonal antibody against the dendritic cell will prove most effective in this application [37].

Conjugated with Toxins or Isotopes

Rather than relying on intrinsic biologic effects of monoclonal antibody directed against lymphocyte surface antigens, it may be useful to employ these to direct toxic substances to the cell [155,158]. For this to work it may be that the antibody must be directed against an antigen that is internalized so that the material will be carried into the cell [38, 156]. It has been suggested that cross-linking on the surface by divalent antibody may be important in this when antireceptor antibody is employed to target the toxin [19,39], although this is not yet certain [90]. Furthermore, it was found that *Pseudomonas* toxin conjugated to anti-interleukin-2 receptor antibody was effective even though this receptor was not expected to undergo modulation [38], so that this apparent requirement may not be absolute. In a contrasting setting, in which a strong effect on the cell surface is desired, coupling to an antibody against an antigen that is not internalized appears to be useful [1]. Another approach might be to conjugate antibodies to short-range radioisotopes [40,46, 170], which should be effective even without internalization.

Thus far the use of conjugated antibodies has not proven as effective in vivo as in vitro [133]. It seems clear that, even if such conjugated antibodies eventually prove to be very effective immunosuppressives, many of the unanswered biologic questions surrounding the use of monoclonal antibodies in vivo will be relevant [170] and must be answered for this approach to achieve its full potential.

FACTORS INFLUENCING MONOCLONAL ANTIBODY EFFECTIVENESS

Antigen Recognized

Whether the antigen recognized by a monoclonal antibody may determine the in vivo effect of the antibody due to simple clearance of the cells opsonized by the antibody, passive inhibition of the function normally served by that antigen on the cell surface, or by stimulating some desired activity on the part of the cell, it should be possible to determine the characteristics and degree of immunosuppression in part by the distribution of the antigen selected. Thus it might be possible to produce either a very generalized immunosuppression, perhaps more like that available with antilymphocyte sera, or a more restricted inhibition of a certain aspect of the response. Lymphocyte function-associated antigen (LFA) is an example of an antigen with very broad representation, and antibody against this can interfere with an antitumor response [48]. Somewhat more selective are the pan-T-cell reagents. Included in this category in the human are OKT3, which is remarkably effective (Chapter 16), and anti-T12, which is apparently effective in some cases [66]. Other antibodies directed against antigens present on all T cells, such as those against the rosette receptor (T11), have not generally been shown to be effective [24,151], although graft-versus-host disease was partially reversed by two antibodies against T11 [121]. The possibility of suppression restricted to the activity of a subset of T lymphocytes seems an appealing potential advantage of monoclonal antibodies, and success with antibody against helper cells has been reported for treatment of graft rejection in monkeys [24,61] and in improving recovery from experimental allergic encephalomyelitis in rodents [14]. The anticytotoxic/suppressor cell antibody Leu 2a was effective against graft rejection in monkeys, but OKT8A was not [24,61]. Whether antibody against cytotoxic T-cell antigens is likely to be effective in graft rejection depends upon whether cytotoxic T lymphocytes play an important role in graft rejection, which is debatable (see Chapter 3) [78,84].

Two aspects of this approach to T-cell subset specificity deserve further study. In the first place, as described in Binding Sites and Affinity, different antibodies against the same antigen can be shown to have different effects, at least in vitro. These differences, based upon functional impairment of the antigen, would be important in cases in which simple clearance of the cells is not an effective mechanism of immunosuppression. Second, there is a strong suspicion that some subset antigens, such as T4 and T8, are coexpressed during activation [15], and that such cells, expressing both T4 and T8, are present in renal allograft biopsies (Chapters 10 and 11). To the extent this is the case, antibody against one antigen should clear cells that coexpress both, but in the opposite situation, in which some functional inhibition rather than simple clearance is the effective mechanism, the antibody would be expected to inhibit only the functions mediated by that antigen, in spite of the coexpression of T4 and T8 on the same cells. As noted above, monoclonal antibodies against host class II (anti-Ia) antigens can produce immunosuppression in vivo, although in one unusual case an anti-Ia antibody actually caused stimulation of cells [64]. It is becoming clear that selecting the appropriate anti-Ia reagent will not be simple. These antigens are different on B cells than on accessory cells [27], and effects on human cells in vitro depend upon whether the antibody recognizes DC, SB, or DR [22,69,111,138, 152]. In addition to these differences due to the complex of genes that comprise this region of the major histocompatibility complex, the final antigen on the cell surface is apparently influenced epigenetically by posttranslational glycosylation enzymes, which attach a remarkable variety of complex carbohydrate [26,28,47] or glycolipid [105] side chains to certain sites on the proteins. In this way the class II antigens may be continuously changing during development and immune activation, which is consistent with the key role played by glycoproteins in interactions between cells [119]. In view of the varied carbohydrate antigens possible, the effects of antibodies against these antigens are likely to vary considerably with regard to the cells and functions with which they interact, depending upon which of the specificities are recognized. Antibodies against Ia and some other antigens on monocytes might be damagingly cross-reactive with epithelium in vivo [53].

A final category of specific antigens that might be considered for immunosuppression, particularly of a response that is already underway, are those that appear during activation. Although antibody against such antigens can block in vitro activities [88,144], there has been only one reported clinical application of an antiblast antibody thus far (CBL1; see Chapter 16).

The effects of a monoclonal antibody in vitro do not necessarily predict the result in vivo. It was shown, for instance, that an IgM monoclonal anti-Thy 1 antibody that had a high titer for complement-dependent cytotoxicity in vitro was without immunosuppressive effect in vivo [106]. In other interesting in vivo experiments, an anti-Thy 1 monoclonal antibody caused a decrease in spontaneous cytotoxic T lymphocytes but an increase in natural killer cell activity in the spleens of treated animals [49]. The most striking example of dissociation between in vivo and in vitro results is perhaps the therapeutic effectiveness of OKT3 in spite of the activation that it can induce in vitro.

Different results can be produced in vivo in mice by treatment with monoclonal antilymphocyte antibodies against different T-cell subsets. In the experiments depicted in Figures 3 and 4, the anti-Lyt 1 and Lyt 2 antibodies evaluated for clearance in the experiments in Figure 1 were used to treat mice in vivo, at the dose found to maximally deplete the peripheral circulation of that lymphocyte subset. As might have been expected, they were not equivalent in their effects on different responses, even though total T cells were markedly depleted by either antibody. The anti-Lyt 1 antibody produced a decreased delayed-type hypersensitivity response (Figure 3) but did not influence the mixed lymphocyte culture generation of lymphocyte-mediated cytotoxicity (LMC) by spleen cells from treated animals (Figure 4). Treatment with anti-Lyt 2, on the other hand, did decrease the splenocyte response in mixed lymphocyte culture. This is not surprising, since the Lyt 1-bearing helper cell subset chould be particularly important in delayed-type hypersensitivity, and the Lyt 2 subset is necessary for the generation of cytotoxicity. It does suggest that the Lyt 1 helper effect in mixed lymphocyte culture (MLC) generation of LMC is in great excess in this system, since depletion of Lyt 1 cells did not suppress this assay. Since a significant depletion of Thy 1-positive (= total T) cells was produced by these reagents, it seems unlikely that the effect was due simply to coating of the cells, but it is evident that further experiments will be required to distinguish with certainty among coating, clearance, and functional alteration, since any of these could produce the specific functional effects found.

We have tested one of the monoclonal anti-human lymphocyte function-associated antigen antibodies produced by fusion of cells from mice immunized with human adherent cells [52], which was cross-reactive for mouse lymphocytes (Table 1). In spite of strong binding to murine lymphocytes, this antibody produced only minimal interference with in vitro assays and was without effect on delayed-type hypersensitivity, even in doses much larger than those used for anti-Lyt 1 (Figure 3). The minimal effect in vitro is interesting since the antibody markedly inhibits human leukocyte functions. This suggests that the antibody-binding site on the murine molecule, which is antigenically similar to the functionally important area on the human molecule, is not a functionally critical area of the murine LFA antigen. This is similar to the epitope diversity for different species described by others [83].

Activation Status of the Immune System Under Treatment

Antigens on cells of the reticuloendothelial system change considerably during maturation [16] and during activation of immune responses [15,67,88,100,144,146,148,150]. Mono-

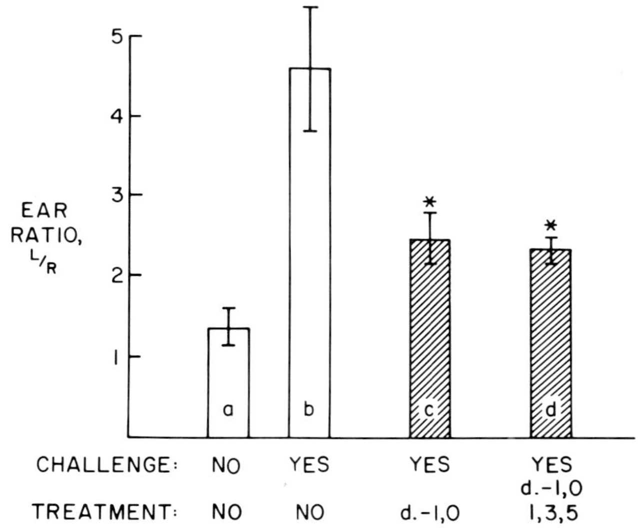

FIGURE 3 The effect of anti-Lyt 1 monoclonal antibody therapy on delayed-type hypersensitivity (DTH) in the mouse. B10.A mice received 2 mg cyclophosphamide intraperitoneally on day −2, sensitization by AKR splenocytes subcutaneously on day 0, intradermal challenge in the ear pinnae plus [^{125}I] iododioxyurodine, on day 6, and ears were removed for γ counting on day 7. Groups C and D received monoclonal antibody as indicated. Results ± standard error of the mean; * = $p < 0.05$ for group B.

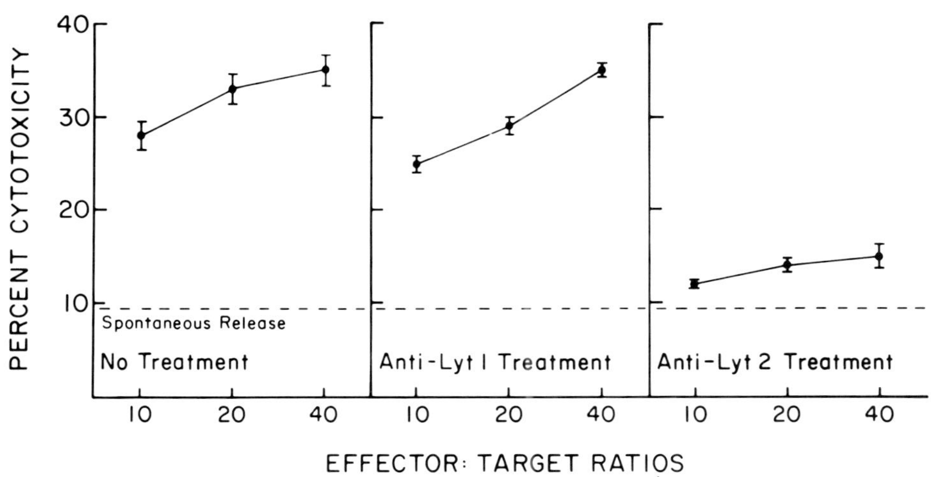

FIGURE 4 Cytotoxicity generated in splenocytes from mice treated with monoclonal antibodies. B10.A mice received the indicated monoclonal antibody intraperitoneally on day −1 and day 0, and then spleen cells were removed and employed as responders to irradiated AKR-stimulating splenocytes. Cytotoxicity that developed in these responders was determined at 6 days using chromium-labeled RDM-4 target cells.

TABLE 1 Species Cross-Reactivity of Mouse Anti-Human LFA and Mac-1

Anti-human reagent	Specificity	Capacity to bind to cells of			In vitro inhibition of		
		Minipigs[a]	Rhesus monkeys[b]	Mice[c]	Minipigs[d]	Rhesus monkeys[e]	Mice[f]
H52	HLFA β	+	+	+	+	–	–7[g]
H5B9	HLFA β	++	+	+	+	n.t.	n.t.
MHM.23	HLFA β	++	+	+	+	n.t.	n.t.
MHM.24	HLFA α	–	–	–	n.t.	n.t.	n.t.
H5A4	HMac-1 α	–	+	±	n.t.	n.t.	n.t.
H4C2	HMac-1 α	n.t.	n.t.	n.t.	n.t.	n.t.	n.t.

[a]Immunoperoxidase and immunoprecipitation techniques (spleen and blood). (Data courtesy of Hildredth and August.)
[b]Immunoperoxidase (spleen). (Data courtesy of Hildredth and August.)
[c]Radioimmunoassay (splenocytes). (Data courtesy of Hildredth and August.)
[d]Mixed lymphocyte culture and T-cell-mediated cytotoxicity. (Data courtesy of Pescovitz and Sachs.)
[e]No effect or stimulation of mixed lymphocyte and mitogen stimulation. (Data courtesy of Thomas.)
[f]Mixed lymphocyte culture generation of cell-mediated cytotoxicity.
[g]Delayed-type hypersensitivity was also not inhibited by H52.
n.t. = Not tested.

cytes [143] and endothelial cells [116], as well as epidermal cells [29], are induced to express Ia by nearby immunologic reactions, perhaps due to γ-interferon [4]. At the least, this might significantly increase the amount of anti-Ia antibody required to reach an effective level as compared with unstimulated animals, and also it might alter the net functional effects of the antibody, if these stimulated cells were to react in some different fashion. Also, T4, T8, and interleukin-2 receptor concentrations increase in amount on activated cells, which might give rise to similar considerations. The presence of Ia is important, particularly for induction of the interleukin-2 mechanism, so that, once this is adequately activated, anti-Ia antisera might no longer block further proliferation [108].

As noted above, we have found evidence that lymphocytes in human renal allograft biopsies may have a high incidence of coexpression of T4 and T8 (see Chapter 10). This is apparently a manifestation of activation [15]. Monoclonal antibody therapy with reagents directed toward one or the other of these antigens would only alter the immune response of these cells in a subset-specific way if a direct effect on the lymphocyte, rather than clearance, were the mechanism of action, since the large fraction of cells that express both would be cleared by antibody against either.

Immunoglobulin Class

A major unsolved question in the design of monoclonal antibodies for use in vivo is the influence of immunoglobulin class. As noted above, the effect of class could be influenced by the antigen against which the antibody was directed, since total cell clearance might be the only possible mechanism by which antibodies against some antigens could mediate immunosuppression, and steric or other functional effects might produce immunosuppression by antibodies against other antigens. Extensive studies of in vivo immunosuppression with a series of monoclonal antibodies, holding the antigen recognized constant and varying the immunoglobulin class widely, have not been done. The best example thus far is the careful study by Opitz and colleagues [106]. Two monoclonal anti-Thy 1 antibodies were studied, one of the IgM and the other of the IgG_{2a} subclass. The IgM antibody, although exhibiting a high titer of complement-dependent cytotoxicity in vitro, produced no effect when administered to mice, but the IgG_{2a}, in spite of a somewhat lower cytotoxic titer, was found to totally block mixed lymphocyte stimulation in splenocytes from treated animals, as well as anti-sheep red blood cell antibody formation and delayed-type hypersensitivity. More comparisons between IgG_{2a}, IgM, and other subclasses are necessary, however, since these two particular antibodies might well recognize different epitopes on Thy 1 and therefore may have had different effects on that basis, unrelated to the immunoglobulin class. The question of whether capacity to fix complement is one of several factors governing the influence of immunoglobulin class is not totally settled by these results. However, the antibodies employed for the experiments in Figures 1, 3, and 4 are interesting in that, in spite of being IgG_{2a}, they do not fix complement. Yet they cause very effective clearance of lymphocytes and at least modest immunosuppression. Other monoclonal antibodies that have proven effective in vivo have been IgG_{2a}, including OKT3, and anti-Lyt 1 [110] reagents. Since the capacity for complement fixation does not appear to be the main determinant of effectiveness in vivo, it may be that the Fc area that determines macrophage uptake is responsible for the effectiveness of IgG_{2a}. As noted above, this mechanism is believed to explain the particular effectiveness of this subclass for immunotherapy of solid tumors. On the other hand, IgG_{2a} antibody may in some instances be ineffective in vivo [11].

Binding Sites and Affinity

Markedly different capacity to block in vitro activity was found for different monoclonal antibodies reactive against the same cell surface structure, human LFA. Those reactive against the α chain will block lymphocyte stimulation, T-cell killing, and tetanus toxoid stimulation but not natural killer cell action or complement receptor function, whereas reagents against the β chain of the same molecule inhibit all these activities [52]. Explanations for this might include the possibility that the α and β chains are not distributed as associated unit molecules equivalently on all cells, or that not all functions of the two-chain unit are equivalently served by the same portions of the molecule. However, it has been shown that the difference, at least with regard to T-cell function and complement binding, stems from the fact that the receptor for the third component of complement (which is Mac-1 in the human) has the same β chain but a different α chain than LFA, so that only antibody against the β chain would be expected to affect all the functions. In other experiments it was found that, for inhibition of cytotoxicity by different monoclonal antibodies, lytic activity was affected differently by the different antibodies against T8 [8,113,157] or against Ti [50]. These are illustrations of the degree to which different monoclonal antibodies against different epitopes on a molecule might produce different results if steric blocking or other interference with function, rather than modulation of the antigen or gross clearance of the cells, is the mechanism of action.

Antibody against one epitope of a complex molecule may cause conformational changes that affect the binding of a second antibody to a different epitope [33,34]. In vivo, it has been shown that, as might be expected, the antitumor effect of a monoclonal antibody varies with the affinity of the antibody [81].

Induction of Modulation

Although it was noted above (Pharmacologic Effect on Lymphocytes or Lymphokines) that modulation can interfere with function and therefore may contribute to the immunosuppressive effect, for instance, of OKT3, modulation might also merely prevent clearance of the cells; such a mechanism seemed to protect leukemia cells from destruction by monoclonal antibody [41,123] and might prevent OKT11A from being immunosuppressive [24]. Conversely, modulation might be useful if toxin-conjugated antibodies were to be employed, as noted in Conjugated with Toxins or Isotopes.

Induction of Anti-idiotype

As part of the antibody response against the foreign protein, anti-idiotypic antibody is formed after treatment of humans with OKT3 (see Chapter 16) and is almost certainly also formed after treatment with many other monoclonal antibodies, although formation of antibody against the monoclonal antibody used for treatment was remarkably absent in other settings [66,98,121,151]. The development of antibody against the monoclonal antibody administered would cause it to be cleared and, therefore, ineffective. On the other hand, because of the important regulatory nature of the idiotype-anti-idiotype mechanism [21], whether the net effect of anti-idiotype might strengthen rather than counteract a desired effect of a given monoclonal antibody in some cases is not certain at present, and questions about this mechanism seem likely to surface commonly during monoclonal antibody therapy.

It has been suggested that monoclonal antibody produced by fusion of a human myeloma line with immunized human cells, to produce a monoclonal antibody consisting of human immunoglobulin, would be an ideal therapeutic agent since it would avoid the problem of anti-mouse antibody, which, for instance, is commonly made by patients treated with OKT3. However, in addition to the possibility of anti-human allotype antibody, to the extent that the treated individual forms anti-idiotype, the potential for immune clearance interfering with a therapeutic effect of monoclonal antibody remains. That this might not be trivial is underscored by the fact that in 2 of 11 patients treated with OKT3, apparently only anti-idiotype was formed [56].

Danger to the Patient

Morbidity due to various factors is theoretically possible; however, many monoclonal antibodies have been given to experimental animals, and some have been given clinically, with remarkably little in the way of side effects. Each monoclonal antibody for which clinical administration is envisioned should be tested extensively for cross-reaction with other human tissues, since the particular epitope against which it is directed might appear on some other, otherwise unrelated, antigen. Some murine monoclonal antibodies against tumor antigens have caused fever during administration to humans [121]. The administration of the first dose of OKT3 has often been accompanied by high fever and bronchospasm, which rarely has been life threatening. This seems unlikely to be simply due to cell clearance and lysis, since other regimens that cause cell clearance do not produce such a noticeable effect. We have evidence that OKT3 causes release of a mediator from lymphocytes that stimulates release of interleukin-1 by monocytes [103]. Since endogenous pyrogen is interleukin-1 (Chapter 4), this provides a specific pharmacologic explanation, at least for the fever produced by OKT3 administration. A similar pharmacologic explanation for the bronchospasm would be interesting, as well as clinically useful. The most severe side effects recorded after experimental administration of monoclonal antibodies for immunosuppression were the deaths, apparently due to anaphylaxis, of several monkeys administered high doses of antiblast antibodies [10]. It is not clear whether this may have been due some impurity rather than the actual immunoglobulin administration, since in other cases, even if a reaction occurs, it is rarely, if ever, a true anaphylactic response. In another report, anti-Thy 1 was evaluated for its effect on three groups of mice with three different autoimmune disorders, and six of eight mice in one group died suddenly after the second dose of antibody [166]. Since the mice in the other groups did not die, some impurity in the preparation is not likely, but anaphylaxis seems similarly unlikely as an explanation for this, and some other pharmacologic effect due to the altered immune system in the particular group suffering fatalities seems more likely.

The greatest risk to the patient is overimmunosuppression, as with all agents that cause immunosuppression not specifically restricted to the alloantigens of the graft. The possibility of treating with antibody against human LFA might be considered particularly prohibitive in this regard; however, kindreds are known whose members lack LFA and Mac 1 due to a lack of the β chain common to this antigen. These individuals survive, at least for years, albeit with severe immunodeficiency [68,135]. Short-term treatment with an antibody against the β chain might mimic this to some degree but would probably not result in more immediately threatening suppression. The possibility of treating with a reagent against the α chain of the human LFA is particularly appealing, since this is not shared by Mac 1 (see Chapter 1), and the effects should therefore be more restricted.

CONSIDERATIONS IN THE GENERATION OF MONOCLONAL REAGENTS

Most experiments and clinical trials thus far have involved the investigation of whatever antibodies happened to arise. Information about characteristics to seek at the time of the "pick," when certain individual clones are chosen for propagation, would greatly facilitate the process. Simple assays that can be completed in a day or two are critical since the logistics do not allow more prolonged culture of all the products of the fusion. However, if a requirement for a particular immunoglobulin subclass or a particular antigen against which the antibody would best be directed were known for certain, it would be possible to incorporate this into the initial selection process. Thus there is an urgent need to systematically determine which of these characteristics are important.

One principle now illustrated in several articles is the use of a surrogate species for testing. For instance, an anti-mouse Ia antibody was found to cross-react with human, rat, rabbit, guinea pig, and dog antigens, and was found to be effective in the pretreatment of dog kidney to remove passenger leukocytes before transplantation [169]. Anti-human reagents often cross-react with cynomolgus or rhesus monkey cells and may be able to be tested, at least for general safety and effectiveness in those species [62], although cost and logistics make this a difficult system for extensive evaluation of basic biologic questions. The large number of monoclonal antibodies that were generated against human monocytes by August and Hildredth (see Chapter 1) were found to react against mouse, cynomolgus, and pig tissue (Table 1). This will allow certain experiments on in vivo effects to be carried out in experimental animals, with the expectation that these results would apply to the human clinical situation. The functional ineffectiveness of the antilymphocyte function antibody in mice described in Antigen Recognized rules out testing in mice, which would have been particularly appealing. However, in vitro functional studies in pigs and monkeys did reveal inhibition in some cases, so that further tests of these reagents in vivo will be able to be done in these species.

Clinical immunosuppression might be aided by using monoclonal antibodies comprised of human, rather than xenogeneic, immunoglobulin [20]. These might be created in the usual way by fusion of a myeloma line, in this case of human origin, with immunized human cells [128]. This has been useful in delineation of clinical autoantibody specificity, but compared with murine monoclonal antibody lacks the advantages offered by rodents of the capacity to intentionally immunize in vivo initially, and the ease of production as ascites [132]. Furthermore, an ideal myeloma line has not been described, and the introduction into a patient of any material from such a tumor line, however purified, is a worrisome prospect. Alternatively, long-term cell lines secreting antibodies may be created by fusion with Epstein-Barr virus-infected cell lines or by a composite technique using Epstein-Barr virus lines and hybridoma fusion [20,70]. Finally, it is now possible to construct chimeric antibodies with an Fc portion derived from human, but with mouse variable region combining sites [101]. Whether the use of human immunoglobulin will be of great benefit in terms of avoiding antibody production by the recipient of the treatment is debatable since a good deal of antibody formed against immunoglobulin may be antiallotype and anti-idiotype.

ACKNOWLEDGMENTS

Supported in part by USPHS grants R01 AI115081 and PO1 AI19373. Valuable discussion with Drs. James Hildreth, Thomas August, and Kimishige Ishizaka, the excellent technical help of Larry Clow, and secretarial assistance of Pamela Creevey are gratefully acknowledged.

REFERENCES

1. Alkan, S. S., Miescher-Granger, S., Braun, D. G., and Hochkeppel, H. K. Antiviral and antiproliferative effects of interferons delivered via monoclonal antibodies. *J. Interferon Res.* 4:355-363, 1984.
2. Bach, F. F. Mechanism and significance of rosette inhibition by antilymphocyte serum. In *International Symposium on Antilymphocyte Serum: Symposia Series in Immunobiological Standardization,* Volume 16, J. F. Bach, J. Dormont, A. Eyquem, M. Raynaud, and R. H. Regamey, eds. Karger, Basel, 1970, pp. 189-198.
3. Badger, C. C., and Bernstein, I. D. Therapy of murine leukemia with monoclonal antibody against a normal differentiation antigen. *J. Exp. Med.* 157:828-842, 1983.
4. Basham, T. Y., Nickoloff, B. J., Merigan, T. C., and Morhenn, V. B. Recombinant gamma interferon induces HLA-DR expression on cultured human keratinocytes. *J. Invest. Dermatol.* 83:88-90, 1984.
5. Bensussan, A., Acuto, O., Hussey, R. E., Milanese, C., and Reinherz, E. L. T3-Ti receptor triggering of T8+ suppressor T cells, leads to unresponsiveness to interleukin-2. *Nature* 311:565-567, 1984.
6. Bernstein, I. D., Tam, M. R., and Nowinski, R. C. Mouse leukemia: Therapy with monoclonal antibodies against a thymus differentiation antigen. *Science* 207:68-71, 1980.
7. Bernstein, I. D., Nowinski, R. C., Tam, M. R., McMaster, B., Houston, L. L., and Clark, E. A. Monoclonal antibody therapy of mouse leukemia. In *Monoclonal Antibodies. Hybridomas: A New Dimension in Biological Analysis,* R. H. Kennett, T. J. McKearn, and K. B. Bechtol, eds. Plenum Press, New York, 1980, pp. 275-291.
8. Biddison, W. E., Rao, P. E., Talle, M. A., Boselli, C. M., and Goldstein, G. Distinct epitopes on the T8 molecule are differentially involved in cytotoxic T cell function. *Hum. Immunol.* 9:117-130, 1984.
9. Biddison, W. E., Shearer, G. M., and Chang, T. W. Regulation of influenza virus-specific cytotoxic T cell responses by monoclonal antibody to a human T cell differentiation antigen. *J. Immunol.* 127:2236-2240, 1981.
10. Billing, R., and Chatterjee, S. Prolongation of skin allograft survival in monkeys treated with anti-Ia and antiblast/monocyte monoclonal antibodies. *Transplant. Proc.* 15:649-650, 1983.
11. Boiocchi, M., and Mondellini, D. Immunotherapy of mouse leukemia with monoclonal antibodies directed against type-C virus structural proteins. *Tumori* 70:9-16, 1984.
12. Bowen, A., Edwards, L. C., Gailiumas, P., and Helderman, J. H. Lymphocyte function in patients treated with monoclonal anti-T3 antibody for acute cadaveric renal allograft rejection. *Transplantation* 38:489-493, 1984.
13. Broder, S., Mann, D. L., and Waldmann, T. A. Participation of suppressor T cells in the immunosuppressive activity of a heteroantiserum to human Ia-like antigens. *J. Exp. Med.* 151:257-262, 1980.
14. Brostoff, S. W., and Mason, D. W. Experimental allergic encephalomyelitis: Successful treatment in vivo with a monoclonal antibody that recognizes T helper cells. *J. Immunol.* 133:1938-1942, 1984.
15. Burns, G. F., Battye, F. L., and Goldstein, G. Surface antigen changes occurring in short-term cultures of activated human T lymphocytes: Analysis by flow cytometry. *Cell. Immunol.* 71:12-26, 1982.
16. Carlsson, S. R., and Stigbrand, T. I. Alterations in expression and glycosylation pattern of the Thy-1 glycoprotein during maturation and transformation of mouse T lymphocytes. *J. Immunol.* 130:1837-1842, 1983.

17. Carroll, A. M., and de Sousa, M. Differential effect of two monoclonal anti-Lyt-1 alloantibodies on lymphocyte distribution in vivo. *Immunology* 52:325-330, 1984.
18. Chang, T-W., and Gingras, S. P. OKT3 monoclonal antibody inhibits cytotoxic T lymphocyte mediated cell lysis. *Int. J. Immunopharmacol.* 3:183-186, 1981.
19. Cobbold, S. P., and Waldmann, H. Therapeutic potential of monovalent monoclonal antibodies. *Nature* 308:460-462, 1984.
20. Cole, S. P. C., Campling, B. G., Atlaw, T., Kozbor, D., and Roder, J. C. Human monoclonal antibodies. *Mol. Cell. Biochem.* 62:109-120, 1984.
21. Coutinho, A., Forni, L., Holmberg, D., Ivars, F., and Vaz, N. From an antigen-centered, clonal perspective of immune response to an organism-centered, network perspective of autonomous activity in a self-referential immune system. *Immunol. Rev.* 79:151-168, 1984.
22. Corte, G., Moretta, A., Cosulich, M. E., Ramarli, D., and Bargellesi, A. A monoclonal anti-DC1 antibody selectively inhibits the generation of effector T cells mediating specific cytolytic acitivty. *J. Exp. Med.* 156:1539-1544, 1982.
23. Cosimi, A. B., Burton, R. C., Kung, P. C., Colvin, R., Goldstein, G., Lifter, J., Rhodes, W., and Russell, P. S. Evaluation of primate renal allograft recipients of monoclonal antibody to human T-cell subclasses. *Transplant Proc.* 13:499-503, 1981.
24. Cosimi, A. B., Colvin, R. B., Jaffers, G. J., Giorgi, J. V., Delmonico, F. L., Fuller, T. C., and Russell, P. S. Immunologic monitoring of monoclonal antibody therapy: Comparison of five antibodies as immunosuppressants of renal allograft rejection. *Transplant. Proc.* 16:1459-1461, 1984.
25. Cosimi, A. B., Skamene, E., Bonney, W. W., and Russell, P. S. Experience with large-dose intravenous antithymocyte globulin in primates and man. *Surgery* 68:54-61, 1970.
26. Cowan, E. P., Cumming, R. D., Schwartz, B. D., and Cullen, S. E. Analysis of murine Ia antigen glycosylation by lectin affinity chromatography. *J. Biol. Chem.* 257:11241-11248, 1982.
27. Cowing, C., and Chapdelaine, J. M. T cells discriminate between Ia antigens expressed on allogeneic accessory cells and B cells: A potential function for carbohydrate side chains on Ia molecules. *Proc. Natl. Acad. Sci. USA* 80:6000-6004, 1982.
28. Cullen, S. E., Kindle, C. S., Shreffler, D. C., and Cowing, C. Differential glycosylation of murine B cell and spleen adherent cell Ia antigens. *J. Immunol.* 127:1478-1484, 1981.
29. Dallman, M. J., and Mason, D. W. Induction of Ia antigens on murine epidermal cells during rejection of skin allografts. *Transplantation* 36:222-224, 1983.
30. Descamps-Latscha, B., Golub, R. M., Ngurjen, A. T., and Feuillet-Fieux, M-N. Monoclonal antibodies against T cell differentiation antigens initiate stimulation of monocyte/macrophage oxidative metabolism. *J. Immunol.* 131:2500-2507, 1983.
31. Dialynas, D. P., Quan, Z. S., Wall, K. A., Pierres, A., Quintans, J., Laken, M. R., Pierres, M., and Fitch, F. W. Characterization of the murine T cell surface molecule, designated L3T4, identified by monoclonal antibody GK1.5: Similarity of L3T4, to the human Leu-3/T4 molecule. *J. Immunol.* 131:2445-2451, 1983.
32. Dillman, R. O., and Royston, I. Applications of monoclonal antibodies in cancer therapy. *Br. Med. Bull.* 40:240-246, 1984.
33. Dongworth, D. W., and McMichael, A. J. Inhibition of human T lymphocyte function. *Br. Med. Bull.* 40:254-261, 1984.
34. Ehrlich, P. H., Moyle, W. R., Moustafa, Z. A., and Canfield, R. E. Mixing two monoclonal antibodies yields enhanced affinity for antigen. *J. Immunol.* 128:2709-2713, 1982.
35. Engelfriet, C. P., von den Borne, A. E. G. Kr., Beckers, D., van der Meulen, F. W., Fleer, A., Roos, D., and Ouwehand, W. H. Immune destruction of red cells. In *A Seminar on Immune Mediated Cell Destruction,* D. Bell, ed. Presented at the 34th

Annual meeting of the American Association of Blood Banks, Chicago, Chapter 5, 1981, pp. 93-130.
36. Fahey, K. J. Studies on goat anti-CBA thymocyte globulin: The large scale preparation, purification and testing of anti-lymphocyte serum and anti-lymphocyte globulin. *Aust. J. Exp. Biol. Med. Sci.* 51:489-499, 1973.
37. Faustman, D. L., Steinman, R. M., Gebel, H. M., Hauptfeld, V., Davie, J. M., and Lacy, P. E. Prevention of rejection of murine islet allograft by pretreatment with antidendritic cell antibody. *Proc. Natl. Acad. Sci. USA* 81:3864-3868, 1984.
38. FitzGerald, D. J. P., Waldmann, T. A., Willingham, M. C., and Pastan, I. *Pseudomonas* exotoxin-anti-TAC. Cell-specific immunotoxin active against cells expressing the human T cell growth factor receptor. *J. Clin. Invest.* 74:966-971, 1984.
39. Glennie, M. J., and Stevenson, G. T. Univalent antibodies kill tumour cells in vitro and in vivo. *Nature* 295:712-714, 1982.
40. Goldenberg, D. M., Sharkey, R. M., Primus, F. J., Mizusawa, E., andHawthorne, M. F. Neutron-capture therapy of human cancer: In vivo results on tumor localization of boron-10-labeled antibodies to carcinoembryonic antigen in the GW-39 tumor model system. *Proc. Natl. Acad. Sci. USA* 81:560-563, 1984.
41. Gordon, J., Abdul-Ahad, A. K., Hamblin, T. J., Stevenson, F. K., and Stevenson, G. T. Mechanisms of tumour cell escape encountered in treating lymphocytic leukaemia with anti-idiotypic antibody. *Br. J. Cancer* 49:547-557, 1984.
42. Granelli-Piperno, A., Andrus, L., and Reich, E. Antibodies to interleukin 2. Effects on immune responses in vitro and in vivo. *J. Exp. Med.* 160:738-750, 1984.
43. Gratama, J. W., Jansen, J., Lipovich, R. A., Tanke, H. J., Goldstein, G., and Zwaan, F. E. Treatment of acute graft-versus-host disease with monoclonal antibody OKT3. *Transplantation* 38:469-474, 1984.
44. Gunter, K. C., Malek, T. R., and Shevach, E. M. T cell-activating properties of an anti-Thy-1 monoclonal antibody. Possible analogy to OKT3/Leu-4. *J. Exp. Med.* 159:716-730, 1984.
45. Haars, R., Rohowsky-Kochan, C., Reed, E., KIng, D. W., and Suciu-Foca, N. Moculation of T-cell antigen receptor on lymphocyte membrane. *Immunogenetics* 20:397-405, 1984.
46. Harrison, A., and Royle, L. Preparation of a At-211 IgG conjugate which is stable in vivo. *Int. J. Appl. Radiat. Isotop.* 35:1005-1008, 1984.
47. Hart, G. W. The role of asparagine-linked oligosaccharides in cellular recognition by thymic lymphocytes. *J. Biol. Chem.* 257:151-158, 1982.
48. Heagy, W., Waltenbaugh, C., and Martz, E. Potent ability of anti-LFA-1 monoclonal antibody to prolong allograft survival. *Transplantation* 37:520-523, 1984.
49. Herbert, A. G., LeGros, G. S., Bidawid, S., and Watson, J. D. In vivo modulation of thymus-derived lymphocytes with monoclonal antibodies in mice. III. Spontaneous and natural cytotoxic effector cells. *Immunology* 51:377-385, 1984.
50. Hercend, T., Meuer, S., Brennan, A., Edson, M. A., Acuto, O., Reinherz, E. L., Schlossman, S. F., and Ritz, J. Natural killer-like function of activated T lymphocytes: Differential blocking effects of monoclonal antibodies specific for a 90-kDa clonotypic structure. *Cell Immunol.* 86:381-392, 1984.
51. Herlyn, D. M., Steplewski, Z., Herlyn, M. F., and Koprowski, H. Inhibition of growth of colorectal carcinoma in nude mice by monoclonal antibody. *Cancer Res.* 40:717-721, 1980.
52. Hildreth, J. E. K., and August, J. T. The human lymphocyte function-associated (HFLA) antigen and a related macrophate differentiation antigen (HMac-1): Functional effects of subunit-specific monoclonal antibodies. *J. Immunol.* 134:3272-3280, 1985.
53. Hogg, N., MacDonald, S., Slusarenko, M., and Beverley, P. C. L. Monoclonal anti-

bodies specific for human monocytes, granulocytes, and endothelium. *Immunology* 53:753-767, 1984.

54. Huber, H., Polley, M. J., Linscott, W. D., Fudenberg, H. H., and Muller-Eberhard, H. H. Human monocytes: Distinct receptor sites for the third component of complement and for immunoglobulin G. *Science* 162:1281-1283, 1968.
55. Hunig, T. Monoclonal anti-Lyt-2.2 antibody blocks lectin-dependent cellular cytotoxicity of H-2-negative target cells. *J. Exp. Med.* 159:551-558, 1984.
56. Jaffers, G. J., Colvin, R. B., Cosimi, A. B., Giorgi, J. V., Goldstein, G., Fuller, T. C., Kurnick, J. T., Lillehei, C., and Russell, P. S. The human immune response to murine OKT3 monoclonal antibody. *Transplant. Proc.* 15:646-648, 1983.
57. Janossy, G. Purging of bone marrow and immunosuppression. *Br. Med. Bull.* 40: 247-253, 1984.
58. Johnson, R. J., Pasternack, G. R., and Shin, H. S. Antibody-mediated suppression of tumor growth. I. Suppression by murine IgG1 isolated from alloantiserum. *J. Immunol.* 118:489-493, 1977.
59. Johnson, R. J., Pasternack, G. R., and Shin, H. S. Antibody-mediated suppression of tumor growth. II. Macrophage and platelet cooperation with murine IgG1 isolated from alloantiserum. *J. Immunol.* 118:494-497.
60. Johnson, R. J., Pasternack, G. R., Drysdale, B. E., and Shin, H. S. Antibody-mediated suppression of tumor growth. III. Molecular assay of murine IgG1 alloantibody required to cause tumor suppression in vivo. *J. Immunol.* 118:498-504, 1977.
61. Jonker, M., Goldstein, G., and Balner, H. Effects of in vivo administration of monoclonal antibodies specific for human T cell subpopulations on the immune system in a rhesus monkey model. *Transplantation* 35:521-526, 1983.
62. Jonker, M., Malissen, B., and Mawas, C. The effect of in vivo application of monoclonal antibodies specific for human cytotoxic T cells in rhesus monkeys. *Transplantation* 35:374-378, 1983.
63. Kaneoka, H., Perez-Rojas, G., Sasasuki, T., Benike, C. J., and Engelman, E. G. Human T lymphocyte proliferation induced by a pan-T monoclonal antibody (anti-Leu 4): Heterogeneity of response is a function of monocytes. *J. Immunol.* 131:158-164, 1983.
64. Kimura, A. K., and Peck, A. B. A novel anti-Ia monoclonal antibody which specifically enhances the corresponding T cell alloreactivity. *J. Immunol.* 133:2360-2364, 1984.
65. Kirch, M. E., and Hammerling, U. Immunotherapy of murine leukemias by monoclonal antibody. I. Effect of passively administered antibody on growth of transplanted tumor cells. *J. Immunol.* 127:805-810, 1981.
66. Kirkman, R. L., Araujo, J. L., Busch, G. J., Carpenter, C. B., Milford, E. L., Reinherz, E. L., Schlossman, S. F., Strom, T. B., and Tilney, N. L. Treatment of acute renal allograft rejection with monoclonal anti-T12 antibody. *Transplantation* 36:620-626, 1983.
67. Koestler, T. P., Rieman, D., Muirhead, K., Greig, R. G., and Poste, G. Identification and characterization of a monoclonal antibody to an antigen expressed on activated macrophages. *Proc. Natl. Acad. Sci. USA* 81:4505-4509, 1984.
68. Kohl, S., Springer, A., Schmalstieg, F. S., Loo, L. S., and Anderson, D. C. Defective natural killer cytotoxicity and polymorphonuclear leukocyte antibody-dependent cellular cytotoxicity in patients with LFA-1/OKM-1 deficiency. *J. Immunol.* 133: 2972-1978, 1984.
69. Koide, Y., Awashima, F., Yoshida, T. O., Takenouchi, T., Wakisaka, A., Moriuchi, J. and Aizawa, M. The role of three distinct Ia-like antigen molecules in human T cell proliferative responses: Effect of monoclonal anti-Ia-like antibodies. *J. Immunol.* 129:1061-1069, 1982.

70. Kozbor, D., Lagarde, A. E., and Roder, J. C. Human hybridomas constructed with antigen-specific Epstein-Barr virus-transformed cell lines. *Proc. Natl. Acad. Sci. USA* 79:6651-6655, 1982.
71. Lakow, E. S., Valentine, M. A., Vaughan, J. H., Tsoukas, C. D., and Carson, D. A. Effects of monoclonal antibodies against lymphocyte surface antigens on interleukin 2 excretion by Epstein-Barr virus-specific human T-cell hybridomas. *Cell. Immunol.* 85:67-74, 1984.
72. Lamb, J. R., Eckels, D. D., Keterer, E. A., Sell, T. W., and Woody, J. N. Antigen-specific human T lymphocyte clones: Mechanisms of inhibition of proliferative responses by xenoantiserum to human nonpolymorphic HLA-DR antigens. *J. Immunol.* 129:1085-1090, 1982.
73. Lance, E. M., Medawar, P. B., and Taub, R. N. Antilymphocyte serum. *Adv. Immunol.* 17:1-92, 1973.
74. Lancki, D. W., Prystowsky, M. B., Vogel, S. N., Beller, D. I., Dialynas, D. P., and Fitch, F. W. Effects of monoclonal antibodies directed against murine T lymphocyte cell surface antigens on lymphokine production by cloned T lymphocytes reactive with class I MHC or Mls alloantigens. *J. Immunol.* 133:2051-2057, 1984.
75. Landegren, U., Andersson, J., and Wigzell, H. Mechanism of T lymphocyte activation by OKT3 antibodies. A general model for T cell induction. *Eur. J. Immunol.* 14:325-328, 1984.
76. Landegren, U., Ramstedt, U., Axberg, I., Ullberg, M., Jondal, M., and Wigzell, H. Selective inhibition of human T cell cytotoxicity at levels of target recognition or initiation of lysis by monoclonal OKT3 and Leu-2a antibodies. *J. Exp. Med.* 155:1579-1584, 1982.
77. Ledbetter, J. A., Evans, R. L., Lipinski, M., Cunningham-Rundles, C., Good, R. A., and Herzenberg, L. A. Evolutionary conservation of surface molecules that distinguish T lymphocyte helper/inducer and cytotoxic/suppressor subpopulations in mouse and man. *J. Exp. Med.* 153:310-323, 1981.
78. LeFrancois, L., and Bevan, M. J. A reexamination of the role of Lyt-2-positive T cells in murine skin graft rejection. *J. Exp. Med.* 159:57-67, 1984.
79. Lefvert, A. K., and Fulpius, B. W. Receptor-like activity of a monoclonal anti-idiotypic antibody against an anti-acetylcholine receptor antibody. *Scand. J. Immunol.* 19:485-489, 1984.
80. Lemonnier, F., Dubreuil, P., and Caillol, D. Inhibition by Fab and Fab′2 monoclonal anti-Ia antibody fragments of T-lymphocyte proliferative responses. *Immunology* 46:533-544, 1982.
81. Lemonnier, F. A., Birnbaum, D. Z., Dubreuil, P. C., and Caillol, D. H. Affinity and inhibitory capacity of T-cell proliferation of monoclonal anti-Ia antibodies. *Scand. J. Immunol* 16:233-241, 1982.
82. Leonard, W. J., Depper, J. M., Uchiyama, T., Smith, K. A., Waldmann, T. A., and Greene, W. C. A monoclonal antibody that appears to recognize the receptor for human T-cell growth factor; partial characterization of the receptor. *Nature* 300:267-269, 1982.
83. Lopez, A. F., Bruns, G. F., and Stanley, I. J. Epitope diversity of monoclonal antibodies revealed by cross-species reactivity. *Mol. Immunol.* 21:371-374, 1984.
84. Loveland, B. E., and McKenzie, I. F. C. Which T cells cause graft rejection? *Transplantation* 33:217-221, 1982.
85. Maier, T., Stammers, A. T., and Levy, J. G. Characterization of a monoclonal antibody directed to a T cell suppressor factor. *J. Immunol.* 131:1843-1848, 1983.
86. Maki, T., Simpson, M., and Monaco, A. P. Development of suppressor T cells by antilymphocyte serum treatment in mice. *Transplantation* 34:376-381, 1982.
87. Malek, T. R., Ortega-R., G., Jakway, J. P., Chan, C., and Shevach, E. M. The murine

IL 2 receptor. II. Monoclonal anti-IL 2 receptor antibodies as specific inhibitor of T cell function in vitro. *J. Immunol.* 133:1976-1982, 1984.

88. Malek, T. R., Robb, R. J., and Shevach, E. M. Identification of a membrane antigen that is distinct from the interleukin 2 receptor and that may be required for interleukin 2-driven proliferative responses. *J. Immunol.* 130:747-755, 1983.
89. Martin, W. J., and Miller, F. J. A. P. Assay for the immunosuppressive capacity of antilymphocyte serum based on its action on thymus-derived cells. *Int. Arch. Allergy Appl. Immunol.* 35:163-178, 1969.
90. Metzger, H. The mechanism of action of antibodies. *Mol. Immunol.* 21:679-79 (1984.
91. Meuer, S. C., Acuto, O., Hussey, R. E., Hodgdon, J. C., Fitzgerald, K. A., Schlossman, S. F., and Reinherz, E. L. Evidence for the T3-associated 90K heterodimer as the T-cell antigen receptor. *Nature* 303:808-810, 1983.
92. Meuer, S. C., Fitzgerald, K. A., Hussey, R. E., Hodgdon, J. C., Schlossman, S. F., and Reinherz, E. L. Clonotypic structures involved in antigen-specific human T cell function. Relationship to the T3 molecular complex. *J. Exp. Med.* 157:705-719, 1983.
93. Meuer, S. C., Hodgdon, J. C., Cooper, D. A., Hussey, R. E., Fitzgerald, K. A., Schlossman, S. F., and Reinherz, E. L. Human cytotoxic T cell clones directed at autologous virus transformed targets: Further evidence for linkage of genetic restriction to T4 and T8 surface glycoproteins. *J. Immunol.* 131:186-190, 1983.
94. Meuer, S. C., Hodgdon, J. C., Hussey, R. E., Protentis, J. P., Schlossman, S. F., and Reinherz, E. Antigen-like effects of monoclonal and antibodies directed at receptors on human T cell clones. *J. Exp. Med.* 158:988-993, 1983.
95. Meuer, S. C., Hussey, R. E., Cantrell, D. A., Hodgdon, J. C., Schlossman, S. F., Smith, K. A., and Reinherz, E. L. Triggering of the T3-Ti antigen-receptor complex results in clonal T-cell proliferation through an interleukin 2-dependent autocrine pathway. *Proc. Natl. Acad. Sci. USA* 81:1509-1513, 1984.
96. Meuer, S. C., Hussey, R. E., Fabbi, M., Fox, D., Acuto, O., Fitzgerald, K. A., Hodgdon, J. C., Protentis, J. P., Schlossman, S. F., and Reinherz, E. L. An alternative pathway of T-cell activation: A functional role for the 50 kd T11 sheep erythrocyte receptor protein. *Cell* 36:897-906, 1984.
97. Michaelides, M., Hogarth, P. M., and McKenzie, I. F. The immunosuppressive effect of monoclonal anti-Lyt-1.1 antibodies in vivo. *Eur. J. Immunol.* 11:1005-1012, 1981.
98. Miller, R. A., Maloney, D. G., McKillop, J., and Levy, R. In vivo effects of murine hybridoma monoclonal antibody in a patient with T-cell leukemia. *Blood* 58:78-86, 1981.
99. Miller, R. A., Maloney, D. G., Warnke, R., and Levy, R. Treatment of B-cell lymphoma with monoclonal anti-idiotype antibody. *N. Engl. J. Med.* 306:517-522, 1981.
100. Milner, J. Different forms of p53 detected by monoclonal antibodies in non-dividing and dividing lymphocytes. *Nature* 310:143-145, 1984.
101. Morrison, S. L., Johnson, M. J., Herzenberg, L. A., and Oi, V. T. Chimeric human antibody molecules: Mouse antigen-binding domains with human constant region domains. *Proc. Natl. Acad. Sci. USA* 81:6851-6855, 1984.
102. Muchmore, A. V., Decker, J. M., and Mann, D. L. Evidence that antisera that react with products of the human HLA-DR locus may block in vitro antigen-induced proliferation by inducing suppression. *J. Immunol.* 128:2063-2066, 1982.
103. Murphy, P. A., Angster, D. F., and Burdick, J. F. Secretion of endogenous pyrogen/interleukin I by human mononuclear cells exposed in vitro to OKT3 antibody. In preparation, 1985.
104. Najarian, J. S., Simmons, R. L., Condie, R. M., Thompson, E. J., Fryd, D. S., Howard,

R. J., Matas, A. J., Sutherland, D. E. R., Ferguson, R. M., and Schmidtke, J. R. Seven years' experience with antilymphoblast globulin for renal transplantation from cadaver donors. *Ann. Surg.* 184:352-368, 1976.

105. O'Neill, H. C., Parish, C. R., and Higgins, T. J. Monoclonal antibody detection of carbohydrate-defined and protein-defined H-2K^k antigens. *Mol. Immunol.* 18: 663-675, 1981.
106. Opitz, H. G., Opitz, U., Hewlett, G., and Schlumberger, H. D. A new model for investigations of T-cell functions in mice: Differential immunosuppressive effects of two monoclonal anti-Thy-1.2 antibodies. *Immunobiology* 160:438-453, 1982.
107. Osawa, H., and Diamantstein, T. Studies on T lymphocyte activation. II. Monoclonal antibody inhibiting the capacity of rat T lymphoblasts to absorb and to respond to IL-2: an anti-IL-2 receptor antibody? *Immunology* 48:617-621, 1983.
108. Palacios, R. Role of individual chains of HLA-DR antigens in activation of T cells induced by alloantigens. *Immunogenetics* 14:309-322, 1981.
109. Palacios, R., and Moller, G. HLA-DR antigens render resting T cells sensitive to interleukin-2 and induce production of the growth factor in the autologous mixed lymphocyte reaction. *Cell. Immunol.* 63:143-153, 1981.
110. Pavlov, H., Hogarth, M., McKenzie, I. F., and Cheers, C. In vivo and in vitro effects of monoclonal antibody to Ly antigens on immunity to infection. *Cell. Immunol.* 71:127-138, 1982.
111. Pawelec, G. P., Shaw, S., Ziegler, A., Muller, C., and Wernet, P. Differential inhibition of HLA-D- or SB-directed secondary lymphoproliferative responses with monoclonal antibodies detecting human Ia-like determinants. *J. Immunol.* 129:1070-1075, 1982.
112. Perry, L. L., and Greene, M. I. Conversion of immunity to suppression by in vivo administration of I-A subregion-specific antibodies. *J. Exp. Med.* 156:480-491, 1982.
113. Pichler, W. J., Wolff-Vorbeck, G., Birke, C., Rieber, P., and Peter, H. H. Comparison of the inhibitory activity of 7 anti-T8 antibodies on specific cellular cytotoxicity. *Immunobiology* 167:376-388, 1984.
114. Pierres, A., Naquet, P., Van Agthoven, A., Bekkhoucha, F., Denizot, F., Mishal, A., Schmitt-Verhulst, A-M., and Pierres, M. A rat anti-mouse T4 monoclonal antibody (H129.19) inhibits the proliferation of Ia-reactive T cell clones and delineates two phenotypically distinct (T4$^+$, Lyt-2,3-, and T4$^-$, Lyt-2,3$^+$) subsets among anti-Ia cytolytic T cell clones. *J. Immunol.* 132:2775-2782, 1984.
115. Plastsoucas, C. D., and Good, R. A. Inhibition of specific cell-mediated cytotoxicity by monoclonal antibodies to human T cell antigens. *Proc. Natl. Acad. Sci. USA* 78:4500-4504, 1981.
116. Pober, J. S., Gimbrone, M. A., Jr., Cotran, R. S., Reiss, C. S., Burakoff, S. J., Fiers, W., and Ault, K. A. Ia expression by vascular endothelium is inducible by activated T cells and by human γ-interferon. *J. Exp. Med.* 157:1339-1353, 1983.
117. Prat, M., Gribaudo, G., Comoglio, P. M., Cavallo, G., and Landolfo, S. Monoclonal antibodies against murine interferon. *Proc. Natl. Acad. Sci. USA* 81:4515-4519, 1984.
118. Rankin, E. M., Hekman, A., Hardeman, M. R., and Hoefnagel, C. A. Dynamic studies of lymphocytes labelled with indium-111 during and after treatment with monoclonal anti-idiotype antibody in advanced B cell lymphoma. *Br. Med. J.* 289: 1097-1100, 1984.
119. Reading, C. L. Carbohydrate structure, biological recognition, and immune function. In *Biology of Glycoproteins,* R. Iratt, ed., Plenum Press, New York, 1984, pp. 235-321.
120. Reinherz, E. L., Meuer, S. C., Fitzgerald, K. A., Hussey, R. E., Hodgdon, J. C., Acuto, O., and Schlossman, S. F. Comparison of T3-associated 49- and 43-kilodalton cell

surface molecules on individual human T-cell clones: Evidence for peptide variability in T-cell receptor structures. *Proc. Natl. Acad. Sci. USA* 80:4104-4108, 1983.

121. Remlinger, K., Martin, P. J., Hansen, J. A., Doney, K. C., Smith, A., Deeg, H. J., Sullivan, K., Storb, R., and Thomas, E. D. Murine monoclonal anti-T cell antibodies for treatment of steroid resistant acute graft-versus-host disease. *Hum. Immunol.* 9: 21-35, 1983.

122. Rinnooy Kan, E. A., Platzer, E., Welte, K., and Wang, C. Y. Modulation induction of the T3 antigen by OKT3 antibody is monocyte dependent. *J. Immunol.* 133: 2979-2985, 1984.

123. Ritz, J., Pesando, J. M., Sallan, S. E., Clavell, L. A., Notis-McConarty, J., Rosenthal, P., and Schlossman, S. F. Serotherapy of acute lymphoblastic leukemia with monoclonal antibody. *Blood* 58:141-152, 1981.

124. Romain, P. L., and Schlossman, S. F. Human T lymphocyte subsets. Functional heterogeneity and surface recognition structures. *J. Clin. Invest.* 74:1559-1565, 1984.

125. Rosenbaum, J. T., Adelman, N. E., and McDevitt, H. O. In vivo effects of antibodies to immune response gene products. I. Haplotype-specific suppression of humoral immune responses with a monoclonal anti-I-A. *J. Exp. Med.* 154:1694-1702, 1981.

126. Russell, P. S. Antilymphocyte sera for immunosuppression: A powerful class of agents awaiting full application to patient care. In *Antibodies in Human Diagnosis and Therapy*, E. Haber and R. M. Krause, eds. Raven Press, New York, 1977, pp. 303-357.

127. Samelson, L. E., and Schwartz, R. H. T cell clone-specific alloantisera that inhibit or stimulate antigen-induced T cell activation. *J. Immunol.* 131:2645-2650, 1983.

128. Schoenfeld, Y., Hsu-Lin, S. C., Gabriels, J. E., Silberstein, L. E., Furie, B. C., Furie, B., Stollar, B. D., and Schwartz, R. S. Production of autoantibodies by human-human hybridoma. *J. Clin. Invest.* 70:205-208, 1982.

129. Shands, J. W. The immunological role of the macrophage. *Mod. Trends Immunol.* 2:86-118, 1968.

130. Sharma, S. D., Budzich, T., Proffitt, M. R., Shepherd, D., and Remington, J. S. Regulation of natural killer cell activity by anti-I-region monoclonal antibodies. *Cell. Immunol.* 85:125-134, 1984.

131. Shouval, D., Shafritz, D. A., Zurawski, V. R., Jr., Isselbacher, K. J., and Wands, J. R. Immunotherapy in nude mice of human hepatoma using monoclonal antibodies against hepatitis B virus. *Nature* 298:567-569, 1982.

132. Sikora, K. Human monoclonal antibodies. *Br. Med. Bull.* 40:209-212, 1984.

133. Sikora, K., Smedley, H., and Thorpe, P. Tumour imaging and drug targeting. *Br. Med. Bull.* 40:233-239, 1984.

134. Simpson, M., and Gozzo, J. J. Studies on the mechanism of action of rabbit anti-mouse thymocyte serum. I. Induction of suppressor cells *Transplantation* 30:64-68, 1980.

135. Springer, T. A., Thompson, W. S., Miller, L. J., Schmalstieg, F. C., and Anderson, D. C. Inherited deficiency of the Mac-1, LFA-1, p150,95 glycoprotein family and its molecular basis. *J. Exp. Med.* 160:1901-1918, 1984.

136. Steplewski, A., Lubeck, M. D., and Koprowski, H. Human macrophages armed with murine immunoglobulin G2a antibodies to tumors destroy human cancer cells. *Science* 221:865-867, 1983.

137. Steplewski, Z., Herlyn, D., Maul, G., and Koprowski, H. Hypothesis: Macrophages as effector cells for human tumor destruction mediated by monoclonal antibody. *Hybridoma* 2:1-5, 1983.

138. Sterkers, G., Henin, Y., Kalil, J., Bagot, M., and Levy, J-P., Influence of HLA class

I- and class II-specific monoclonal antibodies on DR-restricted lymphoproliferative responses. I. Unseparated populations of effector cells. *J. Immunol.* 131:2735-2740, 1983.

139. Sternick, J. L., Viamontes, G. I., Sturmer, A. M., Palladino, M. A., and Shen, E-W. In vivo immunological effects of two monoclonal antibodies of different classes on Lyt-2, T cell subset of the mouse. *Hybridoma* 2:130, 1983.
140. Sternick, J. L., Viamontes, G. I., Sturmer, A. M., Palladino, M. A., and Shen, F.-W. The effects on mice of long-term anti-Lyt-1.2 monoclonal antibody injections. *Hybridoma* 2:129, 1983.
141. Strassman, G., and Bach, F. H. $OKT4^+$ cytotoxic T cells can lyse targets via class I molecules and can be blocked by monoclonal antibody against T4 molecules. *J. Immunol.* 133:1705-1709, 1984.
142. Suthanthiran, M., Williams, P. S., Solomon, S. D., Rubin, A. L., and Stenzel, K. H. Induction of cytolytic activity by anti-T3 monoclonal antibody. Activation of alloimmune memory cells and natural killer cells from normal and immunodeficient individuals. *J. Clin. Invest.* 74:2263-2271, 1984.
143. Sztein, M. B., Steeg, P. S., Johnson, H. M., and Oppenheim, J. J. Regulation of human peripheral blood monocyte DR antigen expression in vitro by lymphokines and recombinant interferons. *J. Clin. Invest.* 73:556-565, 1984.
144. Talle, M. A., Allegar, N., Makowski, M., and Goldstein, G. Distinct classes of human T-cell activation antigens. *Cell. Immunol.* 84:285-298, 1984.
145. Tam, M. R., Bernstein, I. D., and Nowinski, R. C. Alteration of lymphoid cells in AKR mice by treatment with monoclonal antibody against Thy-1 antigen. *Transplantation* 33:269-273, 1982.
146. Tanaka, Y., Tozawa, H., Koyanagi, Y., Yamamoto, N., and Hinuma, Y. A new monoclonal antibody recognizing an antigen of human lymphocytes similar or identical to Tac antigen. *Microbiol. Immunol.* 28:1041-1055, 1984.
147. Tax, W. J. M., Willems, H. W., Reekers, P. P. M., Capel, P. J. A., and Koene, R. A. P. Polymorphism in mitogenic effect of IgG1 monoclonal antibodies against T3 antigen on human T cells. *Nature* 304:445-447, 1983.
148. Thomas, D. B., and Calderon, R. A. T helper cells change their Lyt-1,2 phenotype during an immune response. *Eur. J. Immunol.* 12:16-23, 1982.
149. Thomas, J. M., Carver, F. M., Haisch, C. E., Fahrenbruch, G., Deepe, R. M., and Thomas, F. T. Suppressor cells in rhesus monkeys treated with antithymocyte globulin. *Transplantation* 34:83-89, 1982.
150. Thomas, Y., Rogozinski, L., Rabbani, L., Chess, A., Goldstein, G., and Chess, L. Functional analysis of human T cell subsets defined by monoclonal antibodies. VI. Distinct and opposing immunoregulatory functions within the $OKT8^+$ population. *J. Mol. Cell. Immunol.* 1:103-110, 1984.
151. Thurlow, P. J., Lovering, E., D'Apice, A. J. F., and McKenzie, I. F. C. A monoclonal anti-Pan-T-cell antibody: In vitro and in vivo studies. *Transplantation* 36:293-298, 1983.
152. Todd, R. F., Meuer, S. C., Romain, P. L., and Schlossman, S. F. A monoclonal antibody that blocks class II histocompatibility-related immune interactions. *Hum. Immunol.* 10:23-40, 1984.
153. Tsoukas, C. D., Lambris, J., Lotz, M., Valentine, M. A., Vaughan, J. H., and Carson, D. A. Lymphocyte mitogenesis induced by monoclonal antibodies to the T3 complex. Differential modulation by human IgG. *Cell. Immunol.* 89:66-74, 1984.
154. Tsudo, M., Uchiyama, T., and Uchino, H. Expression of Tac antigen on activated normal human B cells. *J. Exp. Med.* 160:612-617, 1984.
155. Uhr, J. W. A new era in immunopharmacology. *J. Immunol.* 133:i-x, 1984.
156. Vallera, D. A., Quinones, R. R., Azemove, S. M., and Soderling, C. C. B. Monoclo-

nal antibody-toxin conjugates reactive against human T lymphocytes. A comparison of antibody linked to intact ricin toxin with antibody linked to ricin A chain *Transplantation* 37:387-392, 1984.
157. van de Griend, R. J., Giphart, M. J., Van Krimpen, B. A., and Bolhuis, R. L. H. Human T cell clones exerting multiple cytolytic activities show heterogeneity in susceptibility to inhibition by monoclonal antibodies. *J. Immunol.* 133:1222-1229, 1984.
158. Vitetta, E. S., and Uhr, J. W. The potential use of immunotoxins in transplantation, cancer therapy, and immunoregulation. *Transplantation* 37:535-538, 1984.
159. Vitetta, E. S., Uhr, J. W., and Boyse, E. A. Metabolism of H-2 and Thy-1 alloantigens in murine thymocytes. *Eur. J. Immunol.* 4:276-282, 1974.
160. Walder, M. K., Hardy, R. R., Hayakawa, K., Steinman, L., and Herzenberg, L. A. Disappearance and reappearance of B cells after in vivo treatment with monoclonal anti-I-A antibodies. *Proc. Natl. Acad. Sci. USA* 81:2855-2858, 1984.
161. Walker, I. D., Hogarth, P. M., Murray, B. J., Lovering, K. E., Classon, B. J., Chambers, G. W., and McKenzie, I. F. C. Ly antigens associated with T cell recognition and effector function. *Immunol. Rev.* 82:47-77, 1984.
162. Walls, E. V., Borghetti, A. F., Benzie, C. R., and Kay, J. E. Early events during the activation of human lymphocytes by the mitogenic monoclonal antibody OKT3. *Cell. Immunol.* 89:30-38, 1984.
163. Wauwe, J. P., and Goossens, J. G. The mitogenic activity of OKT3 and anti-Leu 4 monoclonal antibodies: A comparative study. *Cell. Immunol.* 77:23-29, 1983.
164. Weiss, A., Imboden, J., Wiskocil, R., and Stobo, J. Role of T3 in the activation of human T cells. *J. Clin. Immunol.* 4:165-173, 1984.
165. Welte, K., Platzer, E., Wang, C. Y., Rinnooy Kan, E. A., Moore, M. A. S., and Mertelsmann, R. OKT8 antibody inhibits OKT3-induced IL 2 production and proliferation in $OKT8^+$ cells. *J. Immunol.* 131:2356-2361, 1983.
166. Wofsy, D., Ledbetter, J. A., Hendler, P. L., and Seaman, W. E. Treatment of murine lupus with monoclonal anti-T cell antibody. *J. Immunol.* 134:852-857, 1985.
167. Wolstenholme, G. E. W., and O'Connor, M., eds. *Antilymphocytic Serum.* Ciba Foundation Study Group. Little, Brown, Boston, 1967.
168. Woodruff, M. F. A., and Anderson, N. F. Effect of lymphocyte depletion by thoracic duct fistula and administration of antilymphocytic serum on the survival of skin homografts in rats. *Nature* 200:702, 1963.
169. Yamamoto, K., Watanabe, T., Otsubo, O., Nakauchi, H., and Okumura, K. Prolonged survival of dog kidney allografts induced by a monoclonal anti-Ia antibody. *Transplantation* 37:419-420, 1984.
170. Zalcberg, J. R., Thompson, C. H., Lichtenstein, M., and McKenzie, I. F. C. Tumor immunotherapy in the mouse with the use of ^{131}I-labelled monoclonal antibodies. *JNCI* 72:697-704, 1984.

16

ANTILYMPHOCYTE ANTIBODY IMMUNOSUPPRESSIVE THERAPY

A. Benedict Cosimi and Francis L. Delmonico
Massachusetts General Hospital and Harvard Medical School, Boston, Massachusetts

The essential role of the immune response is to safeguard and maintain the integrity of the individual, the system's most striking feature being the exquisite specificity of each response. The ultimate objective of immunosuppressive therapy for allograft recipients, therefore, should be to block specifically the host's response to antigenic differences introduced by the graft but spare reactivity to other antigens, such as bacterial and viral organisms. Until recently, the most widely used immunosuppressive protocols employed a combination of cytotoxic agents and steroids as the basic regimen. Although these protocols provided sufficient immunosuppression to make transplantation a routine treatment for many patients with end-stage renal failure, they often exposed allograft recipients to the risk of serious complications. As early investigators recognized the inherent hazards of immunosuppressive therapy, preparations of antilymphocyte antibodies (especially against T lymphocytes) were introduced as "selective" measures of immunosuppression. These preparations were designed to attack principally the infiltrating mononuclear cells observed in allograft biopsies coincident with allograft dysfunction. Such suppression conceptually could retain the host's responses to bacterial infection, since these were attributed to humoral processes independent of T-lymphocyte function. However, with the use of classic techniques to immunize animals and generate these polyclonal products, a heterogeneous group of antibodies were produced not only to T-cell populations, but also to B cells and nonlymphoid cells. It became evident that a global suppression could also result from the administration of antilymphocyte antibodies, not infrequently resulting in opportunistic infections. Hence, the search for even more specific agents continued. A milestone toward that goal occurred when cell hybridization techniques were developed that could yield monoclonal antibodies to single cell membrane determinants [23]. This Nobel prize-winning technology has provided reagents reactive only with T cells, or even more importantly, with specific T-cell subsets [25]. As a result, we have entered a clinical era of investigation in which monoclonal antilymphocyte sera may be used to manipulate selected T-cell populations while leaving intact most of the host's immune competence. This chapter will trace the evolution of these antilymphocyte antibodies (both polyclonal and monoclonal) in the context of their preparation, their prophylactic administration, and their abolition of the rejection reaction.

POLYCLONAL ANTILYMPHOCYTE PREPARATIONS

Initial observations of the destruction of leukocytes by xenotypic antisera were recorded by Elie Metchnikoff near the turn of the century. However, it was only two decades ago that the capacity of antilymphocyte serum (ALS) to interrupt the immune sequence and prolong allograft survival was first reported [44]. Although extensive preclinical investigations since then have consistently demonstrated prolongation of allograft survival by these antibodies, their true clinical value was difficult to establish. Numerous controlled and uncontrolled clinical trials utilizing ALS, ALG, or ATG (antilymphocyte or antithymocyte globulin) have been reported. Several factors, including variability among individual batches of antisera, inadequately controlled studies, limited numbers of evaluable patients, and subtherapeutic dosages, help to explain the inconsistent results observed in many of these trials. However, continued improvements in production techniques and more carefully designed trials, particularly using ATG or ALG for treatment of ongoing rejection, eventually established the clinical usefulness of these agents [6].

Antilymphocyte sera have been administered to allograft recipients either prophylactically to avert rejection or, more recently, for treatment of ongoing rejection episodes. In patients receiving immunosuppression with cytotoxic agents and steroids, one can anticipate that 15-20% of cadaveric renal allograft recipients will never experience severe rejection. With the advent of cyclosporine, this proportion is much higher. Thus, most clinicians now reserve the various preparations of ALS for refractory episodes of acute rejection.

PRODUCTION AND ADMINISTRATION OF POLYCLONAL ANTILYMPHOCYTE ANTIBODIES

Production of antibodies for clinical administration begins with the immunization of an animal using human lymphoid cells. Many cell types have been evaluated. Currently, the most commonly used agents have been produced using cultured lymphoblasts (ALG) or human thymocytes (ATG). Cultured lymphoblasts offer the advantages of ready availability and freedom from contaminating erythrocytes or stromal elements that might induce unwanted antibodies. A possible disadvantage arises from the fact that lymphoblasts are B cells rather than T cells. Human thymus tissue is an excellent source of T-cell antigens reasonably free of contaminating blood cells and stromal tissue. Thus, thymocytes are preferred by most manufacturers of antilymphoid preparations, but adequate amounts of tissue are not always available.

The selection of the heterologous species for immunization is based primarily upon practical considerations, such as cost, animal size, and availability. Experience has indicated that either horses or rabbits can be stimulated to produce potent antilymphocyte antibodies, making these two species the most commonly used.

The immunosuppressive potency of these antisera is confined almost exclusively to the IgG fraction, which is usually isolated for use in humans, although the crude globulin fraction or even whole serum can be successfully administered. Preclinical assessment of immunosuppressive potency has been difficult. To date, no absolutely reliable in vitro test has been identified. Rosette inhibition assays seem to provide the most reasonably consistent means of selecting potent preparations. The capacity of the preparation to prolong allograft survival in nonhuman primates continues to be assessed for some products prior to clinical administration.

In general, it has been found that the route of ALG administration is of relatively little importance in determining the degree of suppression produced. Local inflammatory reactions, however, frequently result from subcutaneous or intramuscular injections. As a result, many clinicians prefer intravenous administration, which has the added advantages of allowing infusion of large individual doses and presentation of the agent via a less immunogenic route.

Prompt and usually profound lymphopenia typically follows the injection of ALS. Although absolute lymphopenia is apparently not necessary for immunosuppression, most effective preparations do provide at least some degree of cell depletion. In addition to the marked decrease in number of T cells, these preparations also produce a decrease in proliferative functions. Upon cessation of treatment, circulating T-cell numbers gradually increase while the proliferative response remains impaired. This observation has been attributed to the development of nonspecific suppressor T cells [41]. It suggests that the initial interruption of cell-mediated graft destruction by ALG results from actual elimination of lymphocytes. The more prolonged suppression is then provided by suppressor cell-mediated inhibition of proliferative responses. Undoubtedly, this sequence is an oversimplification, and a more precise elucidation of the immunosuppressive process will be provided as the functions of specific T-cell subpopulations are better clarified.

USE OF ATG AS A PROPHYLACTIC ADJUNCTIVE AGENT

Patient trials were initially conducted using various "homemade" preparations administered for a period of several days to weeks, as part of a prophylactic suppressive protocol begun at the time of transplantation. In order to limit inconsistent results, which should be anticipated when using many different preparations, we undertook, in 1973, a prospective controlled evaluation of ATG (ATGAM, The Upjohn Company), which was produced in large, pooled lots. Adult recipients of cadaver donor (CD) renal allografts were studied [10]. The control group was treated only with azathioprine and steroids. The study group initially received this same regimen, plus a 14 to 21-day course of ATG beginning at the time of transplantation. This brief course of therapy significantly delayed the onset of acute rejection and reduced the need for high-dose steroid therapy in the early posttransplant period. A significant decrease in the incidence of avascular necrosis of bone was also observed in the ATG group, probably because of the decreased steroid requirement. However, a high incidence of rejection episodes occurred after ATG was stopped. Although long-term allograft survival was 10-13% greater at all time intervals for the ATG group than for the control group (Figure 1), the differences never achieved statistical significance.

Similarly, most other "prophylactic protocol" studies have indicated fewer early rejection episodes and suggested improved allograft survival in the ALG-treated groups. However, like our experience, the difference in long-term function in ATG-treated patients compared with that achieved in conventionally treated patients has often failed to reach statistical significance (Table 1). The multitude of variables involved in such clinical studies and the fairly high rate of survival already attained for kidney transplants using azathioprine and steroids alone help to explain why a statistically significant improvement in survival was inconsistently demonstrated.

TABLE 1 Reports of Randomized Trials Comparing Polyclonal Antilymphocyte Preparations to Conventional "Prophylactic" Immunosuppression in CD Renal Allograft Recipients

Patients treated	1 Year function (%) Control	ATG	Significance ($p < 0.05$)	Reference
100	63	80	+	34
179	55	62	N.S.	39
36	27	62	+	26
66	28	53	+	2
358	46	52	N.S.	43
50	52	79	+	24
67	47	68	+	30
140	50	40	N.S.	1

USE OF ATG AS TREATMENT FOR ACUTE REJECTION

The first clinical trial comparing ATG to high-dose steroids for the treatment of acute renal allograft rejection was reported by Shield et al. in 1979 [35]. Patients experiencing their initial episode of rejection were randomly assigned to treatment with either high-dose steroids or ATG with no increase in steroid dosage. The design of the protocol was to evaluate the use of ATG as the sole agent added to the therapeutic regimen at the time of allograft rejection, thereby making the efficacy of ATG treatment easier to assess. All the patients in this study were living-related donor (LRD) allograft recipients who had been treated with conventional immunosuppression (azathioprine and prednisone) beginning on the day of renal transplantation. Of the recipients treated with steroids for acute rejection, 15% suffered loss of their allografts; in contrast, allograft function returned to normal in all ATG-treated recipients. The incidence of subsequent rejection episodes was noted to be reduced substantially in the ATG-treated patients (25%) compared with the control group (58%).

Many investigators have subsequently reported the efficacy of antilymphocyte sera in the treatment of established episodes of rejection (Table 2). Filo evaluated in CD renal allograft recipients the same ATG preparation we had used [12]. He noted that renal allograft function more rapidly returned to normal with ATG use, and that an improvement in the 1-year allograft survival occurred in ATG-treated patients. Rapid resolution of rejection has similarly been observed following treatment with ALG prepared from cultured lymphoblasts or with ATG produced in rabbits [36,42].

The histopathologic appearance of the allograft may reveal important prognostic information about the reversibility of the rejection process when treated with ALS. Primarily humoral versus primarily cellular events may influence the potential recovery of renal function. The typical acute cellular rejection has been most responsive to ALS treatment even if this process has its onset several months following transplantation. However, "vascular rejection" characterized by a relatively sparse cellular infiltrate and by the predominance of endothelial and glomerular damage may be less amenable to ALS treatment

TABLE 2 Randomized Trials Comparing Steroids to ATG Plus Steroids for Treatment of Acute Renal Allograft Rejection

	Rejection reversal (%)		1-Year function (%)		
Patients treated	Steroids	ATG	Steroids	ATG	Reference
52	62	91	49	74	12
64	75	100	61	82	20
52	75	84	47	73	31
40	65	75	65	70	18
23	83	100	75	91	36
100	64	84	50	78	19

[27]. This pattern of injury presumably involves reactivity of antibody with allograft antigens and may implicate previously established sensitization to the donor. In the many prophylactic trials of ALS or ATG following renal transplantation, it was rare for a recipient to experience an episode of rejection during the period of ATG treatment. When allograft rejection did occur, biopsies not infrequently revealed fibrinoid vascular lesions, again suggesting resistance of this type of rejection to ATG treatment [9].

The current status of the cross-match between recipient serum and donor lymphocytes also provides prognostic information relative to the development of rejection immediately following transplantation and its successful treatment with ALS. In recent years, we and others have had the opportunity to transplant renal allografts to patients with positive historical cross-matches to donor antigens, yet whose current sera were no longer reactive [3,13]. No episodes of hyperacute rejection were observed in our series. Episodes of acute rejection that did occur during the first 2 weeks following transplantation were treated successfully with ATG. A history of sensitization even to the specific donor, therefore, does not necessarily affect adversely the potential recovery from an episode of rejection treated with ATG.

The steroid-sparing effect of ATG is a well-established reason for its selection as treatment for renal allograft rejection. The potency of ATG, without the requirement of high-dose steroids for primary therapy for rejection, has been detailed by Nelson et al. [29]. During the period of ATG therapy, reduction in the daily dose of azathioprine and prednisone was instituted. The ATG protocol consisted of 10-14 daily doses, after which another 7 doses were given every other day, until allograft function returned to normal. Although it was unusual for a LRD allograft recipient to require more than 2 weeks of ATG treatment, it was not uncommon for CD allograft recipients to receive 21 doses of ATG by this protocol. As a result of this experience, we continue to favor immunosuppression with azathioprine and prednisone, with the addition of ATG when necessary for adult recipients of LRD allografts.

Immunologic monitoring of the T-cell levels of peripheral blood lymphocytes has proven useful in the management of patients receiving ATG as primary treatment for allograft rejection [11]. A reduction in the T-cell levels to less than 10% of the pretreatment value has correlated well with improvement in allograft function and with the selection of the appropriate ATG dose.

COMPLICATIONS OF ATG THERAPY

The reported incidence and severity of adverse clinical reactions following ALG administration varies with the preparation being used (Table 3). Fever and chills developing during the initial infusion have been observed in the majority of patients. Rarely, this has been accompanied by bronchospasm. Since subsequent infusions are usually tolerated without incident, it has been suggested that this initial reaction may result from endogenous pyrogens released during rapid lymphocytolysis. Prior to the initial administration of ALG, therefore, many clinicians recommend administration of a single intravenous bolus of methylprednisolone (250-500 mg) plus acetaminophin and diphenylhydramine to ameliorate such reactions.

One of the main concerns during early ALG trials was the possibility that the host's immune response to the foreign protein might result in serum sickness or at least neutralization of the beneficial effects of the antiserum. Though anaphylactic reactions, manifested by hypotension, respiratory distress, and chest or flank pain, must be constantly anticipated, they have been exceedingly rare in ALG-treated patients. Pruritic skin eruptions have been noted in up to 20% of patients. Although this might suggest the onset of serum sickness, the course of therapy has generally been continued without incident using antihistamines to control the skin rash. In fact, demonstration of antibody production to the foreign protein in significant titers has been possible in only a minority of patients receiving intravenous ATG, and numerous patients have been treated with ATG on multiple occasions without adverse effects. The lack of a troublesome immune response to the heterologous IgG is in part due to careful deaggregation and to intravenous administration, both of which present the foreign antigen in a less immunogenic fashion. In addition, ATG suppresses a variety of different lymphocyte populations so that the immune response to the foreign protein itself is also presumably depressed.

TABLE 3 Clinical Toxicity of ALG Therapy

Side-effects	Approximate proportion of patients experiencing effect (%)
Early	
Chills, fever	75-80
Erythema, pruritus	15-20
Thrombocytopenia	50
Local phlebitis	1-25
Herpes labialis infection	50-60
Serum sickness	0-10
Anaphylaxis	<1
Hemolysis	<1
Delayed	
Opportunistic infection	20-25
Neoplasia	No increase
Aseptic necrosis	Decreased

Thrombocytopenia of varying severity has been reported in approximately 50% of patients treated. We have found this generally to be dose related, occurring in patients who require more than 12-15 mg/kg per day to adequately depress T-cell levels. A modest reduction in ATG dosage or further reduction in the azathioprine dosage usually resolves this problem without the need for discontinuing ATG. Although the thrombocytopenia is presumed to result from low levels of antiplatelet antibodies, reversible platelet aggregation within the pulmonary microcirculation has been demonstrated in dogs even in the absence of antiplatelet antibodies [17].

In earlier ATG trials, serious infectious complications, particularly with *Cytomegalovirus,* were encountered. We have found that reduction of the dosage of azathioprine and steroids during ATG therapy to approximately 50% of usually administered levels has resulted in a marked decrease in such infections [33]. The most frequently observed infection in ALG-treated patients is herpes labialis, with approximately 60% of patients developing at least some evidence of this during or immediately after treatment. With the availability of acyclovir therapy, such herpes infections have been easily controlled.

Infection by other opportunistic agents obviously occurs in these patients as well. As noted, however, by carefully limiting the dosages of concomitant immunosuppressive agents administered during ATG therapy, no increased incidence of such infections has been observed. Similarly, the incidence of neoplasia in ATG-treated patients has not been increased over that observed in patients receiving only conventional suppression.

MONOCLONAL ANTILYMPHOCYTE PREPARATIONS

The clinical usefulness and some of the limitations of ALG have been summarized above. Clearly, even the most meticulously prepared polyclonal product cannot be considered a standardized agent, and some variability in immunosuppressive potency and toxicity must be anticipated between batches. More importantly, since ALG necessarily produces a pan-T-cell and some B-cell depletion, these protocols cannot be further refined to achieve more specific immunosuppression.

The stage was set for another advance in this field by the clarification that lymphocytes, far from being identical to one another, can be divided not only into bursa-equivalent (B) cells and thymus-dependent (T) cells but further separated into functionally distinct subpopulations of T cells. In addition, distinctive cell surface antigens have been identified as being associated with the functional capacity of the T cell on which each resides. As a result, an antibody can be prepared against the T-cell subset, for example, which is HLA class II antigen reactive from one individual, anticipating it will react with that same subset in all individuals. Using hybridoma technology, it has been possible to produce such antibodies against many of these specific cell surface antigens.

With this approach, standardized products that react with only selected T-cell populations can be regularly produced without batch-to-batch variability. Because of the purity and specificity of the antibodies, milligram dosages can be expected to provide comparable T-cell depletion to that produced by much larger dosages of ALG. This both simplifies the clinical administration and limits the likelihood of toxic side effects in patients receiving monoclonal antibodies. Perhaps the most important advantage offered by monoclonal antibodies is the opportunity to develop therapeutic protocols in which only selected subpopulations of the T-cell fraction are depleted (Table 4).

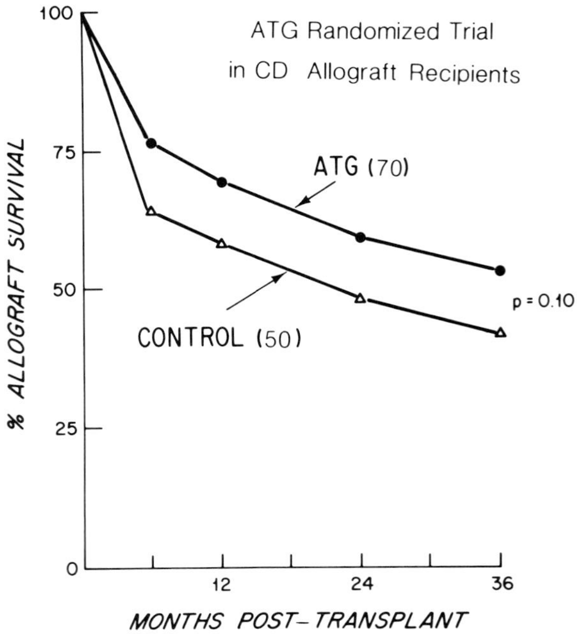

FIGURE 1 Cadaver donor renal allograft survival of recipients randomly treated with azathioprine and prednisone (control) or these agents plus ATG. The proportion of functioning grafts favors the ATG-treated group but does not reach statistical significance. Reproduced with permission from *Controversies in Nephrology,* Georgetown University, Schreiner, G. E., Winchester, J. F., and Mendelson, B. F., eds., p. 352, 1982.

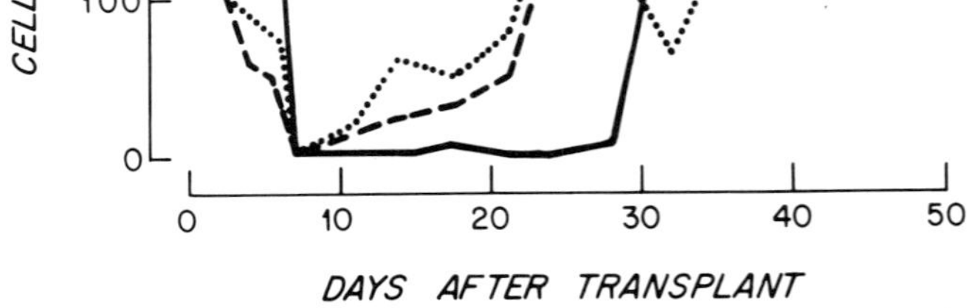

FIGURE 2 Monitoring of peripheral blood lymphocytes of a typical recipient of OKT3 monoclonal antibody. Reproduced with permission from Ref. 40.

TABLE 4 Comparison of Antilymphocyte Preparations

	Polyclonal	Monoclonal
Desired antibodies	Lot-to-lot variability of Ab classes, affinity stability, etc.	Defined, standardized, reproducible
Production	Cumbersome, small batches	"Unlimited" supply
Reactivity	Mixture of antibodies, multiple determinants	Single predetermined specificity
Effective dosage	mg → grams	μg → mg
Lymphocytotoxicity	pan T plus B	Selected subsets possible

PRODUCTION AND ADMINISTRATION OF MONOCLONAL ANTILYMPHOCYTE ANTIBODIES

The steps involved in producing an "immortal" line of cells that will secrete a monomolecular species of antibody combine two previously recognized observations into a single effort. Lymphocytes from immunized animals, when cultured in vitro, can be readily isolated into separate clones, each producing a single antibody. Unfortunately, these clones have a very short life span. In contrast, myeloma cell clones can be grown permanently in culture but produce antibodies with no predefined specificity. When the two types of cells are fused to form a hybridoma, both essential properties—secretion of antibodies with a predefined specificity and permanent growth—are retained. Thus, splenic lymphocytes from mice previously immunized with human T cells are isolated, fused with mouse myeloma cells to obtain hybridomas, and then selected by random cloning to retain only those secreting the desired monoclonal antibodies (Figure 3). A number of these monoclonal antibody preparations, directed against human cell surface antigens, have now become available (Table 5).

The specificity of a monoclonal antibody is due to its purity. This does not preclude cross-reactivity with other cells due to recognition by the antibody of a similar or identical epitope (reactive site) that might be present on different cell surface antigens. As a result, antilymphocyte antibodies must be thoroughly screened prior to their administration to exclude potentially toxic cross-reactivity with other human tissues [14]. On the other hand, cross-reactivity with lymphocytes of nonhuman primates allows preclinical studies of toxicity, efficacy, and mechanisms of action.

We and others have begun to evaluate the immunosuppressive potency of some of these agents administered to allograft recipients. We initially studied the effects of OKT4 treatment of cynomolgus renal allograft recipients [8]. Immunologic monitoring of peripheral blood lymphocytes obtained from these animals revealed complete coating of the OKT4-reactive cells and an excess of OKT4 antibody in the serum of most animals. Nevertheless, the OKT4-reactive cells were not completely removed from the circulation though they were gradually depressed to approximately 20-30% of pretreatment levels. Renal allograft survival was prolonged to as long as 47 days (control, 8-11 days) if the short course of OKT4 treatment had been started prior to transplantation. The trial confirmed that effective immunosuppression could be achieved by depletion of even a single T-cell subpopulation.

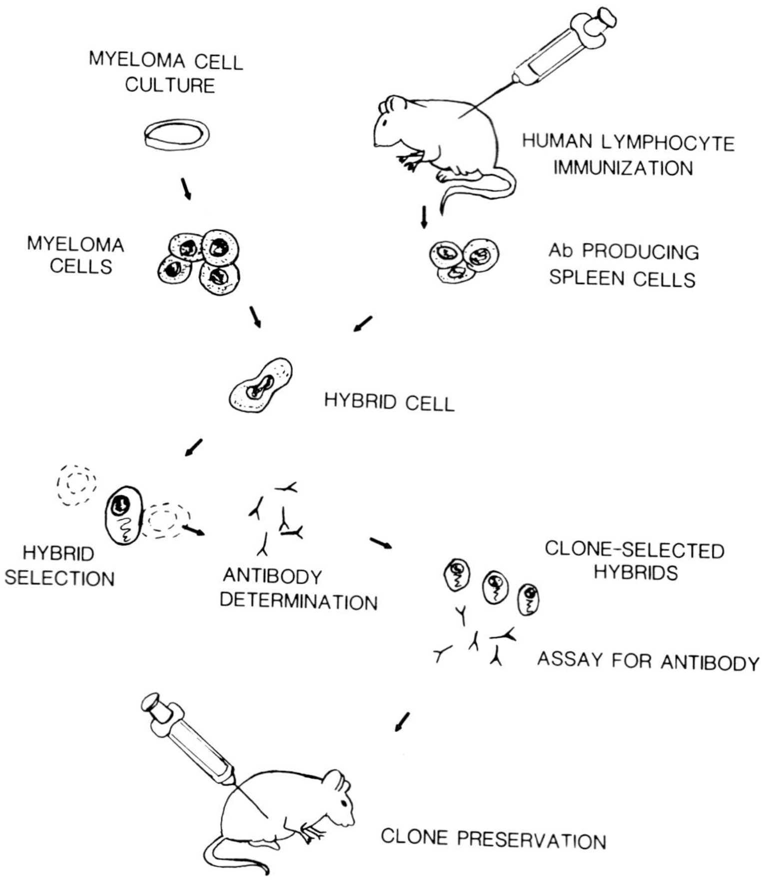

FIGURE 3 Preparation of monoclonal antibody.

We have also treated cynomolgus renal allograft recipients with OKT11A [15]. Following treatment with this antibody, the reactive antigenic site on the peripheral blood lymphocytes was modulated from the cell surface. Essentially no cell depletion occurred. Not unexpectedly, renal allograft survival in these animals was not prolonged, indicating the type of reaction that occurs between the cell membrane antigenic site and administered antibody is crucial in determining immunosuppressive efficacy.

Jonker et al. [21] have confirmed, in rhesus skin allograft recipients, the significant immunosuppressive efficacy of OKT4 and the insignificant prolongation of graft survival by OKT11A. The monoclonal antibody OKT8, specific for HLA class I reactive T cells, was also found to be without immunosuppressive efficacy in the rhesus model. In contrast, we have found treatment with Leu 2a monoclonal antibody (specific for HLA class I reactive T cells) prolongs cynomolgus renal allograft survival to as long as 5 weeks [5].

These studies emphasize that some monoclonal antibodies are more efficient than others in activating mechanisms necessary for effective suppression of the host's response to the allograft. A number of factors, including antibody isotype, antibody affinity with

TABLE 5 Reactivity of Monoclonal Antibodies with Human Peripheral Blood Leukocytes[a]

Antibody	Reactive cell population	% Positive	Cells mm^{-3}
OKT3*, Leu4*, anti-T12[b]	Most circulating T cells	71.1 ± 6.5	1280 ± 380
OKT4*, Leu 3a*	HLA class II antigen reactive T cells	46.7 ± 6.0	791 ± 194
OKT8*, Leu 2a*	HLA class I antigen reactive T cells	28.8 ± 5.1	504 ± 208
Leu 7*	NK subset, some $T8^+$ cells	14.8 ± 4.8	252 ± 114
HLA-DR*	B-cell/monocyte-activated T cells	15.1 ± 4.1	261 ± 106
OKT 11A*, Leu 5*	E-rosetting cells	80 ± 8	1440 ± 460
CBL 1[c]	Activated "blast" cells monocytes	<5	

[a]Asterisk (*) indicates mean standard deviation for 25 normal adult male and females; see Reference 28.
[b]See Reference 22.
[c]See Reference 38.

target antigen, target antigen density, efficiency in activating complement, and mechanism of clearance of coated cells by individual recipients, can be cited as possible explanations for the variable efficacy observed. Continued screening of the numerous agents becoming available, it is hoped, will identify a group of antibodies from this second generation of antilymphocyte preparations that can be effectively incorporated into clinical regimens.

USE OF MONOCLONAL ANTIBODIES AS TREATMENT FOR ACUTE REJECTION

Therapeutic intervention by the intravenous administration of antilymphocyte monoclonal antibodies to human renal allograft recipients has been undertaken to date using three different preparations. We originally reported the use of OKT3, an IgG_{2a} monoclonal antibody, which reacts with an antigenic determinant found on virtually all mature postthymic T cells [7]. Another pilot study has been conducted by Kirkman, utilizing anti-T12, a monoclonal antibody preparation also directed against postthymic T cells [22]. Anti-T12 is an IgM antibody that reacts with a different antigenic determinant than OKT3. Finally, Takahashi has reported the use of another IgM monoclonal antibody, CBL1, prepared against a cultured line of human lymphoblasts [38].

The rationale for initially administering OKT3 at the time of acute rejection was derived from our experience with ATG. The most clear-cut evidence of efficacy would be established if definite reversal of an ongoing rejection reaction could be accomplished. Unfortunately, preclinical trials with this particular antibody were impossible, since it does not react with lymphocytes of any readily available nonhuman species.

To date, a total of 33 CD renal allograft recipients have been evaluated at the Massachusetts General Hospital. These patients were treated from the day of transplantation with standard doses of azathioprine and prednisone. At the onset of biopsy-confirmed acute rejection, OKT3 antibody treatment was the sole addition to their management.

Azathioprine and prednisone dosages were further reduced, based upon the experience gained in the ATG trials. In the first patients treated, the daily dosage of OKT3 antibody was limited to the minimal amount that completely cleared peripheral blood T cells. This usually required 1-2 mg/day. Subsequently, however, we have routinely employed a dosage of 5 mg/day for a total of 10-14 days [40].

In each patient, circulating T-cell numbers plunged to undetectable levels within minutes following the initial OKT3 injection. That the cells had actually been cleared from the circulation was supported by a corresponding fall in total lymphocyte counts and absence of cells bearing other independent T-cell markers. Approximately 5-7 days into the therapeutic course, increasing numbers of cells, nonreactive with OKT3 but reactive with other T-cell markers, became detectable in most patients treated (Figure 2). In vitro incubation of these cells restored OKT3 reactivity, indicating some degree of antigenic modulation had occurred. Modulation of the OKT3 antigen, however, is apparently insufficient to interfere with the therapeutic effect, since in all instances, the established rejection episode was definitively reversed within 2-10 days, without addition of any other immunosuppressive measures.

Despite this striking immunosuppressive efficacy, several limitations to OKT3 monoclonal antibody therapy have been identified. Virtually all patients have experienced chills and a febrile reaction beginning about 40 min after the first injection. Several patients were also noted to have dyspnea and mild bronchospasm. In our experience, all these symptoms have resolved following treatment with antihistamines and antipyretics. Generally, there was no recurrence after the initial infusion. Other investigators, however, have observed even more violent reactions with the initial infusion, and two patients were reported to develop severe bronchospasm and pulmonary edema leading to cardiopulmonary arrest [32].

During the 6- to 48-month follow-up in our study, subsequent rejection episodes have occurred in two-thirds of the patients. Since some of these were irreversible with conventional therapy, long-term graft survival was retained in only 70% of the original group. Hennell has reported a similar incidence of subsequent rejection episodes in 46 recipients of CD renal allografts treated with OKT3 for the initial episode of rejection [16]. Overall, the 1-year graft survival for this group of patients was 70%. Allograft survival was improved to 86% for those patients in whom onset of the second rejection episode was greater than 14 days following completion of the OKT3 therapy. Conversely, if the episode of re-rejection occurred within 14 days of OKT3 therapy, allograft survival was reduced to 56%.

A third possible limitation has been the development of both idiotypic and nonidiotypic antibodies to the OKT3 monoclonal reagent in as many as 85% of treated recipients [16]. Although no clinically evident reactions suggesting anaphylaxis have occurred in our experience, the formation of these anti-mouse antibodies would appear to contraindicate subsequent treatment of these patients with monoclonal antibodies. In an attempt to address these limitations, we have more recently altered the therapeutic protocol by adding increased steroid dosages on the first day of OKT3 therapy, limiting the period of OKT3 treatment to a maximum of 10 days, and administering intravenous cyclophosphamide infusions during the second week of OKT3 therapy. With these changes, we have noted both a marked reduction in the reactions to the initial infusion and decrease in the host's immune response to the infused OKT3 [40].

A multiple-center, prospectively randomized trial comparing OKT3 with high-dose steroids, and ATG if necessary, for reversal of rejection has also been undertaken. Over

100 CD renal allograft recipients were enrolled into this study. The remarkable efficacy of OKT3 in providing rapid depletion of peripheral blood T-cell levels and reversal of established rejection was again demonstrated, with only two rejection episodes in the OKT3-treated group failing to respond [32]. In contrast, only about 70% of rejection reactions responded in the control groups. Although subsequent rejection episodes have claimed some of the allografts in the OKT3 group, graft survival has continued to strongly favor this group because of the high early reversal rate.

Evaluation of the effectiveness of another monoclonal antibody, anti-T12, has been undertaken in a small group of renal allograft recipients [22]. In this trial, 19 patients undergoing acute rejection after either CD or LRD renal transplantation were studied. These patients were initially treated with azathioprine or cyclosporine, and steroids. Rejection was treated with intravenously infused anti-T12 antibody. Only 7 of the recipients had clear-cut reversal of rejection activity. An additional 4 patients had delayed responses after further immunosuppressive therapy had been added to their regimen. A total of 8 patients failed to respond. In contrast to the patients treated with OKT3, no discernible febrile or systemic reactions to the initial infusion of anti-T12 were recorded. One patient did subsequently develop fever, low back pain, and skin rash in association with the development of anti-mouse antibodies. No other significant side effects were identified. Of the 7 patients who had prompt and complete resolution of the rejection episode by the anti-T12 therapy, only 1 required treatment for subsequent rejection activity during a follow-up period of 1-15 months. Further limited trials with this agent have been undertaken, but even less favorable results have been achieved. Thus, its possible role in treatment of renal allograft rejection remains unknown.

A third clinical trial evaluating monoclonal antibody for reversing acute rejection has employed a preparation with more limited T-cell reactivity [38]. In this trial the monoclonal antibody CBL1, which is directed against blast cells, was utilized to test the hypothesis that rejection might be reversed by specific clonal deletion of cells reacting against the graft. The study group included 13 recipients of donor-specific transfusions and LRD allografts and 17 CD allograft recipients. All recipients were initially treated with conventional suppression. At the time of acute rejection, high-dose steroid therapy was administered to many of these patients. When rejection did not reverse after 3-5 days of steroid therapy, monoclonal antibody was added. Intravenous administration of this monoclonal antibody was found to be remarkably nontoxic. None of the patients developed fever, chills, or other significant side effects. There was no evidence of bone marrow toxicity, nor were peripheral blood lymphocyte counts decreased during treatment. Nevertheless, rejection was reversed in 27 of the 30 patients, and subsequent rejection episodes have been infrequent. As in the previous studies, formation of antimouse antibodies was observed in essentially all the patients studied.

PROPHYLACTIC USE OF MONOCLONAL ANTIBODIES

Prophylactic trials employing monoclonal antibody immunosuppression of renal allograft recipients have been conducted with CBL1 and OKT3. CBL1 was not found to be effective in averting episodes of rejection in recipients of LRD renal allografts and prior donor-specific transfusions [37]. Chatenoud has reported the use of OKT3 as the sole immunosuppressive agent in six recipients of CD renal allografts [4]. Without the administration of conventional suppression, these patients were rapidly sensitized to the mouse antibody, as evidenced by the detection of high titers of IgG anti-OKT3 antibodies. This resulted in neutralization of the effect of OKT3 and reappearance of peripheral blood OKT3-reactive cells in five of the six patients prior to the completion of the 14-day course of OKT3 treatment. IgM anti-OKT3 antibodies did not appear to have a similar neutralizing capability. In 11 subsequently treated patients, concomitant administration of azathioprine (3 mg/kg per day) and steroids (0.25 mg/kg per day) delayed the onset of anti-OKT3 antibody production.

From this limited experience, the benefit of administering OKT3 antibody in a prophylactic fashion remains unestablished. With currently existing protocols of immunosuppression, however, the therapeutic advantage of monoclonal antibody treatment would appear to be at the time of allograft rejection.

CURRENT CONCLUSIONS REGARDING ANTILYMPHOCYTE THERAPY

The major complications of pharmacologic immunosuppression have been either infection or incomplete control of rejection. Through refinements in the use of conventional agents, primarily in the limitation of steroid dosages, a decrease in infectious complications and patient mortality has been achieved. The success rate, particularly following CD renal transplantation, however, remained at a marginally acceptable and disturbingly stable level for many years in pateints treated with azathioprine and steroids alone. Further improvement in these results was then achieved for patients in whom ALG or ATG was added to the therapeutic regimen. The efficacy of these polyclonal preparations, especially for reversing acute rejection episodes, has now been firmly established. Despite the usefulness of such preparations, however, they are limited by lot-to-lot variability, contamination by extraneous antibodies, and the inability to refine their application beyond suppression of the entire T-cell response.

The availability of monoclonal antibodies now provides us with agents that may specifically suppress only T cells or even selected T-cell subsets. Initial clinical trials with the pan-T-cell reactive antibodies, OKT3 and anti-T12, have demonstrated truly impressive depletion of peripheral blood T cells and prompt reversal of established rejection episodes following administration of minute dosages. Although the long-term efficacy of these agents remains to be established, these observations have already confirmed the feasibility of using monoclonal antibodies to precisely manipulate T-cell numbers and depress immune responses. An even more exciting aspect of this approach is the possibility of developing protocols directed against only selected T-cell subsets. The recently reported trial using CBL1 antibody is the first clinical venture into this area. Although the observations in these patients are preliminary, they are encouraging.

The tremendous potential of the powerful and sophisticated monoclonal technology has only begun to be applied to transplantation immunology. Undoubtedly, further refinements in the protocols currently being evaluated, as well as trials using other antibodies, will continue. The major question now being addressed is how these agents can or should be incorporated into cyclosporine protocols. With the arrival of both these new immunosuppressive approaches at the same time, it is impossible to predict the precise role each will play in future therapeutic regimens. Because of their already demonstrated effects, however, one can anticipate both increased success rate and decreased toxicity for patients receiving renal allografts.

ACKNOWLEDGMENTS

This work was supported in part by a grant from the United States Public Health Service HL-18646, by funds provided by the Upjohn Company, and the Ortho Pharmaceutical Company. The assistance of Ms. Robyn Keith in the preparation of the manuscript is gratefully acknowledged.

REFERENCES

1. Bell, P. R. F., Blamey, R. W., Briggs, J. D., Castro, J. E., Hamilton, D. N. H., Knapp, M. S., Salaman, J. R., Sells, R. A., Williams, G., Gowans, J. L., Peto, R. R., Richards, S., Phillips, A. W., Weinberg, A. L., and Freestone, D. S. Medical research council trial of antilymphocyte globulin renal transplantation. *Transplantation* 35:539-544, 1983.
2. Butt, K. M. H., Zielinski, C. M., Parsa, I., Elberg, A. J., Wechter, W., and Kountz, S. L. Trends in immunosuppression for kidney transplantation. *Kidney Int.* 13:S95-98, 1978.
3. Cardella, C. J., Folk, J. A., Nicholson, M. J., Harding, M., and Cook, G. T. Successful renal transplantation in patients with T-cell reactivity to donor. *Lancet* 2:1240-1243, 1982.
4. Chatenoud, L., Bandrihaye, M., Kreis, H., Goldstein, G., and Bach, J. F. The restricted human response to the murine monoclonal OKT3 antibody. *Transplant. Proc.* 17:558-559, 1985.
5. Cosimi, A. B. Anti-T-cell monoclonal antibodies in transplantation therapy. *Transplant. Proc.* 15:1889-1892, 1983.
6. Cosimi, A. B. The clinical usefulness of antilymphocyte antibodies. *Transplant. Proc.* 15:583-589, 1983.
7. Cosimi, A. B., Burton, R. C., Colvin, R. B., Goldstein, G., Delmonico, F. L., LaQuaglia, M. P., Tolkoff-Rubin, N., Rubin, R. H., Herrin, J. T., and Russell, P. S. Treatment of acute real allograft rejection with OKT3 monoclonal antibody. *Transplantation* 32: 535-539, 1981.
8. Cosimi, A. B., Burton, R. C., Kung, P. C., Colvin, R., Goldstein, G., Lifter, J., Rhodes, W., and Russell, P. S. Evaluation in primate renal allograft recipients of monoclonal antibody to human T-cell subclasses. *Transplant. Proc.* 13:499-503, 1981.
9. Cosimi, A. B., Wortis, H. H., Delmonico, F. L., and Russell, P. S. Randomized clinical trial of antilymphocytes globulin in cadaver renal allograft recipients: Importance of T-cell monitoring. *Surgery* 80:155-163, 1976.
10. Delmonico, F. L. ATGAM therapy following renal transplantation at the Massachusetts General Hospital. *Transplant. Proc.* 16:979-982, 1984.
11. Delmonico, F. L., Nelson, P. W., Colvin, R. B., and Cosimi, A. B. Immunologic monitoring of ATG treatment for acute allograft rejection. *Transplant. Proc.* 16:1459-1461, 1984.
12. Filo, R. S., Smith, E. J., and Leapman, S. B. Therapy of acute cadaveric renal allograft rejection with adjunctive antithymocyte globulin. *Transplantation* 30:445-449, 1980.
13. Fuller, T. C., Forbes, J. B., and Delmonico, F. L. Renal transplantation with a positive historical donor crossmatch. *Transplant. Proc.* 17:113-114, 1985.
14. Garson, J. S., Beverley, P. C. L., Coakham, H. B., and Harper, E. I. Monoclonal antibodies against human T-lymphocytes label Purkinje neurones of many species. *Nature* 298:375-377, 1982.

15. Giorgi, J. V., Burton, R. C., Barrett, L. V., Delmonico, F. L., Goldstein, G., and Cosimi, A. B. Immunosuppressive effect and immunogenicity of OKT11A monoclonal antibody in monkey allograft recipients. *Transplant. Proc.* 15:639-642, 1983.
16. Norman, D., Barry, J., Hennell, K., Funnell, M. B., Goldstein, G., and Bohannon, L. Reversal of acute allograft rejection with monoclonal antibody. *Transplant. Proc.* 17:39-41, 1985.
17. Henricsson, A., Husberg, B., and Bergentz, S. E. The mechanism behind the effect of ALG on platelets in vivo. *Clin. Exp. Immunol.* 29:515-522, 1977.
18. Hoitsma, A. J., Reekers, P., Kreeftenberg, J. G., van Lier, H. J. J., Chapel, P. J. A., and Koene, R. A. P. Treatment of acute rejection of cadaveric renal allografts with rabbit antithymocyte globulin. *Transplantation* 33:12-16, 1982.
19. Hoitsma, A. J., van Lier, H. J. J., Reckers, P., and Koene, R. A. P. Treatment of acute rejection of cadaveric renal allografts with rabbit antithymocyte globulin. *Transplant. Proc.* 17:72-74, 1985.
20. Howard, R. J., Condie, R. M., Sutherland, D. E. R., Simmons, R. L., and Najarian, J. S. The use of antilymphoblast globulin in the treatment of renal allograft rejection. *Transplant. Proc.* 13:473-474, 1981.
21. Jonker, M., Goldstein, G., and Balner, H. Effects of in vivo administration of monoclonal antibodies specific for human T-cell subpopulations on the immune system in a Rhesus monkey model. *Transplantation* 35:521-526, 1983.
22. Kirkman, R. L., Araujo, J. L., Busch, G. J., Carpenter, C. B., Milford, E. L., Reinherz, E. L., Schlossman, S. F., Strom, T. B., and Tilney, N. L. Treatment of acute renal allograft rejection with monoclonal anti-T12 antibody. *Transplantation* 36:620-626, 1983.
23. Kohler, G., and Milstein, C. Continuous cultures of fused cells secreting antibody of predefined specificity. *Nature* 256:495-497, 1975.
24. Kreis, H., Mansouri, R., Descamps, J. M., Dandavino, R., N'Guyen, A. T., Bach, J. F., and Crosnier, J. Antithymocyte globulin in cadaver kidney transplantation: A randomized trial based on T-cell monitoring. *Kidney Int.* 19:438-444, 1981.
25. Kung, P. C., Goldstein, G., Reinherz, E. L., and Schlossman, S. F. Monoclonal antibodies defining distinctive human T-cell surface antigens. *Science* 206:347-349, 1979.
26. Launois, B., Campion, J. P., Fauchet, R., Kerbaol, M., and Cartier, F. Prospective randomized clinical trial in patients with cadaver-kidney transplants. *Transplant. Proc.* 9:1027-1030, 1977.
27. Matas, A., Sibley, R., Mauer, M., Sutherland, D. E., Simmons, R., and Najarian, S. The value of needle renal allograft biopsy. *Ann. Surg.* 197:226-237, 1983.
28. Moscicki, R., Luttinger, A., and Colvin, R. B. Analysis of human T-cells in blood with monoclonal antibodies and flow cytometry: *Investigation of Cell-mediated Immunity,* T. Yoshida, ed. Churchill-Livingstone, London, 1985, (In Press).
29. Nelson, P. W., Cosimi, A. B., Delmonico, F. L., Rubin, R. H., Tolkoff, Rubin, N. E., Fang, L., and Russell, P. S. Antithymocyte globulin as the primary treatment for renal allograft rejection. *Transplantation* 36:587-588, 1983.
30. Novick, A. C., Braun, W. E., Steinmuller, D., Buszta, C., Greenstreet, R., and Kiser, W. A controlled randomized double-blind study of antilymphoblast globulin in cadaver renal transplantation. *Transplantation* 35:175-179, 1983.
31. Nowygrod, R., Appel, G., and Hardy, M. A. Use of ATG for reversal of acute allograft rejection. *Transplant. Proc.* 13:469-472, 1981.
32. Ortho Multicenter Transplant Study Group. A randomized clinical trial of OKT3 monoclonal antibody for acute rejection of cadaveric renal transplants. *N. Engl. J. Med.* 313:337-342, 1985.
33. Rubin, R. H., Wolfson, J. S., Cosimi, A. B., and Tolkoff-Rubin, N. E. Infection in the renal transplant recipient. *Am. J. Med.* 70:405-411, 1981.

34. Sheil, A. G. R., Kelly, G. E., Storey, B. G., May, J., Kalowski, S., Mears, D., Rogers, J. H., Johnson, J. R., Charlesworth, J., and Stewart, J. H. Controlled clinical trial of antilymphocyte globulin in patients with renal allografts from cadaver donors. *Lancet* 1:359-363, 1971.
35. Shield, C. F., Cosimi, A. B., Tolkoff-Rubin, N., Rubin, R. H., Herrin, J., and Russell, P. S. Use of antithymocyte globulin for reversal of acute allograft rejection. *Transplantation* 28:461-464, 1979.
36. Streem, S. B., Novick, A. C., Braun, W. E., Steinmuller, D., and Greenstreet, R. Low-dose maintenance prednisone and antilymphoblast globulin for the treatment of acute rejection. *Transplantation* 35:420-424, 1983.
37. Takahashi, H., Okazaki, H., Terasaki, P. I., Iwaki, Y., Kinukawa, T., Miura, K., Oguma, S., and Ishigaki, M. Followup on initial trials of kidney transplant rejection reversal by a monoclonal antiblast antibody. *Transplant. Proc.* 17:69-71, 1985.
38. Takahashi, H., Terasaki, P. I., Kinukawa, T., Chia, D., Miura, K., Okazaki, H., Iwaki, Y., Taguchi, Y., Hardiwidjaja, S., Isizaki, M., and Billing, B. Reversal of transplant rejection by monoclonal antiblast antibody. *Lancet* 2:1155-1158, 1983.
39. Taylor, H. E., Ackman, C. F. D., and Horowitz, I. Canadian clinical trial of antilymphocyte globulin in human cadaver renal transplantation. *Can. Med. Assoc. J.* 115:1205-1208, 1976.
40. Thistlethwaite, R., Cosimi, A. B., Delmonico, F. L., Rubin, R. H., Tolkoff-Rubin, N., Fuller, T. C., Neldon, W. W., Fang, L., and Russell, P. S. Evolving use of OKT3 monoclonal antibody for treatment of renal allograft rejection. *Transplantation* 38:695-701, 1984.
41. Thomas, J. M., Carver, F. M., Haisch, C. E., Fahrenbruck, G., Deepe, R. M., and Thomas, F. T. Suppressor cells in Rhesus monkeys treated with antithymocyte globulin. *Transplantation* 34:83-89, 1982.
42. Wakosky, K., and Hall, B. Efficacy of Minnesota antilymphoblast globulin in renal transplantation: A double-blind, randomized, placebo-controlled multicenter trial. *Transplant. Proc.* 17:1304-1311, 1985.
43. Wechter, W. J., Brodie, J. A., Morrell, R. M., Rafi, M., and Schultz, J. R. Antithymocyte globulin (ATGAM) in renal allograft recipients. *Transplantation* 28:294-312, 1979.
44. Woodruff, M. F. A., and Anderson, N. F. Effect of lymphocyte depletion by thoracic duct fistula and administration of antilymphocyte serum on the survival of skin homografts in rats. *Nature (Lond.)* 200:702, 1963.

17

CYCLOSPORINE

Immunobiologic Aspects in Transplantation

Allan D. Hess, Paul M. Colombani, and Ahmed Esa
The Johns Hopkins University School of Medicine, Baltimore, Maryland

HISTORICAL PERSPECTIVES

Since the initial description of the potent immunosuppressive activity of cyclosporin A (CsA) and its apparent selective action on T lymphocytes by Borel [12] and Borel et al. [14] in 1976, considerable interest and enthusiasm has been generated in the application of this nonmyelotoxic agent to clinical transplantation. Initial clinical studies have been encouraging despite the reported toxicities [88,145]. Combined heart and lung transplants, before the advent of CsA fraught with innumerable complications, were now possible [116]. Even high-risk kidney and liver grafts, previously associated with an excessively high rejection rate, showed impressive long-term survival [23,88,101]. Furthermore, clinical trials are underway to determine if CsA will prevent acute graft-versus-host disease (GVHD) in major histocompatibility complex (MHC)-mismatched bone marrow transplants in humans, potentially expanding the application of marrow transplantation as treatment for leukemia [113]. These initial findings have led to the widespread use of CsA in clinical organ grafting with marked success and have recently been extensively reviewed [23,101].

Cyclosporine was initially described as an antifungal metabolite from the soil fungi, *Cylindrocarpon lucidum* Booth and *Tolypocladium inflatum* Gams [112,118]. The chemical and structural properties of CsA have been well characterized. Cyclosporine (Figure 1) is a cyclic endecapeptide with several N-methylated amino acids and a characteristic unsaturated C-9 amino acid that is unique to this substance [112,118].

In early studies, this fungal metabolite was found to have remarkable biologic properties, especially its ability to suppress the immune response without significant myelotoxicity. In a variety of experimental animal systems, administration of CsA resulted in the inhibition of antibody formation to T-dependent antigens, the prolongation of skin graft survival, and the suppression of delayed-type hypersensitivity skin reactions [14,15]. Furthermore, additional studies revealed some selectivity to T-lymphocyte responses since CsA failed to inhibit antibody responses to lipopolysaccharide antigens [14]. From the standpoint of solid organ grafts, CsA was extremely effective at preventing graft rejection [101]. However, no myelotoxicity was observed, which clearly distinguished CsA from other immunosuppressive regimens [14,130]. The absence of myelotoxicity was observed in vivo and confirmed in vitro where CsA had no demon-

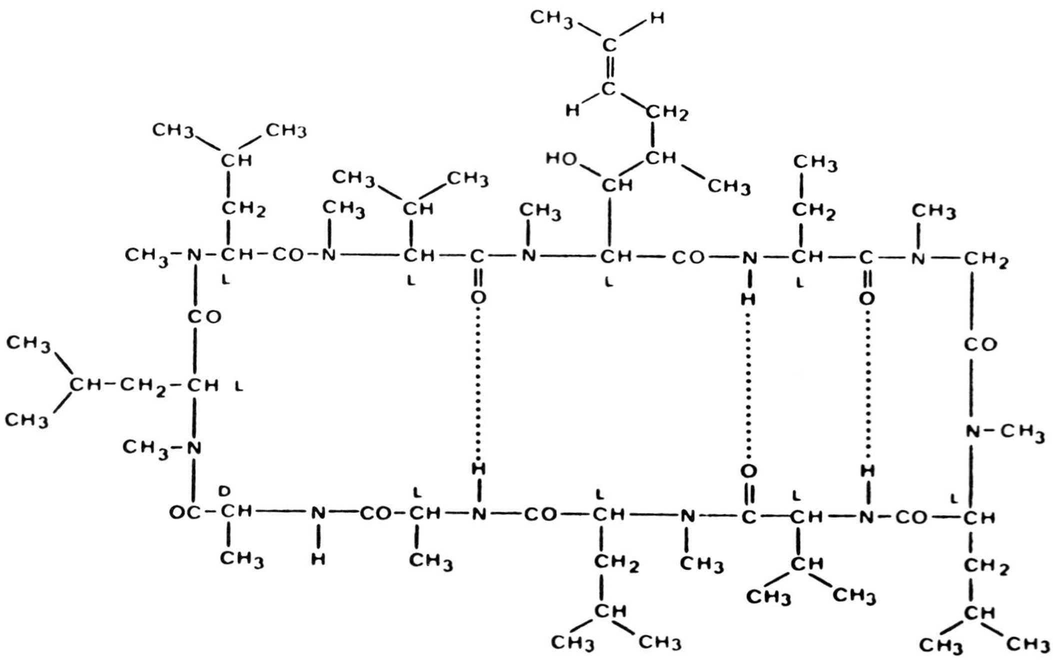

FIGURE 1 Structure of cyclosporine.

strable effect on the growth of hematopoietic progenitor cells in agar [55]. However, most exciting were the observations that CsA facilitated the induction of transplantation tolerance across major histocompatibility complex barriers with only limited postgrafting immunosuppression. Orthotopic renal and cardiac allografts from MHC-mismatched donors were retained indefinitely even after discontinuation of CsA therapy [19,50]. Similarly, rats transplanted with MHC-mismatched bone marrow and treated for a limited period postgrafting with CsA did not develop acute GVHD and showed rapid recovery of immunologic competence and operational tolerance [131,132,134]. Despite the findings in animal systems, CsA for the most part was not able to induce transplantation tolerance in the clinical setting, thus necessitating continued immunosuppressive therapy and potential toxicity. The reason for the failure of tolerance induction in humans remains unknown. Further studies identifying the mode of action of CsA may allow the full realization of tolerance induction to organ allografts in humans.

Numerous additional investigations have been carried out since the initial studies, leading to some understanding of the mechanism of action of this novel agent. A consistent pattern is emerging that suggests that CsA predominantly affects distinct T-lymphocyte subsets that are responsible for graft rejection. In the case of successful tolerance induction. Cyclosporine alters the balance between immunoregulatory suppressor T-cell subsets and the cells required for mediating graft rejection.

This chapter will summarize the current research on CsA and its in vitro and in vivo effect on the complex cellular interactions necessary for a competent allograft response. In addition, recent results regarding the possible mode of action of CsA at the molecular level will be presented.

IN VITRO STUDIES

Inhibition of Lymphoproliferation

Initial studies by several investigators attempted to define the effect of CsA on the in vitro lymphocyte proliferative response to mitogen and alloantigen stimulation [66]. Addition of CsA to the lymphocyte cultures at the beginning of the incubation period resulted in a dose-dependent suppression of the proliferative response to the mitogens, phytohemagglutinin (PHA) and concanavalin A (ConA) and to alloantigens in the primary and secondary mixed lymphocyte culture response (MLR) [66]. Of all the proliferation assays, the primary MLR was the most sensitive to the effects of CsA, whereas the PHA response was the least affected by this agent. In contrast to the ability of CsA to suppress lymphoproliferation, the action of cytolytic effector lymphocytes was not inhibited [66]. Similar dose-dependent suppression of the lymphoproliferative response to mitogen and alloantigen stimulation was observed in humans [61], dogs [31], mice [141], pigs [146], rats [5], and guinea pigs [36]. It is of interest to note that the 50% inhibitory dose of CsA in proliferation assays varied from species to species, which may reflect a differential sensitivity among species to the effects of CsA [13].

These early in vitro studies also revealed several important features of CsA-mediated suppression. First, CsA was not lymphocytotoxic. Incubation of lymphocytes with CsA for 24 hr followed by washing and removal of this agent had no effect on the ability of the lymphocytes to respond to mitogen and/or alloantigen stimulation [61,66]. Similarly, Wang et al. [141] demonstrated that normal MLR and cytotoxic T-lymphocyte responses could be obtained even if CsA was removed as late as 3 days after the beginning of culture. These results clearly indicated that CsA was not lymphocytotoxic and that toxicity could not account for the ability of CsA to inhibit the lymphocyte proliferative response, a feature in marked contrast to other immunosuppressive drugs. The second important feature was the requirement for CsA to be present during the early phase of mitogen and/or alloantigen stimulation. Time-course kinetic studies by several investigators revealed that maximal suppression of mitogen responses occurred when CsA was added within the first 2 hr of culture. Thereafter, addition of CsA yielded intermediate or marginal levels of suppression of the proliferative response [66]. As compared with the mitogen responses, the primary MLR was found to be much less dependent upon the time of addition of CsA after initiation of the culture. Maximal suppression of the lymphocyte proliferative response to alloantigens was observed when CsA was added within the first 72-96 hr of culture. Only marginal suppression of the proliferative response in MLR occurred when CsA was added after this time interval. Further studies [56] revealed, however, that although the proliferative response was inhibited when CsA was added within the first 72-96 hr of culture, the precursor cytotoxic T cell became sensitized and responsive to interleukin-2 (IL-2) within the first 18-24 hr after initiation of culture in the absence of CsA (see below). Taken together, these results clearly suggest that CsA works primarily at an early stage of the immune response in vitro but is also dependent on what assays are used and what parameters are measured. The third important feature was the apparent selectivity of CsA to T-lymphocyte-dependent responses, although this concept has been recently challenged. Initial studies by White et al. [147] demonstrated that CsA failed to inhibit the porcine B-lymphocyte proliferative response to anti-pig IgM, findings in agreement with the original observations of Borel et al. [14], in which this unique agent failed to suppress the antibody response to lipopolysaccharide antigens. Similarly, Burkhardt and Guggenheim [18] showed that CsA did not inhibit the rat B-lymphocyte response to lipopolysaccharide. Further studies by Tosato et al. [129] demonstrated that CsA did not inhibit Epstein-Barr virus (EBV)-induced immunoglobulin synthesis of human lymphocytes. However, recent studies have indicated that CsA can inhibit a subpopulation of B lymphocytes. Kunkl and Klaus [81] and Dongworth and Klaus [35] showed in a murine system that CsA can selectively suppress the antibody response to nonmitogenic T-independent antigens (dinitrophenylated Ficoll, dextran) but does not suppress the response to T-independent mitogenic antigens (dinitrophenylated *Brucella abortus*). Their results suggest the presence of both CsA-sensitive and CsA-resistant B lymphocytes. Such a concept has been recently supported by the observations of Shidani et al. [126], who showed two distinct subsets of memory B lymphocytes based on sensitivity or resistance to CsA. Cyclosporine did not adversely effect the primary or secondary response to trinitrophenyl-lipopolysaccharide (TNP-LPS). In contrast, CsA inhibited the triggering of virgin B lymphocytes and TNP-LPS-induced memory cells by dinitrophenyl-Ficoll. Studies by Muraguchi et al. [102] also demonstrated an effect of CsA on early events in human B-lymphocyte activation with anti-IgM. Although the early studies indicated that CsA predominantly affects T-lymphocyte-dependent responses, recent evidence suggests that CsA does inhibit certain T-independent B-lymphocyte responses, primarily depending on the nature of the antigen used to evoke the response. Clearly, further studies are necessary to clarify the effect of CsA on the response of B lymphocytes.

Effect of Cyclosporine on T-Lymphocyte Cell Subpopulations

Although the initial studies clearly indicated that CsA effectively inhibited the T-lymphocyte proliferative response to mitogen and alloantigen stimulation in a dose-dependent manner, it could not account for the ability of this unique agent to facilitate the induction of transplantation tolerance or for the prolonged survival of allografts after discontinuation of CsA treatment. Similarly, inhibition of lymphocyte proliferation was only a simple measure of the efficacy of this immunosuppressive agent and offered no insight into the effect of CsA on the requisite cell-to-cell collaboration necessary for a competent allograft response. Simplistically, the induction of cytotoxic T lymphocytes that recognize and kill the appropriate target antigen after stimulation in the mixed lymphocyte response, an in vitro model of the allograft response, requires several important steps in addition to antigen recognition: (1) presentation of antigen by macrophages with the subsequent production and release of interleukin-1 (IL-1), (2) activation of precursor cytotoxic T lymphocytes (CTL) with the acquisition of a receptor for interleukin-2 (IL-2), (3) the activation of T-helper lymphocytes with production and release of IL-2 (the production of IL-2 is accentuated by IL-1), (4) the clonal amplification of activated CTL by IL-2, and (5) the activation of suppressor T lymphocytes, which down-regulates or controls this response. The effect of CsA has been studied on several components of this model and has revealed informative data regarding our understanding of the mechanism of action of CsA at the cellular level. However, some controversies still exist and many questions remain unanswered.

Activation of the Precursor Cytotoxic T Lymphocyte

Initial studies by Borel [12], Hess and Tutschka [61], and Wang et al. [141] demonstrated that the in vitro induction of cytolytic T lymphocytes was effectively inhibited by the addition of CsA to a primary MLR. The doses required for complete inhibition of CTL induction were comparable to the levels achieved in vivo ($\geqslant$100 ng/ml) with regimens used for clinical immunosuppression. These observations have since been confirmed by several investigators in vitro and in vivo in different systems, including cytolytic T-lymphocyte responses to viral antigens, including the CTL response to cytomegalovirus, Epstein-Barr virus, and influenza A infected cells [27,28,84,107]. Although CsA effectively inhibits the production of IL-2 (see below), a major question remains whether CsA prevents the activation of the precursor cytolytic lymphocyte. As noted above, the induction of a competent CTL response requires two basic events: (1) the activation and acquisition of a receptor for interleukin-2 and the consequential development of responsiveness to IL-2 and (2) the IL-2-dependent maturation and clonal amplification of the activated CTL. Either the inhibition of IL-2 receptor formation or the inhibition of the response to IL-2 together with the inhibition of IL-2 production by CsA will lead to a compromised cytotoxic T-lymphocyte response.

Initial studies by Larsson in a lectin-dependent system showed that CsA inhibited the acquisition of responsiveness to IL-2, leading to the postulate that CsA inhibits the precursor cytotoxic T lymphocyte from acquiring receptors to this growth factor [86]. The results from Hess et al. [62] using the human MLR system supported this hypothesis. In their studies, exposure of cells harvested from MLR treated with CsA at levels greater than 500 ng/ml to IL-2 did not enhance cytotoxic T-lymphocyte activity after culture. However, culture of primed lymphocytes harvested from MLR treated with levels of CsA at 100 ng/ml did inhibit enhancement of cytotoxic T-lymphocyte activity after culture with interleukin-2. However, in all instances, a proliferative response of the primed lymphocytes from MLR could be demonstrated upon culture with IL-2, indicating that a proportion of cells activated by alloantigen do acquire the ability to functionally respond to interleukin-2. In contrast to these observations, Bunjes et al. [17] demonstrated that addition of exogenous IL-2 to a primary MLR in the presence of CsA could completely restore the proliferative and the cytotoxic T-cell response. The ability of exogenous IL-2 to restore the proliferative response in guinea pig allogeneic MLR were also reported by Dos Reis and Shevach [36], although cytotoxic T-cell activity was not assessed in these cultures. Moreover, in the studies of Dos Reis and Shevach [36], exogenous IL-2 could not restore the primary T-cell proliferative responses to self Ia antigens in the syngeneic mixed leukocyte reaction or to trinitrophenyl-modified syngeneic macrophages. These results suggested the CsA could block the induction of functional IL-2 responsiveness in some systems but not in others. Recent studies by Wagner [139] in a limiting dilution assay system (in the presence of exogenous IL-2) indicated that CsA will prevent naive precursor cytotoxic T-cell activation and the subsequent development of IL-2 responsiveness. Further studies by Hess [56] also provided evidence on the ability of CsA to prevent the development of functional IL-2 responsiveness of the cytotoxic T lymphocyte by CsA in the human MLR system. The results showed that addition of exogenous IL-2 to an MLR containing graded doses of CsA restored the proliferative response to alloantigen challenge in vitro to almost normal levels. In contrast, the effect of exogenous IL-2 on the induction of cytotoxic T lymphocytes in primary MLR in the presence of CsA was completely dependent on the dose of CsA. At the highest doses of CsA (0.5-2.5 μg/ml), no cytotoxic T-cell activity could be detected regardless of the presence of exogenous IL-2. However at a lower dose of CsA (0.1 μg/ml), which routinely resulted in the total inhibition of cytotoxic T-cell induction, addition of exogenous IL-2 resulted in significant levels of detectable cytotoxic T-cell activity, suggesting that the precursor CTL was activated but not clonally amplified due to an absence of IL-2. These results indicated that the effect of CsA on the induction of functional IL-2 responsiveness by the CTL was indeed dose dependent. The studies by Hess [56] also examined the effect of time-sequential addition of CsA or CsA plus exogenous IL-2 to probe the acquisition of functional responsiveness to IL-2 by the precursor cytotoxic T lymphocytes. The results demonstrated that, in the absence of adequate levels of CsA, the precursor cytotoxic T lymphocyte acquires functional IL-2 responsiveness within the first 18 hr of culture after exposure to the alloantigen stimulus, leading to the hypothesis that adequate levels of cyclosporine must be achieved early in vivo to prevent sensitization of the precursor cytotoxic T lymphocyte. This is especially important since CsA will not inhibit the response to IL-2 of lymphocytes that have developed the ability to respond to this lymphokine, findings that have been established in a variety of studies [17,36,62,66,86]. The triggering of IL-2 production by environmental antigens at lower maintenance doses of CsA in clinical transplantation may lead to the initiation of graft rejection if the cytotoxic T lymphocytes have been sensitized since CsA does not block the action of these effector cells [61,66].

The recent development of a monoclonal antibody capable of detecting the IL-2 receptor (TAC) has allowed for the determination of the effect of CsA on IL-2 receptor formation rather than acquisition of functional responsiveness. Recent studies by Miyawaki et al. [98] demonstrated that CsA did not inhibit TAC expression on PHA- or ConA-stimulated human lymphocytes. However, other activation antigens expressed on T lymphocytes, such as class II major histocompatibility antigens or those antigens detected by the OKT9 and OKT10 monoclonal antibodies, were reduced. Comparable observations with no effect of CsA on TAC expression on mitogen-stimulated human lymphocytes were reported by Ryffel et al. [123]. Even though TAC expression was not reduced in cultures with CsA, proliferation was abolished in a dose-dependent manner. In contrast to these findings, Lillehoj et al. [93] demonstrated that CsA inhibited IL-2 receptor formation in mitogen-stimulated murine lymphocytes when tested after 3 days of culture. However, no effect on IL-2 receptor expression was observed when the cells were tested after 24 hr of culture. The cells from these cultures were not responsive to IL-2, a surprising finding since various studies have indicated that CsA does not inhibit primed cells from responding to this soluble factor [17,36,62,66,86]. These studies indicate that the effect of CsA on IL-2 responsiveness and IL-2 receptor formation may be much more complex. Similarly, the expression of TAC antigen and class II major histocompatibility antigen was reduced in CsA-treated human MLR cultures [56,60]. However, it is important to note that TAC expression was not completely abolished in these cultures and probably accounted for the ability of the lymphocytes from the CsA-treated MLR cultures to respond to interleukin-2 [62].

The discrepant results with regard to the effect of CsA on IL-2 receptor expression on mitogen and alloantigen-stimulated cells remains unclear at present. It may be that much higher doses of CsA must be used to prevent TAC expression on mitogen-stimulated T lymphocytes compared with alloantigen-stimulated lymphocytes or that lymphocytes from different species may differ in their sensitivity to the effects of CsA on IL-2 receptor formation. It may also be that activation of lymphocytes by alloantigen (especially the CTL) may require an intricate set of signals and cell-to-cell collaboration, whereas mitogen stimulation may bypass some of the important events required for alloantigen stimulation. CsA may allow the discrimination of signaling events between mitogen and alloantigen stimulation. Such a hypothesis may have some merit since recent studies by Wagner et al. [140] have demonstrated the requirement of a cytotoxic differentiation factor for maturation of the activated precursor cytotoxic T lymphocyte. Lytic function could only be achieved in the presence of this factor. The sensitivity of the production of this factor and of its action to the effects of CsA remains unknown.

Further studies are clearly necessary to establish the effect of CsA on IL-2 receptor expression with regard to alloantigen stimulation versus mitogen stimulation of T lymphocytes and with respect to different functional T-cell subsets. However, these studies clearly indicate that CsA will ultimately be useful as a probe to dissect out signals necessary in the activation of T cells to specific antigen and/or mitogen stimulation.

Effect of Cyclosporine on Suppressor T-Cell Activation

In comparison to the effect of cyclosporine on cytotoxic T-lymphocyte activation, induction of suppressor T lymphocytes in vitro in a variety of model systems was relatively resistant to the effects of this novel immunosuppressive agent. One of the first observations indicating a selective effect between distinct T-lymphocyte subpopulations were the results of Gordon and Singer [51]. They showed in a T-lymphocyte colony-forming assay in agar the inhibition of one type of colony by cyclosporine whereas the other remained unaffected by this agent. The cells that were not affected by CsA were thought to include cells with suppressor characteristics. Relevant to these observations were the studies of Hess and Tutschka [61] in a human primary MLR, which showed that CsA spared the induction of suppressor T lymphocytes activated by alloantigens. At moderate doses of CsA (0.1-1.0 μg/ml), which totally inhibited cytotoxic T-cell induction, cells harvested from these cultures were capable of suppressing in an antigen-nonspecific manner. At higher doses of CsA, the cells harvested from CsA-treated MLR cultures mediated antigen-specific suppressor T-cell function when tested in a fresh MLR. It is important to note that in the MLR there appear to be two distinct types of suppressor T-cell populations, one that acts in an antigen-specific manner and one that suppresses nonspecifically. The latter type of suppressor T cells appears to be transient since it could only be demonstrated at the peak of proliferation or shortly thereafter. It is unknown whether nonspecific suppressor T cells mature into cells that act in an antigen-specific manner or whether there are two distinct types of cells. Nevertheless, CsA spared the induction of suppressor T lymphocytes after alloantigen stimulation in human MLR while totally inhibiting the cytotoxic T-lymphocyte response. Studies by Hess et al. [59] have attempted to characterize the suppressor T lymphocytes activated in MLR in the presence of cyclosporine. Their studies demonstrated that the suppressor T cell had the OKT3$^+$, OKT8$^+$, OKT4$^-$, and OKIa$^+$ phenotype. A similar effect showing that the activation of MLR-generated suppressor cells was more resistant to cyclosporine than cytotoxic T-cell induction was reported by Deeg et al. in dogs [31], by Wang et al. in both an in vitro and in an in vivo MLR system in mice [141], and by Dos Reis and Shevach in guinea pigs [36]. It is of interest to note that in the studies by Dos Reis and Shevach, radiosensitive suppressor T lymphocytes could not be demonstrated in normal MLR cultures (not treated with CsA) but could only be demonstrated after the addition of cyclosporine. This is in contrast to the findings in both murine and human systems in which suppressor T lymphocytes can be routinely demonstrated in control MLR cultures. Moreover, the suppressor T cells from the guinea pig system induced in MLR in the presence of CsA were capable of secreting an antigen-nonspecific suppressor factor that inhibited the proliferative and cytotoxic T-cell response when added to a fresh micro-MLR system [37]. Since these initial observations, many investigators have utilized different systems to demonstrate the inability of cyclosporine to inhibit suppressor T-cell induction. The systems have included ConA-induced suppressor T-cell activity [89], fetal calf serum-induced suppressor T-cell activation, and culture-activated suppressor T lymphocytes [70]. Taken together, the results clearly indicate that in many systems, at least in vitro, CsA spares the activation of suppressor T lymphocytes. In all the above studies in the various systems, CsA by itself did not induce suppressor T-cell function but required the presence of either specific antigen or a specific stimulus. These results ruled out the possibility that CsA triggered suppressor T cells directly in a mitogenic fashion.

One of the important questions was to determine the consequence of the imbalance in the activation of suppressor T cells versus cytotoxic T lymphocytes induced by CsA. Studies by Hess et al. [63] demonstrated that specific tolerance could be induced by treating human MLR with cyclosporine. Cells harvested from CsA-treated cultures were no longer capable of responding to the specific alloantigen used for stimulation. Although a weak secondary proliferative response was observed upon re-exposure to the sensitizing alloantigen, cytotoxic T-cell activity could not be detected. However, the response to third-party alloantigens was normal with respect to both the lymphoproliferative response and the induction of cytotoxic T lymphocytes to the third-party antigens. Fractionation of the specifically tolerant cells from the cyclosporine-treated MLR cultures over nylon wool columns restored their ability to form cytotoxic T lymphocytes to the original sensitizing antigen in a secondary culture. The proliferative response was characteristic of a primary MLR with the peak of proliferation on day 7. The specific tolerant state could be restored by combining the nylon wool-nonadherent fraction with the nylon wool-adherent fraction [66], suggesting that the state of specific tolerance was maintained by a nylon wool-adherent suppressor T lymphocyte. Comparable findings with regard to tolerance induction in vitro were observed by Wang et al. [141] in a murine system that demonstrated that cells from an in vitro and/or an in vivo MLR system treated with CsA were no longer capable of forming cytotoxic T lymphocytes upon re-exposure to the sensitizing alloantigen. However, the in vitro system showed a greater degree of nonspecificity with the inability to form cytotoxic T lymphocytes upon challenge with the third-party alloantigen. This may be the result of the nonspecific suppressor T cells observed in these systems. Taken together, these data indicate that CsA does spare the activation of suppressor T lymphocytes upon exposure to a variety of stimuli, including alloantigens and/or mitogens. The reasons for the apparent differential sensitivity between suppressor T cells and cytotoxic T lymphocytes remains unknown but has been corroborated by in vivo studies, which will be discussed below.

Effect of Cyclosporine on T-Helper Lymphocytes and Lymphokine-Producing Cells

It has been postulated by many investigators that the primary target of cyclosporine has been the T-helper cell, as indicated by the ability of cyclosporine to preferentially inhibit the secretion of interleukin-2 and other lymphokines by this T-cell subset. By far the sensitivity of this specific T-helper cell subset to cyclosporine as determined by the ability of this agent to inhibit production of lymphokines, such as IL-2, compared with other T-cell functions has substantiated this hypothesis to some extent. Initial studies by a variety of investigators have demonstrated that CsA effectively inhibited interleukin-2 production [17,36,56,62]. The inhibition of IL-2 production prevents the clonal expansion of activated T cells that express the receptor for this lymphokine, such as the activated precursor cytotoxic T lymphocyte.

In the human MLR, Hess et al. [56,62] have demonstrated that CsA effectively inhibited IL-2 production after alloantigen stimulation. Since these initial observations, the effect of cyclosporine on interleukin-2 production has been confirmed by a variety of investigators. Bunjes et al. [17] and Wang et al. [142] demonstrated that addition of cyclosporine to lymphocytes stimulated with alloantigen in murine MLR effectively suppressed the production of interleukin-2. Comparable studies were performed by Dos Reis and Shevach [36] in a guinea pig allogeneic MLR system. In addition, Bunjes et al. [17] demonstrated that addition of exogenous IL-1 to CsA-treated cultures of ConA stimulated mouse cells did not result in production of IL-2, indicating that CsA rendered the T-helper cell refractive to the effects of IL-1. Hess et al. [68] demonstrated that addition of exogenous IL-1 to primary human MLR could not overcome the immunosuppressive action of CsA. Similar studies were performed by Palacios and Moller [110], who showed that CsA caused the IL-2-producing T cell to become unresponsive to the monocyte-derived lymphokine, IL-1. This has been further characterized at the clonal level by Palacios [16,109], indicating the absence or down-regulation of the receptor for IL-1 induced by CsA. These initial studies were performed upon primary exposure to alloantigen or mitogens in culture. Andrus and Lafferty [2] showed that CsA was able to inhibit IL-2 production in response to antigen or mitogen restimulation. These cells were sensitized prior to addition of cyclosporine and restimulation with the specific antigen or mitogen. Similar studies utilizing sensitized T lymphocytes were reported by Hess et al. [65] using the human secondary MLR system. Addition of CsA to primed lymphocytes rechallenged with the specific alloantigen resulted in the significant inhibition of IL-2 production. These studies indicated that IL-2 production was not only inhibited in primary responses by CsA but this agent also inhibited production of IL-2 by sensitized lymphocytes upon specific rechallenge with antigen, indicating some efficacy against sensitized cells, findings that were confirmed in vivo [124].

The effect of cyclosporine on T-helper cell function and lymphokine secretion has not been limited to interleukin-2 production. Recent studies by Thomson et al. [128] demonstrated that cyclosporine inhibited the production of T-cell-derived lymphokines affecting macrophage function. Addition of cyclosporine to cultures of spleen cells stimulated with antigen, ConA, or PHA resulted in the inhibition of the production of macrophage procoagulant activity and a lymphocyte-derived macrophage chemotactic factor. Cyclosporine did not, however, affect the response of the macrophage to these soluble factors. Further studies by Block et al. [11] demonstrated that cyclosporine A was able to inhibit the production of migration inhibitory factor (MIF) by human lymphocytes stimulated with ConA. In addition, a recent report has demonstrated that this novel immunosuppressive agent will also inhibit the production of interleukin-3 [85]. Other studies have demonstrated that CsA inhibits the production of γ interferon by lymphocytes that were stimulated by mitogen and/or alloantigen [1,73,115]. On the other hand, production of α or β interferon by human and mouse lymphocytes or fibroblasts was not affected by this agent [73].

Two elegant studies were recently performed, applying techniques used in molecular biology, that may shed some light into the immunosuppressive action of cyclosporine with respect to its effect on lymphokine secretion. Elliott et al. [42] reported that CsA inhibited the induction of interleukin-2 messenger RNA. In their studies, a human and a murine cell line were cultured under conditions in which these cells are normally secreting high levels of interleukin-2 (in the presence of phorbol-12-myristyl-13-acetate). Addition of CsA blocked production of interleukin-2 and was found to be associated with an absence of interleukin-2 messenger RNA accumulation. More recently, studies by Granelli-

Piperno et al. [48] have confirmed and extended these findings. They used as a model system 3-day-old ConA-induced lymphoblasts. Mitogen restimulation of these blast cells resulted in the synthesis of IL-2, interferon, B-cell-stimulating factor, and a cytotoxic differentiation factor. Addition of CsA to this system strongly inhibited production of these lymphokines. They demonstrated that the effect of CsA was to block the induction or production of active lymphokine mRNA as assayed in an oocyte translation system. Even though lymphokine production and lymphokine mRNA was inhibited in these studies, total protein synthesis and proliferation were not affected by the presence of cyclosporine. It is not known whether the effect of CsA was due to an inhibition of mRNA lymphokine transcription or by destabilization of the messenger RNA. Although these results are certainly exciting and provide informative data with regard to the action of cyclosporine on lymphokine production in activated T cells, it remains unknown if the same mechanism of action accounts for the ability of CsA to inhibit T-cell activation. Regardless, the data provided these two studies indicate that CsA can actively suppress lymphokine production in activated cells at the level of messenger RNA production, suggesting that CsA may be an effective suppressive agent for diseases that may be mediated by the production of lymphokines by sensitized T cells, such as rheumatoid arthritis or sarcoidosis.

Taken together, these studies have indicated that cyclosporine A is an effective inhibitor of lymphokine production. The inhibition of these active soluble factors by cyclosporine will lead to a compromised immune response. Inhibition of lymphokine production, such as IL-2, will certainly inhibit the clonal amplification of the cytotoxic T-lymphocyte response and limit delayed-type hypersensitivity immune responses.

In contrast to the effect of cyclosporine on the production of lymphokines that amplify cytotoxic effector and delayed-type hypersensitivity responses, the amplification of the suppressor T-cell arm of the immune response appears to be unimpaired by cyclosporine. Both in vitro and in vivo studies have demonstrated that near-normal levels of suppressor T lymphocytes can be generated in the presence of CsA even in the absence of interleukin-2. These results suggest that the amplification of suppressor T lymphocytes may be, in part, independent of IL-2 production or that there may be alternative mechanisms accounting for suppressor T-cell differentiation and amplification. Initial studies by Hess et al. [60] have demonstrated that, in human MLR, a small percentage of T-helper cells are activated in the presence of CsA, as determined by expression of class II major histocompatibility antigens. These Ia^+ T-helper cells were shown to amplify $OKT8^+$ suppressor T-cell activity. These results suggested that CsA spared the regulatory T-helper cell subset responsible for suppressor T-cell amplification. These studies were confirmed in an elegant series of experiments by Mohagheghpour et al. [100] demonstrating $OKT4^+$ suppressor amplifier cells from CsA-treated human MLR. In their studies, both $OKT8^+$ and $OKT4^+$ subsets derived from the CsA-treated cultures exhibited potent suppressor cell activity. However, the $OKT4^+$ suppressor subset could only mediate suppression if the test system for suppression contained fresh $OKT8^+$ cells, indicating that the $OKT4^+$ cell was an inducer of suppressor cell function. Further studies suggested that the cytotoxic T-cell inducer subset could not be demonstrated from the CsA-treated cultures. These results suggested that the suppressor amplifier T-helper cells were resistant to the effects of CsA, whereas the cytotoxic inducer T-helper cells were sensitive to this agent. Further studies by Hess et al. [59] revealed that the supernatants from CsA-treated MLR cultures that did not contain IL-2 were able to promote enhancement of antigen-specific suppressor T-lymphocyte activity. This soluble factor was not IL-1, IL-2, or α, β, or γ

interferon and stimulated antigen-specific suppressor T-cell function of OKT8$^+$ T lymphocytes harvested from 10-day-old MLR cultures. Furthermore, this soluble factor was able to promote growth of MLR-activated T lymphocytes in a clonogenic agar system. Comparable studies were performed by Converse and Hess [26] utilizing the lymphocyte response to cytomegalovirus antigens. Supernatants from CsA-treated cultures again were found to promote enhancement of antigen-specific suppressor T-cell function. These results were confirmed in mice by Rich et al. [117] utilizing both in vivo and in vitro MLR systems. They demonstrated a soluble factor capable of promoting growth or differentiation of antigen-specific suppressor-T lymphocyte. Initial characterization of this molecule revealed an apparent molecular weight of approximately 21,000 daltons, although a second minor peak of activity was noted at 43,000 daltons. This active factor was apparently derived from the T-helper cell compartment. These studies also suggested that the production of this lymphokine identified in several different systems is resistant to the effects of CsA, in contrast to the production of interleukin-2, interferon, and other T-cell-derived lymphokines, which is CsA sensitive.

These results indicate that the mechanisms (both cellular and soluble factors) accounting for suppressor T-cell amplification are relatively resistant to the effects of cyclosporine and may account for the near-normal levels of suppressor T-cell function induced in the presence of CsA. This pathway may be an alternative mechanism to assure differentiation and amplification of this immunoregulatory subset.

Effects of CsA on Macrophage Functions

Macrophages possess a wide range of activities crucial to host defense mechanisms. Many of these functions stem from the basic ability of the macrophage to phagocytose foreign material. In addition, macrophages are known to be essential for the induction and regulation of the immune response. Our understanding of the role of the macrophage in immunologic responsiveness is still imprecise. Strong experimental evidence indicates that macrophages "process" native antigen into immunogenic moieties and then "present" these moieties, in association with class II determinants (Ia), to the appropriate antigen-reactive lymphocyte subsets [136]. Moreover, macrophages elaborate a number of immunologically important mediators, such as IL-1 [99].

Cyclosporine exerts its immunosuppressive action during the inductive phase of the immune response, at a time when the critical role of the macrophage is well recognized. Whether immunosuppression by CsA is wholly or partially due to changes in macrophage physiology has not been extensively studied. Early studies indicated that CsA did not affect the phagocytic and chemotactic activities of macrophages and did not interfere with enzyme synthesis and secretion [146]. More recent studies suggested that CsA may alter several macrophage functions that are important in the induction of the immune response. Data from several laboratories suggest that CsA, either through inhibition of IL-1 production [17] or interference with the expression of receptors for IL-1, blocks IL-1-dependent activation of T cells [6]. Hellin and Edington [54] have demonstrated that CsA abrogated the synthesis of procoagulant factors by human monocytes. In a recent study, Whisler et al. [144] have found that CsA-treated macrophages produced increased levels of prostaglandin E_2. The accessory role of macrophages in oxidative mitogenesis was also found by Uyemura et al. [137] to be inhibited by CsA treatment.

Experiments performed by Esa et al. provide evidence that CsA inhibits the ability of human monocytes to present antigen (tetanus toxoid and cytomegalovirus) to immuno-component T cells [43]. In these experiments, human monocytes pulsed with antigen in the presence of CsA were significantly reduced in their capacity to trigger T-lymphocyte proliferation. Moreover, lymphocytes cultured with antigen-pulsed monocytes treated with CsA were found to have diminished cytotoxic capacity. In contrast, the generation of suppressor cell activity was not affected by CsA treatment of these monocytes. These effects of CsA on the human monocyte were not apparently dependent on the elaboration of IL-1, since it was not possible to restore normal proliferative responses with exogenous IL-1 after treatment of monocytes with CsA. The mechanism by which CsA inhibits presentation is still obscure. The inability of CsA to impair the activation of suppressor cells suggests that alterations in the expression of class II antigens on the antigen-presenting cell (APC) are involved. Ultraviolet radiation of APC, which leads to diminished Ia expression, has been shown [38] to, as in the case of CsA, selectively block proliferative and cytotoxic responses while leaving the generation of suppressor cells largely unaffected. This suggestion is also indirectly supported by the recent observation that CsA leads to enhanced prostaglandin E_2 (PGE_2) production by monocytes since PGE decreases the expression of Ia [38,144].

Subcellular Action of Cyclosporine

As outlined in the preceding sections of this chapter, T-lymphocyte subset analyses demonstrated that the effect of CsA varied with the subset analyzed, the stimulus provided (alloantigen versus mitogen), and the concentration of CsA utilized. At immunosuppressive, nontoxic levels, CsA appeared to diminish the maturation and proliferation of cytotoxic T cells (possibly by decreasing or eliminating the expression of receptors for interleukin-2) following mitogen or alloantigen stimulation, respectively. The elaboration of lymphokines by T cells, primarily interleukin-2, was diminished. Macrophage production of interleukin-1 and/or antigen presentation may also be diminished [17]. The generation of suppressor-T lymphocytes, however, appeared to be spared. This section will summarize the investigations into the effects of CsA at the subcellular level, primarily on T lymphocytes, and relate these findings to the larger scheme of the effect of CsA on the activation and function of macrophages and the T-lymphocyte subsets.

The initial clue to the subcellular mechanism of action of CsA was the narrow time frame of its effect. The addition of CsA to an established T-cell line did not inhibit proliferation in the presence of growth factors [24]. Similarly, the proliferation of T lymphocytes, as indicated by [^{3}H] thymidine uptake in response to mitogens, was not inhibited by the addition of CsA more than 2 hr following mitogen stimulation and 72-96 hr for alloantigen stimulation [61,143]. From these studies, it appeared that CsA may interfere with the events of T-cell activation prior to DNA synthesis and cell division. Studies by Koponen et al. examining the cell cycle events of T lymphocytes following mitogen stimulation demonstrated that CsA prevented cells from proceeding from the G_0/G_1 phase to S phase in the cell cycle [79,80]. These studies also indicated that CsA acted at a point in the activation sequence that prevented the signals necessary for DNA synthesis and replication.

Studies by Kay et al. investigating messenger RNA and protein synthesis following mitogen stimulation demonstrated that CsA prevented both events [75]. This was consistent with the CsA effect on IL-2 receptor expression since it had been shown that both mRNA transcription and *new* protein synthesis is required for IL-2 receptor expression following activation [34,114]. Fidelius et al. showed that CsA inhibited the induction of ornithine decarboxylase at 4 hr following mitogen stimulation [44,45]. Ornithine decarboxylase is the rate-limiting enzyme step in polyamine synthesis in the nucleus, and the end products of this biosynthetic pathway are necessary for DNA and mRNA synthesis [44,45,78]. All the above studies indicated that CsA acts within the first few hours following stimulation of T lymphocytes to prevent activation signals from reaching the cell's nucleus. Thus, the initiation of mRNA and the new protein synthesis necessary for IL-2 receptor elaboration and lymphokine production, as well as the DNA replication necessary for cell division, was effectively inhibited.

Investigations of the initial membrane and cytoplasmic activation events of T lymphocytes following stimulation in the presence of CsA has followed two directions: studies into the CsA effect on isolated steps in the activation scheme and a search for a receptor for CsA. Both investigative lines are related and can be discussed within the framework of the generally accepted activation scheme of T lymphocytes that proceeds from the cell membrane to the nucleus.

There is ample evidence that binding of cell membrane receptors by mitogens or alloantigen in association with macrophage class II antigen (HLA-DR) creates membrane perturbations allowing for a calcium flux into the cell [9,92]. Initial studies by Palacios et al. hypothesized that CsA may compete for these receptors and thus block this initial membrane activation [16,108,109]. Studies in our laboratory, using a fluorescent, dansylated CsA, demonstrated that CsA did not compete for membrane receptors for such mitogens as phytohemagglutinin, conconavalin A, or the OKT3 monoclonal antibody, the HLA-DR receptor, or the IL-2 receptor [24]. Cyclosporine-binding studies by Ryffel et al. [121] using ^{3}H-labeled CsC and by Colombani et al. [24] using the fluorescent CsA demonstrated that CsA binding to T cells was temperature dependent and saturable following pseudo-first-order kinetics. The apparent dissociation constant for CsA binding to T cells was in the micromolar range from 1×10^{-7} M to 6×10^{-6} M [24,120,121]. In addition, differential binding of fluorescent CsA was found within the T-lymphocyte cell population, which may indicate differential sensitivity to CsA [57]. In studies by LeGrue et al., ^{3}H-labeled CsA, however, was also found to "bind" to liposomes with similar kinetics, and this suggested that membrane binding was passive and probably secondary to the hydrophobic nature of CsA [90,91]. Studies again by Colombani et al. using the fluorescent CsA derivatives, however, demonstrated early membrane binding followed by internalization and increased cytoplasmic fluorescence, which was maximal at 90 min and indicated that CsA may bind and therefore express its activity in the cytoplasm of the cell [24]. A protein had also been isolated by Merker et al. that binds to CsA and was termed "cyclophilin." Cyclophilin, a 17-kilodalton basic protein, was found predominantly in the cytoplasmic fractions from a number of cell types, including T lymphocytes. Much lesser amounts of cyclophilin were found in the membrane and nuclear fractions of the cells studied [53,96]. The identity and significance of cyclophilin remains to be demonstrated. Thus, there is increasing evidence that CsA may act within the cytoplasm of susceptible cells, and one potential protein receptor has been isolated.

The membrane calcium flux and the secondary rise in intracellular calcium has been demonstrated to be critically important to T-cell activation [9,92]. In a study by Kay and Benzie, CsA also inhibited the proliferative response to calcium ionophore A23471, a mitogenic agent that induces this calcium flux [76]. It was hypothesized that receptor-mediated or passive membrane binding of CsA, although not interfering with lectin or alloantigen binding, could interfere with the membrane changes necessary for this calcium in flux [16]. Subsequently, it was demonstrated by Metcalfe that the rise in intracellular calcium secondary to mitogen or Ca ionophore was not affected by CsA, indicating that both receptor binding by mitogens and calcium flux were not influenced by CsA [97].

Studies by Cheung et al. demonstrated that a rise in intracellular calcium was required for mitogen stimulation and proliferation of T cells but not required for B-cell mitogen-induced proliferation. This calcium-dependent T-cell proliferation was prevented by a calmodulin inhibitor (trifluoroperazine) that had no effect on B-cell proliferation [21]. Calmodulin, a 17-kilodalton calcium-dependent regulator protein, has been shown to be critically involved in activating the enzymes necessary for many cellular activities, including cyclic nucleotide turnover, glycogen breakdown and the phosphorylation of enzymes required for ATP production, phospholipid turnover for prostaglandin synthesis, and the phosphorylation of enzymes necessary for mRNA and protein synthesis [3,77,95,150]. Some calmodulin inhibitors may also bind to protein kinase C, a calcium-phospholipid-dependent enzyme, also involved in cell activation [104]. Recent studies by Colombani et al. demonstrated that CsA binds to calmodulin in the presence of calcium with binding kinetics similar to the binding of CsA to intact cells. Cyclosporine also inhibited the ability of calmodulin to activate 3′,5′-cyclic nucleotide phosphodiesterase in an in vitro assay system. Binding of fluorescent CsA to intact cloned T lymphocytes was also competitively inhibited by two calmodulin inhibitors [25]. These competitive binding studies using the calmodulin inhibitors would also, however, implicate protein kinase C as another possible cell receptor for CsA.

Since the calcium-calmodulin complex is involved in the cyclic nucleotide system, particularly cyclic GMP activity, it could be hypothesized that CsA blocks calmodulin elevation of cGMP and subsequent cGMP-dependent events, which have been shown to be involved in T-cell proliferation, cytotoxic T-cell activity, and lymphokine production. This is consistent with the recent studies by Bendtzen et al. that demonstrated that insulin, a cGMP agonist, and two cGMP analogs were able to overcome CsA inhibition of T-cell-derived lymphokine production [6-8]. The calmodulin inhibition by CsA would prevent glycogen breakdown and phosphorylation of kinases necessary for energy production, which is consistent with another recent study that demonstrated ATP depletion in T lymphocytes incubated with CsA [94]. Cyclosporine blockade of calmodulin-related events may, however, allow for a rise in cyclic AMP levels, which has been implicated in suppressor cell generation and the inhibition of T-cell proliferation, cytotoxic T-cell activity, and lymphokine production [22,52,111]. Similar blockade in macrophage function may depress lymphokine production and prevent surface receptor elaboration necessary for antigen presentation. Blockade of calmodulin but not protein kinase C may allow for the activation of protein kinase C since the potentiation of the mitogen response by phorbol esters was not inhibited by CsA [10]. Phorbol esters appear to activate protein kinase C directly and have also been shown to influence a T-cell line to modulate its surface phenotype and or convert to suppressor cell function [122]. Blockade of calcium-calmodulin function may modulate nuclear cAMP production and block the activation of ornithine decarboxylase by a cAMP-dependent protein kinase, which would prevent the mRNA and new protein synthesis necessary for IL-2 receptor elaboration and lymphokine production. Calmodulin has also been found associated with the nuclear matrix and implicated in the process of DNA and mRNA transcription [127]. Direct activation of protein kinase C by phorbol esters may bypass this "normal" activation sequence to raise ornithine decarboxylase activity via cAMP and induce DNA synthesis similar to its tumor-promoting capacity [34,69].

From this review of the T-lymphocyte subcellular events influenced by CsA, a number of facts can be determined, some of which may be applicable to the effect of CsA on macrophages. Cyclosporine did not appear to interfere with mitogen or alloantigen binding to T lymphocytes. The calcium flux secondary to membrane binding was similarly not influenced by CsA. Cyclosporine appeared to have specific saturable receptors, the majority of which appeared to be cytoplasmic in location. One receptor appears to be calmodulin, and other receptors must include "cyclophilin" and possibly protein kinase C until studies are performed to identify cyclophilin or demonstrate binding to protein kinase C. A block of calmodulin activity by CsA would prevent cGMP-activated events and promote cAMP events via protein kinase C or prostaglandin E_2 activation of adenyl cyclase, which would be unopposed. This blockade would prevent the "normal" signals to the nucleus to prepare for and initiate DNA and mRNA synthesis and cell division but may allow for escape secondary to phorbol esters or cAMP-induced generation of suppressor cells. Following activation of the appropriate cyclic nucleotides and enzymes necessary for mRNA, protein, and DNA synthesis, however, CsA at immunosuppressive, nontoxic levels would be ineffective to prevent cell proliferation or the elaboration of lymphokines and receptors necessary for normal T-cell response.

EFFECT OF CYCLOSPORINE ON THE IMMUNE RESPONSE TO TRANSPLANTATION ANTIGENS IN VIVO

The results from the in vitro experiments attempting to dissect out the effect of cyclosporine on T-lymphocyte subsets can be summarized as follows. (1) Cyclosporine appears to inhibit the activation of the precursor cytotoxic T lymphocyte in response to alloantigen stimulation, and CsA appeared to mediate a dose-dependent effect on the ability of the precursor cytotoxic T lymphocyte to acquire functional IL-2 responsiveness, presumably mediated through the inhibition of IL-2 receptor formation. (2) Cyclosporine effectively inhibited the production of lymphokines, especially interleukin-2, that would limit or prevent any clonal expansion of the activated cytotoxic T lymphocytes. (3) Cyclosporine will not inhibit the lytic activity of cytotoxic T cells, nor could CsA inhibit the proliferative response of primed lymphocytes to IL-2. (4) Suppressor T-cell activation was unaffected by cyclosporine as was the mechanisms accounting for maturation or amplification of this immunoregulatory subset. (5) Cyclosporine appeared to inhibit some aspects of macrophage function with respect to antigen presentation but failed to inhibit such macrophage functions as phagocytosis and chemotaxis.

Data from in vivo investigations have corroborated the in vitro findings on the ability of CsA to permit the generation of suppressor T lymphocytes in most instances while inhibiting graft rejection mechanisms. Tutschka et al. [131] showed that CsA led to the establishment of specific donor-to-host tolerance in rats grafted with allogeneic bone marrow. Further studies indicated that the specific tolerance in this bone marrow transplantation model was associated with the rapid development of a specific suppressor T-cell system capable of regulating MLR responses in vitro and could prevent GVHD in new hosts by adoptive transfer of splenocytes [133]. This was in contrast to the normal course of events in the rat model whereby antigen-nonspecific suppressor T cells appear with the abatement of graft-versus-host disease followed by maturation into an antigen-specific suppressor T-cell system, suggesting that CsA accelerated the appearance of the antigen-specific suppressor T cell [135]. Additional studies by Tutschka et al. [133] demonstrated the influence of the thymus on the generation of the tolerance-maintaining suppressor T cells in rats grafted with MHC-incompatible bone marrow and treated with cyclosporine to prevent GVHD. Thymectomized and sham-thymectomized animals showed evidence of GVHD, and suppressor T-cell function could not be demonstrated in the spleens of these animals. In contrast, the sham-thymectomized animals and the animals that were thymectomized and reconstituted with a thymus graft were specifically tolerant even after discontinuation of cyclosporine. Furthermore, specific suppressor cells were detected in the spleens of these animals. These studies suggested that cyclosporine permits the development of antigen-specific suppressor T cells rapidly, cells that maintain transplantation tolerance in the rat lymphohematopoietic chimera. The data also document the thymic requirement for the generation and amplification of these regulatory lymphoid cells in vivo. Similar studies documenting the presence of suppressor lymphocytes in cyclosporine-treated animals grafted with MHC-incompatible tissue have been reported by Hutchinson et al. [71,72]. Suppressor lymphocytes in rat cardiac allograft recipients treated with cyclosporine could be detected by adoptive transfer of splenocytes that prolong cardiac allografts in otherwise unmodified hosts. In addition, the response of spleen cells from the CsA-treated grafted rats in the mixed lymphocyte response was significantly decreased to donor lymphocytes but not against third-party lymphocytes, indicating specificity to this state of immunologic unresponsiveness. In this model, the suppressor T cells were sensitive to treatment with cyclophosphamide [82,83]. Administration of cyclophosphamide (50 mg/kg) and specifically sensitized spleen cells or thoracic duct lymphocytes into CsA-treated and heart-allografted rats resulted in rejection of the foreign heart tissue. Treatment of the animals with lower doses of cyclophosphamide and the sensitized cells did not abrogate the tolerant state. Furthermore, the tolerance-abrogating regimen of treatment with cyclophosphamide and sensitized spleen cells could be restored by addition of spleen cells from untreated CsA-induced tolerant animals. In contrast to the specificity of tolerance induction by CsA in these animal models, Nagao et al. [103] demonstrated a state of unresponsiveness induced by a short course of cyclosporin A utilizing accessory heart allografts in rats. Heart allografts in rats were performed, and a short course of CsA (14 days) was administered. Skin grafts from the heart donor or a third-party donor were performed at several different times after the heart transplantation and discontinuation of CsA therapy, and the fate of the skin and heart grafts were monitored sequentially. The results indicated that there appeared to be three phases of immunologic unresponsiveness in these animals. The first was a stable nonspecific immunosuppression in which skin grafts from both the third party and the donor were accepted early after discontinuation of CsA therapy. A second phase followed of weak, moderately specific immunosuppression in which skin grafts from the original donor were permanently accepted whereas skin grafts from the third-party animals were initially accepted but were eventually rejected. In the third phase, several weeks after CsA therapy was stopped, a strong stable donor-specific immunosuppression was observed in which only the skin graft from the heart donor and the donor heart were permanently accepted. Further studies by this group [146,148] failed to provide evidence for suppressor T cells in vitro, but the in vitro model may not be sensitive enough to detect such cells (see below). These results clearly suggested a phasic maturation of the suppressor T-lymphocyte system or at least the CsA-induced unresponsiveness. Comparable studies on a phase of persistant nonspecific suppression that occurs after a course of cyclosporine was reported by Dunn and colleagues [39,41] in rabbits. In their studies, animals receiving renal grafts and a short course of cyclosporine resulted in long-term allograft acceptance. This graft acceptance was not alloantigen specific since animals in this state can accept second kidney allografts from a new third-party donor without further treatment. Further studies by this group have shown that the state of persistant nonspecific immunosuppression after a course of cyclosporine did not require the initial presence of an allograft [40]. Rabbits treated with cyclosporine for 14 days and then grafted with renal tissue showed significantly enhanced survival of the graft. The results were somewhat contrary to the current thought in cyclosporine research, which assumed that the induction of unresponsiveness required challenge with antigen [61,74, 141]. However, these results may be relevant since it is possible that cyclosporine altered the immunologic status of the recipient by altering the function or maturation of thymic lymphocytes, which results in a situation allowing prolonged allograft survival (see below). In other studies of animals rendered tolerant to histoincompatible organ grafts by cyclosporine, the presence of suppressor cells could not be detected. White et al. [146] reported a failure to detect suppressor regulatory lymphoid cells in pigs tolerant to heart allografts incompatible for the antigens of the major histocompatability complex although these animals showed a decreased responsiveness to donor antigens in MLR. Studies by Norin et al. [105] utilizing lung allografts in dogs yielded similar results. Permanent graft acceptance could be achieved with limited CsA treatment. However, normal reactivity in vitro in MLR to donor antigens was maintained, but significantly reduced lymphocyte-mediated cytotoxicity was observed even after antigen rechallenge of lymphocytes in vitro [106]. Similar observations were initially described by Deeg et al. [33] in canine allogeneic marrow treated with CsA and methotrexate. Mixing experiments with cells from marrow donor and recipient failed to provide evidence for the presence of suppressor T cells in the MLR. However, a recent report by Deeg et al. [32] demonstrated that suppressor-T cells could be detected in canine bone marrow chimeras but only after enrichment on nylon wool, indicating that, at least in this model, suppressor cells were in numbers too low for detection in the usual MLR assay.

A more sensitive system for detection of specific suppressor cells appears to be adoptive transfer, as shown by Tutschka et al. [135]. They showed that, in long-term allogeneic marrow chimeras, antigen-specific suppressor T cells could only be demonstrated by adoptive transfer of splenocytes to new hosts or, in lieu of this maneuver, by giving irradiated lymphoid cells as an antigen rechallenge that raises the activity of numbers of suppressor cells to a level that can be detected in vitro. These data indicate the necessity of appropriate antigen to trigger the amplification of suppressor T cells or maintain adequate levels of suppressor T-cell function so that they can be detected in vitro. These results also implicate that antigen is a necessary requirement for the production and maintenance of antigen-specific suppressor T cells. In an elegant series of experiments by Yasumura and Kahan [149], kidney grafts could be prolonged by a pretransplant treatment of the recipient with donor antigen extract or a donor blood transfusion combined with a short course of cyclosporine. This effect was specific with regard to the source of donor antigen and the donor graft. Their studies also indicated that this preparative regimen prior to transplant accelerated the appearance of antigen-specific suppressor T-cell lymphocytes detectable in vitro. This is a novel approach that must be further pursued if we are to utilize cyclosporine in the most efficient manner in order to establish permanent allograft acceptance with minimal cyclosporine treatment of the recipient.

Taken together, these data clearly indicate that, in many systems, cyclosporine spares the activation of the suppressor T lymphocyte in vivo after grafting with MHC-mismatched tissues. Although the animal data in some experimental model systems suggest that CsA facilitates the induction of transplantation tolerance, permanent graft acceptance without continual cyclosporine therapy has not been achieved in humans or in all animal model systems. Even in such systems as the rabbit, where solid organ allografts such as kidney and heart are permanently accepted, CsA was not effective at producing permanent immunologic unresponsiveness to skin grafts. However, the skin graft was maintained as long as CsA therapy was continued; once CsA therapy was stopped, the skin graft was rejected within 20 days [49]. In the dog, renal and skin grafts remain functional as long as CsA therapy is continued but are rejected after discontinuation of CsA treatment [31]. This is in contrast to permanent acceptance of lung allografts in dogs after limited CsA treatment [105,106]. Comparable anomalies were observed in cynomologus monkeys with prolonged survived of orthotopic cardiac allografts after a 14-day course of CsA treatment, whereas renal allografts were rejected within 10 days after this course of therapy [29,101,116]. These data implicate the efficacy of CsA in preventing the mechanisms accounting for graft rejection while CsA therapy is maintained. However, the reasons for failure of tolerance induction in these systems is unknown. It may relate to the type and density of MHC antigens present on the graft relative to class I and/or class II antigen expression, the relative condition of the thymus (see below), or the pharmacokinetics of CsA administration especially early after grafting. Some potentially informative data regarding the failure of tolerance induction come from the results of Hess [56]. Sensitization of the cytotoxic T lymphocyte as assessed by the development of functional responsiveness to IL-2 can occur at cyclosporine levels of approximately 100 ng/ml. At these low levels, sensitization of the cytotoxic T lymphocyte can occur within 18-24 hr, suggesting that adequate and persistent levels of cyclosporine must be achieved early after allogeneic organ allografts to prevent sensitization of this effector mechanism. This hypothesis has some merit since the results of recent studies by Hess et al. [125] suggest that activated CTL are much less sensitive to the effects of regulatory suppressor cells than naive precursor cytotoxic T lymphocytes. Since CsA permits the activation of suppressor T cells, maximal effect should be achieved at levels of CsA that prevent activation of precursor cytotoxic T cells, thus allowing the development of the potential immunoregulation by suppressor T lymphocytes. Based on these findings, it seems important to establish appropriate dosage and pharmacologic monitoring of CsA levels that are effective in preventing sensitization of the cytotoxic T cell.

One anomalous reaction of CsA must be discussed since it may shed some light on the immunosuppressive action of cyclosporine. Glazier et al. have recently demonstrated that treatment of rats receiving syngeneic bone marrow transplants or autologous marrow reconstitution and treated with cyclosporine for 40 days resulted in the development of a clinical autoimmune syndrome characteristic of graft-versus-host disease 14-28 days after cessation of CsA therapy. The clinical and histologic features of this autoimmune syndrome were indistinguishable from graft-versus-host disease in allogeneic bone marrow transplant recipients [47]. Further studies by Glazier et al. revealed that the induction of the syngeneic GVHD syndrome induced by CsA could be adoptively transferred to naive rats with splenic T lymphocytes. More importantly, the induction of this autoimmune syndrome depended on the integrity of the thymus [46]. Shielding of the thymus during total-body irradiation completely prevented the development of this syngeneic GVHD syndrome, suggesting that the thymus was a critical component in the induction of this clinical autoimmune disorder. Based on the observation that cyclosporine spares the activation of antigen-nonspecific and specific suppressor T cells and the finding [4,119] that CsA decreases medullary thymocytes with an apparent predominance of cortical thymocytes (potential origin of suppressor T lymphocytes), they postulated that the clinical autoimmune disorder induced by cyclosporine in the syngeneic bone marrow transplant setting was the result of an immunologic imbalance favoring the suppressor T lymphocyte. The histologic destruction could have been mediated by release of soluble lymphokines by this T-cell subset. However, recent studies by Hess et al. [58] have shown that the development of the syngeneic graft-versus-host disease is associated with the development of cytotoxic T lymphocytes directed at class II major histocompatibility antigens. The cytotoxic T cell was not restricted by class I MHC antigens and was capable of lysing blast cells from several strains of rats. Cold target inhibition studies suggested that one effector cell was capable of lysing blast cells from the different rat strains that did not share any known class I or II MHC antigens. The effector cell either recognized a common class II determinant shared among many strains of rats (public epitope?) or was polyspecific with respect to "private" class II MHC determinants. The mechanism by which CsA led to syngeneic GVHD and allowed the development of the anti-Ia reactive T cells remains unknown although it may be related to the effect of CsA on thymic tissue. In recent studies by Cheney and Sprent [20] using a murine model of CsA-induced syngeneic GVHD, a striking decrease in overall thymic Ia expression was observed compared with control transplanted animals. The induction of anti-Ia cytotoxic T cells could have eliminated the cells bearing the class II antigens, or more likely, the anti-Ia cytotoxic T cells were generated in an environment of reduced thymic Ia expression. The result would be a failure of the T lymphocyte to recognize self Ia and become tolerant, with the subsequent induction of these Ia-specific cytotoxic T cells. It is tempting to speculate that CsA alters the educational process or accentuates a maturation failure of T lymphocytes in the thymus, allowing for the development of polyclonal or self anti-Ia reactive cells. This data raises important questions with regard to the nonspecific suppression observed after MHC-mismatched allograft transplantation and treatment with cyclosporine [39,40,103]. It is tempting to speculate that CsA leads to the induction of MHC class II-specific cytotoxic T lymphocytes, which would kill activated T cells expressing Ia responding to a foreign allograft. This effect would be related to the function and integrity of the thymus at the time of transplant, especially with regard to class II antigen expression and the action of CsA on thymic tissue. The striking effect of CsA therapy on medullary thymic tissue has been described in early studies by Ryffel et al. [119] and by Baldwin et al. [4] but has failed to generate much research in this area. The effect of CsA on the thymus may readily explain some of the nonspecific immunosuppressive effects of cyclosporine-induced graft acceptance at this level.

SUMMARY AND GENERAL COMMENTS

The available data from in vitro and in vivo investigations strongly suggest that CsA has a sparing effect on the activation and establishment of suppressor cell regulatory mechanisms while inhibiting cytotoxic T-lymphocyte generation in response to transplantation antigens. This imbalance between the regulatory T lymphocytes and cytotoxic effector cells induced by cyclosporine tips the balance toward transplantation tolerance, thus offering the transplantation biologist the ability to operationally direct the immune processes toward immunologic unresponsiveness. The mechanism whereby CsA allows for the induction of transplantation tolerance by creating a disequilibrium between the suppressor and cytotoxic T cells appears to be primarily directed at the level of the precursor cytotoxic T lymphocytes and the T-helper cell subset that secretes lymphokines that amplify the cytotoxic T-effector cell. Table 1 summarizes the CsA-sensitive phases in the activation of cytotoxic T lymphocytes and their amplification and those T-cell functions that are relatively CsA resistant. Cyclosporine not only reduces production of IL-2 and

TABLE 1 Summary of the Effect of CsA on the Cells Required for a Competent Allograft Response

Lymphocyte and/or monocyte subset	Function and/or response	Effectiveness of CsA[a]	Comments
Monocyte/macrophage	Phagocytosis/chemotaxis	Resistant	No effect on phagocytosis or chemotaxis
	Antigen presentation	Sensitive	Apparent abrogation of antigen presentation and production of IL-1
	Production of interleukin-1	Sensitive	
Cytotoxic T lymphocyte			
Precursor-"immature"	Activation after antigen challenge	Sensitive	Dose-dependent inhibition of the activation and maturation of the precursor cytotoxic T cell
	Response/maturation to cytotoxic differentiation factors	Sensitive/unknown	
	Development of receptors to interleukin-2	Sensitive	
	Acquisition of functional responsiveness to interleukin-2	Sensitive	
Activated-mature	Lysis of appropriate target	Resistant	Primed cytotoxic T cells capable of lytic function, which can be clonally amplified by IL-2
	Proliferative response to interleukin-2	Resistant	
Suppressor T lymphocytes			
Precursor-"immature"	Activation after antigen challenge	Resistant	CsA is unable to prevent suppressor T-lymphocyte activation or amplification; suppressor cell differentiation creates an immunologic imbalance between suppressor and cytotoxic effector mechanisms
	Development of receptors for interleukin-2 and factors	Resistant	

Activated-mature	Down-regulate proliferative response via control of interleukin-2 production	Resistant	No effect on suppressor T-cell function or response to soluble lymphokines
	Response to interleukin-2 and suppressor cell differentiation factors	Resistant	
Helper T lymphocytes			
Cytotoxic T cell-amplifier cells	Activation after antigen exposure	Sensitive	The T-helper cell component responsible for production of IL-2 and the subsequent clonal amplification of cytotoxic T cells is effectively inhibited by CsA
	Acquisition of receptors for interleukin-1 accentuating interleukin-2 production	Sensitive	
	Production of interleukin-2	Sensitive	
	Production of cytotoxic differentiation factors	Sensitive?/unknown	
	Development of receptors and functional responsiveness to interleukin-2	Sensitive	
Suppressor T cell-amplifier cells	Activation after antigen exposure	Resistant	The T-helper cell subset that amplifies suppressor T-cell function is relatively resistant to CsA accounting for normal production of soluble factors that mature the suppressor T cell
	Acquisition of receptors for interleukin-1 accentuating production of soluble factors for suppressor T cells?	Resistant?/unknown	
	Production of suppressor cell differentiation factors	Resistant	
	Development of receptors and functional responsiveness to interleukin-2	Resistant	

[a]Resistance or sensitivity to CsA are relative terms, since at high doses (unphysiologic, $>20\ \mu g/ml$) of CsA, most cell functions can be inhibited.

other lymphokines but also inhibits the precursor cytotoxic effector lymphocytes from acquiring the ability to respond to IL-2 in a dose-dependent fashion. Both events are required for the proliferation and maturation of cytotoxic T lymphocytes [30,87,138]. It seems likely, therefore, that the precursor cytotoxic T cell fails to mature and acquire lytic function in the presence of CsA. In contrast, the activation of suppressor T lymphocytes and the apparent amplification mechanisms for suppressor T cells remains unaffected by this novel immunosuppressive agent.

The precise action of cyclosporine in inhibiting maturation of cytolytic effector cells and the inhibition of interleukin-2 production remains unresolved. Recent studies using molecular biology techniques suggest that cyclosporine may inhibit the DNA-RNA transcriptional process required for interleukin-2 production. However, the effect of cyclosporine on the induction of the receptor for IL-2 on the various T-lymphocyte subsets remains controversial. This may be due to the systems utilized for assessing the effect of CsA on IL-2 receptor formation or in fact may represent a subtle difference in the response of lymphocytes to mitogen and alloantigen stimulation. It is known that the induction of cytotoxic T lymphocytes requires several steps, with the production of different lymphokines, including IL-2 and a cytotoxic T-cell differentiation factor, as well as antigen processing and communication between macrophages and/or T initiator lymphocytes. In addition, the effect of CsA on macrophages remains to be fully characterized. These questions still remain unresolved and will require further studies.

On the molecular level, further studies will certainly be informative with regard to the transcription of genes activated upon exposure of T lymphocytes to specific antigen and the role of cyclosporine binding to cell proteins, such as calmodulin, in the reactivation of lymphocytes. It will be important to determine if CsA-resistant cells are activated in a calmodulin-independent fashion whereas CsA-sensitive T cells are totally dependent on calmodulin activity for their activation. Similarly, the role and activity of cyclophilin must be identified.

Although these studies will be clearly important in determining the effect of cyclosporine at the subcellular and cellular level of T-cell activation, the effect of cyclosporine at the level of the entire animal must be further pursued, especially in studies regarding the effect of CsA on the thymus.

Although many questions regarding the mechanism of action of cyclosporine have not been answered, current studies have clarified many of the effects of cyclosporine on the activation of T lymphocytes. Furthermore, the full therapeutic potential of cyclosporine can only be realized when its precise mechanism of action at the subcellular and cellular level as well as at the level of the thymus have been clearly defined. Regardless, the studies to date suggest that CsA is not only a unique effective immunosuppressive agent offering great potential for the control of transplant rejection, but is also a valuable tool in which to probe mechanisms of tolerance induction and suppressor, helper, and cytotoxic T-cell activation.

ACKNOWLEDGMENTS

Supported in part by grants CA 15396 and AI 20990 from the National Institutes of Health, ACS Grant IM 398, and a gift from the Harley W. Howell Foundation. The authors acknowledge the excellent secretarial assistance of Ms. Lisa Alai and the technical assistance of Ms. Pam Engel and Mr. Louis Horwitz.

REFERENCES

1. Abb, J., Abb, H., and Reinhardt, F. Effect of cyclosporin A on the production of interferon by human peripheral blood leukocytes in vitro. *Antiviral Res.* 2:361, 1982.
2. Andrus, L., and Lafferty, K. J. Inhibition of T-cell activity by cyclosporin A. *Scand. J. Immunol.* 15:449, 1981.
3. Bachvaroff, R. J., Miller, F., and Rapaport, F. T. The role of calmodulin in the regulation of human lymphocyte activation. *Cell. Immunol.* 85:135, 1984.
4. Baldwin, W. M., Hutchinson, I. F., Meijer, J. L. M., and Tilney, N. L. Immune responses to organ allografts. III. Marked decrease in medullary thymocytes and splenic T lymphocytes after cyclosporin A treatment. *Transplantation* 31:117, 1981.
5. Belanger, R., Hess, A. D., Tutschka, P. J., and Santos, G. W. The effect of cyclosporine on the rat mixed lymphocyte reaction. *Transplantation* In press, 1985.
6. Bendtzen, K., and Dinarello, C. A. Mechanism of action of cyclosporin A: Effect on T-cell binding of interleukin 1 and antagonizing effect of insulin. *Scand. J. Immunol.* 20:43, 1984.
7. Bendtzen, K., and Petersen, J. Effects of cyclosporin A (CyA) and methylprednisolone (MP) on the immune response. I. T-cell-activating factor abrogates CyA- but not MP-induced lymphokine production. *Immunol. Lett.* 5:79, 1982.
8. Bendtzen, K., Petersen, J., and Soeberg, B. Effects of cyclosporin A (CyA) and methylprednisolone (MP) on the immune response. II. Further studies of the monocyte-T cell interactions leading to lymphokine production. *Acta Pathol. Microbiol. Immunol. Scand.* 91:159, 1983.
9. Birx, D. L., Berger, M., and Fleisher, T. A. The interference of T cell activation by calcium channel blocking agents. *J. Immunol.* 133:2904, 1984.
10. Block, L. H., Siegenthaler, W., and Drew, J. Inhibition of mitogen-induced lymphokine production by cyclosporin A. *Klin. Wochenschr.* 58:739, 1980.
11. Block, L. H., Sutter, P. M., and Mihatsch, M. J. Cyclosporin A: Pharmacologic activity on the immune system and effects in clinical transplantation. *Klin. Wochenschr.* 61:1053, 1983.
12. Borel, J. F. Comparative study of in vitro and in vivo drug effects on cell-mediated cytotoxicity. *Immunology* 31:631, 1976.
13. Borel, J. F. Cyclosporin A-present experimental status. *Transplant. Proc.* 13:344, 1981.
14. Borel, J. F., Feurer, C., Gubler, H. U., and Stahelin, H. Biological effects of cyclosporin A: A new antilymphocytic agent. *Agents Actions* 6:468, 1976.
15. Borel, J. F., Feurer, C., Magnee, C., and Stahelin, H. Effects of the new anti-lymphocyte pepetide cyclosporin A in animals. *Immunology* 32:1017, 1977.
16. Britton, S., and Palacios, R. Cyclosporin A—usefulness, risks, and mechanism of action. *Immunol. Rev.* 65:5, 1982.
17. Bunjes, D., Hardt, C., Rollinghoff, M., and Wagner, H. Cyclosporin A mediates immunosuppression of primary cytotoxic T cell responses by impairing the release of interleukin 1 and interleukin 2. *Eur. J. Immunol.* 8:657, 1981.
18. Burkhardt, J. J., and Guggenheim, B. Cyclosporin A: In vivo and in vitro suppression of rat T-lymphocyte function. *Immunology* 36:753, 1979.
19. Calne, R. Y., White, D. J. C., Roller, K., Smith, D. P., and Herbertson, B. M. Prolonged survival of pig orthotopic heart grafts treated with cyclosporin A. *Lancet* 1:1183, 1978.
20. Cheney, R. T., and Sprent, J. Capacity of cyclosporine to induce autograft-versus-host disease and impair intrathymic T cell differentiation. *Transplant. Proc.* 17:528, 1985.
21. Cheung, R. K., Grinstein, S., and Gelfand, E. W. Permissive role of calcium in the in-

hibition of T cell mitogenesis by calmodulin antagonists. *J. Immunol.* 131:2291, 1983.

22. Coffey, R. G., Hadden, E. M., and Hadden, J. W. Evidence for cyclic GMP and calcium mediation of lymphocyte activation by mitogens. *J. Immunol.* 119:1387, 1977.
23. Cohen, D. J., Loertscher, R., Rubin, M., Tilney, N. L., Carpenter, C. B., and Strom, T. B. Cyclosporine: A new immunosuppressive agent for organ transplantation. *Ann. Intern. Med.* 101:667, 1984.
24. Colombani, P. M., Donnenberg, A. D., Robb, A., and Hess, A. D. Use of T lymphocyte clones to analyze cyclosporine binding. *Transplant. Proc.* 17:1413, 1985.
25. Colombani, P. M., Robb, A., and Hess, A. D. Cyclosporin A binding to calmodulin: A possible site of action on T-lymphocytes. *Science* 228:337, 1985.
26. Converse, P. J., and Hess, A. D. The effect of cyclosporine and interleukin 2 on the restoration of in vitro immune responses to cytomegalovirus. *Scand. J. Immunol.* In press, 1985.
27. Converse, P. J., Hess, A. D., Tutschka, P. J., and Santos, G. W. Effect of cyclosporine on the response of normal human lymphocytes to cytomegalovirus in vitro. *Infect. Immun.* 41:1226, 1983.
28. Cook, R. M. Activity of cyclosporin A in experimental influenza virus infection in mice. *Agents Actions* 13:98, 1983.
29. Cosimi, A. B., Shield, C. F., Peters, C., Burton, R. C., Scott, G., and Russell, P. S. Prolongation of allograft survival by cyclosporin A. *Surg. Form* 30:287, 1978.
30. Davidson, W. F. Cellular requirements for the induction of cytotoxic T cells in vitro. *Immunol. Rev.* 35:263, 1977.
31. Deeg, H. J., Storb, R., Gerhard-Miller, L., Shulman, H. M., Weiden, P. L., and Thomas, E. D. Cyclosporin A, a powerful immunosuppressant in vivo and in vitro in the dog, fails to induce tolerance. *Transplantation* 29:230, 1980.
32. Deeg, H. J., Storb, R., Atkinson, K., Weiden, P. L., Severns, E., and Thomas, E. D. Long-term survival of dogs given unrelated DLA nonidentical marrow grafts and cyclosporin A (CyA) and methotrexate (MTX)—tolerance mediated by a nylon wool adherent suppressor cell. *Exp. Hematol.* 9:94, 1981.
33. Deeg, H. J., Storb, R., Weiden, P. L., Graham, T., Atkinson, K., and Thomas, E. D. Cyclosporin-A: Effect on marrow engraftment and graft-versus-host disease in dogs. *Transplant. Proc.* 13:402, 1981.
34. Depper, J. M., et al. Regulation of interleukin-2 receptor expression: Effects of porbol diester, phospholipase C and reexposure to lectin or antigen. *J. Immunol.* 133:3054, 1984.
35. Dongworth, A. W., and Klaus, G. G. B. Effects of cyclosporin on the immune system of the mouse. I. Evidence for a direct selective effect of cyclosporin A on B cells responding to anti-immunoglobulin antibodies. *Eur. J. Immunol.* 12:1018, 1982.
36. Dos Reis, G. A., and Shevach, E. M. Effect of cyclosporin A on T cell function in vitro: The mechanism of suppression of T cell proliferation depends on the nature of the T cell stimulus as well as the differentiation state of the responding T cell. *J. Immunol.* 129:2360, 1982.
37. Dos Reis, G. A., and Shevach, E. M. Cyclosporin A treated guinea pigs responder cells secrete a genetically restricted factor that suppresses the mixed leukocyte reaction. *J. Clin. Invest.* 71:165, 1983.
38. Drebin, et al. Characterization of ultraviolet radiation induced impairment of antigen-presenting cell at the cellular and molecular levels. In *The Effect of Radiation on the Immune System,* J. A. Parrish, ed. Johnson and Johnson, 1983.
39. Dunn, D. C. The specificity of post cyclosporin "tolerance." *Transplant. Proc.* 13: 383, 1981.

40. Dunn, D. C., White, D. J. G., and Herbertson, B. M. Persistent non-specific immunosuppression after a course of cyclosporin A. *Transplantation* 29:349, 1980.
41. Dunn, D. C., White, D. J. F., Herbertson, B. M., and Wade, J. Prolongation of kidney survival during and after cyclosporin A therapy *Transplantation* 37:359, 1979.
42. Elliott, J. F., Lin, Y., Mizel, S. B., Bleackley, R. C., Harnich, D. G., and Paetkau, V. Induction of interleukin 2 messenger RNA inhibited by cyclosporin A. *Science* 226: 1439, 1984.
43. Esa, A. H., Converse, P. C., and Hess, A. D. Cyclosporin inhibits antigen presentation by human monocytes in vitro. Submitted for publication, 1985.
44. Fidelius, R. K., Laughter, A. H., and Twomey, J. J. The role of mitogens and lymphokines in the induction of ornithine decarboxylase (ODC) in T lymphocytes. *J. Immunol.* 132:1462, 1984.
45. Fidelius, R. K., Laughter, A. H., Twomey, J. J., Taffet, S. M., and Haddox, M. K. The effect of cyclosporine on ornithine decarboxylase induction with mitogens, antigens, and lymphokines. *Transplantation* 37:383, 1984.
46. Glazier, A., Tutschka, P. J., and Farmer, E. R. Studies on the immunobiology of syngeneic and autologous graft-versus-host disease in cyclosporine treated rats. *Transplant. Proc.* 15:3035, 1983.
47. Glazier, A., Tutschka, P. J., Farmer, E. R., and Santos, G. W. Graft-versus-host disease in cyclosporin A treated rats after syngeneic and autologous bone marrow reconstitution. *J. Exp. Med.* 158:1, 1983.
48. Granelli-Piperno, A., Inaba, K., and Steinman, R. Stimulation of lymphokine release from T lymphoblasts. Requirement for mRNA synthesis and inhibition by cyclosporin A. *J. Exp. Med.* 160:1792, 1984.
49. Gratwohl, A., Forster, I., and Speck, B. Skin grafts in rabbits with cyclosporin A. Absence of induction of tolerance and untoward side effects. *Transplantation* 31:436, 1981.
50. Green, C. L., and Allison, A. C. Extensive prolongation of rabbit kidney allograft survival after short-term cyclosporin A treatment. *Lancet* 1:1182, 1978.
51. Gordon, M. Y., and Singer, J. W. Selective effects of cyclosporin A on colony-forming lymphoid and myeloid cells in man. *Nature* 279:433, 1979.
52. Hadden, J. W., Coffey, R. G., Ananthakrishnan, R., and Hadden, E. M. Cyclic nucleotides and calcium in lymphocyte regulation and activation. *Ann. N.Y. Acad. Sci.* 216: 240, 1980.
53. Handschumacher, R. E., Harding, M. W., Rice, J., and Drugge, R. J. Cyclophilin: A specific cytosolic binding protein for cyclosporin A. *Science* 226:544, 1984.
54. Hellin, H. J., and Edington, T. S. Cyclosporin A regulates monocyte/macrophage effector functions by affecting instructor T cells: Inhibition of monocyte procoagulant response to allogeneic stimulation. *J. Immunol.* 132:1074, 1984.
55. Hellman, A., and Goldman, J. M. Effects of cyclosporin A on human granulopoiesis in vitro. *Transplantation* 30:380, 1980.
56. Hess, A. D. Effect of interleukin 2 on the immunosuppressive action of cyclosporine. *Transplantation* 39:62, 1985.
57. Hess, A. D., Colombani, P. M., Donnenberg, A. D., Fischer, A. C., and Ryffel, B. Binding of dansylated cyclosporine discriminates functional T lymphocyte subsets. *Transplant. Proc.* 17(1):1419, 1985.
58. Hess, A. D., Horwitz, L., Beschorner, W. E., and Santos, G. W. Development of graft-vs-host disease-like syndrome in cyclosporine treated rats after syngeneic bone marrow transplantation. I. Development of cytotoxic T lymphocytes with apparent polyclonal anti-Ia specificity including autoreactivity. *J. Exp. Med.* 161:718, 1985.
59. Hess, A. D., Donnenberg, A. D., Engel, P., Tutshcka, P. J., and Santos, G. W. Suppressor-cell amplification circuitry in cyclosporine-treated MLR cultures. *Transplant. Proc.* 15:2343, 1983.

60. Hess, A. D., Donnenberg, A. D., Tutschka, P. J., and Santos, G. W. Effect of cyclosporin A on human lymphocyte responses in vitro. V. Analysis of responding T lymphocytes subpopulations in primary MLR with monoclonal antibodies. *J. Immunol.* 130:717, 1983.
61. Hess, A. D., and Tutschka, P. J. Effects of cyclosporine A on human lymphocyte responses in vitro. I. CsA allows for the expression of alloantigen-activated suppressor cells while preferentially inhibiting the induction of cytolytic effector lymphocytes in MLR. *J. Immunol.* 124:2601, 1980.
62. Hess, A. D., Tutschka, P. J., Pu, Z., and Santos, G. W. Effect of cyclosporin A on human lymphocyte responses in vitro. IV. Production of T cell stimulatory growth factors and development of responsiveness to these growth factors in CsA-treated primary MLR cultures. *J. Immunol.* 128:360, 1982.
63. Hess, A. D., Tuschka, P. J., and Santos, G. W. Effect of cyclosporin A on human lymphocyte responses in vitro. II. Induction of specific alloantigen unresponsiveness mediated by a nylon wool adherent suppressor cell. *J. Immunol.* 126:961, 1981.
64. Hess, A. D., Tutshcka, P. J., and Santos, G. W. In vitro activation of human suppressor cells: Relative quantitation and specificity of suppressor cells generated in primary and secondary mixed lymphocyte cultures. *Exp. Hematol.* 9:415, 1981.
65. Hess, A. D., Tutschka, P. J., and Santos, G. W. Effect of cyclosporin on human lymphocyte response in vitro. III. CsA inhibits the production of T lymphocyte growth factors in secondary mixed lymphocyte responses but does not inhibit the response of primed lymphocytes to TCFG. *J. Immunol.* 128:355, 1982.
66. Hess, A. D., Tutschka, P. J., and Santos, G. W. The effect of cyclosporin a on T-lymphocyte subpopulations. In *Cyclosporin A,* D. J. G. White, ed. Elsevier Biomedical Press, Amsterdam, 1982, p. 209.
67. Hess, A. D., Tutschka, P. J., and Santos, G. W. Cyclosporine induced tolerance: Mechanism of maintaining specific immunologic unresponsiveness. *Transplant. Proc.* 15:539, 1983.
68. Hess, A. D., Tutschka, P. J., and Santos, G. W. Effect of cyclosporine on the induction of cytotoxic T lymphocytes: Role of interleukin 1 and interleukin 2. *Transplant. Proc.* 15:2248, 1983.
69. Hirano, T., Fujimoto, K., Teranishi, T., Nishino, N., Omoue, K., Maeda, S., and Shimada, K. Phorbol ester increases the level of interleukin-2 mRNA in mitogen-stimulated human lymphocytes. *J. Immunol.* 132:2165-2167, 1984.
70. Hutchings, P. A., Cooke, A., and Gunn, H. C. Murine T cell suppression demonstrable in the absence of cytotoxicity and the effect of cyclosporin A on this system. *J. Immunol.* 130:1071, 1983.
71. Hutchinson, I. F., Shadur, C. A., Duarte, J. S. A., Strom, T. B., and Tilney, N. L. Cyclosporin A spares selectively lymphocytes with donor-specific suppressor characteristics. *Transplantation* 32:210, 1981.
72. Hutchinson, I. F., Shadur, C. A., Baldwin, W. M., Strom, T. B., and Tilney, N. L. Mechanisms of cardiac allograft prolongation by cyclosporin A. *Transplant. Proc.* 13: 412, 1981.
73. Kalman, V. K., and Klimpel, G. R. Cyclosporin A inhibits the production of gamma interferon (IFN) but does not inhibit production of virus induced IFN. *Cell. Immunol.* 78:122, 1983.
74. Kasahara, K., White, D. J. G., and Calne, R. Y. Antigen dependence of cyclosporin A induced allograft response. *Transplantation* 34:216, 1982.
75. Kay, J. E., Benzie, C. R., and Borghetti, A. F. Effect of cyclosporin A on lymphocyte activation by the calcium ionophore A23187. *Immunology* 50:441, 1983.
76. Kay, J. E., and Benzie, C. R. Effects of cyclosporin A on the metabolism of unstimulated and mitogen activated lymphocytes. *Immunology* 49:153, 1983.

77. Klee, C. B., and Vanaman, T. C. Calmodulin. *Adv. Protein Chem.* 35:213-321, 1982.
78. Klimpel, G. R., Byus, C. V., Russell, D. H., and Lucas, D. O. Cyclic AMP-dependent protein kinase activation and the induction of ornithine decarboxylase during lymphocyte mitogenesis. *J. Immunol.* 123:817, 1979.
79. Koponen, M., Grieder, A., and Loor, F. The effects of cyclosporine on the cell cycle of T-lymphocyte cell lines. *Exp. Cell Res.* 140:237-250, 1982.
80. Koponen, M., and Loor, F. T cell lines as a tool to study the mechanism of action of cyclosporine. In *Transplantation and Clinical Immunology,* Vol. 13. Elsevier-North Holland, New York, 1982, p. 7.
81. Kunkl, A., and Klaus, G. G. B. Selective effects of cyclosporine A on functional B cell subsets in the mouse. *J. Immunol.* 125:2526, 1980.
82. Kupiec-Weglinski, J. W., Lear, P. A., Strom, T. B., and Tilney, N. L. Population of cyclophosphamide-sensitive T supprssor cells maintain cyclosporine-induced allograft survival. *Transplant. Proc.* 15:2357, 1983.
83. Kupiec-Weglinski, J. W., Filho, M. A., Strom, T. B., and Tilney, N. L. Sparing of suppressor cells: A critical action of cyclosporine. *Transplantation* 38:97, 1984.
84. Kurtz, J. B., and Homan, W. P. Murine cytomegalovirus infection and cyclosporin A. *Transplantation* 34:215, 1982.
85. Lafferty, K. J., Borel, J. F., and Hodgkin, P. Cyclosporine-A (CsA): Models for the mechanism of action. *Transplant. Proc.* 15:2242, 1983.
86. Larsson, E. L. Cyclosporin A and dexamethasone suppress T cell responses by selectively acting at distinct sites of the triggering process. *J. Immunol.* 124:2828, 1980.
87. Larsson, E. L., Coutinho, A., and Martinez, C. A suggested mechanism for T lymphocyte activation: Implications on the acquisition of functional reactivities. *Immunol. Rev.* 51:61, 1980.
88. Laupacis, A., Keown, P. A., Ulan, R. A., McKenzie, N., and Stiller, C. R. Cyclosporin A: A powerful immunosuppressant. *Can. Med. Assoc.* 126:1041, 1982.
89. Leapman, S. B., Filo, R. S., Smith, E. J., and Smith, P. G. In vitro effects of cyclosporin A on lymphocyte subpopulations. I. Suppressor cell sparing by cyclosporin A. *Transplantation* 30:404, 1980.
90. Legrue, S. J., Friedman, A. W., and Kahan, B. D. Lack of evidence for a cyclosporine receptor on human lymphocyte membranes. *Transplant. Proc.* 15:2259, 1983.
91. Legrue, S. J., Friedman, A. W., and Kahan, B. D. Binding of cyclosporine by human lymphocytes and phospholipid vesicles. *J. Immunol.* 131:712, 1983.
92. Lichtman, A. H., Segal, G. B., and Lichtman, M. A. The role of calcium in lymphocyte proliferation (an interpretive review). *Blood* 61:413, 1983.
93. Lillehoj, H. S., Malek, T. R., and Shevach, E. M. Differential effect of cyclosporin A on the expression of T and B lymphocyte activation antigens. *J. Immunol.* 133:244, 1984.
94. Lum, C. T., Wanner, F. J., Tilberg, A. F., and Robertson, C. A. Cyclosporine-induced adenosine triphosphate depletion in murine T and B lymphocytes. *Surgery* 96:256, 1984.
95. Means, A. R., Lagace, L., Guerrieo, V., and Chafouleas, J. G. Calmodulin as a mediator of hormone action and cell regulation. *J. Cell. Biochem.* 20:317, 1982.
96. Merker, M. M., and Handschumacher, R. E. Uptake and nature of the intracellular binding of cyclosporin A in a murine thymoma cell line BN5147. *J. Immunol.* 132:3064, 1984.
97. Metcalfe, S. Cyclosporine does not prevent cytoplasmic calcium changes associated with lymphocyte activation. *Transplantation* 38:161, 1984.
98. Miyawaki, T., Yachie, A., Ohzeki, S., Nagaoki, T., and Taniguchi, N. Cyclosporin A does not prevent expression of TAC antigen, a probable TCGF receptor molecule on mitogen stimulated human T cells. *J. Immunol.* 130:2737, 1983.

99. Mizel, S. B. Interleukin-1 and T cell activation. *Immunol. Rev.* 63:51, 1982.
100. Mohagheghpour, N., Benike, C. J., Kansas, G., Bieber, C., and Engleman, E. G. Activation of antigen-specific suppressor T cells in the presence of cyclosporin requires interactions between T cells of inducer and suppressor lineage. *J. Clin. Invest.* 71: 165, 1983.
101. Morris, P. J. Cyclosporin A. *Transplantation* 32:349, 1981.
102. Muraguchi, A., Butler, J. L., Kehrl, J. N., Falkoff, R. J. M., and Fauci, A. S. Selective suppression of an early step in human B cell activation by cyclosporin A. *J. Exp. Med.* 158:690, 1983.
103. Nagao, T., White, D. J. G., and Calne, R. Y. Kinetics of unresponsiveness induced by a short course of cyclosporin A. *Transplantation* 33:31, 1982.
104. Nishizuka, Y. The role of protein kinase C in cell surface signal transduction and tumour promotion. *Nature* 308:693, 1984.
105. Norin, A. J., Emeson, E. E., Kamholz, S. L., Pinsker, K. L., Montefusco, C. M., Matas, A. J., and Veith, F. J. Cyclosporin A as the initial immunosuppressive agent for canine lung transplantation. *Transplantation* 34:372, 1982.
106. Norin, A. J., Emeson, E. E., Pinsker, K. L., Kamholz, S. L., and Veith, F. J. Studies with T cells from long-term surviving canine lung allograft recipients: Reduced lymphocyte-mediated cytotoxicity but not reduced mixed lymphocyte reactivity. *Transplant. Proc.* 15:2979, 1983.
107. Palacios, R. Cyclosporin A abrogates proliferation of T cells and generation of suppressor and cytotoxic T-cell function induced by Epstein-Barr Virus. *Immunobiology* 160:321, 1981.
108. Palacios, R. Conconavalin A triggers T lymphocytes by directly interacting with their receptors for activation. *J. Immunol.* 128:337, 1982.
109. Palacios, R. Mechanism of T cell activation. Role and functional relationship of HLA-DR antigen and interleukins. *Immunol. Rev.* 63:73, 1982.
110. Palacios, R., and Moller, G. Cyclosporin A blocks receptors for HLA-DR antigens on T cells. *Nature* 290:792, 1981.
111. Parker, C. W. Role of cyclic nucleotides in regulating lymphocytes. *Ann. N.Y. Acad. Sci.* 332:255, 1979.
112. Petcher, T. J., Weber, H. P., and Ruegger, A. Crystal and molecular structure of an iodo-derivative of the cyclic undecapeptide cyclosprin. *Helv. Chim. Acta* 59:1480, 1976.
113. Powles, R. L., and Morgenstein, G. R. Allogeneic bone marrow transplantation using mismatched family donors. In *Cyclosporin A,* D. J. G. White, ed. Elsevier Biomedical Press, Amsterdam, 1982, p. 539.
114. Redelman, D., Bluestein, H. G., Cohen, A. H., Depper, J. M., and Warmsley, S. Deoxyadenosine (AdR) inhibition of newly activated lymphocytes blockade at the G_0-G_1 interface. *J. Immunol.* 132:2030-2038, 1984.
115. Reem, G. H., Cook, L. A., and Vilck, J. Gamma interferon synthesis by human thymocytes and T lymphocytes by cyclosporin A. *Science* 221:63, 1983.
116. Reitz, B. A., Bieber, C. P., Raney, A. A., Pennock, J. L., Jamieson, S. W., Oyer, P. E., and Stinson, E. B. Orthotopic heart and combined heart and lung transplantation with cyclosporin A immune suppression. *Transplant. Proc.* 13:393, 1981.
117. Rich, S., Carpino, M. R., and Arhelger, C. Suppressor T cell growth and differentiation: Identification of a cofactor required for suppressor T cell function and distinct from interleukin 2. *J. Exp. Med.* 159:1473, 1984.
118. Ruegger, A., Kuhn, M., Lichti, H., Loosli, H-R., Huguenin, R., Quiquerez, C., and von Wartburg, A. Cyclosporin A, ein immunosuppressio wirksamer peptidmetabolit aus *Trichoderma polysporium* (Link ex Pers). *Rafai. Helv. Chim. Acta* 59:1075, 1976.

119. Ryffel, B., Deyssenroth, and Borel, J. F. Cyclosporin A: Effects on the mouse thymus. *Agents Actions* 11:373, 1981.
120. Ryffel, B., Willard-Gallo, K. E., Tammi, K., and Loken, M. R. Quantitative fluorescence analysis of cyclosporine binding to human leukocytes. *Transplantation* 37: 276, 1984.
121. Ryffel, B., Gotz, U., and Heuberger, B. Cyclosporin receptors on human lymphocytes. *J. Immunol.* 129:1978, 1982.
122. Ryffel, B., Henning, C. B., and Huberman, E. Differentiation of human T lymphoid leukemia cells into cells that have a suppressor phenotype is induced by PMA. *Proc. Natl. Acad. Sci. USA* 79(12):7336, 1982.
123. Ryffel, B., Tammi, K., Greider, A., and Hess, A. D. Effects of cyclosporine on human T cell activation. *Transplant. Proc.* 17:1268, 1985.
124. Schulak, J. A., Monson, D., Shelby, J., and Carry, R. J. Abrogation of second-set rejection with cyclosporine. *Transplantation* 36:289, 1983.
125. Schwartz, A., Sutton, S. L., and Gershon, R. K. Regulation of in vitro cytotoxic T lymphocyte generation. I. Evidence that killer cell precursors differentiate to effector cells in two steps. *J. Exp. Med.* 155:783, 1982.
126. Shidani, B., Colle, J. H., Motta, I., and Trufta-Bachi, P. Effect of cyclosporin on the induction and activation of B memory cells by thymus-independent antigens in mice. *Eur. J. Immunol.* 13:359, 1983.
127. Simmen, R. C., Dunbar, B. S., Guerriers, Y., Chafoulea, J. G., Clark, J. H., and Means, A. R. Estrogen stimulates the transient association of calmodulin and myosin kinase with the chicken liver nuclear light chain matrix. *J. Cell Biol.* 99:588, 1984.
128. Thomson, A. W., Moon, D. K., and Nelson, D. S. Suppression of delayed type hypersensitivity reactions and lymphokine production by cyclosporin A in the mouse. *Clin. Exp. Immunol.* 52:599, 1983.
129. Tosato, G., Pike, S. E., Koski, I. R., and Blaese, R. M. Selective inhibition of immunoregulatory cell functions by cyclosporin A. *J. Immunol.* 128:1986.
130. Tutschka, P. J. Cyclosporin A–a new outlook for immunosuppression in clinical transplantation. *Blut* 39:81, 1979.
131. Tutschka, P. J., Beschorner, W. E., Allison, A. C., Burns, W. H., and Santos, G. W. Use of cyclosporin A in allogeneic bone marrow transplantation (BMT) in the rat. *Nature* 280:5718, 1979.
132. Tutschka, P. J., Beschorner, W. E., and Hess, A. D. Use of cyclosporin A (CsA) to prevent graft-versus-host disease (GVHD) in a rat model of allogeneic marrow transplantation. *Blut.* (*Suppl.*) 25:241, 1980.
133. Tutschka, P. J., Hess, A. D., Beschorner, W. E., Korbling, M., and Santos, G. W. Cyclosporin A in bone marrow transplantation–Baltimore experience in preclinical studies. In *Experimental Hematology Today,* F. S. Baum and G. D. Ledney, eds. Springer-Verlag, New York, 1981, p. 99.
134. Tutschka, P. J., Hess, A. D., Beschorner, W. E., and Santos, G. W. Cyclosporin A in allogeneic bone marrow transplantation: Preclinical and clinical studies. In *Cyclosporin A,* D. J. G. White, ed. Elsevier Biomedical Press, Amsterdam, 1982, p. 519.
135. Tutschka, P. J., Ping Ki, Beschorner, W. E., Hess, A. D., and Santos, G. W. Suppressor cells in transplantation tolerance. II. Maturation of suppressor cells in the bone marrow chimera. *Transplantation* 32:321, 1985.
136. Unanue, E. R., Beller, D. I., Lu, C. Y., and Allen, P. A. Antigen presentation: Comments on its regulation and mechanism. *J. Immunol.* 132:1, 1984.
137. Uyemura, K., Dixon, J. F. P., and Parker, J. W. Inhibitory effect of cyclosporine on adherent cells in the oxidation-induced lymphocyte mitogenesis. *Transplant. Proc.* 15:2376, 1983.

138. Von Boehmer, N., Hengartner, H., Nabholz, M., Lernhardt, W., Schreier, M. N., and Haas, W. Fine specificity of a continuously growing killer cell clone specific for H-Y antigen. *Eur. J. Immunol.* 9:592, 1979.
139. Wagner, H. Cyclosporin A: Mechanism of action. *Transplant. Proc.* 15:523, 1983.
140. Wagner, H., Hardt, C., Rouse, B., Rollinghoff, M., Scheurich, P., and Pfizermaier, F. Dissection of the proliferative and differentiative signals controlling murine cytotoxic T lymphocyte responses. *J. Exp. Med.* 155:1876, 1982.
141. Wang, B. S., Heacock, E. H., Collins, K. H., Hutchinson, I. F., Tilney, N. L., and Mannick, J. A. Suppressive effects of cyclosporin A on the induction of alloreactivity in vitro and in vivo. *J. Immunol.* 127:89, 1981.
142. Wang, B. S., Zheng, C., Heacock, E. H., Tilney, N. L., Strom, T. B., and Mannick, J. A. Inhibition of the production of a soluble helper mediator by cyclosporin A results in the failure to generate alloreactive cytolytic cells in mixed-lymphocyte culture. *Clin. Immunol. Immunopathol.* 27:160, 1983.
143. Weisinger, D., and Borel, J. F. Studies on the mechanism of action of cyclosporine A. *Immunobiology* 156:454, 1979.
144. Whisler, R. L., Lindsey, J. A., Proctor, K. V. W., Morisaki, N., and Cornwell, D. G. Characteristics of cyclosporine induction of increased prostaglandin levels from human peripheral blood monocytes. *Transplantation* 38:377, 1984.
145. White, D. J. G. Cyclosporin A: Clinical pharmacology and therapeutic potential. *Drugs* 24:322, 1982.
146. White, D. J. G., Calne, R. Y., and Plumb, A. Mode of action of cyclosporin A: A new immunosuppressive agent. *Transplant. Proc.* 11:855, 1979.
147. White, D. J. G., Plumb, A. M., Pawelec, G., and Brons, G. Cyclosporin A: An Immunosuppressive agent preferentially active against proliferating cells. *Transplantation* 27:55, 1979.
148. White, D. J. G., Timmerman, W., Davies, HffS, Nagao, T., Kasahara, K., and Plumb, A. Properties of cyclosporin-A-induced graft acceptance. *Transplant. Proc.* 13:379, 1981.
149. Yasumura, T., and Kahan, B. D. Prolongation of rat kidney allografts by pretransplant administration of donor antigen extract on whole blood transfusion combined with a short course of cyclosporine. *Transplantation* 36:603, 1983.
150. Ying, M. L. Calmodulin. *Mol. Cell. Biochem.* 45:101-112, 1982.

18
EXPERIMENTAL CYCLOSPORINE NEPHROTOXICITY

Bernhard Ryffel and Helen Siegl
Sandoz Ltd., Basel, Switzerland

Gilbert Thiel and Michael J. Mihatsch
University of Basel, Basel, Switzerland

Cyclosporine (CsA) is successfully used in organ transplantation. The major side effect of this immunosuppressive agent in patients is renal dysfunction. In the acute phase it is characterized by dose-dependent and reversible blood urea nitrogen (BUN) and creatinine increases and a moderate reduction of the glomerular filtration rate (GFR) [5,25,43,44]. The major concern, however is the possible long-term consequence of CsA therapy on kidney function and morphology. The histologic findings of renal biopsies from kidney transplant patients treated with either CsA or conventional immunosuppressive therapy were summarized in a recent symposium [26]. At the high CsA doses initially used, proximal tubular lesions were found and interpreted as signs of nephrotoxicity [27]; occasionally, arteriolar [27] and glomerular lesions [38] were reported, which might be causally related to interstitial fibrosis [22,27].

These findings in patients were, however, not completely unexpected, since nephrotoxicity was also observed in the toxicologic studies performed in our laboratory [34]. As shown in Table 1, nephrotoxicity was found in rats and cynomolgus monkeys, whereas no renal adverse effects were found in dogs, rhesus monkeys, and mice. Based on these experiments, the rat was considered the ideal species for experimental studies on CsA nephropathy. It must be emphasized, however, that the dose of CsA needed to induce renal dysfunction was high compared with the immunosuppressive dose in the same species.

SENSITIVITY OF VARIOUS STRAINS OF RATS

Cyclosporine was tested at high doses (100 mg/kg per day PO for 10 days) in the following strains: spontaneously hypertensive, Sprague-Dawley, Wistar, and Fischer rats. As can be seen in Table 2, decreased gain or loss of body weight and mortality were observed. Serum BUN and, to a lesser extent, creatinine were increased and GFR measured by the clearance of creatinine reduced. Histologically, tubular alterations of varying degree were observed in all strains. Glomerular lesions were not present, but in spontaneously hypertensive rats the development of arteriolar lesions was accelerated. Based on these results, the following rank order for sensitivity to CsA effects in these strains can be pro-

TABLE 1 Toxicologic Studies with Cyclosporine[a]

Species	Strain	Duration (weeks)	Doses (mg/kg per day)	Route	Mortality[b]	Nephrotoxicity[c]
Monkey	Rhesus	13	0, 20, 60, 200	PO	0/3	–
Monkey	Cynomolgus	4	0, 5, 25, 45	IV	3/8	+
Rat	SD (OFA)	13	0, 14, 45, 90	Feed	18/20	+
Rat	WSA	13	0, 4, 12, 36	PO	2/10	+
Rat	CD	4	0, 6, 24, 48	IV	9/20	+
Dog	Beagle	52	0, 5, 15, 45	PO	0/8	–
Rat	SD (OFA)	104	0, 0.5, 2, 8	Feed	86/100[d]	+
Mouse	OF1	78	0, 1, 4, 16	Feed	56/100[d]	–

[a]SD = Sprague-Dawley; WSA = Wistar;
[b]Number of animals dying during the experiment per total number of animal of the high-dose group.
[c]Nephrotoxicity was indicated by BUN increases or renal morphologic changes.
[d]Mortality of control groups was 68/100 (rats) and 43/100 (mice).

posed: spontaneously hypertensive > Fischer > Wistar > Sprague-Dawley. Generally, female rats were more resistant to CsA nephrotoxicity.

Whiting et al. [49] and Blair et al. [6] reported similar renal functional and morphologic changes in male Sprague-Dawley rats using rather high CsA doses (50 and 100 mg/kg per day given for 2-3 weeks). No vascular or glomerular changes were found in this strain.

Farthing et al. [15] observed CsA nephrotoxicity in male Wister hooded rats. However, the main finding in their study was general toxicity as shown by body weight loss and increased protein catabolism, especially at the 50 mg/kg per day dose.

Based on these results it is concluded that a variety of different rat strains display CsA nephrotoxicity. Extrarenal signs of toxicity should not be omitted in reviewing renal toxicity.

CsA NEPHROPATHY IN SPONTANEOUSLY HYPERTENSIVE RATS

The rationale for using spontaneously hypertensive rats for the further investigation of CsA nephropathy was

1. The high sensitivity of this strain as shown by previous experiments.
2. The presence of arteriolar changes, which were not found in other rat strains, and may occur in humans.
3. The hypertensive effect of CsA in this strain, which is similar to that observed in bone marrow and heart transplant patients [20,31].
4. The observed increase in plasma renin activity (PRA) after CsA. This effect is seen in both rats and dogs [39,40].
5. That hypertension in spontaneously hypertensive rats is caused by increased vascular resistance due to neurogenic and local membrane factors. Thus, stimulation of the renin-angiotensin-aldosterone system (RAAS) by CsA might accelerate the development of hypertension [32].

TABLE 2 Susceptibility of Various Strains of Rats[a]

Strain	CsA	N	ΔBw^b (g)	Mortality (%)	BUN (mg per 100 ml)	Creatinine (ml per 100 ml)	Tubulopathy[c] V	I	C	Arteriolopathy
SH	-	4	30	0	15.9 ± 0.5	0.48 ± 0.08	0	0	0	0
	+	8	-10	12	30.1 ± 5.9	0.62 ± 0.10	1.5	3.75	0	2.75
SD	-	4	72	0	20.2 ± 2.5	0.39 ± 0.04	0	0	0	0
	+	8	12	0	27.2 ± 0.7	0.52 ± 0.07	1	3	1	0
WSA	-	4	48	0	20.9 ± 0.1	0.49 ± 0.02	0	0.75	0	0
	+	8	9	0	34.7 ± 6.3	0.52 ± 0.08	1.5	3.5	1.5	0
FIS	-	4	44	0	16.1 ± 1.8	0.46 ± 0.07	0	2	0	0
	+	8	-8	50	29.1 ± 3.4	0.67 ± 0.08	3	4	0	0

[a]CsA (100 mg/kg per day) was given orally for 10 days to male rats of the following strains: spontaneously hypertensive (SH), Sprague-Dawley (SD), Wistar (WSA), and Fischer (FIS). Control rats received the vehicle only (olive oil, 2 ml/kg).
[b]Body weight change (g) during the experimental period; the initial body weight was 160-180 g.
[c]Renal morphologic changes. Tubulopathy (V, vacuolization; I, inclusion bodies; C, calcification) and arteriolopathy were estimated by a score (0-4+); mean values of four rats per group are given.

TABLE 3 Pilot Study in Spontaneously Hypertensive Rats

Sex	CsA[a] (mg/kg per day)	Duration (weeks)	Body weight (g)	BUN (mg/100 ml)	Creatinine (mg/100 ml)	Creatinine clearance (ml/hr)	PRA (ng/ml per hr)	Arteriolopathy[b] (% affected arterioles)
♂	0	4	265	18.0 ± 2.3	0.54 ± 0.05	1.14 ± 0.16	4.14 ± 0.28	13.3 ± 3.3
	20	4	220	62.3 ± 1.9[c]	1.07 ± 0.12[c]	0.45 ± 0.07[c]	25.07 ± 4.82[c]	38.4 ± 0.8[c]
	0	8	280	28.5 ± 7.3	0.74 ± 0.08	0.83 ± 0.11	11.7 ± 2.55	78.0 ± 6.0[c]
	20	8	248	50.7 ± 8.6[c]	0.95 ± 0.06[c]	0.43 ± 0.24[c]	8.20 ± 3.29	50.3 ± 11.0[c]
♀	0	4	192	18.4 ± 1.2	0.55 ± 0.07	0.78 ± 0.01	6.52 ± 0.22	8.3 ± 4.6
	20	4	185	22.9 ± 8.2	0.64 ± 0.14	0.64 ± 0.15	6.20 ± 0.30[c]	30.6 ± 8.2[c]
	0	8	210	15.4 ± 2.1	0.57 ± 0.03	0.85 ± 0.05	2.20 ± 0.34	10.8 ± 2.2
	20	8	190	26.2 ± 9.1	0.72 ± 0.16	0.60 ± 0.25	9.70 ± 3.56[c]	38.3 ± 4.2[c]

[a]Cyclosporine was given daily PO for 4 (n = 6) or 8 weeks (n = 3) to spontaneously hypertensive rats of both sexes.
[b]Arteriolopathy: number of affected arterioles per 100 evaluated arterioles in renal sections.
[c]Differences to untreated controls at 4 weeks, Student's t test, $p < 0.01$.

In a pilot experiment male and female spontaneously hypertensive rats were given CsA, 20 mg/kg per day orally for 4 weeks, when half the animals were killed; the remainder of the animals were treated for an additional 4 weeks. The dose of 20 mg/kg is about twice the therapeutic dose used in renal transplant patients. The results of this study (Table 3) were as follows:

1. Male rats were more sensitive than females.
2. Serum creatinine and urea nitrogen levels were increased; clearance of creatinine decreased.
3. Arteriolar changes were more pronounced in spontaneously hypertensive rats after 4 weeks of CsA treatment.
4. Plasma renin activity and aldosterone (not shown) were increased in CsA- treated rats, except for the treated male rats at 8 weeks.
5. In addition, the vascular changes were not detectably different in treated male rats and controls at 8 weeks, mainly because vessels were difficult to identify in heavily scarred kidneys.

These findings stimulated a second experiment in order to monitor CsA effects on blood pressure. Thus, young spontaneously hypertensive rats, which had not yet developed sustained hypertension (8-10 weeks) and older rats with established hypertension (12 weeks), were given CsA (20 mg/kg per day) for 4 weeks. Blood pressure was recorded with a tail cuff sphygmomanometer at weekly intervals.

In both age groups a significant blood pressure increase was evident within 2 weeks of drug administration. In addition, tachycardia, hyperglycemia, and increased PRA were observed. Nephrotoxicity was reflected by BUN and creatinine increases as well as by morphologic changes [40].

From these experiments it was evident that the spontaneously hypertensive rat has many features in common with the adverse reactions observed in CsA-treated patients. Thus, the morphologic and functional changes were investigated in more detail, as well as dose and time dependency.

MORPHOLOGIC CHANGES

Tubular Changes

Cyclosporin A induced characteristic lesions in the proximal tubule. The tubular lesions consisted of irregular (small to large) cytoplasmic vacuolization, inclusion bodies, and microcalcification (dystrophic type), as shown in Figure 1 (see Color Plate 6 in color section following page 252). The inclusion bodies may reach the size of the cell nucleus and stain red with the chromotrope aniline blue stain [36]. Electron microscopy (Figure 2) revealed dilation of the endoplasmatic reticulum, giant mitochrondria, and enlarged lysosomes corresponding to the inclusion bodies observed with light microscopy. Myelin bodies, which commonly occur in aminoglycoside nephrotoxicity, were never present [33].

These tubular changes were seen by light microscopy mainly at high doses and are considered indicators of CsA overdosage. Though distinct degenerative changes of the proximal tubular epithelium with increased organelle turnover were present, tubular necrosis was not a common feature even at high doses of CsA. A slight, focal interstitial infiltration with lymphocytes and histiocytes was occasionally observed.

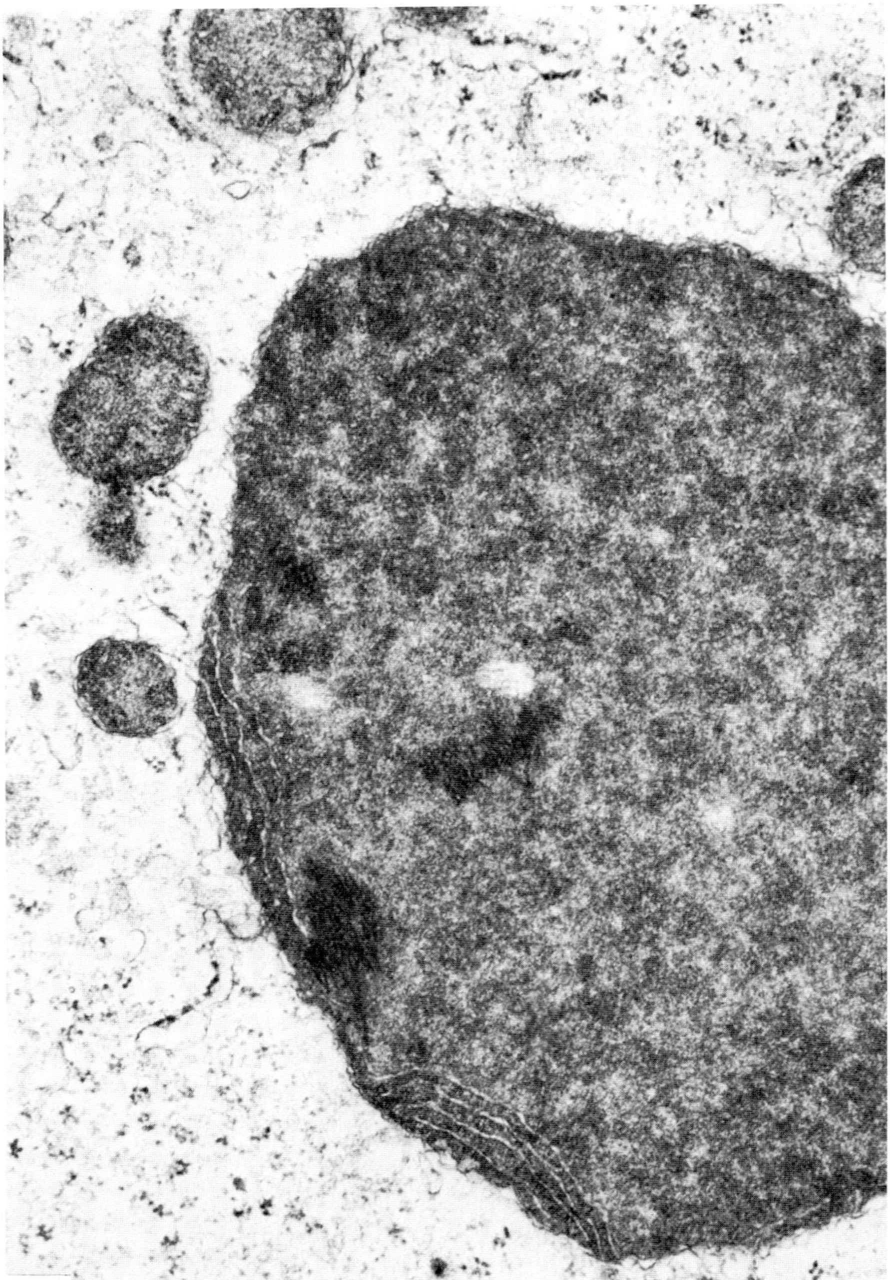
A

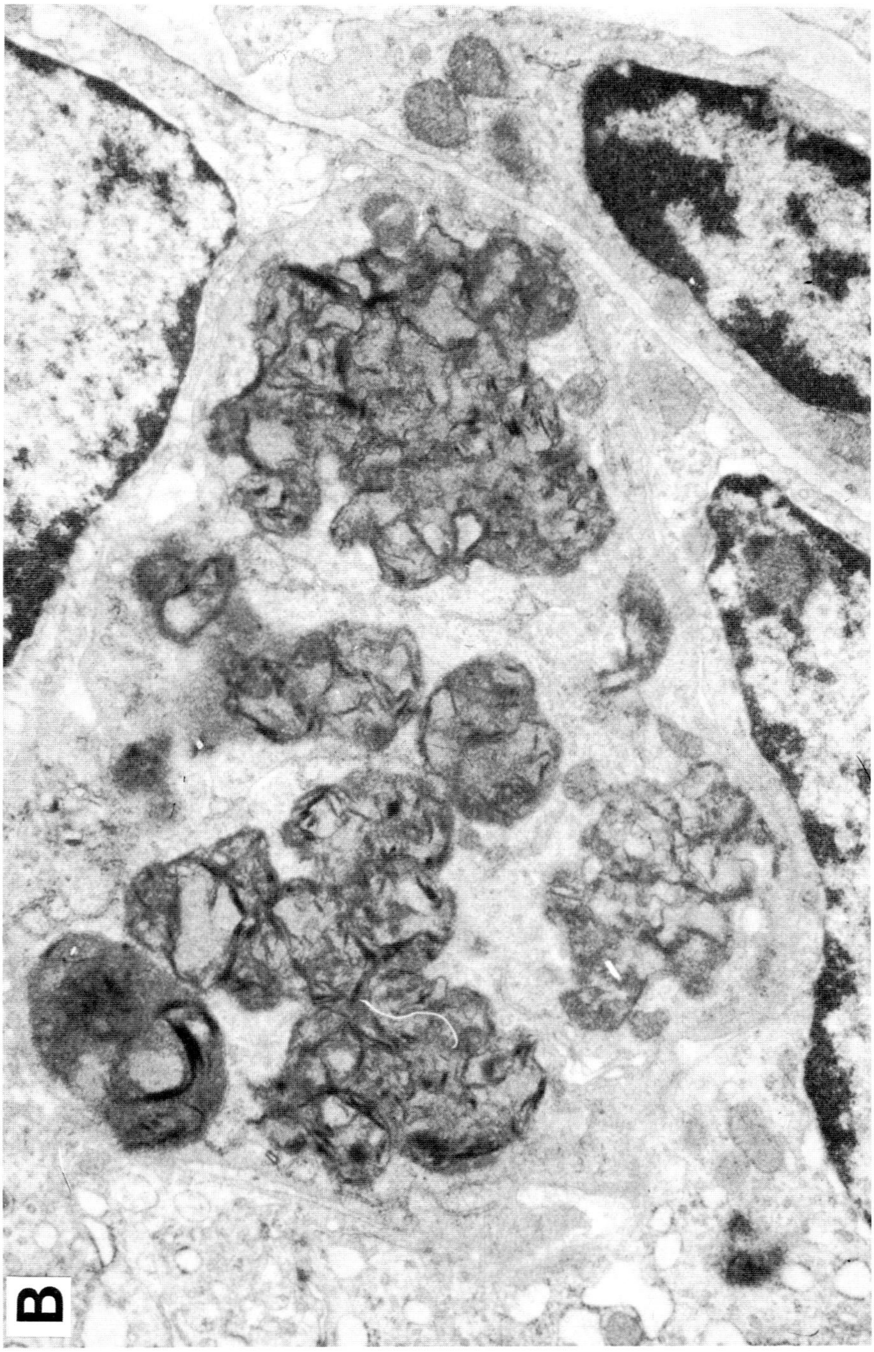

FIGURE 2 Electron microscopy of proximal tubular epithelium with giant mitochondrion (A) and bizarrely shaped lysosome (B).

Arteriolar Changes

Histologically typical arteriolar changes were observed that were more distinct in older, CsA-treated spontaneously hypertensive rats. At low CsA doses a more exudative form with fibrinoid necrosis of the media [Figure 3a (Color Plate 7)] was present, whereas at higher doses or after prolonged CsA administration a more proliferative form of arteriolopathy with obliteration of the vessel lumen predominated [Figure 3 b (see Color Plate 7)]. Immunofluorescence revealed only fibrin in the vessel walls. These arteriolar changes were progressive, resulting in renal scarring.

In conclusion, tubular and arteriolar changes occur in CsA-treated spontaneously hypertensive rats. Similar if not identical renal morphologic changes have been reported in CsA-treated patients [27].

TIME AND DOSE DEPENDENCY AND REVERSIBILITY

The time dependency of the tubular changes was investigated in more detail in normotensive Wistar rats. As shown in Table 4, detectable changes occurred after 3 days at 50 mg/kg and after 2 days at 100 mg/kg CsA. These changes progressed further during the 10 days of the experiment. After a 10-day recovery period, most of the tubular changes proved to be reversible. Dose-dependent tubular lesions were also observed in rats given continuous intravenous infusions of CsA [27].

The arteriolar changes developed at the earliest within 10 days in spontaneously hypertensive rats (at a dose of 50 mg/kg per day). However, arteriolopathy can also be induced at the 20 mg/kg CsA dose when given over a 4-week period.

Since arteriolopathy is a progressive disease that also develops in untreated spontaneously hypertensive rats, the lesions are most likely not reversible.

TABLE 4 Tubular Changes in Wistar Rats: Kinetics and Reversibility

Duration of CSA administration (days)[a]	50 mg/kg per day[b]			100 mg/kg per day[b]		
	I	V	C	I	V	C
1	0	0	0	0	0	0
2	0	1	0	2	2	0
3	2.5	2	0	3.5	4	0
5	3	1.5	0	6.5	4.5	0
7	3	1.5	2	6.5	4.5	2
10	2.5	1.5	2.5	4	5	2
20[c]	0	0	1	0	0	0.5

[a]Male Wistar rats (two per group) were given CsA (50 or 100 mg/kg daily PO up to 10 days.

[b]Histologic tubular changes (I = inclusion bodies, V = vacuolization, and C = calcification) are given as a cumulative score (0-4+), two animals per time point.

[c]Recovery group: After 10 days of CsA administration, these rats were killed 10 days later (n = 4).

FUNCTIONAL CHANGES

Male spontaneously hypertensive rats were given various doses of CsA (0-100 mg/kg per day) for 4 weeks. The main findings were

1. A dose-dependent decrease in body weight gain (> 10 mg/kg per day) or even body weight loss at the higher doses of 50 and 100 mg/kg per day. Food intake (⩾50 mg/kg per day) and water intake were decreased except for the 10 and 20 mg/kg dose groups. At the 100 mg/kg dose, central nervous toxicity became apparent (hyperreactivity and convulsions), and 50% of the rats died.
2. Serum chemistry showed dose-dependent blood urea nitrogen and creatinine increases (Table 5). Hyperglycemia, hypoalbuminemia, and distinct changes in serum electrolytes ($Na^+\downarrow$, $K^+\uparrow$. $Ca^{2+}\downarrow$, $PO_4^{3-}\uparrow$) were observed.
3. Urinalysis (Figure 4) revealed dose-dependent aciduria, slightly increased volume with calciuria, sodium retention, and decreased osmolality. The GFR as measured by the creatinine or inulin clearances was decreased in a dose-dependent manner. The osmolar and negative free water clearance (T_c H_2O) were decreased, however. Microscopic examination of the urine sediment was normal.
4. The effect of CsA on blood pressure and heart rate is shown in Figure 5. Whereas low doses caused hypertension and tachycardia, blood pressure and heart rate were normalized or even lower than controls at high doses.
5. Cyclosporin A trough levels were in the microgram per milliliter range and correlated fairly well with the administered doses.
6. The effect of CsA on PRA followed roughly that of blood pressure. Thus at the lower doses of PRA was increased, whereas at high doses PRA was in the control range or even decreased. The normalization of PRA at the higher doses was rather unexpected since these rats were most likely volume and salt depleted (Table 5). By contrast, aldosterone serum levels were increased in a dose-dependent fashion.

Impaired electrolyte transport might be an early sign of CsA nephrotoxicity in rats. Direct evidence for decreased Na^+ reabsorption in the proximal tubule was presented by Gutsche et al. [19] using micropuncture techniques in the rat. A decreased NaCl reabsorption in the ascending limb of the Henle's loop would stimulate the tubuloglomerular-feedback (TGF) mechanism resulting in GFR reduction.

Dieperink et al. [11] found in male Sprague-Dawley rats (12.5, 25, and 50 mg/kg per day given for 14 days) a dose-dependent reduction of the clearance of lithium, which is a measure of proximal tubular Na^+ and water reabsorption. In that study the fractional delivery of Na^+ and K^+ to the distal tubule was increased.

Distal tubular function may also be altered, as reported by Battle et al. [2], who showed a decreased capacity to acidify urine in CsA-treated rats (25 mg/kg per day for 8 days) after a NH_4Cl load, whereas no change of K^+ excretion was found after K^+ loading. The conclusion from this study was that a defective H^+ secretion might be an early sign of CsA nephropathy.

Clinically, a significant hyperkalemia and hyperchloremic acidosis were observed in CsA-treated renal transplant patients by Adu et al. [1]. Hyperkalemia was inappropriate for the GFR reduction. Despite hyperkalemia, aldosterone serum levels were in the low to normal range. Adu et al. concluded that CsA might cause hypoaldosteronism and defective tubular secretion of K^+ and H^+, resulting in hyperkalemic, hyperchloremic acidosis.

TABLE 5 Serum Chemistry in Spontaneously Hypertensive Rats Given CsA for 4 Weeks[a]

CsA (mg/kg per day)	Δ BW[b] (g)	Na^+ (mEq/liter)	K^+ (mEq/liter)	Ca^{2+} (mEq/liter)	PRA (ng/ml per hr)	Aldosterone (pg/ml)	Glucose (mg per 100 ml)	BUN (mg per 100 ml)	Creatinine (mg per 100 ml)	CsA (μg/ml)
0	+20	140 ± 1.4	5.4 ± 0.1	5.4 ± 0.1	4.75 ± 1.70	136 ± 31	108 ± 44	15.3 ± 0.9	0.47 ± 0.1	–
20	+17	131 ± 6**	5.7 ± 0.9	5.1 ± 0.1	21.42 ± 13.30**	216 ± 52**	181 ± 44**	22.0 ± 2.4*	0.68 ± 0.2	4.14 ± 0.88
50	+9	133 ± 2.5**	6.8 ± 0.7**	4.9 ± 0.1**	9.51 ± 3.58*	260 ± 3.58*	220 ± 49**	38.0 ± 5.5**	0.76 ± 0.2*	5.95 ± 2.30
100	-33	134 ± 1.0**	6.7 ± 0.4**	4.7 ± 0.2**	5.59 ± 3.67	285 ± 120	259 ± 97**	39.0 ± 2.5**	1.06 ± 0.2**	14.47 ± 4.79

[a]Male rats were treated with various doses of CsA (0-100 mg/kg per day) for 28 days. Control rats received the vehicle (5 ml/kg olive oil) only.
[b]Body weight changes (Δ BW) during the experiment; the initial body weights were 285 ± 8 g.
[c]Differences from controls were calculated by test of variance and Student's t-ests: $* < 0.05$, $** < 0.01$.

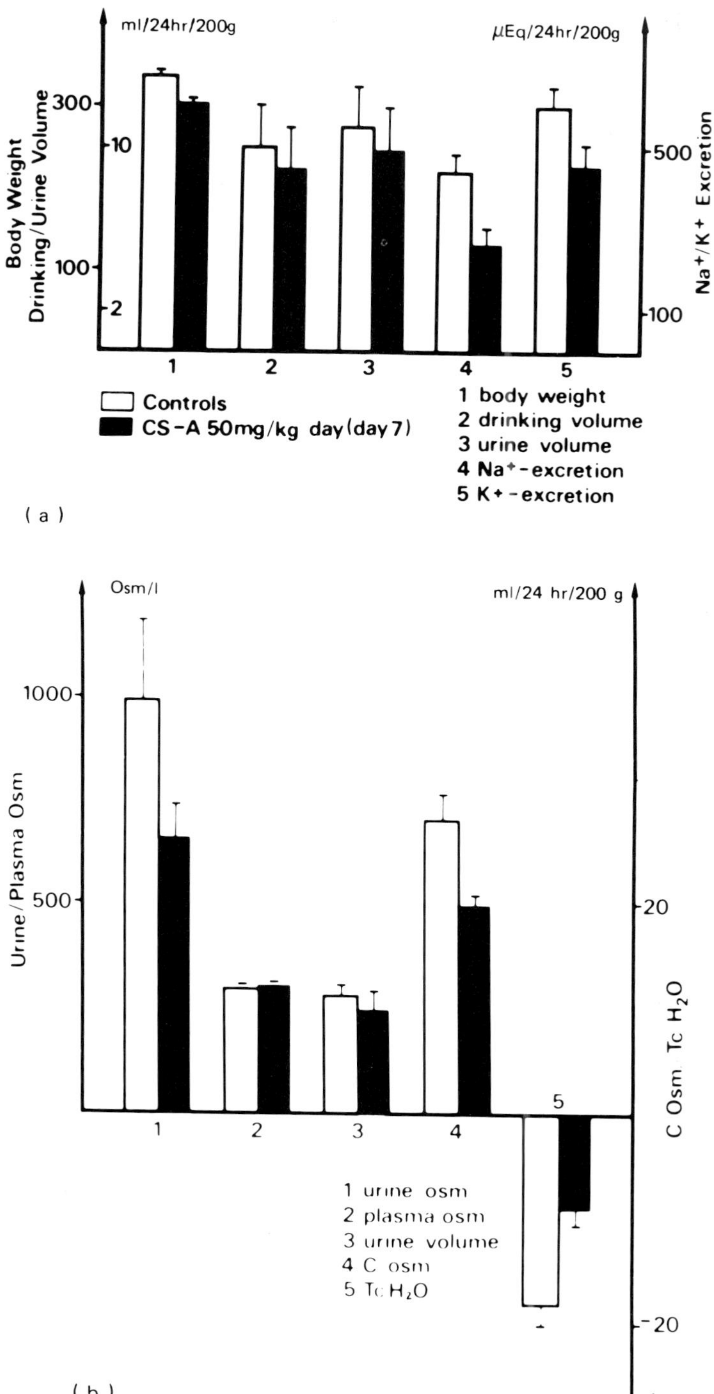

FIGURE 4 Renal functional changes in spontaneously hypertensive rats treated with CsA, 50 mg/kg per day for 7 days. Mean values ± SD are shown.

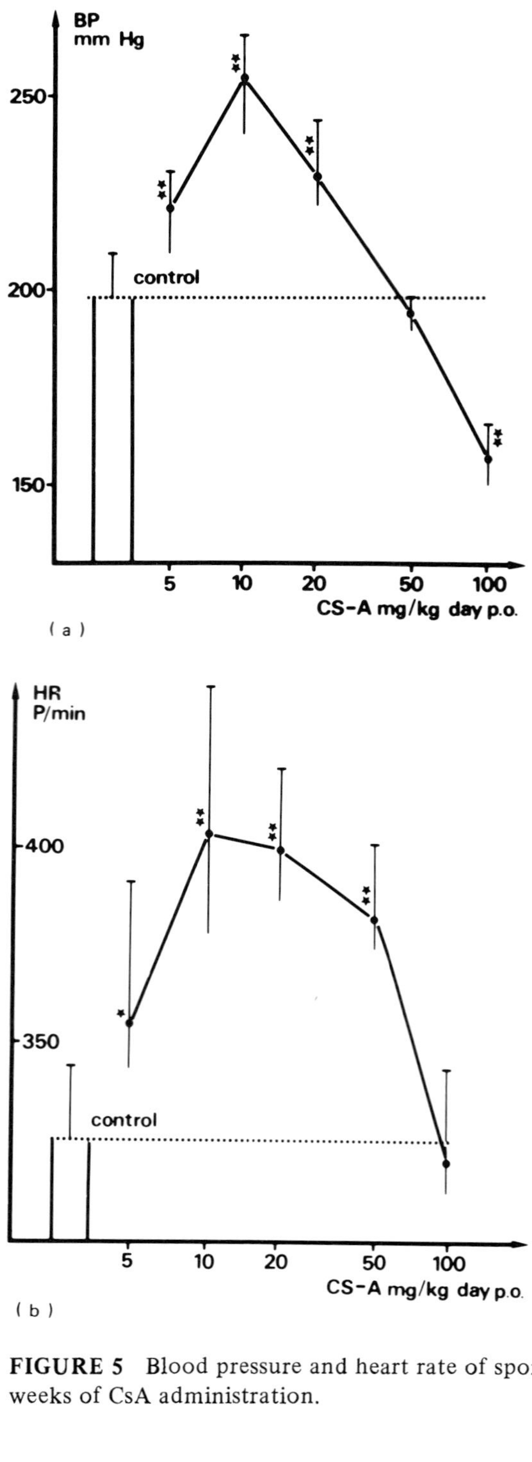

FIGURE 5 Blood pressure and heart rate of spontaneously hypertensive rats after 4 weeks of CsA administration.

These data indicating hypoaldosteronism are difficult to reconcile with the experimental findings in rats (Table 5). However, it should be remembered that most of the patients reported by Adu et al. were treated for hypertension with β blockers, which inhibit PRA and might explain partially the low aldosterone levels.

In conclusion, CsA nephropathy in rats is initially characterized by tubular dysfunction and reduced GFR. The relationship between these two factors has yet to be clarified.

CsA PHARMACOKINETICS

In order to validate an experimental system, such pharmacokinetic parameters as absorption, distribution, metabolism and excretion of a compound must be compared with data obtained in humans. Detection of CsA in blood or serum was made possible by the development of a radioimmunoassay (RIA) and a liquid chromatographic technique (HPLC) [12,29]. Since the antibody used in the RIA cross-reacts with metabolites, this method overestimates levels of the parent molecule at least twofold.

1. Absorption. Orally administered CsA—resistant to the gastrointestinal enzymes—is readily absorbed from the gastrointestinal tract, reaching peak serum levels at 4-6 hr as detected by RIA (Figure 6). About 50% of an oral dose is absorbed. Repeated administration results in higher peak and trough levels, indicating a slight accumulation in the serum. The vehicle seems not to be important since CsA may also be given in a feed mixture, which results in comparable serum levels (unpublished).
2. Distribution. Studies with radiolabeled CsA were performed that indicated drug accumulation in liver, kidney, fat, lymphoid tissue, and skin, whereas almost no

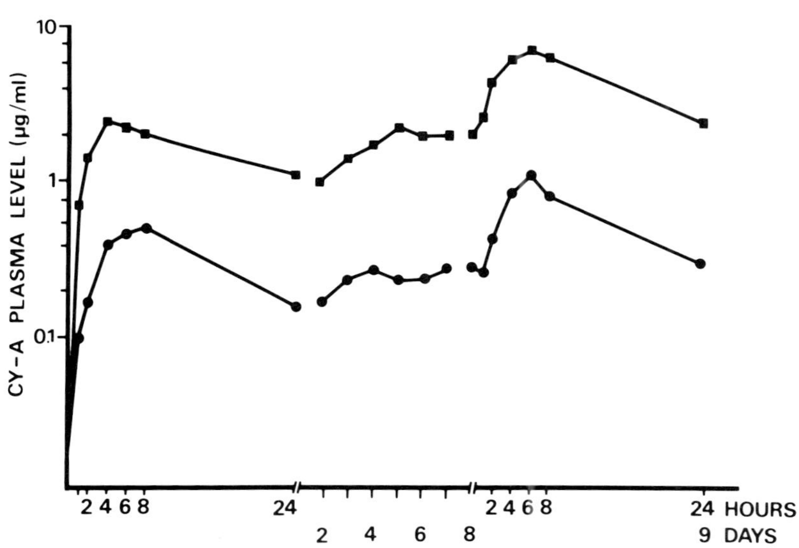

FIGURE 6 Pharmacokinetics after a single or repeated oral doses of CsA (10 and 30 mg/kg per day) in Wistar rats.

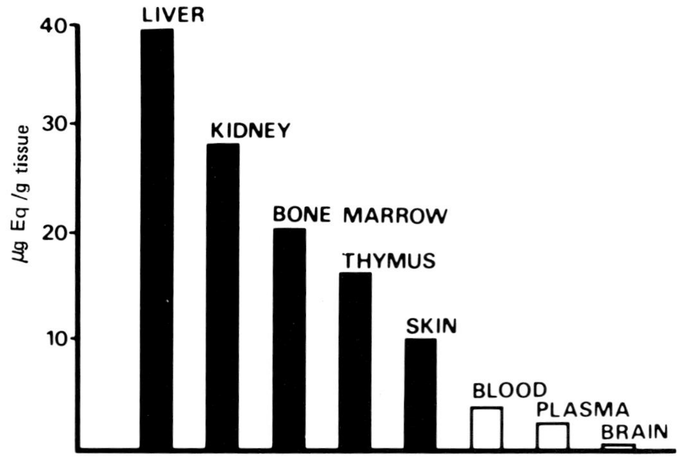

FIGURE 7 Distribution of total radioactivity in several organs in Wistar rats given [^{3}H] CsA (G. Maurer and O. Wagner, unpublished).

radioactivity was detected in whole-brain homogenate (Figure 7). The high tissue affinity of the drug was reflected in tissue/blood ratios of 2-10.

3. Metabolism. Extensive metabolism occurs in the liver, which includes hydroxylation and N-demethylation, resulting in more than 10 metabolites that all preserve the peptide ring structure [24]. Preliminary experiments indicate that most of the metabolites have little or no immunosuppressive activity.
4. Elimination. After an oral dose of CsA most is eliminated by the bile into the feces, with only about 5% eliminated by the urine.
5. Bioavailability after various routes of administration. In order to determine the effect of various routes of administration on serum levels and toxicity, Wistar rats were given 50 mg/kg per day for 10 days, PO, SC, or IP (Table 6). Cyclosporin A trough levels were higher in intraperitoneally administered rats. Renal and general toxicity was in the same range for all treatment groups.
6. Tubular accumulation of CsA. von Willebrand and Häyry were able to detect material in human tubular cells that reacted with the antibody used in the RIA [52]. It was assumed that this finding meant CsA accumulation in tubular cells, indicating CsA nephrotoxicity [53]. Using the identical technique we were unable to demonstrate CsA-reactive material in rat or in human renal tissue. However, by use of radioactive CsA, some preferential accumulation of the compound in the outer stripe of the outer medulla was observed after in vitro incubation of rat kidney sections (unpublished).
7. Toxicity of metabolites. Cunningham et al. [7] reported experimental data that indicate that induction of hepatic cytochrome P_{450} in rats by aroclor results in accelerated metabolism, decreased levels, and reduced nephrotoxicity of CsA. These results indicate that the parent molecule, rather than a metabolite, is responsible for the nephrotoxicity. This is further supported by results from rats given a major metabolite (OL17), which was completely devoid of toxicity (Table 7). By contrast, inhibition and/or interaction of the cytochrome P_{450} system by

TABLE 6 Effects of CsA Given by Various Routes to Wistar Rats

CsA[a] (50 mg/kg per day)	Body weight (g)	BUN (mg/100 ml)	Total protein (mg/100 ml)	CsA level[b] μg/ml)	Urine: Volume (ml/24 hr)	Urine: Na^+ (mEq/24 hr)	Urine: K^+ (mEq/24 hr)	Urine: Ca^{2+} (μmol/24 hr)	Renal tubular changes[c]
-	271 ± 8	16.3 ± 1.9	5.72 ± 0.36	-	26 ± 11	0.38	0.74	10.4	0.8
PO	240 ± 15	21.2 ± 2.4*	4.98 ± 0.08	1.32 ± 0.49	31 ± 14	0.73	1.37*	31.9*	3.9
SC	253 ± 12	2.20 ± 1.2*	4.80 ± 0.21	1.91 ± 0.87	25 ± 13	0.37	0.90	10.4	3.3
IP	228 ± 11	17.9 ± 3.8	4.70 ± 0.35*	7.87 ± 1.69*	32 ± 8	0.34	1.08	14.5	3.6

[a]Male rats (body weight 244 ± 7 g) received CsA (50 mg/kg per day) for 10 days, n = 5 rats per group.
[b]CsA level 24 hr after last administration (RIA).
[c]Cumulative mean score (0-4+) of tubular lesions (inclusion bodies, vacuolization, and calcification).

TABLE 7 Absence of Nephrotoxicity in Wistar Rats Given the Major Metabolite (OL 17)

Administration[a] (50 mg/kg per day)	BUN (mg/100 ml)	Creatinine clearance (ml/min)	Serum: Protein (mg/100 ml)	Serum: Bilirubin (mg/100 ml)	Urine: Volume (ml/24 hr)	Urine: Ca^{2+} (μmol/24 hr)	Tubulopathy[b]
Olive oil	13.9 ± 2.1	0.69 ± 15	6.6 ± 0.2	0.20 ± 0.03	28 ± 10	21.2 ± 17.2	0.1
CsA	25.6 ± 6.8[b]	0.39 ± 0.13[b]	4.3 ± 0.3[b]	0.48 ± 0.13[b]	18 ± 14	50.9 ± 56.5	2.2
OL 17	13.5 ± 1.8	0.81 ± 0.17	6.2 ± 0.2	0.25 ± 0.05	25 ± 13	22.7 ± 14.7	0.2

[a]Male Wistar (five rats per group) were treated for 28 days PO.
[b]Cumulative mean score (0-4+) of tubular changes (vacuolization, inclusion bodies, and calcification).

ketoconazole, for example, results in higher CsA serum levels and increased toxicity [48].

In conclusion, CsA is readily absorbed from the gastrointestinal tract, extensively metabolized in the liver, and eliminated via bile. Toxicity is most likely due to the parent molecule. Interference with hepatic metabolism may change bioavailability, resulting in altered pharmacokinetics.

Finally, comparison of rat findings with human data indicate that pharmacokinetic parameters correlate fairly well between the two species [4,24], the differences being quantitative rather than qualitative in nature.

SENSITIZING FACTORS FOR NEPHROTOXICITY

A variety of factors that increase the detrimental effect of CsA on renal function were investigated in rats.

1. Ischemia. Thiel et al. [45] reported that warm ischemia in rats enhanced nephrotoxicity. Similar data were obtained in dogs [9], but not in rabbits [10].
2. Heminephrectomy. Another factor that increases nephrotoxicity of CsA is heminephrectomy. As shown in Table 8, heminephrectomized rats given CsA had higher BUN and creatinine levels and more distinct morphologic signs of nephrotoxicity than sham-operated controls. Similar findings have been reported by others [17,37], indicating that renal adaptation to a CsA insult is impaired after heminephrectomy.
3. NaCl load. In order to evaluate effects of sodium loading, spontaneously hypertensive rats were given 0.9% NaCl as drinking solution (ad libitum). Sodium loading to CsA-treated rats caused deterioration of both functional and morphologic renal parameters compared with rats receiving tap water and CsA [41].
4. Irradiation. Local single kidney irradiation with 1500 rads accentuated the morphologic changes in CsA-treated rats (unpublished).
5. Nonsteroidal anti-inflammatory drugs (NSAID). Inhibition of the prostaglandin (PG) synthesis with the cyclo-oxygenase inhibitor indomethacin enhanced CsA toxicity (unpublished). These results indicate that the PG system is important in protecting against CsA nephrotoxicity.
6. Dehydration. In the late stage of CsA intoxication, volume depletion may be important as indicated by a decreased urine volume and water intake. Thus, administration of diuretics for a prolonged period may enhance general toxicity. Furosemide has been shown to increase CsA toxicity in rats, possibly due to Na^+ depletion and dehydration [51].
7. Chemotherapeutics. Concomitant administration of antibiotics with a nephrotoxic potential may be hazardous in CsA-treated animals. Thus, concomitant administration of gentamicin and CsA at high doses clearly has a detrimental effect on renal function [50]. However, therapeutic doses of both CsA and various chemotherapeutics, such as gentamicin, amphotericin B, and ketoconazole, in healthy, normotensive Wistar rats do not potentiate CsA nephropathy [35].

In conclusion, various risk factors for CsA nephropathy have been identified that should—if possible—be avoided in patients receiving the drug.

TABLE 8 Comparison of CsA Nephropathy in Intact and Heminephrectomized (Hnx) Wistar Rats[a]

Experimental day	Finding	Controls		CsA 50	
		Intact	Hnx	Intact	Hnx
7	Urine volume (ml per 24 hr per 200 g)	11 ± 4	7 ± 2	10 ± 4	13 ± 7
	Na^+ excretion (μEq per 24 hr per 200 g)	336 ± 79	296 ± 76	259 ± 84	163 ± 29
	K^+ excretion (μEq per 24 hr per 200 g)	607 ± 101	504 ± 90	461 ± 127	324 ± 72
	Tc H_2O (ml per 24 hr per 200 g)	-18.2 ± 4.4	-17.7 ± 3.2	-9.5 ± 3.2	-5.1 ± 5.4
14	C in (ml/min per 100 g)	0.49 ± 0.07	0.40 ± 0.10	0.23 ± 0.06	0.11 ± 0.04
	CsA (24 hr) level (μg/ml)	-	-	8.78 ± 1.69	5.88 ± 2.75
28	BUN (mg per 100 ml)	15.2 ± 1.5	19.9 ± 2.1	28.4 ± 4.5	58.4 ± 29.1
	Creatinine (mg per 100 ml)	0.71 ± 0.16	0.84 ± 0.02	1.15 ± 0.10	1.34 ± 0.14
	Tubular lesions	0.2	0.2	1.9	2.2

[a]Male Wistar rats (five rats per group) were treated for 4 weeks with CsA, 50 mg/kg per day or the vehicle (olive oil). Heminephrectomy (Hnx) was performed under ether anesthesia.

PREVENTION OF CsA NEPHROTOXICITY

Various strategies for reducing CsA nephrotoxicity were investigated. Only a few of these experiments are summarized.

1. Probenecid. Renal tubular accumulation of various antibiotics was reported to be reduced by probenecid, a known blocker of the organic anion transport system [47]. We gave Wistar rats treated with high-dose CsA probenecid concomitantly. Except for a slight decrease in BUN levels, probenecid altered neither the pharmacokinetic profile nor nephrotoxicity (Table 9).
2. Prostaglandin (PGE_2). Administration of dimethyl-PGE_2 decreased CsA toxicity in Wistar-Furth rats [23]. Our experiments, however, indicated that dimethyl-PGE_2 reduced the bioavailability of orally administered CsA, which might explain the preventive effect (Ryffel, submitted).

TABLE 9 Effects of Probenecid on CsA Nephropathy in Wistar Rats[a]

CsA (mg/kg per day)	Probenecid (mg/kg per day)	BUN (mg per 100 ml)	Creatinine (mg per 100 ml)	Inulin clearance (ml/hr)	CsA level[b]		Renal changes[c]
					4 hr	24 hr	
-	-	11.6 ± 1.1	0.47 ± 0.08	43.4 ± 6.6	-	-	0.3
-	2 X 100	9.6 ± 1.1	0.54 ± 0.06	39.2 ± 8.8	-	-	1.2
100	-	24.3 ± 12.2	0.80 ± 0.14	28.8 ± 6.9	21.1 ± 5.6	8.4 ± 1.2	2.9
100	2 X 100	15.0 ± 6.9	0.89 ± 0.22	25.8 ± 8.3	29.7 ± 10.7	7.9 ± 1.7	2.8

[a]Male Wistar rats (five rats per group) were treated for 7 days; CsA was given orally (100 mg/kg per day) in olive oil; probenecid was given in two divided doses (8 a.m. and 4 p.m.) PO.
[b]Cyclosporin plasma levels (RIA) 4 and 24 hr after the last administration.
[c]Cumulative mean score (0-4+) of tubular lesions (inclusion bodies and vacuolization).

TABLE 10 Effects of a Ca^{2+} Antagonist and Diuretics on CsA Nephropathy in Spontaneously Hypertensive Rats[a]

Experimental groups	Dose, (mg/kg per day, PO)	Body weight (g)	Blood pressure (mm Hg)	Heart rate (P/min)	PRA (ng/ml per hr)	BUN (mg/100 ml)	Serum creatinine (mg/100 ml)	Glucose (mg/100 ml)	Renal morphology[b] TP	AP	n
Control	-	259 ± 9	187 ± 13	354 ± 13	3.6 ± 1.9	16.4 ± 1.3	0.45 ± 0.09	96 ± 12	0.1 ± 0.1	0.2 ± 0.2	18
CsA	20	243 ± 11	213 ± 12	394 ± 28	7.9 ± 3.2	22.1 ± 3.1	0.48 ± 0.07	243 ± 15	1.4 ± 0.7	1.4 ± 0.4	18
CsA + verapamil	20 20	255 ± 17	211 ± 14	377 ± 28	5.2 ± 1.9	22.6 ± 3.8	0.44 ± 0.03	251 ± 52	0.5 ± 0.6	0.2 ± 0.2	6
CsA + spironolactone	20 50	262 ±21	192 ± 8	348 ± 44	8.7 ± 3.8	18.9 ± 2.1	0.42 ± 0.06	98 ± 10	0.5 ± 0.5	0.5 ± 0.5	6
CsA + clopamide	20 1	224 ± 4	182 ± 9	365 ± 25	46.7 ± 28.2	20.0 ± 3.4	0.48 ± 0.19	Not measured	0.4 ± 0.5	0.4 ± 0.5	6

[a]Male rats were treated with CsA alone or CsA with verapamil, spironolactone or clopamide for 4 weeks.
[b]Renal changes (TP = tubulopathy, AP = arteriolopathy) are given as a mean score ($0\text{-}4^{+}$).

3. Glucose. Administration of 5% glucose as drinking solution to normotensive and hypertensive rats diminished general and renal toxicity. This might be due to a rehydration and increased caloric intake. Gerkens et al. [18] showed that a NaCl drinking solution in Na^+-depleted normotensive rats decreased nephrotoxicity, which might be also due to rehydration.
4. Calcium antagonist and diuretics. The aim of the investigation in male, not yet hypertensively stable spontaneously hypertensive rats was to prevent CsA nephrotoxicity and general adverse reactions in a 4-week experiment by concomitant administration of the calcium antagonist verapamil or the diuretics spironolactone and clopamide. The results are given in Table 10.

   Simultaneous administration of verapamil (20 mg/kg per day admixed with the food) did not inhibit blood pressure increases or affect clinical serum parameters. A slight inhibition of CsA-induced tachycardia and PRA increases were observed. The histopathologic changes, especially the arteriolar lesions, were reduced, however.

   The aldosterone antagonist spironolactone (50 mg/kg per day) reduced blood pressure and improved CsA-induced morphologic damage of the kidneys (Table 10).

   Finally, the salidiuretic drug clopamaide (1 mg/kg per day, given in the drinking fluid) provided a certain protection against CsA adverse reactions.

   Based on these results it is concluded that Na^+ and Ca^{2+} ions might play an important role in the mechanism responsible for CsA-induced general and renal adverse reactions.

DRUG INTERACTIONS

Clinically, a variety of drugs given concomitantly with CsA have been shown to interfere with the metabolism of CsA. The antifungal agent ketoconazole decreases CsA elimination at the level of the hepatic cytochrome P_{450} system [16]. By contrast, phenytoin and rifampicin enhance CsA elimination by stimulation of the microsomal cytochrome P_{450} system [8,21]. In both situations, the CsA dose must be adapted to the altered metabolism of the immunosuppressant. Effects of CsA on the metabolism of other compounds was observed for prednisolone, where a decreased clearance of this drug in CsA-treated patients was observed [30].

Another type of interaction occurs with trimethoprim and cotrimoxazole, which given alone have no overt effect on renal function, but which, given with CsA, enhance CsA nephropathy [46]. Furthermore, there is a suspicion from clinical studies that NSAIDs might increase general adverse reactions, especially potentiating arterial hypertension (unpublished).

COMPARISON WITH GENTAMICIN NEPHROTOXICITY

The nephrotoxic potential of CsA was compared with that of gentamicin [33] in rats, as shown in Table 11. Whereas gentamicin induced acute renal failure with distinct BUN and creatinine increases,CsA had only minor effects on these parameters. Extensive tubular necrosis was never seen after CsA (Figure 8).

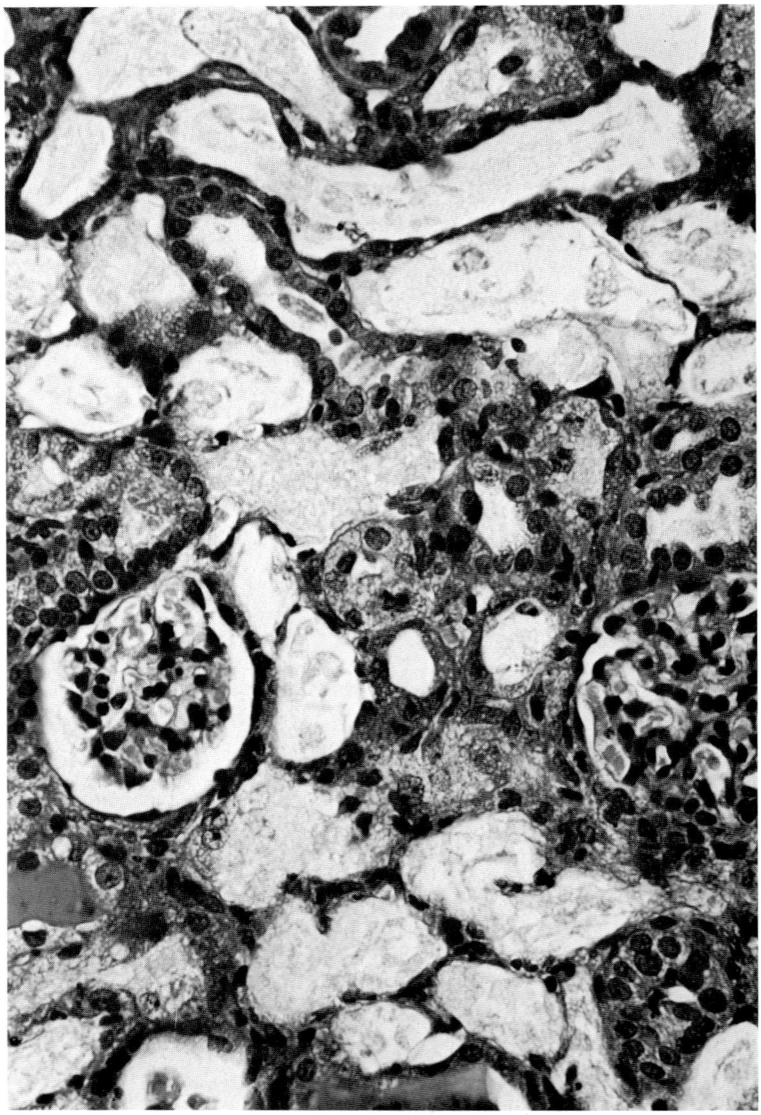

(A)

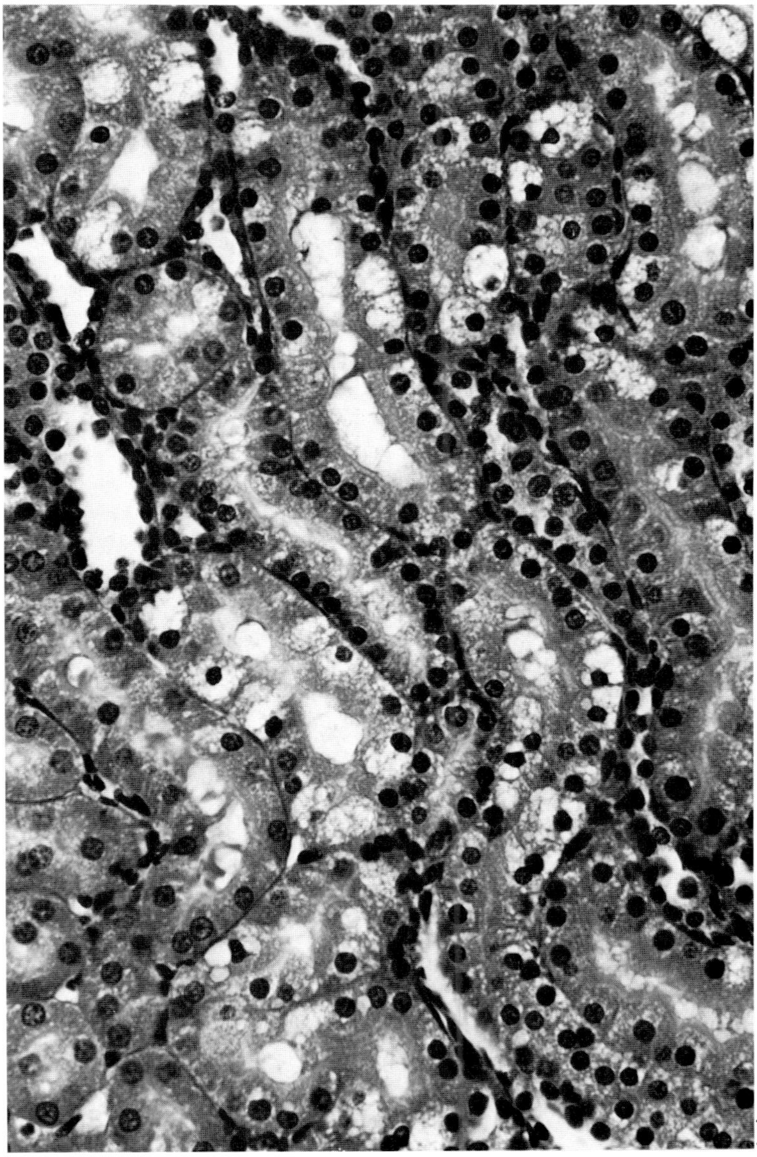

(B)

FIGURE 8 Comparison of gentamicin and CsA-induced tubular lesions. Tubular necrosis after gentamicin (A) and CsA-associated tubulopathy (B). (Hematoxylin and eosin.)

TABLE 11 Comparison of CsA and Gentamicin Nephrotoxicity[a]

Dose (mg/kg per day)	Route	BUN (mg/100 ml)	Creatinine (mg/100 ml)	Tubular changes V	N	I
Solvent (oil)	PO	26.1 ± 4.5	0.72 ± 0.11	0	0	0
CsA 100	PO	35.1 ± 5.6	0.69 ± 0.07	2.5	0	0
Gentamicin 50	SC	105.1 ± 22.8	2.80 ± 0.44	0	3	2
Gentamicin 100	SC	186.7 ± 59.6	6.32 ± 2.08	0	4	3

[a]Male Wistar rats, 200 g, were treated for 10 days; five rats per group. Morphologic changes (vacuolization, necrosis, and lymphocytic infiltrates), score: 0-4, mean of five rats.

SPECULATIONS ON THE MECHANISMS OF CsA NEPHROPATHY

The present data allow some speculations on the mechanisms of CsA nephropathy. Taking all experimental findings in consideration it is postulated that extrarenal factors (anorexia, blood pressure, and extracellular volume changes) contribute to a great extent to CsA nephropathy. Assuming that renal and extrarenal changes (Table 12) are interrelated, a viscious circle may ensue.

Schematically four components of CsA nephrotoxicity can be distinguished: renal vasoconstriction, tubulotoxicity, arteriolotoxicity, and extrarenal changes.

Reductions of GFR and RBF are dose-dependent and are early signs of CsA nephrotoxicity. GFR reduction is most likely due to *preglomerular vasoconstriction.* The following possibilities may be causally related to GFR reduction:

1. Direct vasoconstrictor effect of CsA; no experimental findings thus far support this mechanism.
2. Activation of the renin-angiotensin system; the following experimental findings support this hypothesis:
   a. Stimulation of the tubulo-glomerular feed back system due to increased Na^+ and/or Cl-delivery at the macula densa [11,19].

TABLE 12 Overview of Renal and Extrarenal Findings in CsA Treated Animals

Symptoms	Anorexia, decreased body weight gain BP↑, HR↑ CNS effects
Serum	BUN↑, creatinine↑, Na^+↓, K^+↑, Ca^{2+}↓, PO_4^{2-}↑, glucose↑, uric acid↑, bilirubin↑, PRA↑, aldosterone↑
Urine	volume↓, pH↓, Na^+↓, K^+↓↓, Na^+/K^+↑, PG↓, Ca^{2+}↑
Clearances	C_{in}↓, C_{pah}↓, C_{osm}↓, TC_{H2O}↓
Pathology	Tubular and arteriolar lesions

   b. Direct effect of CsA on PRA release, as suggested by in vitro experiments [3]
   c. Decreased vascular reactivity to pressor effects as shown in anesthesized and ganglion-blocked spontaneously hypertensive rats treated with CsA [42]
   d. Extracellular volume depletion due to anorexia and decreased thirst
3. Changes in the production and/or release of prostaglandins (PG), which play an important role in the regulation of the vascular tone [14]. In favor of dysregulated PG production are:
   a. Reduced prostacyclin stimulating factor (PSF), which is essential for prostacyclin synthesis, was found in CsA-treated rabbits [28].
   b. The PG synthesis inhibitor indomethacin increased CsA nephropathy in both dogs and rats [40].
   c. Decreased renal PG production was measured in CsA-treated spontaneously hypertensive rats (Stahl, unpublished), which was, however, not observed in normotensive rats after a single high dose [13].

The relative importance of the various mechanisms for the vasoconstriction resulting in GFR reduction is unknown and has to be established by further experiments.

Tubulotoxicity is a characteristic lesion of the proximal tubule occurring only at high CsA doses (> 50 mg/kg) and must be distinguished from tubular necrosis as seen in the aminoglycoside toxicity. The proximal tubular changes may be associated with defects of tubular functions e.g., gluconeogenesis, transport of amino acids, phosphate, calcium, etc. (Beck, V., et al., submitted). In addition, distal tubular dysfunction has been reported [2].

Arteriolotoxicity as observed occasionally in CsA-treated patients was never found in a variety of normotensive strains of rats. Experimental manipulation such as local irradiation, five-sixths nephrectomy and Goldblatt hypertension, did not result in excess arteriolar changes after CsA (Thiel, G., *Clinical Nephrology*, in press). Vascular thrombosis was reported in CsA-treated rabbits in a model of experimental serum sickness, lesions which may resemble the hemolytic uremic syndrome observed occasionally in CsA-treated patients [26]. The SH rat was the only strain of rats which developed arteriolar alterations with low CsA doses (10-20 mg/kg). In addition to the effects on the arterioles CsA accelerated the development of arterial hypertension in SH rats.

Extrarenal effects of CsA occurring in various strains of rats and especially in spontaneously hypertensive rats should be considered, such as tachycardia, accelerated development of hypertension, and hyperglycemia–indicating increased sympathetic nerve activity –as well as malnutrition, dehydration, changes in intra- and extracellular electrolyte concentrations, and metabolic acidosis. All these extrarenal changes might cause further deterioration in renal function.

In summary, the rat may not be the ideal, but is at present the best available animal model of CsA nephropathy. This species, especially the spontaneously hypertensive strain, reflected to some extent renal and extrarenal (hypertension) changes occurring in CsA-treated patients. Finally, the morphologic alterations were similar in both species. This experimental model allows further investigations on the pathogenic mechanisms, which are elusive at the present time.

REFERENCES

1. Adu, D., Turney, J., Michael, J., and McMaster, P. Hyperkalaemia in cyclosporin-treated renal allograft recipients. *Lancet* 2:370-372, 1983.

2. Battle, D. C., Gutterman, C., and Tarka, J. Cyclosporin A and distal tubular dysfunction (abstract). IX Int. Congress of Nephrology, 1984, Los Angeles.
3. Baxter, C. R., Duggin, G. G., Willis, N. S., Hall, B. M., Horvath, J. S., and Tiller, D. J. Cyclosporin A-induced increases in renin storage and release. *Res. Commun. Chem. Pathol. Pharmacol.* 37:305-311, 1982.
4. Beveridge, T., Gratwohl, A., Michot, F., Niederberger, W., and Nüesch, E. Cyclosporin A: Pharmacokinetics after a single dose in man and serum levels after multiple dosing in recipients of allogeneic bone-marrow grafts. *Curr. Ther. Res.* 30:5-16, 1981.
5. Beveridge, T., Maurer, W., Poole, T. W., Wiskott, E., and Wood, A. J. Cyclosporin in cadaveric renal transplantation: One year follow-up of a multicentre trial. *Lancet* 2: 986-989, 1983.
6. Blair, J. T., Thomson, A. W., Whiting, P. H., Davidson, R. J. L., and Simpson, J. G. Toxicity of the immune suppressant cyclosporin A in the rat. *J. Pathol.* 138:163-178, 1982.
7. Cunningham, C., Whiting, P. H., Burke, M. D., Wheatley, D. N., and Simpson, J. G. Increasing the hepatic metabolism of cyclosporine abolishes nephrotoxicity. In *Cyclosporine,* B. D. Kahan, ed. Grune and Stratton, New York, 1983, p. 496.
8. Daniels, N. J., Dover, J. S., and Schachter, R. K. Interaction between cyclosporin and rifampicin. *Lancet* 2:639, 1984.
9. Devineni, R., McKenzie, N., Keown, P., and Stiller, C. Renal effects of cyclosporine: Clinical and experimental observations. In *Cyclosporine,* B. D. Kahan, eds. Grune and Stratton, New York, 1983, p. 479.
10. Dieperink, H., and Starklint, H. Effect of cyclosporin A on ischaemically damaged rabbit kidneys. *Dan. Med. Bull.* 30:278-280, 1983.
11. Dieperink, H., Starklint, H., and Leyssac, P. P. Nephrotoxicity of cyclosporine–an animal model: Study of the nephrotoxic effect of cyclosporine on overall renal and tubular function in conscious rats. In *Cyclosporine,* B. D. Kahan, ed. Grune and Stratton, New York, 1983, p. 520.
12. Donatsch, P., Abisch, E., Homberger, M., Traber, R., Trapp, M., and Voges, R. A radioimmunoassay to measure cyclosporin A in plasma and serum samples. *J. Immunoassay* 2:19-32, 1981.
13. Duggin, G. G., Baxter, C. R., Hall, B. M., Horvath, J. S., and Tiller, D. J. Cyclosporin A–effects on renal renin and prostaglandins. *Hum. Toxicol.* (in press) 1984.
14. Dunn, M. J. Nonsteroidal antiinflammatory drugs and renal function. *Annu. Rev. Med.* 35:411-428, 1984.
15. Farthing, M. J. G., Clark, M. L., Pendry, A., Sloane, J., and Alexander, P. Nature of the toxicity of cyclosporin A in the rat. *Biochem. Pharmacol.* 30:3311-3316, 1981.
16. Ferguson, R. M., Sutherland, D. E. R., Simmons, R. L., and Najarian, J. S. Ketoconazole, cyclosporin metabolism, and renal transplantation. *Lancet* 2:882-883, 1982.
17. Gavin, M. P., Whiting, P. H., Simpson, J. G., Asfar, S. K., Heys, S. D., and Thomson, A. W. Renal function in rats treated with cyclosporin following unilateral nephrectomy. *Nephron* (in press).
18. Gerkens, J. F., Bhagwandeen, S. B., Dosen, P. J., and Smith, A. J. The effect of salt intake on cyclosporine-induced impairment of renal function in rats. *Transplantation* 38:412-417, 1984.
19. Gutsche, H. U., Delz, E., Lüneburg, M., Gnutzman, K. H., and Niedermayer, W. Effect of cyclosporine on the proximal tubular function of the rat kidney (abstract). *Kidney Internatl.* 26:637, 1984.
20. Hows, J. M., Yin, J. L., Chipping, P. M., Fairhead, S. M. Postgraft immunosuppression with cyclosporine in allogeneic bone marrow transplantation for severe aplastic anemia. In *Cyclosporine,* B. D. Kahan, ed. Grune and Stratton, New York, 1983, p. 418.

21. Keown, P. A., Laupacis, A., Carruthers, G., Stawecki, M., and Koegler, J. Interaction between phenytoin and cyclosporine following organ transplantation. *Transplantation* 38:304-305, 1984.
22. Klintmalm, G., Bohman, S. O., Stundelin, B., and Wilczek, H. Interstitial fibrosis in renal allografts after 12 to 46 months of cyclosporin treatment: Beneficial effect of low doses in early post-transplantation period. *Lancet* 2:950-953, 1984.
23. Makowka, L., Gilas, T., Hoffat, F., Falk, J. A., and Falk, R. E. The prevention of cyclosporine induced nephrotoxicity by 16, 16- dimethyl-prostaglandin E_2. *Transplant. Proc.* in press, 1984.
24. Maurer, G., Loosli, H. R., Schreier, E., and Keller, B. Disposition of cyclosporine in several animal species and man. *Drug Metabol. Dispos.* 12:120-126, 1984.
25. Merion, R. M., White, D. J. G., Thiru, S., Evans, D. B., and Calne, R. Y. Cyclosporine: Five years' experience in cadaveric renal transplantation. *N. Engl. J. Med.* 310:148-154, 1984.
26. Mihatsch, M. International workshop on cyclosporine nephropathy. *Clin. Nephrol.* *24*:107-119, 1985.
27. Mihatsch, M. J., Thiel, G., Spichtin, H. P., Harder, F., and Torhorst, J. Morphological findings in kidney transplants after treatment with cyclosporine. *Transplant. Proc.* 15: 2821-2821, 1983.
28. Neild, G. H., Rocchi, G., Imbert, L., Fumagalli, F., and Brown, Z. Effect of cyclosporine on prostacyclin synthesis by vascular tissue in rabbits. In *Cyclosporine,* B. D. Kahan, ed. Grune and Stratton, New York, 1983, p. 182.
29. Nussbaumer, K., Niederberger, W., and Keller, H. P. Determination of cyclosporin A in blood and plasma by column switching-HPLC after rapid sample preparation. *J. High Resol. Chromatogr. Chromatogr. Commun.* 5:424-427, 1982.
30. Oest, L. Effects of cyclosporin on prednisdone metabolism. *Lancet* 2:451, 1984.
31. Oyer, P. E., Stinson, E. B., Jamieson, S. W., Hunt, S. A., and Perlroth, M. Cyclosporine in cardiac transplantation. In *Cyclosporine,* B. D. Kahan, ed. Grune and Stratton, New York, 1983, p. 330.
32. Phelan, E. L., and Simpson, F. O. Grenetic hypertension in the rat. In *Hypertension in the Young and Old,* G. Onesti and K. E. Kim, eds. 1981, p. 92.
33. Porter, G. A., and Bennet, W. M. Nephrotoxic acute renal failure due to common drugs. *Am. J. Physiol.* 241:1-8, 1981.
34. Ryffel, B., Donatsch, P., Madörin, M., Matter, B. E., and Rüttimann, G. Toxicological evaluation of cyclosporin A. *Arch. Toxicol.* 53:107-141, 1983.
35. Ryffel, B., Siegl, H., Müller, A. M., and Mihatsch, M. J. Experimental cyclosporine nephrotoxicity: Risk of concomitant chemotherapy. IX Int. Congress of Nephrology 1984.
36. Scheuer, P. J. *Liver Biopsy Interpretation,* 3rd ed. Baillière, London, 1978.
37. Schurek, H. J., Neumann, K. H., Jesinghaus, W. P., Aeikens, B., and Wonigkeit, K. Single nephron function after heminephrectomy (HX) in rats with cyclosporine A (CyA). IX Int. Congress of Nephrology 1984.
38. Shulman, H., Striker, G., Deeg, H. J., Kennedy, M., and Storg, R. Nephrotoxicity of cyclosporin A after allogeneic marrow transplantation. *N. Engl. J. Med.* 305:1392-1395, 1981.
39. Siegl, H., and Ryffel, B. Effect of cyclosporine on renin-angiotensin-aldosterone system. *Lancet* 2:1274, 1982.
40. Siegl, H., Ryffel, B., Petric, R., Shoemaker, P., and Muller, A. Cyclosporine, the renin-angiotensin-aldosterone system, and renal adverse reactions. *Transplant. Proc.* 15:2719-2785, 1983.
41. Siegl, H., Ryffel, B., Petric, R., Donatsch, P., and Mihatsch, M. Cyclosporine nephrotoxicity in spontaneously hypertensive rats: The influence of sodium chloride. IX Int. Congress of Nephrology 1984.

42. Siegl, H., Ryffel, B., and Donatsch, P. The anesthetized, chlorisondamine (Ecolid) treated, spontaneously hypertensive rat (SHR) as a useful model to study cyclosporine A (CSA) nephrotoxicity. *Hum. Toxicol.* 3:418, 1984.
43. Stiller, C. R. A randomized clinical trial of cyclosporine in cadaveric renal transplantation. *N. Engl. J. Med.* 309:809-815, 1983.
44. Thiel, G., Harder, F., Loertscher, R., Brünisholz, M., and Landmann, J. Cyclosporin A used alone or in combination with low-dose steroids in cadaveric renal transplantation. *Klin. Wochenschr.* 61:991-1000, 1983.
45. Thiel, G., Torhorst, J., and Brunner, F. P. Renal toxicity of cyclosporin A in the rat. *Proc. Clin. Dial. Transplant. Forum* 10:62-65, 1980.
46. Thompson, J. F., Chalmers, D. H. K., Hunnisett, A. G. W., Wood, R. F. M., and Morris, P. J. Nephrotoxicity of Trimethoprim and cotrimoxazole in renal allograft recipients treated with cyclosporine. *Transplantation* 36:204-206, 1983.
47. Tune, B. M. Nephrotoxicity of cephalosporin antibiotics: Mechanisms and Modifying factors. In *Nephrotoxic Mechanisms of Drugs and Environmental Toxins,* G. A. Porter, ed. Plenum Medical Book Company, p. 151.
48. White, D. J. G., Blatchford, N. R., and Cauwenbergh, G. Cyclosporine and ketoconazole. *Transplantation* 37:214-215, 1984.
49. Whiting, P. H., Thomson, A. W., Blair, J. T., and Simpson, J. G. Experimental cyclosporine A nephrotoxicity. *Br. J. Exp. Pathol.* 63:88-94, 1982.
50. Whiting, P. H., Simpson, J. G., and Thomson, A. W. Nephrotoxicity of cyclosporine in combination with aminoglycoside and cephalosporin antibiotics. In *Cyclosporine,* B. D. Kahan, ed. Grune and Stratton, New York, 1983, p. 486.
51. Whiting, P. H., Cunningham, C., Thomson, A. W., and Simpson, J. G. Enhancement of high dose cyclosporine A toxicity by frusemide. *Biochem. Pharmacol.* 33:1075-1079, 1984.
52. von Willebrand, E., Häyry, P., and Ahonen, J. Differential diagnosis of cyclosporin (CyA) nephrotoxicity versus rejection by fine needle aspiration biopsy (FNAB), (abstract). *Kidney Int.* 24:418, 1983.
53. von Willebrand, E., and Häyry, P. Cyclosporine A deposits in renal allografts. *Lancet* 2:189-192, 1983.

19

ALLOGRAFT REJECTION IN RENAL ALLOGRAFT RECIPIENTS UNDER CYCLOSPORINE-PREDNISONE IMMUNOSUPPRESSIVE THERAPY

Barry D. Kahan, Charles T. Van Buren, Stuart M. Flechner, Carol A. Wideman, and Ronald H. Kerman
University of Texas Medical School at Houston, Houston, Texas

The introduction of cyclosporine (CsA), a cyclic endecapeptide of novel chemical structure, has improved the survival rate of renal allografts due to more effective immunosuppression than had been heretofore obtained with the purine analog azathioprine (Aza) [2]. Multicenter reports of the outcome of primary cadaveric renal allografts in patients under Aza-prednisone (Pred) by Opelz et al. [16] and MacDonald et al. [14] revealed less than half the primary cadaveric renal allografts were functioning at the end of the first postoperative year. On the other hand, Starzl et al. [18] demonstrated the benefit of the combination of CsA-Pred therapy, namely, 80% 1-year survival of cadaveric grafts. In the full report of his initial 66 consecutive renal allografts, Starzl et al. [19] noted 80.7% actuarial graft survival of primary and 60% of secondary grafts, with only two in the former and three in the latter group lost to rejection, although 50% of recipients underwent rejection therapy. Whereas administration of antithymocyte (ATG) [3] or antilymphoblast (ALS) globulin may achieve similar levels of 1-year graft survival as CsA-Pred, these regimens are associated with a higher incidence of rejection episodes (58% versus 31% of CsA patients, a highly significant difference), and pretransplant conditioning with bilateral nephrectomy, splenectomy, and 10 blood transfusions may be necessary [6,15].

The efficacy of CsA as a single immunosuppressive agent probably relates to its relatively selective effect to inhibit T-lymphocyte functions while sparing B cells and myeloid elements [1]. Furthermore, there appears to be inhibition of T-helper, with sparing of T-suppressor, cells in human renal allograft recipients [20]. Although particularly efficacious in animal models, the immunosuppressive potency of the drug may be limited by at least three factors: (1) failure to inhibit primed T cells, thus not impairing secondary responses [1]; (2) variable pharmacokinetics due to impaired absorption or enhanced drug elimination [9]; and (3) inconsistent pharmacodynamic action as has been assessed by the in vitro inhibitory activity of patient sera upon third-party mixed lymphocyte reactions by normal cells [17]. Therefore, as in the Aza era, rejection remains the most common cause of graft loss; however, its incidence, severity, and prognosis are attenuated by CsA therapy.

IMMUNOSUPPRESSIVE REGIMEN

A group of 300 consecutive patients receiving renal allografts under CsA immunosuppression from September 1980 through September 1984 included 90 living related donor (LRD) and 210 cadaveric donor (CD) recipients. All LRD transplants except 1 were first grafts, but 46 of 210 recipients of CD kidneys had received previous transplants. The CsA regimen began at 14 mg/kg orally each of the first 7 days supplemented with an intravenous 2.5 mg/kg slowly over 4 hr on the first 2 days. The immunosuppressive protocol tapered to 12 mg CsA per kilogram on days 8-14 and 10 mg/kg days 14-28, reaching 7 mg/kg by day 60 and 5 mg/kg by day 180. The CsA dose was reduced if trough serum CsA levels as determined by radioimmunoassay (RIA) exceeded 250 ng/ml in the presence of renal dysfunction [7]. Two initial Pred regimens were utilized, both beginning at 120 mg daily: the high-dose program tapered by 10 mg/day; the low-dose program tapered by 20 mg/day. The former regimen reached 30 mg at day 60, the latter at day 6. The former regimen reached 15 mg Pred at day 180, the latter at day 120. These regimens were compared in concurrent, overlapping fashion. Therapy for rejection episodes occurring during the first month included three (but for later episodes only one) 500-mg bolus of methylprednisolone followed by steroid recycling according to the high-dose regimen [8].

DIAGNOSIS OF ALLOGRAFT REJECTION EPISODES

Because of the complicating factor of CsA nephrotoxicity, the diagnosis of rejection is more difficult to establish in CsA than in Aza-treated patients. Our previous analysis [4] suggested that the following factors favor the diagnosis of rejection: >50% decreased urine output, reduced blood flow on ^{99m}technetium radionuclide renal scans, fever, and an abundant interstitial cellular infiltrate on renal biopsy. Almost every patient had a renal biopsy prior to institution of antirejection therapy. Although there are no absolute histopathologic features of rejection versus nephrotoxicity, certain patterns are suggestive. In cellular rejection there tends to be an intense lymphocytic cellular infiltrate, particularly invading tubules accompanied by marked edema. The CsA lesion in the first 30-60 days tends to show a slight and patchy lymphoid infiltrate, isometric tubular cell vacuolization, and calcification with only mild edema. The diagnosis of acute cellular rejection versus CsA nephrotoxicity is obfuscated by common factors: hypertension, reduced urinary sodium, decreased creatinine clearance, and tubular proteinuria. Acute humoral rejection and CsA arteriolopathy show numerous features in common with subendothelial deposits, granulocyte platelet aggregates, and fibrin thrombi. Further, the triggering of allograft thrombosis by thrombotic complications of CsA [21] imitates irreversible rejection. In addition, there remains considerable confusion to distinguish the chronic injury of CsA from that of rejection, due to the presence of interstitial fibrosis and glomerular sclerosis common to both. Since the determination of a "rejection" episode represents a complex, multifactorial decision, the clinical and histologic findings of all cases presented herein were reviewed by the entire team, in order to amend and correct previous analyses that had defined rejection solely based on the administration of steroid therapy. Of course, determination of the exact date of rejection was impossible; the days cited herein refer only to the date on which therapy was initiated.

INCIDENCE OF REJECTION

The 300 consecutive renal allografts performed and followed at this center for up to 4 years showed an overall mortality rate of 5.7%, including 2.2% in recipients of LRD and 7.1% for CD grafts (Table 1) [10]. Individual survival rates in patients with primary or retransplants, live or cadaver donors, and ages under 14 or over 55 years have been recently published [12]. None of the 16 recipients of HLA-identical kidneys under CsA therapy suffered a rejection episode, but one diabetic patient succumbed to fungal sepsis.

TABLE 1 Overall Results of 300 Renal Allografts Followed for 6-54 Months Recipients Treated with CsA-Pred

	LRD (total, n = 90)		CD (total, n = 210)		Total	
Causes of death						
Sepsis	2		11		13	
ASCVD	0		3		3	
Other	0		1		1	
Total	2	(2.2%)	15	(7.1%)	17	(5.7%)
Causes of graft loss						
Causes other than rejection						
Death	2		15		17	
Abandoned–sepsis	1		6		7	
Thrombosis	0		6		6	
Recurrent disease	1		1		2	
Technical	1		1		2	
Primary nonfunction	0		3		3	
Total	5		32		38	
Rejection related						
Rejection under CsA-Pred therapy:						
Hyperacute rejection	(0)		(6)		(6)	
Accelerated	(3)		(3)		(6)	
Early acute	(1)		(7)		(8)	
Delayed acute	(0)		(3)		(3)	
Chronic	(1)		(9)		(10)	
Total	5		28		33	
Prednisone withdrawal	2		0		2	
After conversion to Azathioprine	1		5		6	
Total grafts lost	13	(14%)	65	(31%)	78	(26%)

Although rejection was the major single cause of graft loss, namely, 41 cases, 53% of lost grafts and 14% of all grafts (Table 1), the majority of CsA-treated patients never experienced a rejection-related problem or were even treated with increased steroids, namely, 50.5% of the CD group and 56% of the LRD group. In addition to the 33 cases of loss due to allograft rejection under CsA-Pred therapy, 2 kidneys were lost after withdrawal of corticosteroids, according to a protocol described elsewhere [5], and 6 lost due to irreversible rejection after conversion to Aza for suspected CsA-induced nephrotoxicity. Among the grafts rejected in patients maintained on CsA-Pred, 5 were from haploidentical LRD and 28 from CD, reflecting a loss rate of 6 and 13%, respectively. The 47 recipients of multiple transplants showed 13 rejection losses (28% of the entire group): all 6 CD grafts lost to hyperacute rejection, 2 irreversible acute, 1 chronic rejection, and 4 of the 6 kidneys lost after conversion to Aza. On the other hand, the 253 primary transplant recipients included 20 cases of graft loss due to rejection (8% of the entire group), 16 deaths, 10 losses to sepsis, 5 thromboses, 2 technical errors, 1 recurrent disease, 1 primary nonfunction, and 1 lost to other causes. Thus, even under CsA therapy retransplantation is associated with a markedly increased risk of allograft loss due to rejection.

OVERALL CLINICAL FEATURES OF REJECTION

Hyperacute Form

There were six cases of hyperacute rejection, all of which occurred in retransplants and were refractory to corticosteroid therapy (Table 2). Hyperacute rejection was signaled by oliguria and fever in almost all cases. Although the vain hope that the impaired function was due to secondary acute tubular necrosis related to CsA delayed transplant nephrectomy in a few cases, most kidneys were removed within 1 month.

Accelerated Form

Of the 15 episodes of accelerated rejection, 6 (40%) were irreversible with steroid therapy and 7 reversible. This high rate of graft loss is consistent with the limited potency of CsA to affect primed T-helper cells. In addition, one patient erroneously diagnosed as accelerated rejection and treated with steroid therapy for secondary deterioration in renal function failed to improve and suffered lethal disseminated candidiasis. One patient's graft was abandoned without therapy due to obvious enteric infection. All six irreversible episodes occurred in primary graft patients; only one of the reversible episodes occurred in a secondary patient. Of the seven patients whose initial episode remitted, three suffered recurrent rejection episodes within the first 30 days, but only one of them emerged with unequivocal chronic rejection with compromised function in the second year. Patients suffering accelerated rejection tended to display prominent clinical features: weight gain most commonly followed by fever and never proteinuria. Radionuclide renal scans showed marked deterioration in renal blood flow in all cases.

Acute Form

Of the 44 patients suffering acute rejection episodes, 41 individuals were treated with only 8 (20%) having irreversible courses, and 33 (80%) were reversible with corticosteroid therapy. Only one of the lost grafts was from an LRD. Of the eight irreversible acute rejections, half occurred in secondary transplants, two of which were due to recurrent patient

TABLE 2 Types of Rejection Episodes Encountered in 300 Patients Under CsA-Pred Therapy

Type of rejection	Total number	Day	Reversed	Probable nephrotoxicity	Both	Lost	Abandoned
Hyperacute	6	0-2	0	0	0	6	0
Accelerated	15	3-5	7	1	0	6	1
Early acute	71	0-30	33	27	0	8	3
Delayed acute	16	30-60	6	5	2	3	0
Chronic	32	>60	17	1	4	10	0
Total	140		63	34	6	33	4

noncompliance leading to steroid-resistant rejection. Two primary graft patients experienced rejection concealed by the marginal function of their allografts, and the remaining two lost their grafts after an unfortunate delay in initiation of therapy due to confusion with nephrotoxicity

Of the 33 reversible episodes, 13 occurred in LRD and 20 in CD kidneys. There were almost always two and usually three major clinical features suggesting rejection: fever, graft swelling, greater than 50% decreased urine output, and weight gain were equal in prevalence. Because CsA administration may cause hypertension, this sign has little significance. Only 5 patients suffering acute rejection failed to show a significant decrease in blood flow upon renal scan. In 7 cases there were precipitating causes for the rejection episodes: overly enthusiastic reduction of CsA dosage to treat mild nephrotoxicity, or of prednisone dosage because of acute duodenal ulceration. In 1 case, transplant pyelonephritis appeared to trigger the process. Most acute rejections occurred during the second week (16 of 40), with 10 during the third, 6 during the fourth week, and 8 acute rejections by day 40. Following successful therapy, 6 patients showed a second acute rejection episode during the first year, and 3 individuals suffered frank chronic rejection by 8 months. A single patient had one recurrent, but almost totally reversed, rejection episode, and 2 patients suffered recurrent acute rejection episodes during the first year, leaving permanent residual deficits.

The major problem in the management of acute rejection in CsA-treated patients was a high incidence of misdiagnosis with consequent unnecessary steroid therapy. Misdiagnosis occurred in 8 LRD and 19 CD graft recipients, representing almost 10% of patients in each group. The cardinal features distinguishing pure nephrotoxicity were the combination of no response to steroid therapy with unequivocal improvement in renal function after CsA dose reduction, as observed in 12 patients, representing 18% of the 68 steroid-treated recipients. Contributing to the clinical picture of nephrotoxicity in the other 15 patients were latent cytomegalovirus (CMV) infections in 9 instances, other forms of sepsis (3 cases), acute tubular necrosis (1 case), and/or technical complications (2 cases). Of these 27 erroneously treated patients, intensified steroid therapy precipitated or unmasked frank septic episodes in 13 cases (48%), with 5 deaths, demonstrating the hazard of overtreatment of an adequately immunosuppressed patient. In an additional 3 patients, serious infection was noted at the time of diagnosis of rejection, increased steroid therapy was withheld, with survival of all patients but none of their grafts. Therefore since the risk of graft loss due to acute rejection is but 20% (8 of 41) and since the risk of significant morbidity or mortality by misdiagnosis is high (48%), caution must be exercised to firmly establish the diagnosis of rejection before initiation of increased corticosteroid therapy.

Delayed Acute Rejection

A group of 16 patients were treated for acute rejection episodes occurring between days 40 and 90. Of the three lost grafts, one patient had recurrent acute rejection crises and two patients experienced sudden irreversible deterioration of renal function between days 60 and 90; neither admitted noncompliance to the CsA regimen. Of 13 additional patients who received steroid therapy, 6 rejections were readily reversed without graft loss and 7 patients only showed improvement after CsA dose reduction. Retrospective analysis suggested 2 patients had combined rejection and nephrotoxicity, and 5 solely toxicity.

Chronic Form

After 3 months, only 32 patients, that is, 12% of the 266 grafts at risk, required rejection therapy. Only 4 patients experienced rejection episodes that had no antecedent cause: a previous rejection episode had occurred in the 8 cases who required retreatment, and 20 patients had noncompliance either due to self-discontinuation of drug administration (9 patients) or to overzealous drug tapering due to a misperception by the physician that renal dysfunction was due to nephrotoxicity rather than rejection (11 patients). After the first 90 days, 10 grafts were lost, namely, at 126, 226, 391, 422, 440, 456, 520, 568, 650, and 1041 days. Of these 10 grafts, patient noncompliance was associated with 3 instances, and iatrogenic underdosage due to overzealous attempts to improve modestly impaired renal function attributed to nephrotoxicity in 5 cases. In addition, reversible rejection episodes occurred in 17 other patients at 96, 106, 130, 143, 145, 151, 223, 275, 299, 306, 307, 353, 371, 385, 532, 548, and 1095 days. Among the reversed rejection episodes, only 5 patients were noncompliant to CsA therapy; 6 patients had iatrogenic decreased CsA doses. A single patient was noncompliant to steroid therapy. In 6 patients, insufficient immunosuppressive drugs could not be implicated. In addition, 5 treated patients did not obtain benefit from steroid therapy, but only 1 individual suffered a clinically overt, but reversible, CMV infection thereafter. The other 4 patients experienced some improvement in serum creatinine level after subsequent CsA dose reduction; however, they all had persistent dysfunction, suggesting an irreversible component of rejection and/or nephrotoxicity. There were few clinical features, including fever, change in graft size, tenderness, or altered urine output, a finding akin to that in Aza-treated patients.

RELATION OF REJECTION EPISODES TO SERUM TROUGH LEVELS

Because of the variable absorption and elimination of CsA, both serial trough values and pharmacokinetic profiles were performed, in order to identify patients at risk for a poor immunosuppressive effect. Half of the 10 patients experiencing accelerated rejection episodes during the first week displayed either impaired absorption or rapid elimination of CsA on pharmacokinetic analysis. However, 3 of these patients kept their grafts after steroid therapy of rejection, accompanied by readjustment of the CsA regimen. If the patient displayed poor absorption as assessed by bioavailability determinations after oral

TABLE 3 Correlation of Rejection Episodes and CsA Trough Levels

	Patients with serial trough levels[b]		
Rejection episode[a]	<100 ng/ml	>100 ng/ml	Total
+	7	15	22
–	9	87	96
Total	16	102	118[c]

[a]Rejection episode defined as any patient who underwent steroid recycling as antirejection therapy.
[b]Maximum trough level observed during first two weeks after transplantation.
[c]p value of significance by Fisher exact test <0.05.

and intravenous doses, the drug was delivered solely intravenously by continuous infusion until the oral bioavailability was documented to be above 10%. If the patient displayed rapid CsA elimination, the dosing frequency was increased to twice or thrice a day. In addition, 4 of the 6 cases of recurrent acute rejection displayed abnormalities either in CsA absorption or in CsA clearance, apparently related to coexistent administration of multiple medications.

Most patients in this series underwent serial therapeutic drug monitoring of daily serum trough CsA levels. Low values were demonstrated to predict rejection. First, the incidence of rejection progressively increased in patients with CsA levels <100 ng/ml for 5 days (10%), 10 days (20%), or >14 days (33%), suggesting that early adequate drug levels are necessary for effective prophylaxis of rejection. Second, there was a significant association between levels >100 ng/ml and absence of allograft rejection in a group of 118 patients who had serial CsA serum trough levels determined by RIA (Table 3).

IMMUNOLOGIC INDICES OF REJECTION

In order to detect early rejection with the first 40 days, each patient underwent serial posttransplant immune monitoring of the three indices: (1) T-cell subsets, determined by the reaction of OKT (Ortho) monoclonal antibodies as assessed by the fluorescence-activated cell sorter; (2) enumeration of actively rosetting T cells; and (3) measurement of spontaneous whole-blood blastogenesis, performed 5 days weekly during hospitalizations using methods previously described in detail [13]. Of the 300 patients, 239 had sufficient immune monitoring data to be useful. Table 4 shows the incidence of various immunologic findings in 34 acute allograft rejection episodes, 52 CsA-induced nephrotoxic episodes, 56 other complications, such as acute tubular necrosis, false corticosteroid therapy, blood transfusions, and infection, compared with 97 totally benign initial 30-day posttransplant courses. An increased T4/T8 ratio was the most useful single index (A.4 and B.4) to distinguish rejection from nephrotoxicity, from a benign course, or from the effects of other immunostimulatory conditions, such as infection or blood transfusion. Of interest was the low incidence of nephrotoxic patients who displayed elevated T4/T8 (8 of 52; 15%), consistent with the hypothesis that adequate CsA immunosuppression is associated with depressed T4/T8 ratios [20]. On the other hand, as a single index neither spontaneous blastogenesis nor the number of active or total T cells was helpful. Table 5 reveals that

TABLE 4 Correlation of Nonspecific Immunologic Monitoring Indices with Various Clinical Conditions Occurring During the First 40 Posttransplant Days

	Immune findings[b]				Clinical conditions			
	SB	AT	TT	4/8	Rejection n = 34	Nephrotoxicity n = 52	Benign n = 97	Other complications n = 56
A.	All ⊕ tests:							
1.	↑				79[a]	63	39	88
2.		↓			59	38	31	86
3.			↓		29	23	24	57
4.				↑	61	8	15	33
5.	↓				3	6	3	4
6.		↑			0	10	7	0
7.			↑		15	21	12	19
8.				↓	6	6	2	6
B.	Sole ⊕ test							
1.	↑				6	16	5	9
2.		↓			0	0	1	4
3.			↓		0	0	0	0
4.				↑	10	2	3	2
C.	Combinations of two tests							
1.	↑	↓			55	35	27	77
2.	↑		↓		27	18	22	54
3.	↑			↑	56	4	5	29
4.		↓	↓		29	21	22	57
5.		↓		↑	43	2	4	27
6.			↓	↑	29	2	5	20
D.	Combinations of three tests							
1.	↑	↓	↓		30	22	20	56
2.	↑		↓	↑	26	0	3	20
3.		↓	↓	↑	26	0	3	20
4.	↑	↓		↑	44	2	3	29
5.	↓	↑		↓	0	0	0	0

[a]Percentage of patients showing the change in immune index.
[b]SB = spontaneous blastogenesis, AT = activated T cells, TT = total T cells, 4/8 = T4/T8 ratio.

TABLE 5 Statistical Significance of Immunologic Indices to Distinguish Rejection Episodes from Other Posttransplant Conditions

Index[b]				Statistical significance distinguishing rejection from			
SB	AT	TT	4/8	Nephrotoxicity	Benign course	Infection	Blood transfusion
			↑	<0.005 (24.7)[a]	<0.005 (16.6)	<0.01 (7.8)	<0.005 (8.5)
↑				NS	<0.005 (10.5)	NS	NS
↑			↑	<0.005 (22.7)	<0.005 (20.9)	<0.005 (8.6)	NS
	↓		↑	<0.005 (18.7)	<0.005 (19.9)	NS	NS
		↓	↑	<0.005 (9.9)	NS	NS	NS
↑	↓			NS	NS	NS	NS
↑		↓	↑	<0.01 (7.8)	NS	NS	NS
	↓	↓	↑	<0.005 (8.0)	NS	NS	NS
↑	↓		↑	<0.005 (18.4)	<0.005 (19.2)	<0.025 (5.2)	NS

[a]p values determined upon 2 X 2 analysis by Fisher exact test (with χ^2 value in parentheses).
[b]Abbreviations as in Table 4.

the best combination of indices to distinguish rejection from quiescence was elevated spontaneous blastogenesis (↑ SB) with ↑ T4/T8 ($p < 0.005$, $\chi^2 = 20.9$). The combination of depressed (↓) active T and ↑ T4/T8 did not discriminate rejection from infection. The performance of hemodialysis treatments by themselves caused ↑SB ($p < 0.025$, $\chi^2 = 5.4$) and ↑SB with ↓ activated T cells (AT) ($p < 0.01$, $\chi^2 = 7.7$) without change in T4/T8 (data not shown). Infection was significantly associated with sole increases in total -T ($p < 0.005$, $\chi^2 = 9.6$), SB, ↓AT ($p < 0.025$, $\chi^2 = 5.6$), ↑SB with ↓AT ($p < 0.025$, $\chi^2 = 6.3$), but not with significant associative changes in SB alone or in T4/T8 ratios (Table 5). Thus, infection was best distinguished from rejection by the lack of ↑T4/T8 in patients with ↑SB ($p < 0.005$, $\chi^2 = 8.5$). The alloantigenic stimulus of a blood transfusion led to ↑SB, ↓AT, and ↑T4/T8 compared with quiescent patients at a $p < 0.005$ significance value ($\chi^2 = 10.7$) but was distinguished from rejection, although with greater difficulty, by the number of patients showing only ↑T4/T8 without changes in the other parameters ($p < 0.005$, $\chi^2 = 8.5$). In conclusion, ↑T4/T8 appears to be the best, although imperfect, immunologic index in the CsA-treated patient with a 39% false-negative rate (Table 4, A.4) and a 20% (37 of 205) false-positive rate.

COMMENTS

The results reported herein clearly reflect the first stages of developing a rational strategy toward CsA patient management. They reveal several issues requiring further assessment: first, the pharmacology of CsA must be better understood to predict aberrant reactions of some patients on a pharmacokinetic or a pharmacodynamic basis. Because of the ability to measure CsA and a limited range of its metabolites, and because the mechanism of action of CsA on interleukin-2 generation is now appreciated, there should be a unique opportunity to precisely assess drug action. Second, there is a need to develop exact criteria to discern nephrotoxicity from other causes of renal dysfunction. Isolated reports estimating CsA content in renal biopsies or claiming the differential diagnostic import of enzymuria have not been confirmed. The diagnosis remains a clinical impression. In the appropriate setting, T4/T8 ratios seem helpful, although not always reliable: a persistently low ratio is rarely seen in patients suffering allograft rejection. The third area for further investigation is the most appropriate therapy of rejection in the CsA-treated patient, specifically the question of whether antilymphocyte sera affords rejection reversal and is steroid sparing. Thus although CsA has markedly reduced the incidence of rejection, better understanding of this complication is a compelling problem due to difficulties in discerning it from nephrotoxicity and the high penalty of erroneous therapy.

Since CsA appears to have the potential to provide effective control of early rejection episodes, it affords an interval for the implementation of strategies to achieve donor-specific unresponsiveness. In the prior era of Aza therapy, the almost inevitable occurrence of an early acute rejection episode demanded that immunosuppressive strategies achieve not only durable, but also early, control of alloimmunity. The capacity of CsA to forestall this serious complication should provide the necessary time even in cadaver donor transplantation to engineer the host's immune system to accept the graft. In experimental systems, multiple immunologic vectors have been demonstrated to prolong allograft survival, such as suppressor T cells, anti-idiotypic antibodies, and immunodepletion with irradiation. Induction of a true unresponsive state might reduce the dosage or mitigate the need for chronic CsA therapy, thereby minimizing the long-term complications of nephrotoxicity, hepatotoxicity, and predilection to infection and neoplasia. Therefore, continued research should in the future reduce CsA to a drug exploited in short-term use for the prophylaxis of allograft rejection.

SUMMARY

Experience with allograft rejection in 300 consecutive renal allograft recipients followed for up to 4 years reveals not only a modest incidence of graft loss due to rejection (11%), but also a low incidence (32%) of rejection episodes requiring steroid therapy. These estimates include 22 patients noncompliant to CsA therapy due to gastrointestinal or other side effects (11 patients) or due to inappropriate physician reduction of the dosage (11 patients). Therefore, CsA affords effective prophylaxis of rejection. At least half of the accelerated and early acute rejection episodes occur in patients displaying poor pharmacokinetic or pharmacodynamic responses to CsA. Therefore, a prospective trial is underway to assess whether early recognition of these abnormalities prevents or reduces the severity of rejection episodes. Indeed, the generally excellent level of immunosuppression presents a particularly great hazard of 48% incidence of sepsis if intensified steroid therapy is administered due to an erroneous diagnosis of rejection. With the effective early control of rejection afforded by CsA, renewed attention can now be directed to immunologic engineering approaches leading to true allogeneic unresponsiveness.

REFERENCES

1. Borel, J. F. Comparative study of in vitro and in vivo drug effects on cell-mediated cytotoxicity. *Immunology* 31:631-641, 1976.
2. Calne, R. Y., Rolles, K., Thiru, S., McMaster, P., Craddock, G. N., Azia, S., White, D. J. G., Evans, D. B., Dunn, D. C., Henderson, R. G., and Lewis, P. Cyclosporin A

initially as the only immunosuppressant in 34 recipients of cadaveric organs: 32 kidneys, 2 pancreases, and 2 livers. *Lancet* 1:1033-1036, 1979.

3. Filo, R. S., Smith, E. J., and Leapman, S. B. Reversal of acute renal allograft rejection with adjunctive ATG therapy. *Transplant. Proc.* 13:482-491, 1981.
4. Flechner, S., Van Buren, C. T., Kerman, R. H., and Kahan, B. D. The nephrotoxicity of cyclosporine in renal transplant recipients. *Transplant. Proc.* 15(4):2689-2694, 1983.
5. Flechner, S. M., Kerman, R. H., Van Buren, C. T., Epps, L., and Kahan, B. D. The use of cyclosporine in living related renal transplantation: Donor specific hyporesponsiveness and steroid withdrawal. *Transplantation* 38:685-691, 1984.
6. Halloran, P. F., Lien, J., Aprile, M., and White, N. Preliminary results of a randomized comparison of cyclosporine and Minnesota and antilymphoblast globulin. *Transplant. Proc.* 14:627-630, 1982.
7. Kahan, B. D., Van Buren, C. T., Lin, S., Ono, Y., Agostino, G., LeGrue, S. J., Boileau, M., Payne, W. D., and Kerman, R. H. Immunopharmacologic monitoring of cyclosporin A treated recipients of cadaveric kidney allografts. *Transplantation* 34:36-45, 1982.
8. Kahan, B. D., and Peters, C. Transplantation of organs. In *Lewis Practice of Surgery*, H. Goldsmith, ed. Harper and Row, Hagerstown, Maryland, 1983, pp. 1-38.
9. Kahan, B. D., Ried, M., and Newburger, J. Pharmacokinetics of cyclosporine in human renal transplantation. *Transplant. Proc.* 15:446-453, 1983.
10. Kahan, B. D., Van Buren, C., Flechner, S., Payne, W. D., Boileau, M., and Kerman, R. Cyclosporine immunosuppression mitigates immunologic risk factors in renal allograft transplantation. *Transplant. Proc.* 15(4):2469-2478, 1983.
11. Kahan, B. D., Van Buren, C. T., Flechner, S., Jarowenko, M., Yasumura, T., Rogers, A. J., Yoshimura, N., LeGrue, S., Drath, D. B., and Kerman, R. H. Clinical and experimental studies using cyclosporine in renal transplantation. *Surgery* 97:125-140, 1985.
12. Kahan, B. D., Kerman, R. H., Wideman, C. A., Flechner, S. M., Jarowenko, M., and Van Buren, C. T. Impact of cyclosporine on renal transplant practice at the University of Texas Medical School at Houston. *Am. J. Kidney Dis.* 5:288-295, 1985.
13. Kerman, R. H., and Kahan, B. D. Immunological evaluation of transplant rejection: Pre and postoperative indices detecting immune responsiveness. *Ann. Clin. Res.* 13: 244-263, 1981.
14. MacDonald, J. C., Vaughn, W., Filo, R. S., Picon, G. M., Niblack, G., Spees, E. K., and Williams, G. M. Cadaver donor renal transplantation by centers of the southeastern organ procurement foundation. *Ann. Surg.* 193:1-8, 1981.
15. Najarian, J. S., Ferguson, R. M., Sutherland, D. E. R., Rynasiewicz, J. J., and Simmons, R. L. A prospective trial of the efficacy of cyclosporine in renal transplantation at the University of Minnesota. *Transplant. Proc.* 15:438-441, 1983.
16. Opelz, G., Mickey, M. R., and Terasaki, P. I. HLA matching and cadaver transplant survival in North America. *Transplantation* 23:490-497, 1977.
17. Rogers, A. J., Yoshimura, N., Kerman, R. H., and Kahan, B. D. Immunopharmacodynamic evaluation of cyclosporine-treated renal allograft recipients. *Transplantation* 38:657-664, 1984.
18. Starzl, T. E., Weil, R. III, Iwatsuki, S., Klintmalm, G., Schroter, G. P. J., Koep, L. J., Iwaki, Y., and Terasaki, P. I. The use of cyclosporin A and prednisone in cadaver kidney transplantation. *Surg. Gynecol. Obstet.* 151:17-26, 1980.
19. Starzl, T. E., Klintmalm, G. B. G., Weil, R. III, Porter, K. A., Iwatsuki, S., Schroter, G. P. J., Fernandez-Bueno, C., and MacHugh, N. Cyclosporin A and steroid therapy in sixty-six cadaver kidney recipients. *Surg. Gynecol. Obstet.* 153:486-494, 1981.

20. Van Buren, C., Kerman, R., Agostino, G., Payne, W., Flechner, S., and Kahan, B. D. The cellular target of cyclosporin A action in humans. *Surgery* 92:167-174, 1982.
21. Van Buren, D., Van Buren, C. T., Flechner, S. M., Maddox, A. M., Verani, R., and Kahan, B. D. De novo hemolytic uremic syndrome in renal transplant recipients immunosuppressed with cyclosporine. *Surgery* 98:54-62, 1985.

20

NEPHROTOXICITY OF CYCLOSPORIN A

Paul A. Keown, Calvin R. Stiller, and A. Cameron Wallace
University Hospital, University of Western Ontario, London, Ontario, Canada

In contradistinction to conventional immunosuppressive agents, cyclosporin A (CsA) does not limit global myeloproliferation but inhibits the immune response by a direct effect on helper/inducer T-cell function [29]. At this level, the production of colony stimulating factor (CSF) and interleukin-1 and 2 is inhibited, interrupting cell-cell communication, and the liberation of lymphokines such as macrophage migration-inhibition factor (MIF), macrophage-activating factor (MAF), and macrophage procoagulant activity (MPCA) is impaired, limiting amplification of the inflammatory response [82,89]. This unique selectivity renders CsA particularly attractive for manipulation of the immune response in the intact organism.

In vivo studies have confirmed the potent immunosuppressive effect of CsA observed in vitro. Antibody formation and cell-mediated immunity were effectively inhibited in all species examined, and CsA was highly effective in preventing allograft rejection following skin, solid organ, or bone marrow transplantation without myelosuppression [5,8,28]. Concomitant toxicologic studies demonstrated that CsA possessed a high therapeutic/toxic ratio. Renal toxicity was evident in rodents only at high doses, exceeding by sixfold those required to induce immunosuppression, and consisted of mild vacuolization and degeneration of epithelial cells in the proximal renal tubules. Studies in the dog and primate using doses of CsA up to 200 mg/kg per day revealed no biochemical or histologic evidence of organotoxicity [64].

The nephrotoxicity observed upon initial use of CsA in humans was thus both unexpected and disappointing. Following cadaveric renal transplantation, the incidence and duration of initial graft nonfunction were increased and glomerular filtration was compromised in those grafts in which function was established [6]. Disorders of tubular function characterized by hyperkalemia and renal tubular acidosis were accompanied by histologic evidence of tubular epithelial cell damage, and nephrotoxicity was occasionally so severe following bone marrow transplantation as to produce complete and irreversible cessation of renal function, necessitating hemodialysis [13].

With increasing experience in the use of CsA, however, and the adoption of lower and more appropriate dosage schedules, the incidence and severity of renal damage have diminished appreciably. The introduction of therapeutic drug monitoring, enabling direct measurement of CsA concentrations in the blood compartment by radioimmunoassay (RIA) or high-performance liquid chromatography (HPLC), has considerably facilitated therapy, permitting individualization of treatment to reflect the variation in bioavailability and metabolism and minimize the risk of overdosage [35,38,85]. The adverse effect of CsA on the kidney, however, remains an intriguing and important consideration in the clinical use of this highly effective immunosuppressant. In this chapter we will review the etiology, pathogenesis, and morphology of this effect, define those risk factors that predispose to or accentuate the nephrotoxicity of CsA, and examine the therapeutic strategies available for minimization of such renal toxicity.

PATHOGENESIS OF CYCLOSPORINE NEPHROTOXICITY

Despite the clinical importance of CsA nephrotoxicity, no satisfactory unifying mechanism has been established to explain this complication. Rather, the diversity of functional and histologic changes observed suggest that CsA has a multifactorial influence, producing an alteration in renal hemodynamics, accelerated platelet activation on the vessel wall and causing direct renal tubular cell toxicity (Table 1). These physiologic effects underlie the acute functional changes observed on administration of CsA, while progression to chronic nephropathy is determined by the interaction of multiple risk factors, among which the dosage and duration of administration are of critical importance.

Physiologic Effects

Studies in the experimental animal and in the human indicate that CsA has a dose-dependent effect upon renal function. In excess of a certain threshold, CsA results in a marked reduction of glomerular filtration with oliguria, an elevation in the ratio of blood urea nitrogen (BUN) to creatinine, and the virtual disappearance of sodium from the urine, reflecting increased proximal tubular reabsorption [15,17]. This functional effect is rapidly reversible upon drug withdrawal, suggesting an acute alteration in glomerular capillary perfusion. Studies in the rat and dog using radiolabeled microspheres have shown that CsA causes an acute decrease in both renal cortical and medullary blood flow, which is sustained throughout the duration of treatment [46,58]. Decreased perfusion also occurs in other vital organs, predominantly the pancreas, liver, and lung, although it is not a ubiquitous feature [46,58]. Investigations conducted by Myers et al. suggest that these observations may pertain also in humans; renal plasma flow is significantly diminished in CsA-treated cardiac allograft recipients with renal functional impairment [53].

Regulation of renal blood flow is dependent upon a complex interaction between several systems. The first of these and most carefully examined has been the renin-angiotensin-aldosterone system (RAAS) [44]. Renin, secreted by the juxtaglomerular apparatus of the juxtamedullary glomeruli, acts upon the hepatic-derived α_{II}-globulin angiotensinogen to form the decapeptide angiotensin I, which in turn is cleaved to the nonapeptide angiotensin II. This hormone has a potent direct vasoconstrictor effect on the preglomerular afferent arteriole, reducing glomerular blood flow and, hence, glomerular filtration [44]. In the spontaneously hypertensive rat, CsA has a dose-dependent, bidirectional effect upon plasma renin activity (PRA), producing maximum stimulation at a dose of 20 mg/kg per day with a subsequent decrease to baseline at high doses [71]. Plasma aldosterone is also increased, although this effect is not sustained and observed only at higher doses (100 mg/kg per day). In the dog, CsA also causes an acute increase in PRA, although whether this is sustained is not yet known [71]. In the human, hyperreninemia accom-

TABLE 1 Mechanisms of Action and Physiologic Consequences of CsA on the Kidney

Physiologic mechanism	Site of action	Physiopathologic effect
1. Vasoconstriction: PG/TxA_2 imbalance or RAAS activation	Renal cortical and medullary vessels	Azotemia, antidiuresis, antinatriuresis, hyperkalemia, hypertension
2. Platelet activation: PSF depletion and TxA_2 production	Afferent arterioles and glomerular capillaries	Platelet clumping, endovascular microthrombus formation, fibrin deposition
3. Direct toxicity: direct effect or inhibition of mitochondrial respiration	Straight and convoluted proximal	Diuresis, natriuresis, tubular cell vacuolization and death, azotemia

panies the acute renal insufficiency observed immediately following cardiac transplantation with CsA, but long-term CsA administration is in general characterized by low levels of plasma renin [16].

Closely linked to the RAAS in regulation of renal blood flow is the prostaglandin-thromboxane system [30]. Prostaglandins are unsaturated fatty acid compounds derived from 20-carbon essential fatty acids, the most important of these precursors in the human being arachidonic acid. Prostaglandins are ubiquitous in their distribution throughout the body and are produced at many sites within the kidney at the level of both cortex and medulla [43]. These compounds participate in several physiologic processes within the kidney, including autoregulation of renal blood flow and glomerular filtration, modulation of renin release, tubular ion transport, and water metabolism [43]. Prostaglandins PGE_2, PGD_2, and PGI_2 are potent vasodilators, modulating tone in the pre- and postglomerular arterioles to reduce total renal resistance and increase renal blood flow [27]. Glomerular filtration increases in parallel, and both fractional water and sodium excretion are enhanced due to decreased reabsorption in the proximal tubule [66]. Prostaglandins, particularly PGD_2, PGE_2, and PGI_2, play an important role in mediating renal renin release, thus resetting vasomotor tone and facilitating sodium and potassium exchange in the distal nephron through enhanced aldosterone production [94]. In contrast, other metabolites of arachidonic acid appear to exert opposing effects. Thromboxane A_2 (TxA_2) is a potent vasoconstrictor in many tissues and may contribute to the intense renovascular constriction and impaired glomerular filtration observed in many pathologic states [50,93].

Vasodilatory prostaglandin act locally within the kidney to prevent a deleterious effect of vasoconstriction on renal function, particularly under conditions of volume depletion, hyperreninemia, and diminution of functional renal reserve [43]. Under such conditions, inhibition of prostaglandins synthesis by indomethacin or other nonsteroidal anti-inflammatory drugs causes an acute decrease in renal perfusion and glomerular filtration, accompanied by oliguria with a decreased fractional sodium excretion, hyporeninemic hypoaldosteronism with decreased sodium-potassium exchange in the distal nephron and consequent hyperkalemia, and hypertension [12,18,43]. These physiologic changes are identical to those observed following low-dose CsA administration, and the parallel kinetics of functional deterioration and recovery following drug withdrawal are compatible with a common pathogenic mechanism. Cyclosporin A has been shown to suppress prostaglandin synthesis in vitro by inhibition of phospholipase A_2 activity [19]. In vivo, CsA decreases prostaglandin production in renal cortical slices and inhibits prostacyclin production by blocking the generation of prostacyclin-stimulating factor [57]. In addition, we have shown that thromboxane synthesis is enhanced in the CsA-treated experimental animal with acute impairment of renal function [58]. These observations thus support the concept that the acute and reversible functional changes accompanying CsA nephrotoxicity result from a decrease in renal glomerular capillary perfusion secondary to a disturbance of the balanced interaction among individual arachidonate metabolites.

In addition to its vasoconstrictor properties, TxA_2 is a strong inducer of platelet aggregation, an effect directly antagonized by vasodilatory prostaglandins, particularly PGI_2 [31]. A failure of vascular PGI_2 synthesis has been demonstrated in patients with the hemolytic uremic syndrome and eclampsia, disorders characterized histologically by acute renal failure with platelet clumping and microthrombosis [87]. In the rabbit, Neild et al. have shown that CsA treatment causes depletion of prostacyclin-stimulating factor in the serum [57], and subsequent vessel wall injury by immune complexes or endotoxin precipitates microvascular thrombosis and acute vasculopathy [55]. It is conceivable that the acute vasculopathy observed in the human in the immediate posttransplant period is precipitated by a similar imbalance between endovascular PGI_2 and TxA_2 production and that the progressive vascular damage with intimal injury and luminal occlusion seen later posttransplant may reflect continuing low-grade platelet activation on the vessel wall.

It is clear, however, that the effects of CsA on the kidney are not explained entirely by platelet activation or a reversible decrease in renal blood flow. The enzymuria, progressive loss of concentrating ability and renal tubular sodium reabsorption, and epithelial vacuolization and cell death in the convoluted and straight segments of the proximal tubule observed with the administration of high doses of CsA indicate a direct toxic effect on the renal tubule analogous to that produced by known direct nephrotoxins [14,74]. Cyclosporin A is taken up into the tubular cell (although the mechanism of this still remains unknown), where toxic damage may occur via two potential mechanisms. Cyclosporin A may accumulate in the lysosomes within the epithelial cell, resulting in loss of lysosomal integrity with the accumulation of intracellular toxins, or saturation of lysosomal storage with accumulation of CsA in the cytosol where it could effect other intracellular organelles [60]. Second, CsA may impair proximal tubular cell respiration by inhibition of oxidative phosphorylation through uncoupling of electron transport and by blocking of mitochondrial electron transport and dinitrophenyl (DNP)-uncoupled respiration [73].

Progressive Renal Injury

Continuing renal damage in patients receiving CsA is characterized by progressive deterioration in glomerular filtration, frequently accompanied by hypertension of increasing severity. Proteinuria is absent or of tubular origin, and continuing tubular damage is further emphasized by a persistent elevation in urinary enzyme excretion and impairment of tubular acidification [1]. Characteristic structural changes accompany this progressive functional deterioration. Vasculopathy is evident, with intimal proliferation, luminal narrowing, and medial hypertrophy and sclerosis. In addition, chronic tubulointerstitial damage is observed with epithelial cell vacuolization, tubular atrophy, and diffuse interstitial fibrosis [78].

Elucidation of the mechanisms involved in this progression is difficult in the absence of a satisfactory experimental model. Clinical and histologic evidence in humans, however, permit the development of an operational hypothesis. Persistent renal vasoconstriction and sodium retention, triggered by the physiologic events previously described, lead to sustained low-renin hypertension. This, in combination with chronic endothelial damage of immunologic origin or due to low-grade platelet activation on the vessel wall secondary to dysregulation of prostaglandin-thromboxane metabolism, results in ischemia of the renal parenchyma with characteristic degenerative changes in the nephron and interstitium. Concomitant and synergistic tubular toxicity in the presence of high concentrations of CsA, indicated by persistent functional and histologic evidence of tubular damage, results in atrophic degeneration of the nephron and progressive interstitial fibrosis.

CLINICAL SYNDROMES ASSOCIATED WITH CsA NEPHROTOXICITY

Careful analysis of the effect of CsA on the native and allografted kidney indicates that four discrete clinicopathologic syndromes may be discerned: (1) delayed renal allograft function, (2) acute, reversible renal functional impairment, (3) acute vasculopathy, and (4) chronic nephropathy with interstitial fibrosis.

Delayed Renal Allograft Function

The detrimental effect of CsA on initial graft function following renal allotransplantation was reported in initial pilot studies of this drug, with an apparent increase in the incidence of delayed function due to acute tubular necrosis (ATN) ranging from 19 to 40% and acute secondary oliguria in up to 30% of cases [6,7,67]. The clinical impact of this effect was so impressive that establishment of initial diuresis was considered essential in some centers prior to commencement of CsA therapy [6]. The comparative incidence and duration of delayed graft function following renal transplantation in controlled studies is shown in Table 2. There is a wide center-to-center variation in initial nonfunction rate in patients receiving nonnephrotoxic conventional immunosuppressive agents (12-60%) [9,21,24,68, 80], reflecting among other factors the harvesting technique employed and the type and duration of organ storage. The range of initial nonfunction in patients receiving CsA is similarly broad (19-83%), but there is a clear trend toward a higher incidence of nonfunction in these patients [9,21,24,68,80]. No controlled data are currently available to demonstrate convincingly that the duration of nonfunction is prolonged in patients receiving CsA. However, the accumulating evidence provided by individual patients with protracted graft nonfunction in whom conversion to alternative immunosuppression was followed almost immediately by brisk diureses and establishment of satisfactory graft function strongly supports the clinical impression that CsA delays recovery from vasomotor nephropathy, perhaps by a mechanism related to inhibition of prostaglandin secretion [63].

Analysis of the randomized study performed by the Canadian Multicentre Transplant Study Group (CMTSG) defined certain risk factors that predisposed to delayed graft function in patients receiving CsA [9,68]. The subgroup of patients who received a kidney with a long machine perfusion time (>24 hr) had an incidence of initial nonfunction of 77%, compared with 29% in those in whom the perfusion time was less than 24 hr. The incidence of initial graft nonfunction was also higher in patients in whom the surgical reanastomosis time exceeded 45 min (59%) compared with those with shorter reanastomosis time (44%). In patients who received a kidney perfused more than 24 hr, the incidence of nonfunction was unrelated to the serum CsA level achieved postoperatively. When the perfusion time was less than 24 hr, however, the mean serum trough level of CsA during the first 3 days

TABLE 2 Incidence and Duration of Initial Graft Nonfunction Following Renal Transplantation in Patients Receiving Cyclosporine or Conventional Immunosuppression

		Incidence (%)			Duration	
Study		CIS[a]	CsA	Δ	CIS	CsA
Basel	62	19	20	+1	(6)[b]	(7)
Minneapolis	100	12	19	+7	23.5[c]	23.0
Houston	114	22	28	+6	(4)	(4)
Birmingham	70	40	44	+4	(2.0)	(2.6)
Canada	210	39	52	+13	10.7	15.8
Australia	60	60	83	+23	13.0	23.0

[a]Conventional immunosuppression.
[b]Mean number of dialyses.
[c]Days.

TABLE 3 Incidence of Initial Graft Nonfunction and Graft Survival in Relation to Duration of Hypothermic Graft Storage in Patients Receiving Cyclosporine

	Primary graft			Multiple graft		
Duration of cold storage (hr)	Number	INF (%)[a]	GS (%)[b]	Number	INF (%)	GS (%)
0-12	82	29	82	23	52	78
12-24	96	24	87	22	59	62
24-36	26	35	81	5	100	40
36	9	44	44	0	–	–

[a]Initial nonfunction.
[b]Graft survival, 3 months.
Source: Derived from Beltizsky et al. [50].

after transplantation correlated closely with the incidence of nonfunction: with mean serum trough levels of less than 200 ng/ml, less than 20% of kidneys exhibited initial graft nonfunction, whereas the incidence of anuria rose to over 50% with CsA levels in excess of 400 ng/ml.

The influence of simple hypothermic storage upon graft function and viability was examined in an expanded subset of the pooled CMTSG data by Belitzsky et al. [3]. As shown in Table 3, the incidence of initial nonfunction was low (<30%) in first renal graft recipients in whom the kidney was stored in the cold for less than 24 hr and graft survival was excellent, exceeding 80%. With longer storage, however, the incidence of initial nonfunction increased, and graft survival was decreased in those kidneys stored for greater than 36 hr by this method. The incidence of initial graft nonfunction in patients receiving second or subsequent transplants was unexpectedly high, exceeding 52% even with kidneys stored for less than 24 hr.

TABLE 4 Influence of Initial Graft Function on Graft Survival in Patients Receiving Cyclosporine: Primary Cadaver Grafts Stored by Simple Hypothermia or Pulsatile Perfusion

Method of graft storage	Initial function		Initial nonfunction	
	Number	GS (%)[a]	Number	GS (%)
Hypothermic storage	153	87	60	71
Pulsatile perfusion	81	90	35	62

[a]Graft survival, 3 month.
Source: Derived from Belitzsky et al. [50].

Although graft function is ultimately established in the majority of patients, primary graft nonfunction is not entirely benign. Patient management is rendered more complex by the need for repeated dialysis, and clinical indices of graft rejection are eliminated, rendering early diagnosis more difficult and increasing the possibility of irreversible graft damage from this process. Patients with initial graft nonfunction had a longer hospital stay (44 versus 30 days, $P = 0.005$), an increased number of treated "rejection episodes" (1.29 versus 0.80, $P = 0.001$), and a higher cumulative steroid dose (2.74 versus 1.56 g, $P = 0.005$) [76]. Serum creatinine 6 months posttransplantation was also higher than in those patients with initial graft function (208 ± 83 versus 171 ± 62 μM) [76]. Of greater concern, however, is the apparent adverse influence of initial nonfunction upon subsequent graft survival, an effect independent of storage modality (Table 4). In primary graft recipients who had initial function posttransplant, 3-month graft survival exceeded 87%, whereas survival was between 62 and 71% in those whose function was delayed [3].

Acute Reversible Renal Functional Impairment

In the experimental animal, administration of immunosuppressive doses of CsA causes a fall in glomerular filtration, urine volume, and fractional excretion of sodium and potassium with consequent hyperkalemia [15,17]. With increasingly toxic doses (50 mg/kg), despite continuing impairment of GFR, sodium excretion increases accompanied by polyuria, and there is evidence of severe renal tubular injury [17,58].

The counterpart of these effects is observed in the human kidney. Acute impairment in renal function in patients receiving CsA following bone marrow transplantation was first reported by Powles et al. [62]. In these patients, CsA was often used in high doses (20 mg/kg per day) parenterally, often in combination with other known nephrotoxins, and renal functional impairment was characteristically observed with enormously high CsA serum levels, exceeding 1000 ng/ml [13,62]. Renal functional impairment was occasionally dramatic, requiring dialysis, and sometimes protracted or irreversible [13,62]. In the cardiac allograft recipient, acute oliguria frequently occurs within the first 96 hr posttransplant, characterized by avid renal tubular sodium reabsorption and a urinary sodium less than 5 mmol/liter (Figure 1) [16]. Oliguria is normally self-limiting, with normal urine volumes re-established by day 5. Peak serum creatinine posttransplant coincides temporally with peak serum CsA levels during the first week, but no direct correlation between the two is demonstrable. In contrast, the deterioration in renal function correlates most closely with impaired renal function prior to cardiac transplantation, sug-

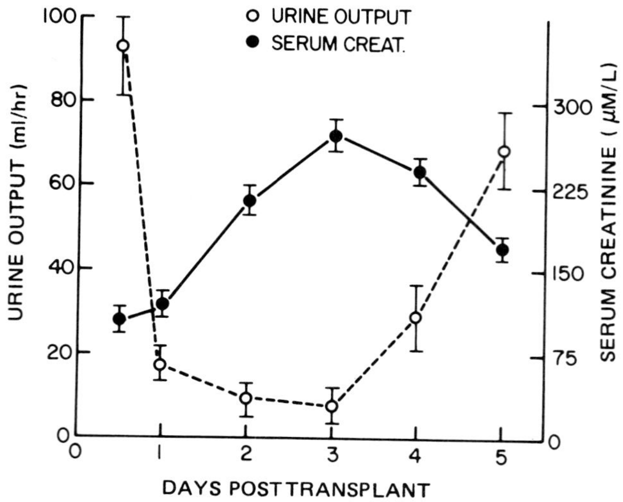

FIGURE 1 Acute reversible renal insufficiency following cardiac transplantation in patients receiving CsA. (Courtesy Dr. N. F. McKenzie.)

gesting that those with inadequate renal reserve are most susceptible to the functional deterioration precipitated by this drug. Acute renal dysfunction has also been reported following hepatic transplantation, particularly with the use of intravenous CsA [61].

Although acute CsA nephrotoxicity in the transplanted kidney is characterized by similar pathophysiologic events, the use of lower doses of CsA has gradually modified the clinical presentation. The GFR decreases slowly and progressively: the mean daily increase in serum creatinine with acute toxicity in the first month is 38 ± 30 μM although in later periods the rate of rise is proportionately slower [41]. Many episodes of acute toxicity are accompanied by only a small change in urinary volume, with oliguria occurring in less than 10% of cases. Weight gain is uncommon, as is hypertension or fever [41]. Renal dysfunction is accompanied by hyperchloremia, hyperkalemia, and increased urinary excretion of *N*-acetyl β-glucosaminidase.

The relationship between acute CsA nephrotoxicity and blood levels of the drug has been the subject of much debate. However, acute nephrotoxicity is generally observed in association with rising or elevated serum CsA levels exceeding 200 ng/ml, and is frequent with levels exceeding 400 ng/ml [35,37]. Toxicity due to CsA alone is rarely observed in the early posttransplant period with serum CsA levels of less than 200 ng/ml [35,37].

The nephrotoxicity of CsA may be enhanced by drug interactions, of which two broad groups may be defined. Pharmacokinetic interactions result in the accumulation of CsA due to impairment of metabolism or elimination. Such an effect is produced by the antifungal agent ketoconazole [23], which inhibits microsomal oxidase activity, and erythromycin, by a similar potential effect. Although it has not been unequivocally established, cimetidine may exert a similar action by a direct inhibition of hepatic cytochrome P_{450} enzyme activity, or by reduction in hepatic blood flow resulting in a global decrease in drug metabolism. Hepatic dysfunction secondary to pharmacologic or other agents may exert a similar effect. Pharmacodynamic interactions, in contrast, result from a synergistic toxicity at the level of the end organ. Such interactions have been described with aminoglycoside antibiotics, trimethoprim, vancomycin, amphotericin B, and furosemide and, as we have observed, with nonsteroidal anti-inflammatory drugs [34,36,83,91, 92].

Distinction between CsA nephrotoxicity and acute rejection is frequently difficult in the transplanted kidney. The characteristic clinical features of rejection are muted in patients receiving CsA, such that graft tenderness, fever, and leukocytosis are less frequent. Klintmalm, Flechner, and others have compared the clinical characteristics of the two processes [25,41]. Acute CsA nephrotoxicity occurs in approximately 25-40% of patients posttransplant; acute rejection is seen in between 12 and 52% of recipients. Both occur with greatest frequency in the first 4 months posttransplant, but acute graft rejection is subsequently rare. The increase in serum creatinine accompanying CsA toxicity is generally slow, rising to 25% above baseline by approximately 1 week. Oliguria is less common, and fever is highly unusual. In contrast, at least one of the following findings is normally seen during rejection episodes: a decrease in urine volume of greater than 500 ml/day, an increase in weight of greater than 0.5 kg, fever exceeding 37.5°C, or a rapidly increasing serum creatinine level (>30 μM/day). CsA serum levels are generally higher during acute nephrotoxicity (>200 mg/ml) and have frequently risen prior to the deterioration in renal function. In contrast, levels tend to be lower during acute rejection (<150 ng/ml) and have fallen preceding this time. The mean trough serum level during acute rejection within the first 90 days posttransplant in our own series was 165 ng/ml, compared with 210 ng/ml during clinical and immunologic quiescence [37].

Additional procedures have been employed to distinguish between these entities. Acute CsA nephrotoxicity is not associated with severe interstitial edema in the grafted organ, and intracapsular pressure is therefore low. Acute rejection, in contrast, is associated with intense inflammation and interstitial edema, and the elevated interstitial pressure may be detected by manometry [65]. Fine needle aspiration biopsy also permits the determination of an inflammatory process within the graft by examination of the infiltrating cells [33]. In patients with good graft function, tubular epithelial cell morphology appears normal, and according to von Willebrand there is no or only faint deposition of CsA in this site as determined by immunofluorescence. In cases of indisputable nephrotoxicity with poor graft function and rising serum creatinine, there is clear evidence of destructive changes in the tubular epithelial cells with prominent deposition of CsA [88]. In contrast, during episodes of rejection, there is a distinct inflammatory response within the interstitium, including the presence of activated T lymphocytes, B lymphocytes, and macrophages. Finally, the direct measurement of donor-specific immune responses, such as complement-dependent cytotoxicity and lymphocyte-mediated cytotoxicity, may be of assistance in demonstrating immunologic activity toward the graft [79]. Discrimination, however, often depends upon a diagnostic test of therapy. A reduction in the dose of CsA with a resultant fall in creatinine suggests drug toxicity; a satisfactory response following the administration of steroids or antilymphocyte globulin is suggestive of rejection.

Acute Vasculopathy

The development of an acute vasculopathy in patients receiving CsA was first described by Schulman following bone marrow transplantation [69]. This devastating complication occurred immediately posttransplant and was characterized clinically by thrombocytopenia, red cell fragmentation, hyperbilirubinemia, and acute renal failure associated with a coagu-

TABLE 5 Discriminant Factors in the Differential Diagnosis of CsA Nephrotoxicity and Acute Renal Allograft Rejection[a]

Parameter	CsA nephrotoxicity	Acute rejection	Reference
Clinical			
Time of onset	>30 days	<60 days	53, 63
Fever (>37.5°C)	0	25%	
Weight gain (>0.5 kg)	25%	50%	
Decreased urine volume (>500 ml)	12%	56%	
Biochemical			
Rise in serum creatinine	<25%	>25%	53, 63
Rate of rise	7.4 days	3.6 days	
Pathology			
Histology	Tubular injury	Heavy cellular infiltrate and edema	65, 82, 83, 85
Cytology	Tubular cell injury	Mononuclear infiltrate	
Intracapsular pressure	<40 mm Hg	>40 mm Hg	
Immunology			
Antidonor immune response	Negative	CDC/LMC + VE	10-12
Trough serum CsA level	<200 ng/ml	>100 ng/ml	

[a]Complement-dependent cytotoxicity (CDC) and lymphocyte-mediated cytotoxicity (LMC).

lative vasculopathy. A similar clinical entity has been observed following kidney and heart transplantation, and Leithner et al. have described the recurrence of a hemolytic uremic syndrome following cadaveric renal transplantation in a patient receiving high-dose CsA [42].

Studies in the experimental animal indicate a causative relationship between CsA and acute vasculopathy. In a rabbit model of acute serum sickness induced by bovine serum albumin (BSA) and endotoxin, the concomitant administration of high-dose CsA (25/kg) causes acute renal failure due to thrombotic occlusion of glomerular capillaries, with afferent arteriolar necrosis and deposition of fibrin and amorphous eosinophilic material, similar to that seen in the hemolytic-uremic syndrome [55].

Acute vasculopathy in the transplanted kidney, although not the focus of major attention until recently, has been clearly described [75]. In general, this has been assumed to reflect acute vascular rejection, but Neild et al. have reported such changes in the kidney in patients with high CsA levels without clear evidence of rejection [56]. Ferguson et al. similarly observed the development of acute vascular lesions comparable histologically to those described above in 8% of patients receiving CsA following renal allotransplantation [22]. The histologic picture is attended by rapid deterioration in renal function, usually within the first 3 weeks posttransplant. The vasculopathy occurs in the absence of histologic evidence of cellular rejection, as evidenced by interstitial infiltration and edema, and is accompanied by avid platelet consumption within the graft as demonstrated by indium-labeled platelet studies. The renal dysfunction is poorly responsive to conventional antirejection therapy, but in limited studies has responded to heparin or streptokinase infusion with discontinuation of CsA.

On reviewing our own experience, we have documented 16 cases of comparable acute vasculopathy in patients transplanted over a period of 2½ years (Table 6). Acute functional deterioration occurred within the first weeks posttransplant: satisfactory graft function was sustained in 4 cases; graft loss occurred in the remaining 12. All cases revealed histologic deposition of immunoglobulin within the vessel wall, and all were accompanied by mild to severe interstitial cellular infiltration, suggesting acute rejection. In addition, 14 of the 16 patients had demonstrable evidence of donor-specific humoral or cell-mediated immunologic activity preceding or accompanying functional deteriora-

TABLE 6 Acute Vasculopathy in Patients Receiving CsA Following Renal Transplantation: Measurement of the Direct Antidonor Immune Response and Quantitative Histology[a]

Graft outcome	Number	Antidonor immune response				Histologic features		
		CDC	LMC	Both	Neither	Vasculopathy	Ig	Cellular rejection
Sustained function	4	3	4	3	0	+/+++	+/+++	+/+++
Graft loss	12	7	8	5	2	++/+++	+/+++	+/+++

[a]+, Mild; ++, moderate; +++, severe.

ation and the appearance of acute vasculopathy. It is thus difficult to determine whether the acute vascular lesions described may occur independently following renal transplantation. However, it is possible that endothelial damage from graft-directed immunologic effector mechanisms may trigger accelerated platelet deposition and permit continuing acute vascular damage.

Chronic Nephropathy with Interstitial Fibrosis

In contradistinction to the acute effects of CsA described above, which can be seen in appropriate experimental animal models, chronic CsA nephrotoxicity has been observed solely in the human. Early studies of renal transplantation in patients receiving CsA, frequently at higher doses than currently employed, documented that allograft function was inferior to that in patients receiving conventional immunosuppression and reported progressive deterioration of renal function, which was unresponsive to additional immunosuppression or steroid therapy, in a variable proportion of cases [32,40]. Histologic examination of such grafts revealed tubular atrophy, moderate to severe interstitial fibrosis, and progressive vascular thickening with medial sclerosis and luminal narrowing. A clear clinical example of severe chronic nephrotoxicity is shown in Figure 2. Following renal transplantation and establishment of satisfactory renal function, a progressive rise in creatinine ensued that was unresponsive to therapy. Biopsy showed the histologic pattern described above, which was erroneously interpreted as chronic graft rejection. Progres-

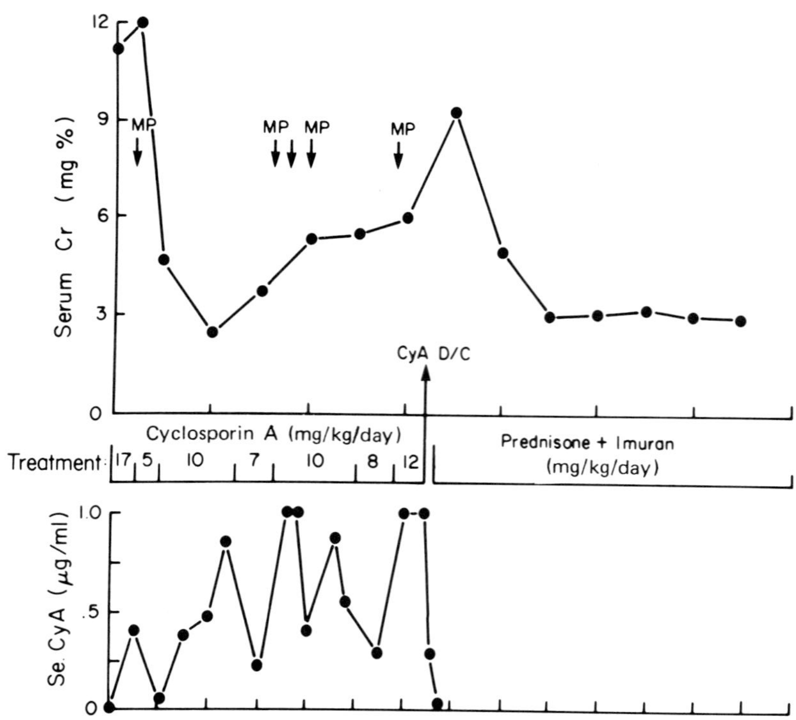

FIGURE 2 Severe chronic CsA nephrotoxicity with resolution of renal dysfunction following conversion to azathioprine immunosuppression.

TABLE 7 Allograft Function Following Renal Transplantation in Patients Receiving CsA Within the CMTSG Study

Months	3	6	12	18	24
Graft survival[a]					
CsA	89	81	78	76	74
I & P[b]	71	67	66	64	62
Graft function (creatinine μM/l)					
CsA	206	185	193	205	204
I & P	170	146	160	168	186

[a]% Actuarial.
[b]Imuran and prednisone.

sive renal dysfunction was accompanied by severe hypertension requiring quadruple-agent therapy. Upon withdrawal of CsA, renal function improved dramatically, with a fall in creatinine from 800 to 200 μM, and has remained stable at this level for 3 subsequent years.

With more careful control of the CsA dosage employed and pharmacologic monitoring of blood CsA levels, the incidence of such overwhelming chronic toxicity has decreased markedly. As shown in Table 7, however, the mean serum creatinine in patients receiving CsA immunosuppression following renal transplantation is normally higher than in controls receiving conventional therapy. The rise in serum creatinine is most marked during the first 12 months but then appears to reach a plateau and remain stable. Patients can be clinically divided into three groups on the basis of long-term renal function [37]. The first, representing the majority of patients, experience no change in GFR and the serum creatinine remains stable, although elevated, throughout the transplant course. In the second group, there is a slow and progressive rise in creatinine, which generally responds to a decrease in the CsA dose with a subsequent fall in serum level and may then remain constant. The third group, however, is characterized by a marked progressive rise in serum creatinine despite a reduction in CsA to levels that no longer ensure satisfactory immunosuppression. Such patients represent approximately 10% of those receiving CsA. Analysis of the clinical course in such patients indicates that many have sustained prior graft damage in the form of protracted perfusion or warm ischemia and have unacceptably high blood CsA levels during the first weeks of therapy (Table 8) [37]. In addition, the hypertension that accompanies chronic nephrotoxicity may perpetuate renal dysfunction by increasing renal ischemia. It is increasingly evident that long-term susceptibility to the nephrotoxic effects of CsA is occasioned by events that occur in the perioperative or immediate postoperative period [39].

HISTOLOGIC CHARACTERISTICS OF CYCLOSPORINE NEPHROTOXICITY

Interpretation of the histologic changes caused by CsA is constrained by three major limitations. First, as is the case clinically and biochemically, there is a serious problem in distinguishing certain alleged "cyclosporine lesions" from those due to rejection or idiopathic acute tubular necrosis. These conditions may coexist in the same patient, and composite lesions may thus be produced, obscuring interpretation. Second, the number of serial

TABLE 8 Characteristics of Organ Storage, Serum CsA Levels, and Early Graft Function in Patients with Chronic CsA Nephrotoxicity

Months	0.5	1	4	6	8	12
Nephrotoxicity						
Serum creatinine (μM/l)	590	361	264	282	317	264
Trough serum CsA (ng/ml)	530	272	195	210	248 //	138[a]
Mean perfusion time: 32 hr						
Mean anastomosis time: 49 min						
Stable function						
Serum creatinine (μM/l)	290	150	150	150	150	158
Trough serum CsA (ng/ml)	231	208	184	201	133	147
Mean perfusion time: 17.9 hr						
Mean anastomosis time: 39 min						

[a]Cyclosporin A discontinued (//) and recommenced at 50% of dose.

biopsies that may be performed during the transplant course is limited, rendering true sequential analysis of the evolution of these changes impossible. Repeated fine needle aspiration has been claimed to overcome this difficulty, but the procedure has not yet found general acceptance as an alternative [33]. The only way to secure continuous biopsy information at present is with animal models, which do not completely parallel the human picture. Third, the lesions thus far ascribed to CsA are not diagnostic in the sense that simple qualitative appraisal is sufficient: most of the lesions cited are suggestive of toxicity only when present to a greater degree than in other conditions, and quantitative evaluation is needed if the morphologic diagnosis of CsA toxicity is to be established. Adequate criteria have not yet been defined or accepted, a recent workshop on CsA lesions making it obvious that different centers have focused their attention on varying aspects of the subject [72]. There are at present a small number of lesions generally agreed to be typical of CsA toxicity, a number of others cited by individual centers to be strongly in favor of that diagnosis, and there are no lesions considered diagnostic by any pathologist. Those to which we will direct our attention can be divided into four categories: acute tubular necrosis, acute tubulointerstitial injury, acute vasculopathy, and interstitial fibrosis.

Acute Tubular Necrosis (ATN)

The pathology of this condition in the native kidney was first described in detail by Lucke in patients suffering severe shock, crushing injuries, and other similar insults [45]. At that time, extensive necrosis of distal tubules with "tubulorrhexis" was believed to be the diagnostic feature. Although severe lesions of the foregoing type can still be encountered (sometimes presenting at a late stage with tubular calcification), it has become obvious in recent years that acute renal failure of tubular origin may present minimal pathologic features by light microscopy and only loss of the brush-border surface and mild signs of epithelial damage by electron microscopy [75].

Following renal transplantation in patients receiving conventional, nonnephrotoxic immunosuppressive agents, initial graft nonfunction not clearly attributable to immunologic mechanisms is observed in 10-60% of patients [9,21,24,47,68,80]. The changes ob-

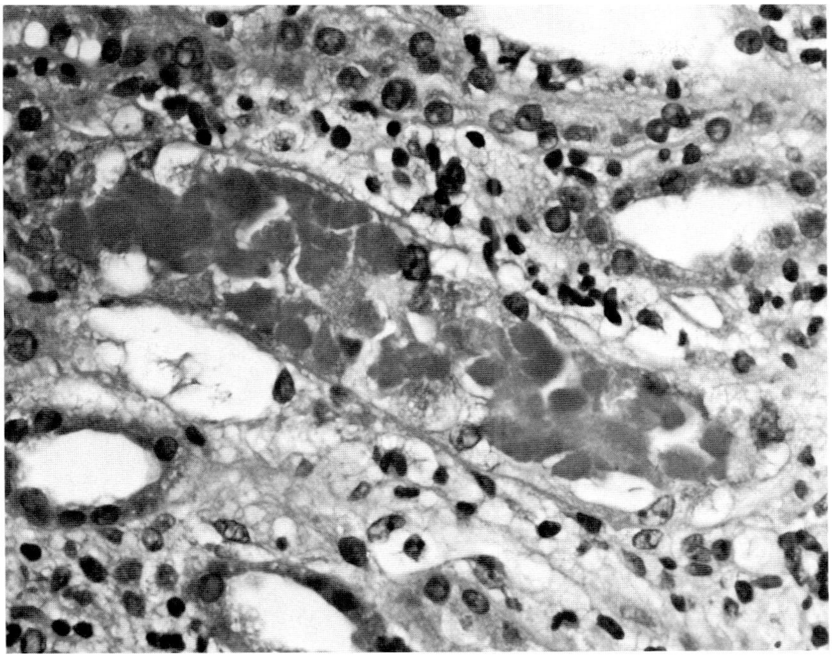

FIGURE 3 Section of renal cortex showing severe acute tubular necrosis 9 days after transplantation; on CsA therapy. Kidney did not function up to biopsy date. The tubule in the center shows necrosis with sloughing of dead epithelial cells into the lumen. Some interstitial lymphocyte infiltration and edema are present. Cyclosporin A toxicity is difficult to exclude as an additional factor, but the early nonfunction favors ischemic ATN. (H&E, X450.)

served histologically within the grafted kidney parallel those in classic ATN, exhibiting a range of severity. Mild changes are characterized by flattening of the tubular epithelium, vacuolar degeneration, and patchy individual cell necrosis. Signs of regeneration, characterized by mitotic figures within the epithelial cells and irregularity of tubular lining, are often observed. The most severe state is characterized by extensive tubular epithelial necrosis, sloughing of cells into the lumen, the presence of hyaline, cellular, and granular casts in the lumen, and extensive calcification (Figures 3 and 4). These changes may occasionally be accompanied by mild interstitial edema and focal infiltration of mononuclear cells, occurring either secondary to the tubulointerstitial damage or reflecting a mild and clinically undetected immune response against the allograft.

Initial graft nonfunction in the patient receiving CsA is characterized by a similar range of histologic features [72]. No specific lesions may be isolated that clearly identify CsA toxicity in this early stage, although with increasing time the appearance of giant mitochondria and other features described below may be more suggestive of CsA effect. The difficulty in separating ATN from mild tubulointerstitial nephritis has been clearly emphasized, and with certain types of drug-induced tubular damage the two conditions may exist simultaneously [75]. The mild, focal interstitial mononuclear cell infiltrate observed during this period in some patients receiving CsA may thus similarly be drug de-

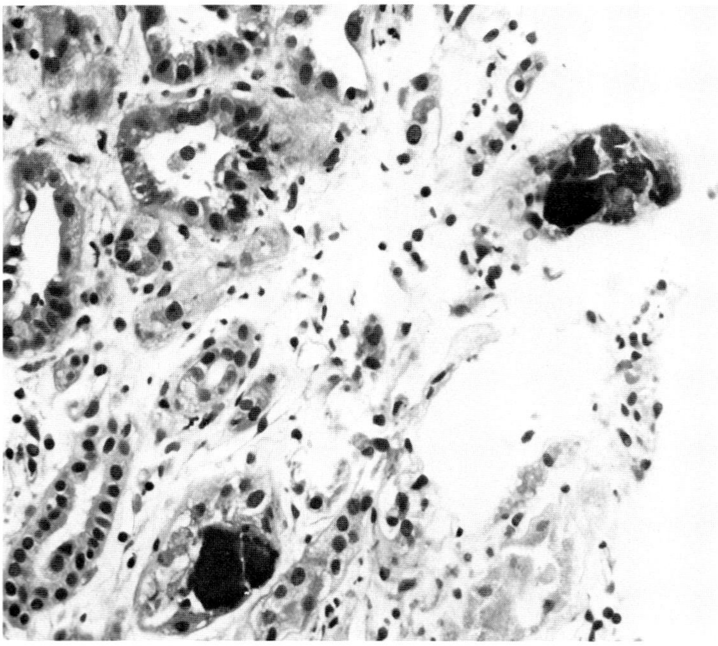

FIGURE 4 Renal tubular calcification at a late stage of tubular necrosis. Minor degrees are common in acute tubular necrosis and may be impossible to distinguish from mild CsA lesions. (H&E, X290.)

pendent or secondary to nonspecific tubular injury or mild immunologic activity within the graft.

The Acute Tubulointerstitial Lesions of CsA Toxicity

The similarity between early lesions of CsA toxicity and ATN has been mentioned. Within the first 5-10 days posttransplant, the morphology of a nonfunctioning graft may be difficult to categorize because of the presence of both conditions, and this diagnostic problem is often resolved only by analysis of the clinical course.

From the first 5 days to several weeks posttransplant, there may be a much greater problem in distinguishing between mild rejection and CsA toxicity, and many workers concluded that a correct diagnosis is not always possible. Two groups of lesions characteristic of CsA nephrotoxicity have been reported in the early transplant phase. The first is a vasculitis and will be considered separately in the following section. The other group consists of a mild interstitial nephritis with tubular damage. The pathologic picture is one of mild interstitial edema, focal lymphocyte infiltration, and a variety of tubular lesions, which are often very slight. Mihatsch et al. [49] have produced convincing evidence that three such tubular changes are highly characteristic of CsA toxicity. (1) Giant mitochondria are present in the convoluted portion of the proximal tubule (Figures 5 and 6). These can be seen by light microscopy using chromotrope aniline blue (CAB) stain or in plastic sections with toluidine blue but are easily missed with most preparations. They are readily seen by

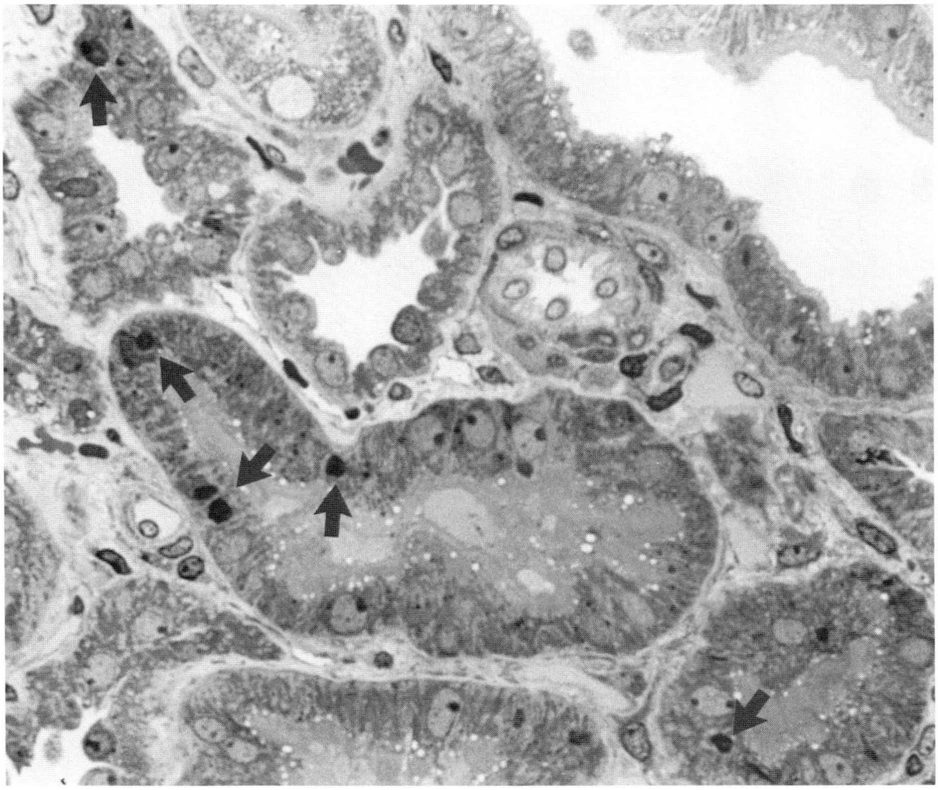

FIGURE 5 Renal transplant biopsy at 13 days; clinical course consistent with CsA nephrotoxicity. Light microscopic view of giant mitochondria in proximal tubules (arrows). This toluidine blue stain on 1-μm plastic sections reveals the structures very easily. They range in size up to about one-half the size of the nuclei (X680).

electron microscopy and not easily confused with other tubular components. (2) There is isometric vacuolation in the straight portion of the proximal tubules (Figure 7). This appears to be similar to the "vacuolar degeneration" commonly encountered in many types of tubular damage. (3) Tubular calcification occurs in foci of damaged tubules, probably representing a dystrophic calcification in necrotic cells.

The discriminative value of these changes is not universally accepted, however [20, 70]. Giant mitochondria may be more numerous in CsA-treated cases [20] but in our own experience are infrequent, despite routine examination of the tubules by electron microscopy. Sibley et al., using a somewhat demanding type of morphometry, have shown that the best discriminator between CsA toxicity and rejection is the predominance of intracapillary lymphocytes around the tubules in CsA toxicity, rather than an extravascular (interstitial) infiltrate, which predominates in acute rejection (Figures 8 and 9) [70]. Both the Sibley and the Wallace groups reported that the finding of large numbers of lysozomes in proximal and distal tubules was significantly more common in CsA toxicity than rejection [70,90] (Figure 10). This has not been confirmed by others, although it has

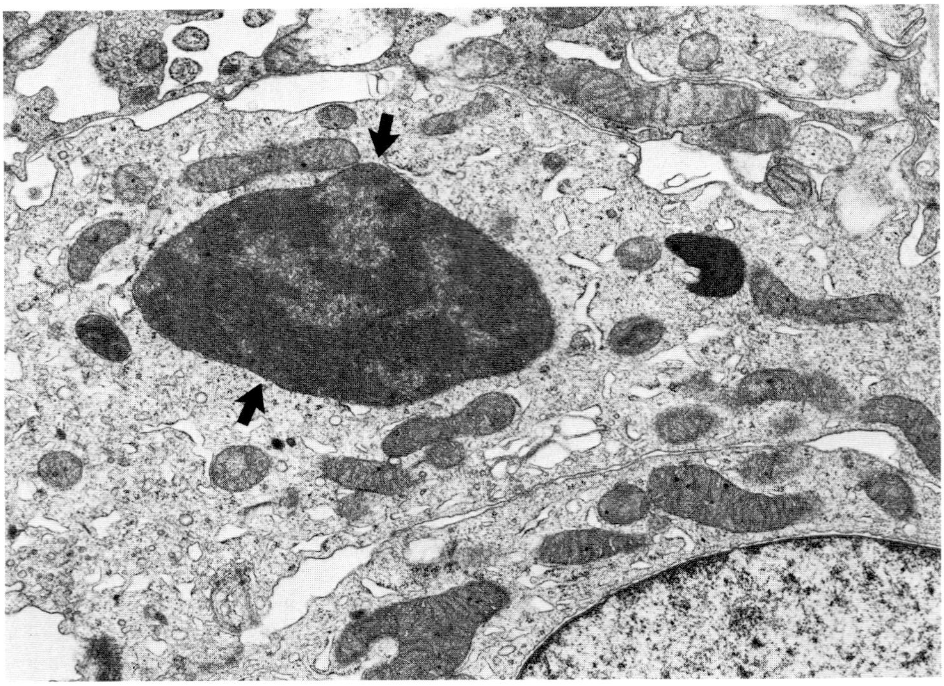

FIGURE 6 Giant mitochondrion from same biopsy as Figure 5. The double membrane (arrows) confirm the identity of the organelles (EM X23,760).

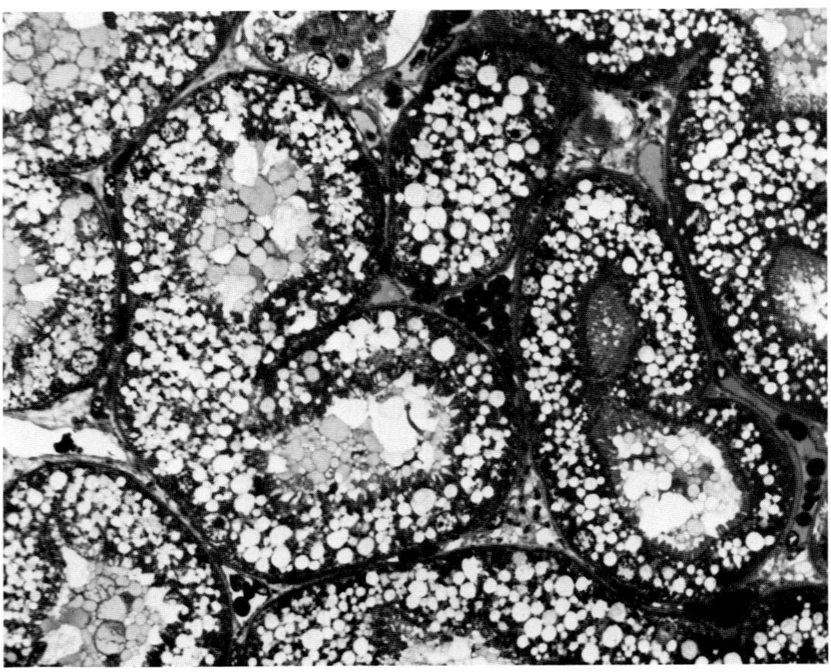

FIGURE 7 Isometric vacuolation in epithelium of proximal convoluted tubules in patient with clinical evidence of CsA toxicity. Note intact brush borders. This change is a nonspecific and common lesion, but characteristic of CsA, especially in experimental toxicity. (Toluidine blue, X450.)

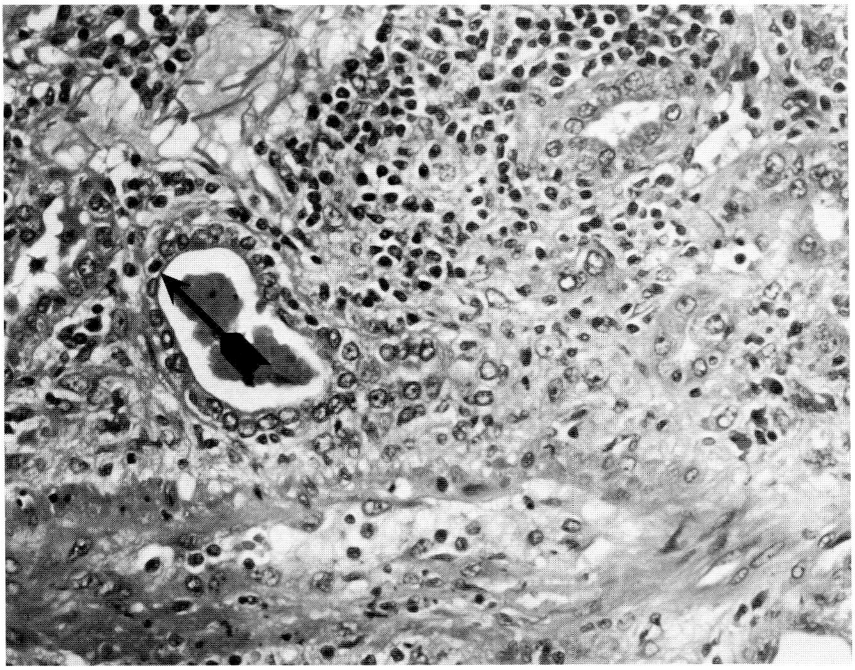

FIGURE 8 Renal transplant biopsy at 30 days showing typical lesions of severe acute cellular rejection. The features here usually accepted (but not universally) as typical of rejection are marked interstitial edema; diffuse and extensive lymphocyte interstitial infiltration; acute vasculitis (bottom of figure); and infiltration of tubules by lymphocytes (arrow). (H&E, X290.)

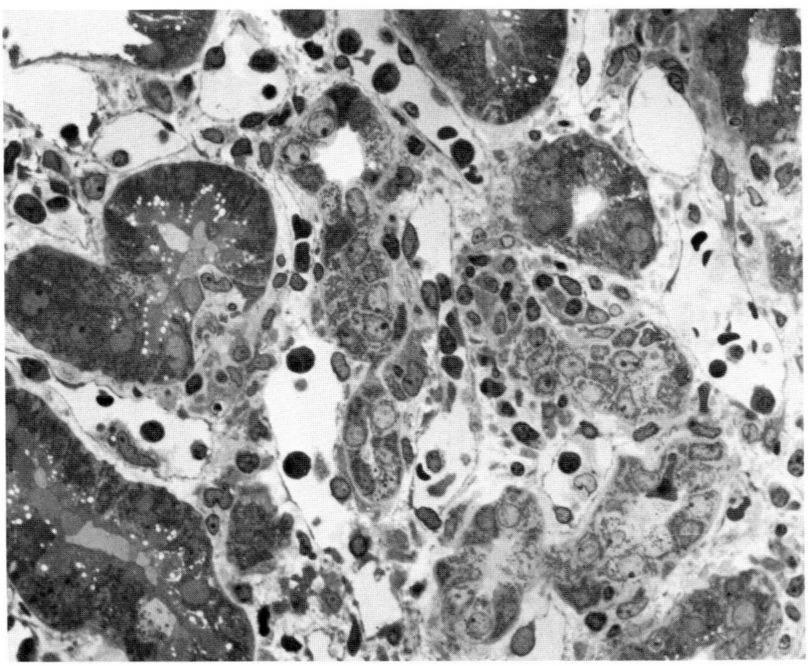

FIGURE 9 Transplant biopsy showing mild inflammatory cell accumulation with only minimal edema. Most of the leukocytes are in peritubular capillaries rather than in the interstitium. These features are claimed to be in favor of CsA toxicity over mild rejection. (H&E, X450.)

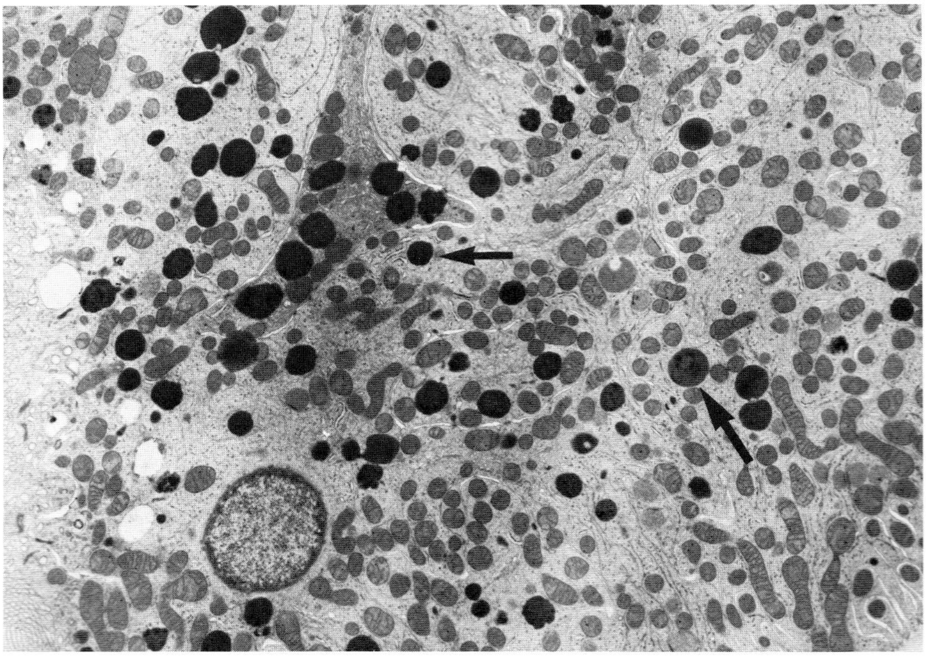

FIGURE 10 Proximal tubular cells in CsA-treated patient 60 days after transplant. The numerous dark lysozomes (arrows) are a nonspecific finding with many causes, but were the most consistent finding in our own blind comparison of CsA and non-CsA transplant cases (EM X11,200).

been reported with animal experiments. In reviewing the results from various centers, it becomes clear that considerable attention must be paid to CsA dosages and trough levels. It may be possible that some centers seldom encounter certain lesions commonly reported elsewhere in the past simply because of lower dosages used.

There appears to be a consensus that very marked edema, intense lymphocyte infiltration, and direct invasion of tubules ("tubulitis") and of glomeruli ("glomerulitis") (Figures 11 and 12) represent rejection rather than CsA toxicity [49]. Yet even these points are disputed. Morris reported that in some cases of apparent CsA toxicity the renal biopsy tissue "looked like a lymph node," a picture we have never encountered [51]. Farnsworth found neither the degree of edema nor the intensity of lymphocyte infiltration to be of value in diagnosis, and Sibley reported that tubulitis was not a useful discriminator between rejection and CsA toxicity [20,70].

It has been the hope of nephropathologists that phenotypic analysis of cell populations by surface markers would provide a simple and accurate method of distinguishing between graft rejection and a "toxic" interstitial reaction. Unfortunately, the situation has remained confused, complicated, among other things, by difficulties in performing accurate counts on the cells in the biopsy. Some workers have found that OKT8 cells are proportionally higher in the graft when rejection is present, and Sibley's group provide strong evidence that a high OKT8/OKT4 ratio is indicative of rejection [59,86]. Others, however, report no consistent patterns that reliably aid discrimination [26,84]. One com-

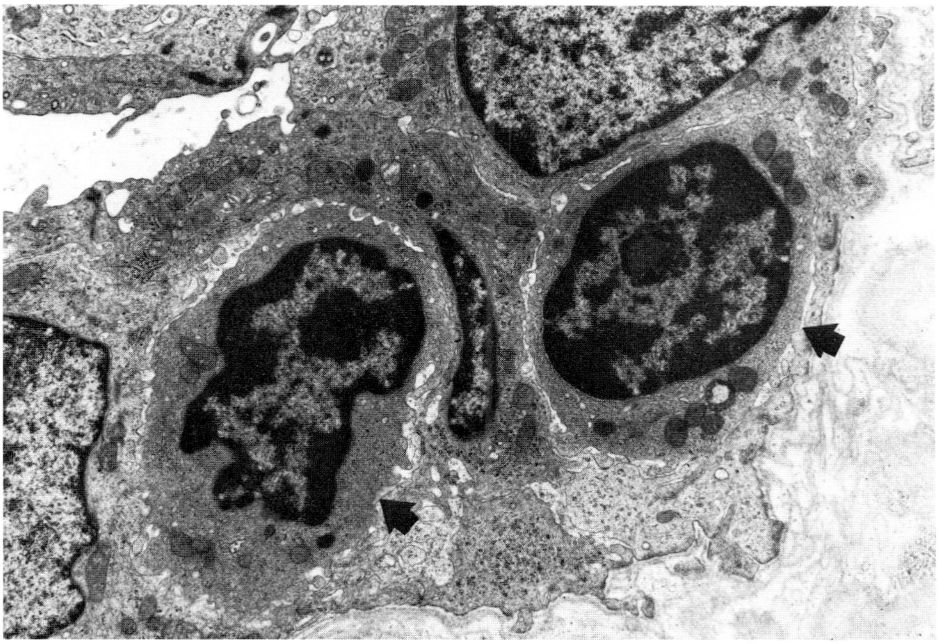

FIGURE 11 Distal tubular epithelium from a patient with acute cellular rejection, not on CsA therapy. The invasion of epithelium by large lymphocytes (arrows) is accompanied by distortion of the epithelium, and usually epithelial necrosis is present, eventually in association with this. The phenomenon can be seen by light microscopy (see Figure 8) (EM X9100).

pelling need in more useful analysis of the infiltrates is an antibody panel that distinguishes between suppressor and cytotoxic cells, both of which are positive for OKT8 surface antigen. It appears likely, however, that T-cell subset analysis performed under stringent conditions may yield at least supportive information in distinguishing rejection and CsA toxicity, or may at times confirm the simultaneous occurrence of both processes.

Vascular Lesions of Cyclosporine Toxicity

A number of reports have appeared in the last 5 years of an acute syndrome characterized by renal failure, microangiopathic hemolytic anemia, and thrombocytopenia occurring in patients with bone marrow allografts who received CsA [2,69]. The morphology of these syndromes has not been described completely in many instances but includes the presence of microthrombi in renal vessels, particularly glomerular capillaries, and in some instances thrombotic lesions in lung and brain. Fibrin and platelets were seen in vessels by electron microscopy, and there were signs of endothelial damage. The condition was classified either as a hemolytic-uremic syndrome or thrombotic thrombocytopenic purpura. It should be noted that these two conditions morphologically may be nearly identical: in each there may be endothelial damage with lifting of the endothelium and subendothelial deposits of granular material, white cell and platelet aggregation, and fibrin thrombi (Figures 13 and 14).

Precisely the same changes may be found in severe acute vascular rejection, and we

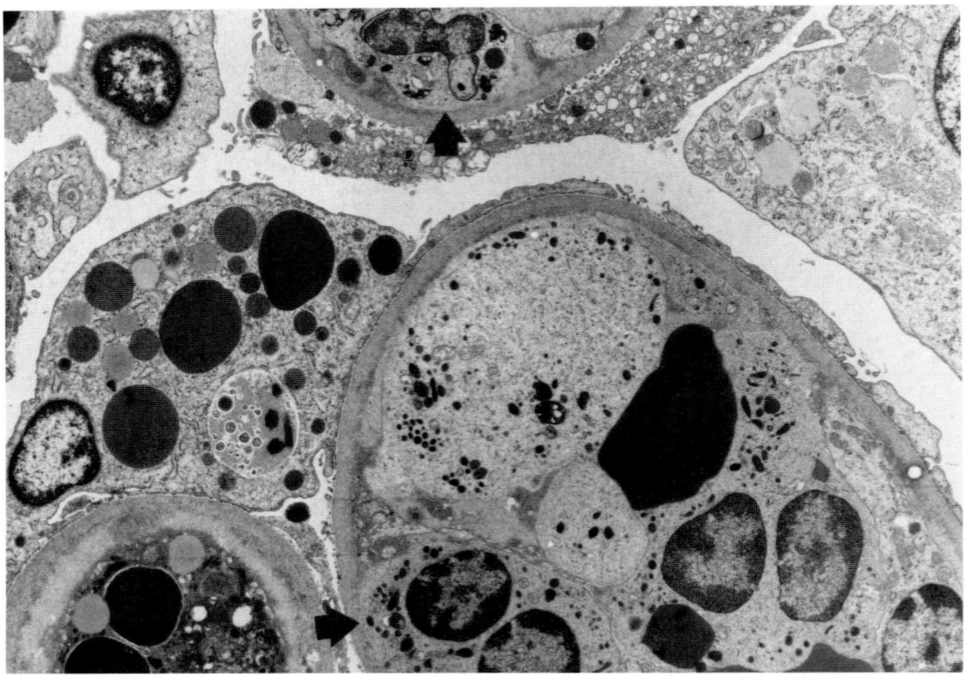

FIGURE 12 Acute glomerulitis in rejecting kidney, non-CsA patient. The glomeruli are filled with lymphocytes and granulocytes that obstruct the lumen. There is loss of endolium in some areas (arrows) (EM X5040).

have seen a number of such cases in patients never exposed to CsA (Figure 15). In bone marrow transplantation, an immunologic etiology is less likely, suggesting that this lesion also occurs as a result of rejection and of CsA toxicity. It is possible that these changes have not been generally attributed to CsA following renal transplantation because of the difficulty of distinguishing them with confidence from acute vascular rejection [20, 70,81]. As reported earlier, we have observed these lesions in a small proportion of our patients receiving this drug. In all cases there was associated evidence of acute cellular rejection or immunoglobulin deposition on the vessel wall, and all cases except two exhibited evidence of an established humoral or cell-mediated response to donor antigens compatible with acute rejection.

A slightly different type of renal vascular lesion has been described by Mihatsch et al. (Figures 16 and 17) [49]. Mihatsch has described a spectrum of arteriolar and small arterial lesions varying from fairly acute vasculitis with necrosis (which he likened to HUS but did not indicate as including capillary thrombi), to a bland, more chronic type of lesion consisting of increased hyaline material in the media with production of nodular "mucoid" masses in the media and subintima (see also Color Plates 2 and 7 in center of book) [49]. These lesions differed from rejection in involving small arteries and arterioles only in not showing the typical intimal hyperplasia and hypercellularity commonly associated with thrombosis. Thiru has described a similar "peculiar insudative lesion" in arterioles in patients receiving CsA but has not given a detailed report on the lesions [81]. It is possible that these diverse vascular lesions may represent a pathologic spectrum deriving from a common toxic effect, the primary event being endothelial injury. These vascular lesions

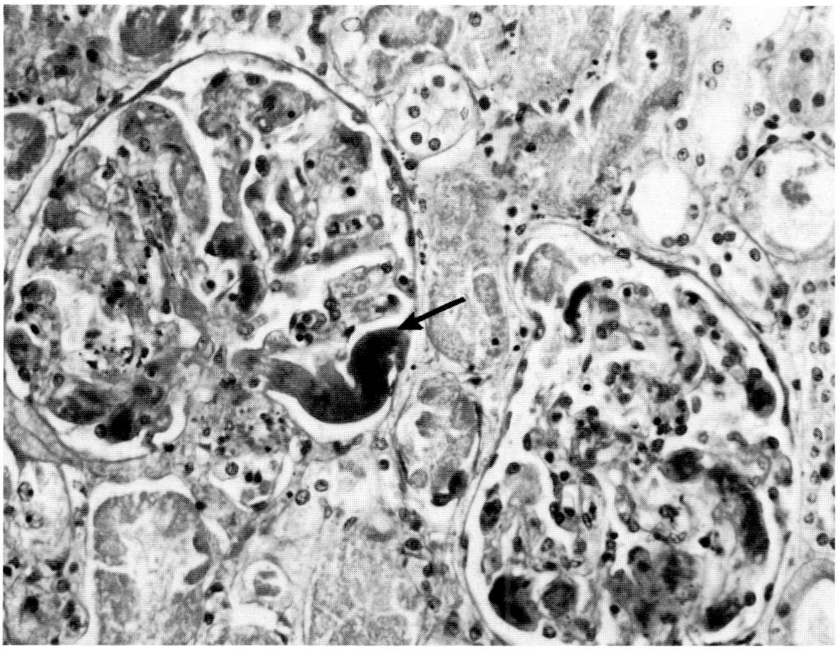

FIGURE 13 Paraffin section of a glomerulus from a patient with hemolytic-uremic syndrome (native kidney, not a transplant). The dark areas in glomerular capillaries (arrow) are stained for fibrin. A similar picture can occur with acute rejection, DIC, and TTP. (MSB stain, ×260.)

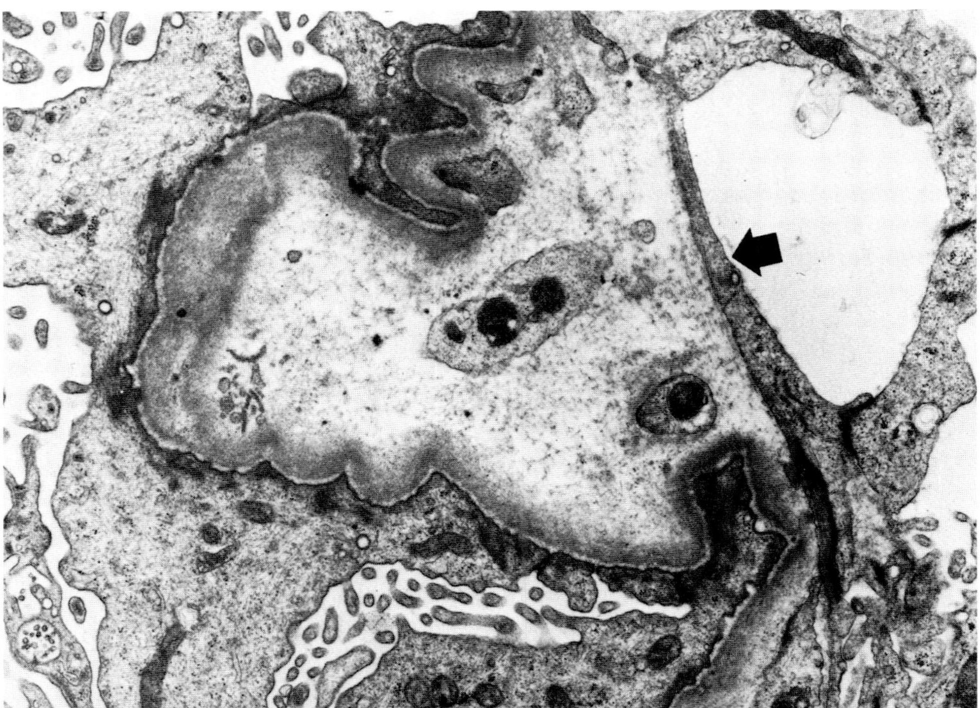

FIGURE 14 Ultrastructure of same biopsy as Figure 13. There is lifting of the endothelium from basement membrane (arrow) and deposition of fluffy protein material between endothelium and basement membrane (EM ×7125).

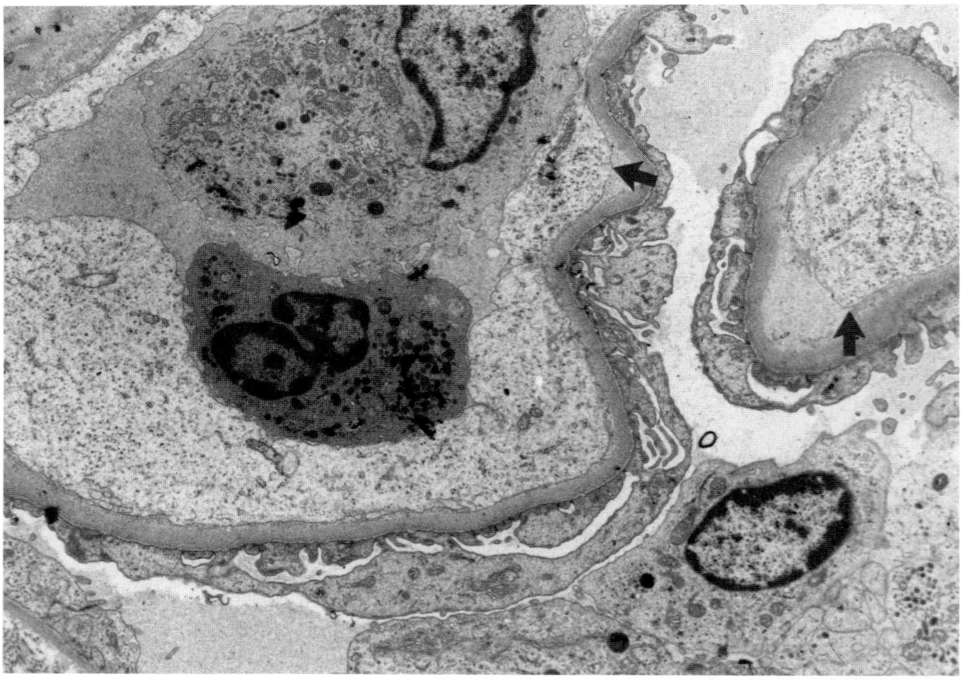

FIGURE 15 Glomerular capillary from a case of severe acute rejection at 30 days, not on CsA. Endothelial cells are swollen and are lifted from basement membrane in same way as in Figure 14 (arrows). Thus an identical picture can result from immunologic rejection as from toxic effects on endothelium; in each case, severe endothelial injury is probably the primary lesion (EM X5040).

may produce a permanent vasculopathy accompanied by interstitial fibrosis. Again, chronic rejection with slow vascular sclerosis may result in a very similar pattern. An added diagnostic problem in lesions at this stage is that hypertension, irrespective of its origin, may result in hyaline vascular lesions similar to those described.

Interstitial Fibrosis

This condition is characterized by an increase in connective tissue in the interstitial compartment of the kidney (that area not occupied by tubules, glomeruli, or blood vessels) and is almost universally accompanied by tubular atrophy and thickening of tubular basement membranes. In contrast to interstitial edema, in which both hematoxylin and eosin and trichrome stains show a pale background, interstitial fibrosis is evidenced by an increase in trichrome-positive material. Although the basic lesion is totally nonspecific, being encountered as a sequel of many destructive renal processes, including glomerulonephritis, pyelonephritis, and nephrosclerosis, it is generally accepted as one of the most characteristic lesions of long-term CsA therapy [20,49,70,81].

Some writers have ascribed the fibrosis to the general fibrogenic stimulus of CsA in promoting fibroblast activity; others have suggested it may be, at least partially, secondary to the acute and chronic vascular lesions. Mihatsch et al. have reported that a "striped"

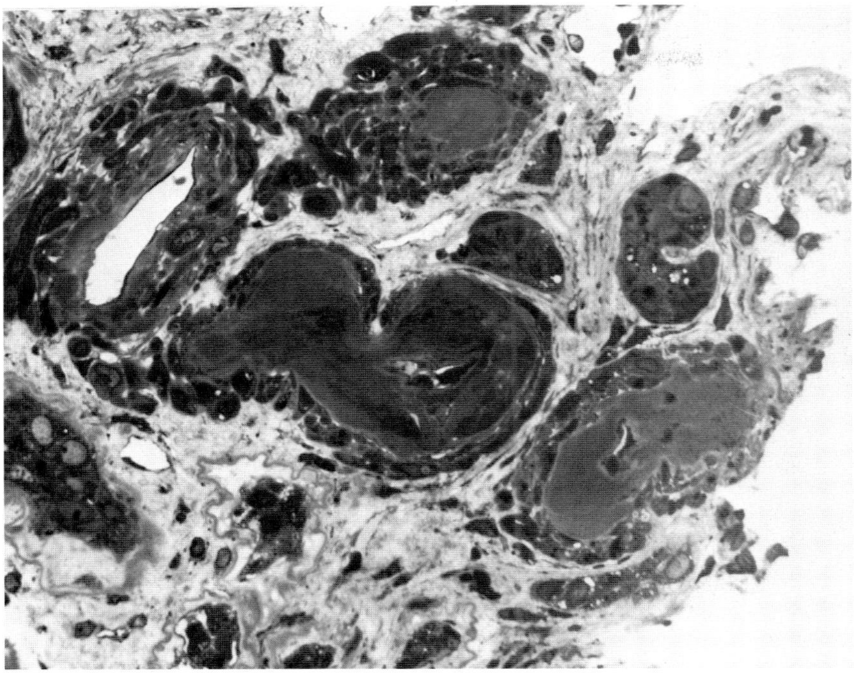

FIGURE 16 Small arteries in a renal biopsy from a patient with a heart transplant, on CsA for 440 days, developing hypertension and mild renal failure. Nodular deposits are present with a "hyaline" or "mucinous" appearance. (Toluidine blue, X470.)

or segmental distribution is more typical of CsA therapy than diffuse fibrosis, although others have failed to associate this pattern with CsA [20,49,70]. Such a striped distribution could result from ischemic fibrosis secondary to vascular stenosis, as is sometimes seen with the variable vascular lesions in nephrosclerosis.

That interstitial renal fibrosis has been demonstrated in patients with heart transplants is strong evidence that it is due to CsA therapy rather than chronic rejection (Figure 18) [16,53]. Nonetheless, it is a common lesion in chronic rejection and was described long before CsA immunosuppression was introduced into the transplant field (Figure 19).

The numerous reports by Bohle on glomerular disease emphasize that, irrespective of its cause, interstitial fibrosis is nearly always accompanied by decreased renal function [4]. It is probable that the fixed and irreversible component of renal dysfunction observed in some patients receiving long-term CsA therapy is attributable to this lesion.

MANAGEMENT OF CYCLOSPORINE NEPHROTOXICITY

The prevention and management of CsA nephrotoxicity is most easily considered in relation to early graft function, acute nephrotoxicity, and chronic nephrotoxicity. An algorithm may be derived for therapy and is depicted in Table 9.

The risk factors predisposing to delayed graft function have been described and include prolonged cold and warm ischemia. In addition, we have shown that donor age appears an important variable, graft survival being impaired in kidneys from donors over the age of 50

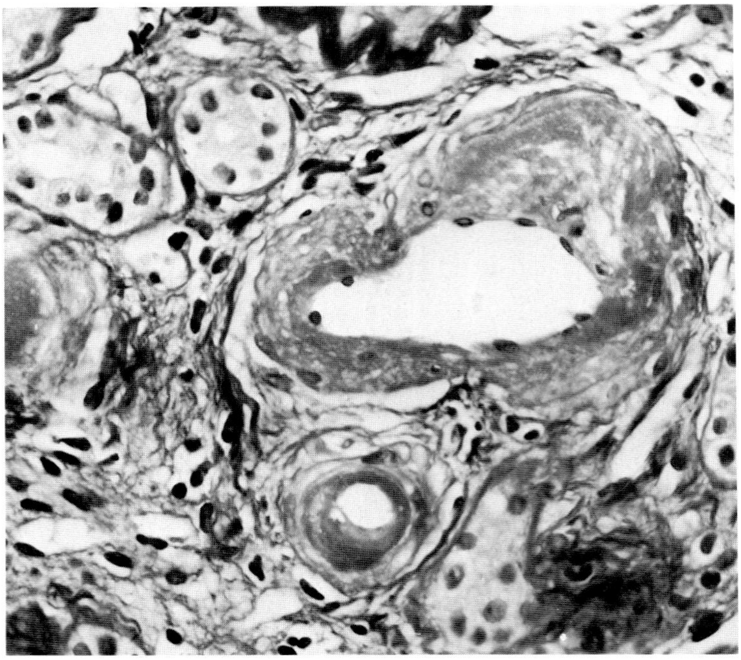

FIGURE 17 Arteriole and small artery; same biopsy as Figure 16. The hyaline lesions are nonspecific in appearance, and it is not clear whether these particular ones are CsA induced or related to the developing hypertension. (H&E, X425.)

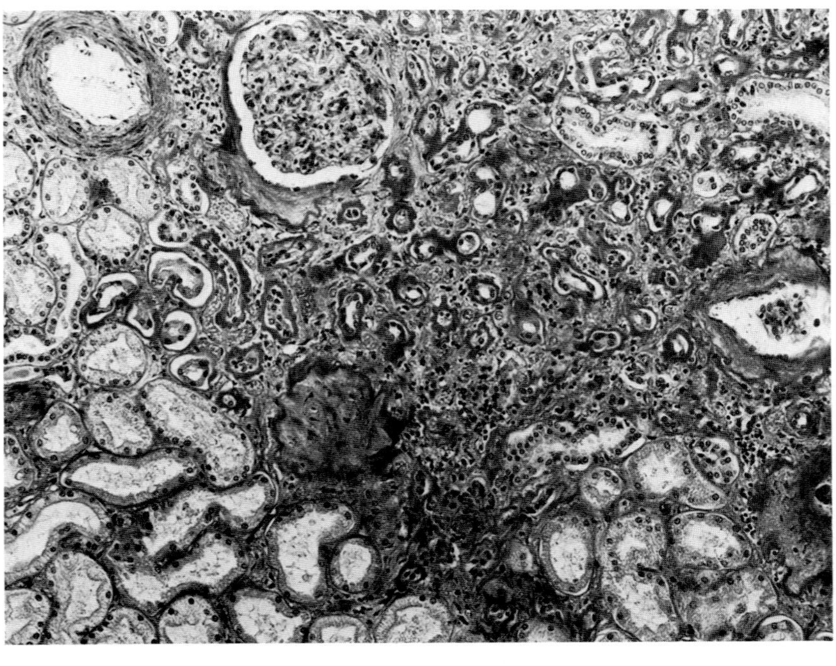

FIGURE 18 Interstitial fibrosis of a "striped" or segmental type claimed to be typical of CsA toxicity. Areas of fibrosis, tubular basement membrane thickening, and tubular atrophy are interspersed with relatively normal areas. Renal biopsy in a heart transplant patient on CsA for 80 weeks. (Trichrome, X105.)

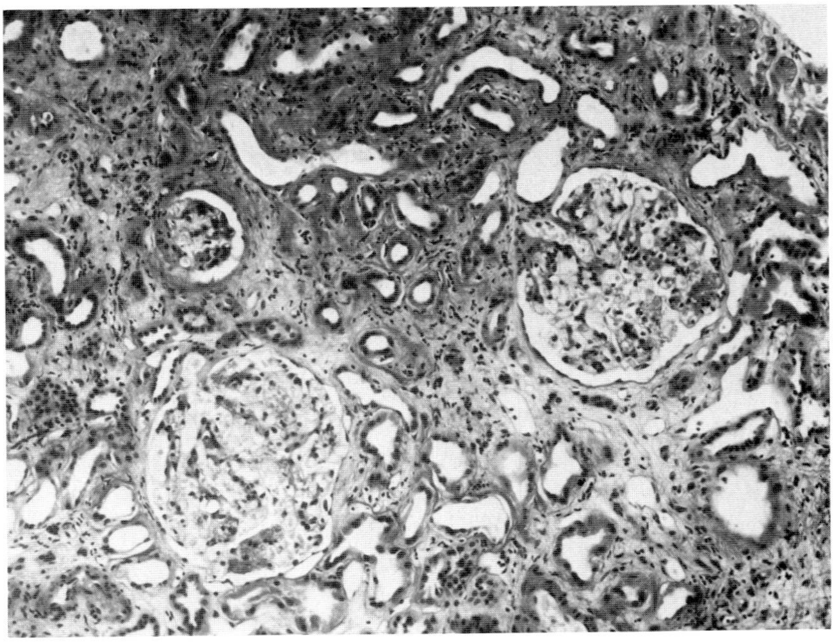

FIGURE 19 Severe interstitial fibrosis of long-standing chronic rejection; biopsy 2 years after transplant, no CsA therapy. These sorts of lesions may be more diffuse than CsA-induced fibrosis, and vessels may not show the "hyalinosis" described with CsA, but a distinction between rejection and CsA fibrosis is nonetheless difficult. (Trichrome, ×105.)

years. In the absence of these factors, CsA-induced delayed function is uncommon, and CsA may be administered in normal doses from the time of surgery. When such risk factors are present, however, CsA may be administered by low-dose continuous infusion at a rate of 4-5 mg/kg per 24 hr, maintaining constant serum levels in the range of 200 ng/ml. Such parenteral infusion is associated with little toxicity and facilitates maintenance of desired levels, avoiding the vagaries of intestinal absorption in the immediate postoperative period. Alternative immunosuppressive therapy may also be employed until graft function is clearly established. Two approaches have been adopted, the use of azathioprine or antilymphocyte globulin (ALG). It is clear that the former is a less effective immunosuppressive than CsA and is no longer considered the therapy of choice by most centers. Short-term sequential therapy with ALG administered for a period of 5 days has been employed by ourselves and others with efficacy and safety, with conversion to CsA once graft function is established. Administration of a full 3-week course of ALG prior to conversion has been associated with severe complications of sepsis and malignancy resulting from over immunosuppression, and is to be discouraged [10]. If graft function is therefore not established before this time, we electively continue sequential therapy with azathioprine rather than CsA.

Acute deterioration in renal allograft function within the first 3 months posttransplant represents a diagnostic and therapeutic exercise. Such episodes may be divided into three subgroups on the basis of clinical, biochemical, histologic, and immunologic data. Those

TABLE 9 Algorithm for the Clinical Use of CsA in Renal Transplantation

Allograft dysfunction	Diagnostic category	Characteristic features	Therapeutic approach
Initial graft nonfunction	"High risk"	Donor > 50 years PT > 24 hr RT > 45 min	ALG 5-10 days; if function, switch to CsA; if no function, consider full course ALG and maintenance azathioprine
	"Low risk"	Donor < 50 years PT < 24 hr RT < 45 min	CsA IV X 3-5 days, then PO
Acute graft dysfunction	Acute rejection	Fever, oliguria, weight gain; diffuse infiltration; immunology + ve	↑ CsA levels to 200 ng/ml, with MP 250 mg IV X 3 days; if no response, ALG X 5-7 days or monoclonal
	Uncertain	Combined features of rejection and toxicity	↓ CsA to 100 ng/ml; if no response, MP 250 mg IV X 3 days
	Nephrotoxicity	Mild focal infiltrate, tubular injury; immunology – ve	↓CsA to 100 ng/ml
Chronic graft dysfunction	Chronic toxicity	Hypertension, interstitial fibrosis, tubular injury	↓ CsA to 50 ng/ml; resolution, maintain therapy; rejection, switch to azathioprine ± CsA (low dose)
	Chronic rejection	Vascular thickening, intimal proliferation, interstitial fibrosis, unresponsive to CsA	No clearly beneficial therapy; commence low-protein diet, avoid overimmunosuppression, and prepare for retransplant

that clearly reflect acute rejection require appropriate antirejection therapy, which generally consists of intravenous methylprednisolone or an increase in oral prednisone dose, and if proven refractory to this treatment, a course of antilymphocyte product may be instituted. A second group represents clear nephrotoxicity, unaccompanied by features of graft rejection. Such episodes normally respond satisfactorily to a stepwise reduction in CsA dose to reduce serum trough levels to the range of 150-200 ng/ml. The third category consists of episodes that cannot be clearly classified as rejection or nephrotoxicity, and under certain conditions features of both may coexist. Such episodes may respond to a trial of therapy, in which antirejection therapy is initiated, with a simultaneous or sequential reduction in CsA dose to achieve serum trough levels in the range of 150-200 ng/ml.

Chronic progressive nephrotoxicity is uncommon but occurs predominantly in those patients receiving high-risk grafts or having been exposed to high CsA levels following transplantation [37,39]. The CsA dose is first reduced stepwise to produce the lowest trough serum level compatible with adequate immunosuppression. This range is normally between 50 and 100 ng/ml [37]. It is essential to be cautious in this reduction, because acute rejection may only ensue several weeks after trough serum levels have been reduced to clearly subtherapeutic levels, perhaps reflecting transient immunologic hyporesponsiveness due to host-graft adaptation. In the majority of patients, such a reduction in CsA dose is adequate to eliminate continuing toxicity and achieve a fall or plateau in the serum creatinine. In a small proportion of patients, however, progressive renal dysfunction is observed even following reduction of CsA to a dose that is no longer optimally immunosuppressive [37]. In such patients, conversion to alternative therapy may be achieved, although not with safety in all cases [11,76]. Azathioprine is normally commenced 1-5 days prior to discontinuation of CsA to ensure adequate effect and subsequently titrated to the white count. Such conversion of therapy, whether done preventatively or interventionally, is attended by the risk of acute rejection in approximately 10% of cases [52]. The majority of these respond to appropriate therapy, but graft loss has been described. In an effort to avoid this outcome, combination therapy is currently being investigated in certain centers. A combination of low-dose CsA and azathioprine has been successful in maintaining immunosuppression in this setting in a limited series with a low incidence of acute rejection.

OVERVIEW

Cyclosporin A is a major development in pharmacologic manipulation of the immune response and has permitted a major advance in organ transplantation, decreasing patient morbidity and mortality and significantly increasing graft survival. Because of its immunosuppressive efficacy there is a marked reduction in steroid requirement, and long-term steroid therapy may ultimately prove to be unnecessary in the majority of patients [77, 95]. The duration of hospitalization, the incidence of infection, and consequently the cost of transplantation are reduced [54].

The undesirable effect of CsA on the kidney must thus be considered within this context. As indicated, the acute functional effect observed to some degree in most patients receiving this drug is rapidly reversible and unaccompanied by long-term detriment in studies now followed for up to 5 years [48]. Progressive deterioration of renal function occurs in a small proportion of patients, often associated with therapeutic doses that currently would now be considered unacceptably high, and may in some cases be eliminated or reversed by carefully controlled conversion to alternative immunosuppression.

Cyclosporin A is a highly effective immunosuppressant that has raised the bench mark for organ transplantation, and potentially for immune manipulation in autoimmune disease, to a new threshold. The challenge that now remains is to utilize this agent, either alone or in combination, in the most appropriate fashion to minimize its adverse effects.

REFERENCES

1. Adu, D., Turney, J., Michael, J., and McMaster, P. Hyperkalaemia in cyclosporin-treated renal allograft recipients. *Lancet* 2:370-371, 1983.
2. Atkinson, K., Biggs, J. C., Hayes, J., Ralston, M., Dodds, A. J., Concannon, A. J., and Nardoo, D. Cyclosporin A associated nephrotoxicity in the first 100 days after allogeneic bone marrow transplantation: Three distinct syndromes. *Br. J. Haematol.* 54: 59-67, 1983.

3. Belitzsky, P., for the Canadian Transplant Study Group. Initial nonfunction of cyclosporine treated cadaver renal allografts preserved by simple cold storage. *Transplant. Proc.* 17:1485-1488, 1985.
4. Bohle, A., Bader, R., Grund, K. E., Machensen, S., and Neunhoeffer, J. Serum creatinine concentration and renal interstitial volume. *Virchows Arch.* [*Pathol. Anat.*] 375:87-96, 1977.
5. Borel, J. F., and Meszaros, J. Skin transplantation in mice and dogs. Effect of cyclosporin A and dihydrocyclosporin C. *Transplantation* 29:161-162, 1980.
6. Calne, R. Y., Rolles, K., White, D. J., Thiru, S., Evans, D. B., McMaster, P., Dunn, D. C., Craddock, G. N., Henderson, R. G., Aziz, S., and Lewis, P. Cyclosporin A initially as the only immunosuppressant in 34 recipients of cadaveric organs: 32 kidneys, 2 pancreases and 2 livers. *Lancet* 2:1033-1034, 1979.
7. Calne, R. Y., White, D. J. G., Evans, D. B., and Wight, C. Three years' experience with cyclosporin A in clinical cadaveric kidney transplantation. In *Cyclosporin A*, D. J. G. White, ed. Elsevier Biomedical Press, Amsterdam, 1982, p. 379.
8. Calne, R. Y., White, D. J. G., Rolles, K., and Smith, D. P. Prolonged survival of pig orthotopic heart grafts treated with cyclosporin A. *Lancet* 1:1183-1185, 1978.
9. Canadian Multicentre Transplant Study Group. A randomized clinical trial of cyclosporine in cadaveric renal transplantation. *N. Engl. J. Med.* 309:809-815, 1983.
10. Canadian Multicentre Transplant Study Group. Comparison of ALG-imuran-cyclosporine and Alg-cyclosporine for cadaver renal transplantation. *Transplant. Proc.* 17: 1201-1203, 1985.
11. Canafax, D. M., Sutherland, D. E. R., Ascher, N. L., Simmons, R. L., and Najarian, J. S. Cyclosporine nephrotoxicity in renal allograft recipients: Conversion to azathioprine to improve renal function. In *Cyclosporine: Biological Activity and Clinical Applications*, B. C. Kahan, ed. Grune and Stratton, Orlando, Florida, 1984, p. 658.
12. Clive, D. M., and Stoff, J. S. Renal syndromes associated with nonsteroidal anti-inflammatory drugs. *N. Engl. J. Med.* 310:563-572, 1984.
13. Gluckman, E., Devergie, A., Lokeic, F., Poirier, O., and Baumelou, A. Nephrotoxicity of cyclosporin A in bone-marrow transplantation. *Lancet* 2:144-145, 1981.
14. Cronin, R. E. Aminoglycoside nephrotoxicity: Pathogenesis and prevention. *Clin. Nephrol.* 11:251-256, 1979.
15. Devineni, R., McKenzie, N., Duplan, J., Keown, P., Stiller, C., and Wallace, A. C. Renal effects of cyclosporine: Clinical and experimental observations. In *Cyclosporine: Biological Activity and Clinical Applications*, B. C. Kahan, ed. Grune and Stratton, Orlando, Florida, 1984, p. 479.
16. Devineni, R., McKenzie, N., Wall, W., Campbell, C., Stiller, C., Keown, P., and Kostuk, W. Renal function in patients receiving cyclosporine for orthotopic cardiac transplantation. *Transplant. Proc.* 17:1256-1257, 1985.
17. Dieperink, H., Staklint, H., and Leyssac, P. P. Study of the nephrotoxic effect of cyclosporine on overall renal and tubular function in conscious rats. In *Cyclosporine: Biological Activity and Clinical Applications*, B. C. Kahan, ed. Grune and Stratton, Orlando, Florida, 1984, p. 520.
18. Donker, A. J. M., Arisz, L., Brentjens, J. R., van der Hem, G. K., and Hollemans, H. J. The effect of indomethacin on kidney function and plasma renin activity in man. *Nephron* 17:288-296, 1976.
19. Fan, T.-P. D., and Lewis, G. P. Mechanism of cyclosporin A induced inhibition of prostanoid synthesis by macrophages. IUPAHAR Ninth International Congress of Pharmacology, London, 1984, Abstract 54.
20. Farnsworth, A., Hall, B. M., Ng, A. B. P., Duggin, G. G., Horvath, J. S., Sheil, A. G. R., and Tillen, D. J. Renal biopsy morphology in renal transplantation. *Am. J. Surg. Pathol.* 8:243-252, 1984.

21. Ferguson, R. M., Rynasiewicz, J. J., Sutherland, D. E. R., Simmons, R. L., and Najarian, J. S. Cyclosporin A in renal transplantation: A prospective randomized trial. *Surgery* 92:175-182, 1982.
22. Ferguson, R., Sharma, J., and Sommer, B. Cyclosporine associated arteriopathy: A significant cause of allograft loss after renal transplantation. *Transplantation* in press.
23. Ferguson, R. M., Sutherland, D. E. R., Simmons, R. L., and Najarian, J. S. Ketoconazole, cyclosporin metabolism and renal transplantation. *Lancet* 2:882-883, 1982.
24. Flechner, S. M., Payne, W. D., Van Buren, C. T., Kerman, R., and Kahan, B. D. The effect of cyclosporine on early graft function in human renal transplantation. *Transplantation* 36:268-272, 1983.
25. Flechner, S. M., Van Buren, C., Kerman, R. H., and Kahan, B. D. The nephrotoxicity of cyclosporine in renal transplant recipients. In *Cyclosporine: Biological Activity and Clinical Applications,* B. C. Kahan, ed. Grune and Stratton, Orlando, Florida, 1984, p. 473.
26. Forsum, U., Claesson, K., Frodin, L., Parra-Karlsson, A., Klareskog, L., Odlund, B., Stenkvist, B., and Tufveson, S. Methods for monitoring T-lymphocyte subsets in renal allografts. *Transplant. Proc.* 15:1178-1181, 1983.
27. Gerber, J. G., Branch, R. A., Nies, A. S., Gerkens, J. F., Shand, D. G., Hollifield, J., and Cares, J. A. Prostaglandin release II. Assessment of renin secretion following infusion of PGE_2, I_2 and D_2 into the renal artery of anesthetized dogs. *Prostaglandins* 15:81-88, 1978.
28. Gluckman, E., Arcese, W., Devergie, A., and Boiron, M. Cyclosporin-A prophylactic treatment of graft-versus-host disease in human allogeneic bone marrow transplantation: preliminary results. *Transplant. Proc.* 13:368-370, 1981.
29. Gordon, M. Y., and Singer, J. W. Selective effects of cyclosporin A on colony-forming lymphoid and myeloid cells in man. *Nature* 279:433-434, 1979.
30. Halulska, P. V., Dollery, C. T., and MacDermot, J. Thromboxane and prostaglandin in disease: a review. *Q. J. Med (New Series)* 52:461-471, 1983.
31. Hamberg, M., Svenson, I., and Samuelsson, B. Thromboxanes, a new group of biologically active compounds derived from prostaglandin endoperoxides. *Proc. Natl. Acad. Sci. USA* 71:3400-3404, 1975.
32. Hamilton, D. V., Evans, D. B., Henderson, R. G., Thiru, S., Calne, R. Y., and White, D. J. G. Long-term nephrotoxicity of cyclosporin A in transplantation. *Dial. Transplant.* 11:158-160, 1982.
33. Hayry, P., and von Willibrand, E. Practical guidelines for fine needle aspiration biopsy of human renal allografts. *Ann. Clin. Res.* 13:288-306, 1981.
34. Kahan, B. D. Cyclosporine: A powerful addition to the immunosuppressive armamentarium. *Am. J. Kidney Dis.* 3:444-455, 1984.
35. Kahan, B. D., Reid, M., and Newburger, J. Pharmacokinetics of cyclosporin A in human transplantation. *Transplant. Proc.* 15:446-453, 1983.
36. Kennedy, M. S., Deeg, H. J., Siegel, M., Crowley, J. J., Storb, R., and Thomas, E. D. Acute renal toxicity with combined use of amphotericin B and cyclosporine after bone marrow transplantation. *Transplantation* 35:211-213, 1983.
37. Keown, P. A., Stiller, C. R., Sinclair, N. R., Carruthers, G., Howson, W., Stawecki, M., McMichael, J., Koegler, J., McKenzie, N., and Wall, W. The clinical relevance if cyclosporine blood levels as measured by radioimmunoassay. In *Cyclosporine: Biological Activity and Clinical Applications,* B. C. Kahan, ed. Grune and Stratton, Orlando, Florida, 1984, p. 222.
38. Keown, P. A., Stiller, C. R., Ulan, R. A., Sinclair, N. R., Wall, W. J., and Carruthers, G. Immunological and pharmacological monitoring in the clinical use of cyclosporin A. *Lancet* 1:686-689, 1981.

39. Klintmalm, G., Bohman, S.-O., Sundelin, B., and Wilczek, H. Interstitial fibrosis in renal allografts after 12 to 46 months of cyclosporin treatment: Beneficial effect of low doses in early post-transplantation period. *Lancet* 2:950-953, 1984.
40. Klintmalm, G. B. G., Iwatsuki, S., and Starzl, T. E. Nephrotoxicity of cyclosporin A in liver and kidney transplant patients. *Lancet* 1:470-471, 1981.
41. Klintmalm, G., Ringden, O., and Groth, C. G. Clinical and laboratory signs in nephrotoxicity and rejection in cyclosporine-treated renal allograft recipients. In *Cyclosporine: Biological Activity and Clinical Applications,* B. C. Kahan, ed. Grune and Stratton, Orlando, Florida, 1984, p. 599.
42. Leithner, C., Sinzinger, H., Pohanka, E., Schwarz, M., Kretschmer, G., and Syre, G. Occurrence of hemolytic uremic syndrome under cyclosporine treatment: Accident or possible side effect mediated by a lack of prostacyclin-stimulating plasma factor? In *Cyclosporine: Biological Activity and Clinical Applications,* B. C. Kahan, ed. Grune and Stratton, Orlando, Florida, 1984, p. 571.
43. Levenson, D. J., Simmons, C. E., and Brenner, B. M. Arachidonic acid metabolism, prostaglandins and the kidney. *Am. J. Med.* 72:354-374, 1982.
44. Lifschitz, M. D., and Stein, J. H. Renal vasoactive hormones. In *The Kidney,* vol. 1, B. M. Brenner and F. C. Rector, eds. W. B. Saunders, Philadelphia, 1981, p. 650.
45. Lucke, B. Lower nephron nephrosis: The renal lesions of the Crush syndrome, of burns, transfusions and other conditions affecting the lower segments of the nephrons. *Milit. Surg.* 99:371-376, 1946.
46. McKenzie, N., Devineni, R., Vezina, W., Keown, P., and Stiller, C. The effect of cyclosporine on organ blood flow. *Transplant. Proc.* in press, 1986.
47. McMaster, P., Haynes, I. G., Michael, J., Adu, D., Vlassis, T., Roger, S., Turney, J., Stock, S., Buckels, J., Mackintosh, P., and Ezzibdeh, M. Cyclosporine in cadaveric renal transplantation: A prospective randomized trial. In *Cyclosporine: Biological Activity and Clinical Applications,* B. C. Kahan, ed. Grune and Stratton, Orlando, Florida, 1984, p. 307.
48. Merion, R. M., White, D. J. G., Thiru, S., Evans, D. B., and Calne, R. Y. Cyclosporine: Five years' experience in cadaveric renal transplantation. *N. Engl. J. Med.* 310:148-154, 1984.
49. Mihatsch, M. J., Thiel, G., Spichtin, H. P., Oberholzer, M., Brunner, F. P., Harder, F., Olivieri, V., Bremer, R., Ryffel, B., Stocklin, E., Torhorst, J., Gudat, F., Zollinger, H. U., and Loershter, R. Morphological findings in kidney transplants after treatment with cyclosporine. *Transplant. Proc.* 15(Suppl. 1):2821-2835, 1983.
50. Moncada, S., and Vane, J. P. Pharmacology and endogenous roles of prostaglandin endoperoxides, thromboxane A_2 and prostacyclin. *Pharmacol. Rev.* 30:293-331, 1979.
51. Morris, P. in discussion of Calne, R. Y., and White, D. J. S. The use of cyclosporine A in clinical organ grafting. *Ann. Surg.* 196:330-337, 1982.
52. Morris, P. J., French, M. E., Dunnill, M. S., Hunnisette, A. G. W., Ting, A., Thompson, J. F., and Wood, R. F. M. A controlled trial of cyclosporine in renal transplantation with conversion to azathioprine and prednisolone after three months. *Transplantation* 36:273-277, 1983.
53. Myers, B. D., Ross, J., Newton, L., Luetscher, J., and Perlroth, M. Cyclosporine-associated chronic nephropathy. *N. Engl. J. Med.* 311:699-705, 1984.
54. Najarian, J. S., Strand, M., Fryd, D. S., Ferguson, R. M., Simmons, R. L., Ascher, N. L., and Sutherland, D. E. R. Comaprison of cyclosporine versus azathioprine-antilymphocyte globulin in renal transplantation. In *Cyclosporine: Biological Activity and Clinical Applications,* B. C. Kahan, ed. Grune and Stratton, Orlando, Florida, 1984, p. 247.
55. Neild, G. H., Ivory, K., and Williams, D. G. Glomerular thrombi and infarction in

rabbits with serum sickness following cyclosporine therapy. In *Cyclosporine: Biological Activity and Clinical Applications,* B. C. Kahan, ed. Grune and Stratton, Orlando, Florida, 1984, p. 566.

56. Neild, G., Reuben, R., Hartley, B., and Cameron, J. S. Glomerular thrombi in renal allografts associated with cyclosporin therapy. *Am. Soc. Nephrol. Abs.* 247A, 1984.
57. Neild, G. H., Rocchi, G., Imberti, L., Fumagalli, F., Brown, A., Remuzzi, G., and Williams, D. G. Effect of cyclosporine on prostacycline synthesis by vascular tissue in rabbits. In *Cyclosporine: Biological Activity and Clinical Applications,* B. C. Orlando, ed. Grune and Stratton, Orlando, Florida, 1984, p. 182.
58. Petric, R., Keown, P. A., McDonald, J., and Stiller, C. R. Cyclosporine Nephrotoxicity, renal blood flow and thromboxane release. *Transplant. Proc.* (in press).
59. Platt, J. L., Ferguson, R. M., Sibley, R. K., Gajl-Peclzalska, K. J., and Michael, A. F. Renal interstition cell populations in cyclosporine nephrotoxicity. Identification using monoclonal antibodies. *Transplantation* 36:343-346, 1983.
60. Porter, G. A., and Bennett, W. M. Nephrotoxin induced acute renal failure. In *Acute Renal Failure,* B. M. Brenner and J. Stein, eds. Churchill-Livingstone, New York, 1980, p. 123.
61. Powell-Jackson, P. R., Young, B., Calne, R. Y., and Williams, R. Nephrotoxicity of parenterally administered cyclosporine after orthotopic liver transplantation. *Transplantation* 36:505-508, 1983.
62. Powles, R. L., Barrett, A. J., Clink, H., Kay, H. E. M., Sloane, J., and McElwain, T. J. Cyclosporin A for the treatment of graft-versus-host disease in man. *Lancet* 2:1327-1231, 1978.
63. Rocher, L. L., Milford, E. L., Kirkman, R. L., Carpenter, C. B., Strom, T. B., and Tilney, L. N. Conversion from cyclosporine to azathioprine in renal allograft recipients. *Transplantation* 38:669-674, 1984.
64. Ryffel, B., Donatsch, P., Madorin, M., Matter, B. E., Ruttiman, G., Schon, H., Stoll, R., and Wilson, J. Toxicological evaluation of cyclosporin A. *Arch. Toxicol.* 53:107-141, 1983.
65. Salaman, J. R., and Griffin, P. J. Fine-needle intrarenal manometry: A new test for rejection in cyclosporin-treated recipients of kidney transplants. *Lancet* 2:709-711, 1983.
66. Schor, N., Ichikawa, I., and Brenner, B. M. Mechanisms of action of various hormones and vasoactive substances on glomerular ultrafiltration in the rat. *Kidney Int.* 20:442-451, 1981.
67. Sheil, A. G. R., Hall, B. M., Tiller, D. J., Duggin, G. G., Stephen, M. S., Thompson, J. F., Horvath, J. S., Johnson, J. R., May, J., Rogers, J. R., and Boulas, J. Pre-operative administration of cyclosporin A to cadaveric donor renal allograft recipients (preliminary report from a controlled clinical trial). In *Cyclosporin A,* D. J. G. White, ed. Elsevier Biomedical Press, Amsterdam, 1982, p. 387.
68. Sheil, A. G. R., Hall, B. M., Tiller, D. J., Stephen, M. S., Harris, J. P., Duggin, G. G., Horvath, J. S., Johnson, J. R., Rogers, J. R., and Boulas, J. Australian trial of cyclosporine (CsA) in cadaveric donor renal transplantation. In *Cyclosporine: Biological Activity and Clinical Applications,* B. C. Kahan, ed. Grune and Stratton, Orlando, Florida, 1984, p. 307.
69. Shulman, H., Striker, G., Deeg, H. J., Kennedy, M., Storb, R., and Thomas, E. D. Nephrotoxicity of cyclosporin A after allogeneic marrow transplantation. Glomerular thromboses and tubular injury. *N. Engl. J. Med.* 305:1392-1395, 1981.
70. Sibley, R. K., Rynasiewicz, J., Ferguson, R. M., Fryd, D., Sutherland, D. E. R., Simmons, R. L., and Najarian, J. S. Morphology of cyclosporine nephrotoxicity and acute rejection in patients immunosuppressed with cyclosporine and prednisone. *Surgery* 94:225-234, 1983.

71. Siegle, H., Ryffel, R., Petric, R., Shoemaker, P., Muller, A., Donatsch, P., and Mihatsch, M. Cyclosporine, the renin-angiotension-aldosterone system, and renal adverse reactions. In *Cyclosporine: Biological Activity and Clinical Applications,* B. C. Kahan, ed. Grune and Stratton, Orlando, Florida, 1984, p. 503.
72. Sibley, R. K., Bergstrand, A., Bohmar, S., Fransworth, A., Krause, P., Lange, W., Mihatsch, M., Oppedal, B., Ruffel, S., Sell, S., Thiel, G., Thiru, S., Wallace, A., Wonergert, K., and Zollinger, H. Renal histopathology in kidney transplants and patients immunosuppressed with cyclosporine (CYA). X Int. Cong. of Transplant. Soc. Minneapolis 62, 1984.
73. Simmons, C. F., Bogusky, R. T., and Humes, H. D. Acute renal failure by diethylaminoethyl dextran: Importance of cationic charge. *Kidney Int.* 19:424-430, 1981.
74. Soberon, L., Bowman, R. L., Pastoriza, E. M., and Kaloyanides, G. J. Comparative nephrotoxicities of gentamicin and amikacin. *Johns Hopkins Med. J.* 142:85-90, 1978.
75. Solez, K. Acute renal failure: Acute tubular necrosis, infarction and cortical necrosis. In *Pathology of the Kidney,* Vol. 2, 3rd edition, R. H. Hepinstall, ed. Little, Brown, Boston, 1983, p. 1069.
76. Stiller, C., for The Canadian Transplant Study Group. The Canadian Trial of cyclosporine: Cyclosporine therapy compared to standard immunosuppression in renal transplants. An exploration of nephrotoxicity. In *Cyclosporine: Biological Activity and Clinical Applications,* B. C. Kahan, ed. Grune and Stratton, Orlando, Florida, 1984, p. 263.
77. Stiller, C., for The Canadian Transplant Study Group. The requirements for maintenance steroids in cyclosporine-treated renal transplant recipients. In *Cyclosporine: Biological Activity and Clinical Applications,* B. C. Kahan, ed. Grune and Stratton, Orlando, Florida, 1984, p. 274.
78. Stiller, C. R., Keown, P. A., Sinclair, N. R., and Ulan, R. A. Immune responses and pharmacokinetics in the human renal allograft recipient treated with cyclosporin A. In *Cyclosporin A,* D. J. G. White, ed. Elsevier Biomedical Press, Amsterdam, 1982, p. 379.
79. Stiller, C. R., Sinclair, N. R., Abrahams, S., McGirr, D., Singh, H., Howson, W. T., and Ulan, R. A. Anti-donor immune responses in prediction of transplant rejection. *N. Engl. J. Med.* 294:978-982, 1976.
80. Thiel, G., Harder, R., Lortscher, R., Brunisholz, M., Landmann, J., Brunner, F., Follath, F., Wenk, M., and Mihatsch, M. Cyclosporin A used alone or in combination with low-dose steroids in cadaveric renal transplantation. *Klin. Wochenschr.* 61: 991-1000, 1983.
81. Thiru, S., Mahes, E. R., Hamilton, D. V., Evans, D. B., and Calne, R. Y. Tubular changes in renal transplant recipients on cyclosporine. *Transplant. Proc.* 15(Suppl. 1): 2846-2851, 1983.
82. Thompson, A. W., Moon, D. K., Geczy, G. L., and Nelson, D. S. Cyclosporin A inhibits lymphokine production but not the responses of macrophages to lymphokines. *Immunology* 48:291-299, 1983.
83. Thompson, J. F., Chalmers, D. H., Hunnisett, A. G., Wood, R. F., and Morris, P. J. Nephrotoxicity of trimethoprim and cotrimoxazole in renal allograft recipients treated with cyclosporine. *Transplantation* 36:204-206, 1983.
84. Tomaszewski, J. E., Kornstein, M., Brooks, J., and Zmijewski, C. M. T lymphocyte distribution in rejected allografts. *Lab. Invest.* 48:86A, 1983.
85. Totterman, T. H., Nisell, J., Killander, A., Gharton, G., and Lonnqvist, B. Cyclosporin blood levels do correlate with clinical complictions. *Lancet* 2:692-693, 1984.
86. Van Es, A., Meyer, C. J. L. M., Oljans, P. J., Tanke, H. J., and Van Es, L. A. Mononuclear cells in renal allografts. *Transplantation* 37:134-139, 1984.

87. Vermylen, J., Badenhorst, P. N., Deckmyn, H., and Arnout, J. Normal mechanisms of platelet function. In *Clinics in Hematology,* L. A. Harker and T. S. Zimmermann, eds. L. B. Saunders, LOndon, 1983, p. 107.
88. von Willebrand, E., and Hayry, P. Cyclosporin-A deposits in renal allografts. *Lancet* 2:189-192, 1983.
89. Wagner, H. Cyclosporin A: Mechanism of action. *Transplant. Proc.* 15:523-526, 1983.
90. Wallace, A. C., Shum, D. T. W., Stiller, C. R., Keown, P. A., and Ulan, R. A. Pathology of renal transplants on patients receiving cyclosporin A. *Can. Cong. Lab. Med.,* Abstract, 1981.
91. Whiting, P. H., Simpson, J. G., Davidson, R. J. L., and Thomson, A. W. The toxic effects of combined administration of cyclosporin A and gentamicin. *Br. J. Exp. Pathol.* 63:554-561, 1982.
92. Whiting, P. H., Cunningham, C., Thomson, A. W., and Simpson, J. G. Enhancement of high dose cyclosporin A toxicity by frusemide. *Biochem. Pharmacol.* 33:1075-1079, 1984.
93. Yarger, W. E., Schocken, D. D., and Harris, R. H. Obstructive nephropathy in the rat. Possible roles for the renin-angiotension system, prostaglandins and thromboxanes in post-obstructive renal function. *J. Clin. Invest.* 65:400-412, 1980.
94. Yun, J., Kelly, G., Bartter, F. C., and Smith, H., Jr. Role of prostaglandins in the control of renin secretion in the dog. *Circ. Res.* 40:459-464, 1977.
95. Cyclosporin A as sole immunosuppressive agent in recipients of kidney allografts from cadaver donors. Preliminary results of a European Multicentre Trial. *Lancet* 2:57-63, 1982.

21

CANCER IN RECIPIENTS OF ORGAN ALLOGRAFTS

Douglas W. Hanto* and Richard L. Simmons
University of Minnesota Health Sciences Center, Minneapolis, Minnesota

It is now well recognized that immunodeficiencies of various types predispose to the development of de novo cancers. McKhann [71] and Penn et al. [84] independently first reported an association between cancer and immunosuppression in renal allograft recipients in 1969. The reported incidence of cancer arising in individuals with genetically determined immunodeficiency diseases is 4% [107]. In immunosuppressed renal allograft recipients, the incidence ranges from 1 to 16% at different centers [5,51,83,88-90], averaging 4% [89], far greater than that in the general population matched for age [105]. The most frequent neoplasms in genetically affected patients are those of the lymphoreticular system [21,107] and, in transplant recipients, nonmelanotic skin and lip cancer, followed by lymphoproliferative diseases [82,87,89].

In 2139 organ transplant recipients reported to the Cincinnati Transplant Registry (Table 1) [89], skin and lip cancer, malignant lymphomas, and squamous cell carcinoma of the cervix accounted for 59% of the total cancers (Figure 1). By excluding the recipients with nonmelanotic skin cancer and cervical carcinoma in situ, we can compare the remaining results with cancer statistics from the general population [106]. Malignant lymphomas and leukemias account for 16% of the tumors in transplant recipients, compared with 7-8% in the general population [106]. Conversely, carcinoma of the prostate accounts for 19% of cancers in males in the general population, but for less than 1% of the cancers in transplant recipients. Similarly, carcinoma of the colon and rectum, carcinoma of the female breast, and lung cancer account for 15, 13, and 16% of all cancers in the general population [106], but only 4, 3, and 4% of the tumors in transplant recipients [89]. These differences are related in part to the relative youth of transplant recipients (average age in mid-30s), but may have another explanation in the probable different pathogenesis of cancer following transplantation. However, for whatever reason, transplant patients do not frequently develop the common solid tumors more prevalent with advanced age.

Systematic investigation has been difficult because of the sporadic nature of the problem. Several theories have been proposed for the increased incidence of cancer in immune-deficient individuals, however, including impaired immune surveillance mechan-

**Present affiliation*: Washington University School of Medicine, St. Louis, Missouri.

TABLE 1 De Novo Malignancies in Organ Allograft Recipients

Type of tumor	No. of patients[a]
Cancers of skin and lips	880
Lymphomas	316
Carcinomas of uterus	151
Cervix, 136	
Body, 15	
Carcinomas of the lung	101
Carcinomas of colon and rectum	83
Kaposi's sarcomas	80
Carcinomas of breast	74
Carcinomas of kidney	63
Host kidney, 58	
Allograft kidney, 5	
Carcinomas of the vulva, perineum, penis, or scrotum	63
Leukemias	57
Metastatic carcinomas (primary site unknown)	56
Carcinomas of the head and neck (excluding thyroid parathyroid and eye)	55
Carcinomas of urinary bladder	42
Carcinomas of liver and bile ducts	37
Carcinomas of thyroid	32
Soft tissue sarcomas	30
Cancers of stomach (two carcinoid tumors)	28
Ovarian cancers	23
Testicular carcinomas	23
Carcinomas of prostate gland	23
Cancers of the pancreas	20
Brain neoplasms (excluding lymphomas)	13
Miscellaneous neoplasms	33
Total	2283

[a]There were 2139 patients, of whom 137 (6.4%) had two or more distinct tumor types involving different organ systems. Of these, 7 patients each had three separate types of cancer. Patients: kidney (2079), heart (41), bone marrow (8), liver (6), pancreas (3), and heart and lung (2).

Source: Reproduced from I. Penn, Risk of cancer in the transplant patient. In *Principles of Organ Transplantation,* M. W. Flye, ed. W. B. Saunders, Philadelphia (in press, 1985). (By permission of the publisher.)

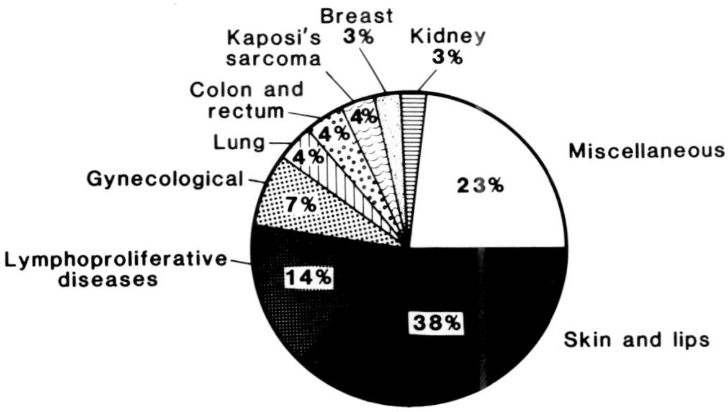

FIGURE 1 Distribution of the most common malignancies arising in organ transplant recipients.

isms [55], chronic antigenic stimulation [29], reactivation of latent oncogenic viruses [69], and direct oncogenic effects of immunosuppressive drugs [89,90]. Some of these theories will be discussed in this chapter, as we examine the different types of malignant neoplasms found in transplant recipients.

SKIN AND LIP CANCER

Skin cancers are the most common malignant neoplasms. Nonmelanoma skin cancer accounts for approximately 30% of all new cancers in the United States [98,105]. In transplant recipients, approximately 38% of de novo cancers are of the skin and lips, and the risk increases with the duration of immunosuppression (Figure 1) [44,85,89]. There is also an increased frequency of premalignant actinic keratoses among transplant patients [67], and these lesions may develop into carcinomas more rapidly. Furthermore, the skin cancers are commonly multiple and metastasize more frequently. Although skin cancer probably accounts for less than 1-2% of all transplant deaths [44,54,89,101], it causes significant morbidity as reflected in loss of limbs and disfigurement (Figure 2). Squamous cell and basal cell carcinomas are the most common types of skin and lip cancers (Table 2).

Incidence and Risk Factors

The incidence of nonmelanotic skin cancer is determined by the amount of exposure to ultraviolet light, which depends on latitude, altitude, occupation, clothing, and outdoor recreational activities [110]. When exposure is equal, fair-skinned people are more likely to develop skin cancer than those with dark skin. Other risk factors include exposure to chemical carcinogens (e.g., arsenic and organic hydrocarbons), x-rays and γ rays, chronic scars, ulcers, and sinus tracts.

In the general population, the incidence of nonmelanotic skin cancer varies from 0.15% per year in Minnesota to 0.38% per year in Texas [98]. The first report of new skin cancer in renal transplant patients came from Sydney, Australia, and showed a 14% incidence

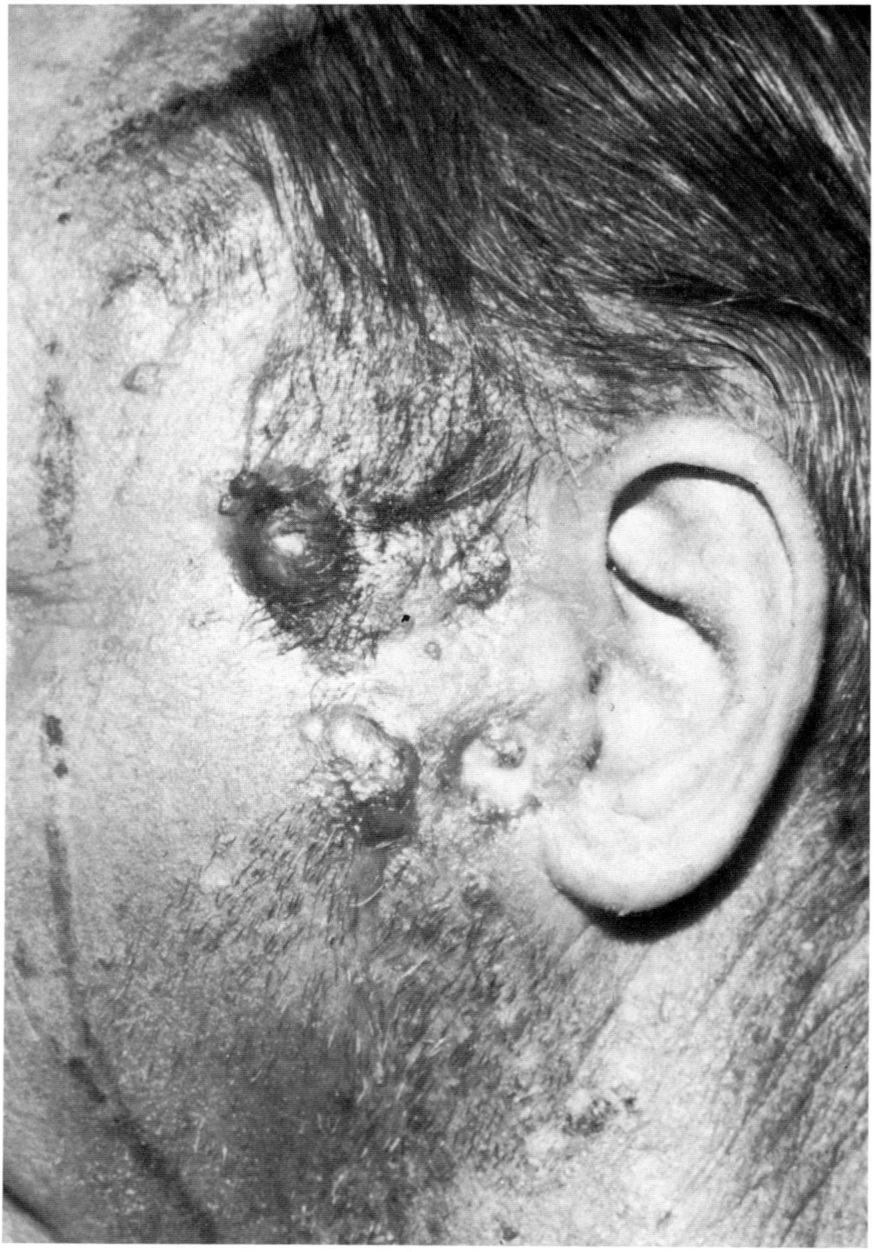

FIGURE 2 Multiple recurrent squamous cell carcinomas of the face.

TABLE 2 Carcinomas of the Skin and Lips

Type of neoplasm	No. of patients
Squamous cell carcinomas	461
Basal cell carcinomas	241
Squamous and basal cell carcinomas	115
Malignant melanoma	45[a]
Unclassified	11
Merkel's cell carcinoma	4[b]
Malignant sweat gland carcinoma	2[c]
Intracystic sebaceous gland carcinoma	1
Total	880

[a]Fifteen patients also had squamous or basal cell carcinomas.
[b]One patient also had squamous and basal cell carcinomas.
[c]Two patients also had squamous or basal cell carcinomas.
Source: Reproduced from *Principles of Organ Transplantation,* M. W. Flye, ed. W. B. Saunders, Philadelphia (in press, 1985). (By permission of the publisher.)

[116]. Since then, several reports have emphasized the increased incidence of skin and lip carcinoma in these patients, ranging from 1.4% in Minnesota to 5-14% in Australia and New Zealand [3,44,49,54,57,77,85,88,100-102,118].

Hoxtell et al. [49] reported that in the University of Minnesota renal transplant series the risk of skin cancer was 7.1 times that in the general population. Squamous cell carcinoma was 36.4 times normal. A significantly increased risk of basal cell carcinoma was found only in women. A fourfold increase in squamous cell carcinoma was reported from the United Kingdom [54]. A sevenfold increase in skin cancer was reported from Sweden but in contrast to other series was due to an increase in basal cell carcinoma [6]. From Melbourne, a 5% overall incidence of skin cancer was reported [67], which was translated into a risk factor of 20.6 times that of the general population, 18 times for males and 24.5 times for females [44].

In the Brisbane series the incidence of all types of cancer was 9.3% and 7% reported from all of Australia and New Zealand [100,101], which can be explained by the higher incidence of skin cancer. Skin cancer made up 93% of the total cancers in Brisbane [44], 77% in Australia and New Zealand [100,101], and 38% in the Cincinnati Transplant Tumor Registry [89].

The incidence of skin cancer after transplantation increases with time [44,67,101]. An overall incidence of 5% was found in one series, but when compared with patients who survived 1 and 4 years with a functioning graft, the figures were 8 and 17%, respectively [67]. Furthermore, premalignant skin lesions were found in 28% of patients who survived for four years. Similar figures were found in the combined Australia and New Zealand series [101]. With an estimated incidence of about 5% per year in one series, at 5 years the incidence was 23% and at 9 years, 44% [44]. The incidence is much lower in the northern United States [49].

Age and Sex

In the general population the average age at the time of diagnosis of skin cancer is approximately 64 years [85], but the peak incidence is between 75 and 84 years of age. In transplant recipients the diagnosis is usually made during the early 40s [44,67,77,101,116]. Children as young as 13 have had squamous cell carcinoma of the face [85].

The male/female ratio for skin cancer in the general population is approximately 3:1 for squamous cell carcinoma and 2:1 for basal cell carcinoma. In transplant recipients, the male predominance persists, with the overall ratios of 1.5:1 [44] to 3:1 [85]. The increase in risk is greater for females (24.5 times) than males (18 times) [44].

Interval from Transplantation to Diagnosis

In immunosuppressed patients cancer can develop within 2 months [85], although longer intervals, from 43 to 58 months [49,77], are the average in the United States. In Australia the average interval is 18 [116] to 34 months [44], probably the result of more intense sun exposure in a susceptible population.

Cell Type, Location, and Multiple Tumors

The most common tumors are squamous cell and basal cell carcinomas. In the general population the basal cell to squamous cell carcinoma ratio varies from 3:1 (Texas) to 6:1 (Minnesota) [49]. In the transplant population this ratio is changed to 1:1.9 because of the increased incidence of squamous cell carcinoma (52% of the total) without a significant change in the incidence of basal cell carcinoma (27% of the total) (Table 2) [44,83, 85]. Both types of tumors occurred in 13% of patients.

Most lesions are located on the sun-exposed areas of the head, neck, lips (vermillion border of the lower lip exclusively), and upper extremities (especially dorsal surfaces of the forearm, hands, and fingers) [44,85]. According to a report from the Cincinnati Registry [89] of 880 patients with skin cancer, 727 had involvement of the skin only, 86 had squamous cell carcinoma of the lips only, and 67 had skin and lip involvement (Table 2). Extensive actinic damage is common, and premalignant actinic keratoses probably progress to invasive squamous cell carcinoma more frequently in transplant patients [67]. There also appears to be more rapid progression from actinic keratosis, keratoacanthoma, and Bowen's disease to invasive squamous cell carcinoma.

According to the Cincinnati Registry, 43% of patients had multiple skin cancers [89], as did 75% of the Australian patients [44]. Of the Australian cases, 50% had more than one lesion at initial diagnosis. Others have reported the development of up to 40 primary skin carcinomas, some of them in young patients with multiple warts [77,85,118]. A viral etiology and link to epidermodysplasia verruciformis has been postulated [77].

Diagnosis, Treatment, and Prognosis

Frequent skin examinations and self-examination, particularly of skin exposed to sun, should be regular features of posttransplant care. Because the differential diagnosis of skin lesions in these patients by gross examination alone is often misleading, a biopsy should be performed on all new lesions. For example, carcinoma of the lip often appears as a superficial ulcerated lesion without other characteristics of cancer and is frequently misdiagnosed as a herpes simplex "cold sore." If a cold sore persists for 3-4 weeks, a biopsy should be performed [85]. Other unrelated neoplasms must be looked for because the relative risk is increased 11 times [44]. All patients should be instructed in the diligent use of sun screen when outdoors.

Conventional therapy usually includes local excision, cryosurgery, radiotherapy, or topical 5-fluorouracil cream, depending upon the size, location, and extent of the lesion. There is no evidence that reduction of immunosuppressive medications causes spontaneous regression or delays spread of this cancer or reduces the incidence of new lesions.

In the immunocompromised host, squamous cell carcinoma appears to be more virulent than in the general population [44,65,85]. Although local recurrence is unusual, the Cincinnati Registry notes that 12% (56 patients) of transplant patients with squamous cell carcinoma had regional lymph node or distant metastases [89]. In the general population the incidence of metastases of squamous cell carcinomas that arise in actinic damaged skin is 0.1-0.5% [31,61]. In contrast, squamous cell carcinoma of the lip has a high risk of metastases (5-37%) in both groups [110]. At the University of Minnesota, we have seen six patients with squamous cell carcinomas of the lip, of whom two (33%) developed regional lymph node metastases (unpublished observations). One died of an aggressive squamous cell carcinoma that metastasized to the lung. Because we cannot predict which tumors will metastasize, all patients with squamous cell carcinoma of the lip must be evaluated regularly.

Although few transplant patients die because of skin cancer, a 10-fold increase in the risk of death from squamous cell carcinoma of the skin has been reported [54]. Hardie reported 2 deaths in 24 patients with skin cancer, 1 from cell carcinoma, and 1 from a melanoma, 2.4% of the transplant deaths in his series [44]. In the Cincinnati Registry, 4% of patients with skin cancer died of metastatic disease [89].

Pathogenesis

Many factors interact to cause the increased incidence of skin and lip carcinoma in immunosuppressed transplant recipients. Both epidemiologic and experimental evidence implicate ultraviolet light in the pathogenesis of skin carcinoma in the general population and immunocompromised patients [32,110]. Tobacco exposure is an important risk factor in lip cancer [14]. Other factors that may also be important, either alone or in combination, include impaired immune surveillance mechanisms, chronic antigenic stimulation from the transplanted allograft, reactivation of latent oncogenic viruses, and direct oncogenic effects of immunosuppressive drugs.

Although none of these has been proved, a few clues are available. Hairless mice, a strain prone to the development of ultraviolet light-induced skin cancer, develop skin cancer with greater frequency when exposed to a combination of ultraviolet light and azathioprine [56]. Thymectomy plus the chemical carcinogen 3,4-benzopyrene will produce a higher incidence of skin tumors in mice than 3,4-benzopyrene alone [74]. Furthermore, under certain circumstances, herpesviruses are oncogenic viruses. Ultraviolet-irradiated herpes simplex virus type 1 transforms both the mouse L cell [78] and hamster embryo fibroblasts [92] and can cause chromosomal changes in vitro [79,115]. This ability of ultraviolet light to change this virus from the infectious to the oncogenic form is intriguing because (1) most skin cancers occur on sun-exposed areas of the body and (2) the lower lip is a frequent location of both herpes simplex type 1 infection and squamous cell carcinoma in transplant patients. A case of squamous cell carcinoma of the lower lip that developed at the site of a chronic herpes simplex infection has been reported in a nonimmunosuppressed patient [11]. Eglin et al. have detected RNA complementary to herpes simplex virus in 14 of 24 human oral squamous cell carcinomas [19]. However, they do not state how many were positive for HSV-1 or HSV-2, although both were tested. Thus, lip cancer in transplant patients might be related to a combination of herpes simplex virus infection, immunosuppression, and ultraviolet light. Evidence also exists that suggests an oncogenic role for human papilloma virus (HPV) [7,62-64]. Patients with the rare, chronic flat wart disease, epidermodysplasia verruciformis, have detectable HPV in skin lesions [81]. Squamous cell carcinoma develops in 35% of these patients during the second and third decade, usually on sun-exposed skin [50,93,94]. Anogenital neoplasias have also been linked to HPV [121].

OTHER CANCERS INVOLVING THE SKIN

Melanoma

The risk of melanoma after organ transplantation is unclear because the patient population is small [89,120]. The Cincinnati Registry has accumulated data on 45 patients with melanoma (5.1% of all patients with skin cancer [89] compared to 2.7% in the general population) [105]. Hardie reported two patients with melanoma [44], one of whom had done well for 9 months with no evidence of recurrent disease; the other, with two melanomas, died of metastatic disease 2 years after appearance of the second tumor. There is some evidence to suggest that melanoma in some of these patients may evolve from dysplastic nevi [33] and may have enhanced malignant growth potential with increased immunosuppression [108]. Other reports have cited the development of melanoma after the use of immunosuppressive therapy not associated with transplantation [8,12,66].

Kaposi's Sarcoma

Kaposi's sarcoma is a rare tumor that comprises only 0.6% of all cancers in the general population in the United States [15,83]; although a recent outbreak has been reported in homosexual men with the acquired immune deficiency syndrome (AIDS) [9,18,24,25,99]. This disease seems at least in part to result from an immunodeficiency induced by T-cell infection with human T-cell leukemia virus (HTLV III). A total of 80 cases (3.5%) of Kaposi's sarcoma in organ transplant recipients were reported to the Cincinnati Registry [89]. Harwood et al. [46] reported 4 cases of Kaposi's sarcoma in 100 renal transplant recipients, which represented a 400- to 500-fold greater incidence than in a controlled population in Toronto. Penn reviewed 20 cases of Kaposi's sarcoma arising in organ transplant recipients [86]. Their average age at the time of transplantation was 42 years, and the diagnosis was made an average of 16 months later. This is a shorter interval than is usually seen with other de novo neoplasms in transplant patients (37 months). The male/female ratio was 2:1, compared with 9:1-15:1 in the general population.

Kaposi's sarcoma is an angiomatous neoplasm derived from vasoformative mesenchyma, which primarily involves the skin [1]. On gross examination the characteristic lesions are multiple, irregular, bluish dermal plaques or nodules, which occasionally resemble raised pyogenic granulomas. Although the disease usually begins on the feet and legs, the lesions can be found on the mucous membranes of the mouth and oropharynx. The skin is almost always involved, and visceral involvement, particularly the gastrointestinal tract, can also occur [103]. The diagnosis of Kaposi's sarcoma is made primarily on gross appearance and histologic confirmation.

Treatment usually involves reduction in immunosuppression [45,59,86], radiotherapy [45,60,86], or chemotherapy [45,58,86]. In one series, 8 of 11 patients with nonvisceral involvement had complete regression of their disease after a change or reduction in their immunosuppressive medication [86]. Two additional patients had partial remission, and one was not treated (outcome not stated). The results are difficult to interpret because several patients did receive radiotherapy, chemotherapy, or both, and two patients merely had cyclophosphamide substituted for azathioprine with no reduction in the corticosteroid dosage. However, two patients with skin involvement had total remission of the disease after discontinuation of azathioprine only.

Of 13 patients with visceral involvement by Kaposi's sarcoma, 9 died [86]. In this series, complete remission occurred in only 1 patient after chemotherapy, a reduction in steroids, and substitution of cyclophosphamide for azathioprine. A second patient had a partial response to a combination of chemotherapy, radiotherapy, and a reduction in azathioprine; a third showed no improvement after a reduction in azathioprine alone.

Few details are available regarding the subsequent changes in renal function in these patients. Of 12 patients who had a change in their immunosuppressive medications, 7 (58%) had no change in renal function, whereas 5 had a reduction in renal function. The cause of this disorder is obscure, although a viral etiology has been proposed. Cytomegalovirus (CMV) has been isolated in an in vitro established tumor cell line [27]. A serologic association between American Kaposi's sarcoma (but not the African form) and cytomegalovirus has been reported [28]. This is of interest because of the high incidence of CMV infection soon after transplantation and the relatively short interval between transplantation and diagnosis. An association between CMV and Kaposi's sarcoma is also suggested by the demonstration of CMV antigens by immunofluorescence and CMV RNA by in situ hybridization in tumor biopsy specimens [17].

LYMPHOPROLIFERATIVE DISEASES

General Considerations

"Malignant lymphomas" are the second most common malignancy after skin and lip carcinoma and make up 14% of the total (Figure 1). The risk of a renal allograft recipient developing malignant lymphoma is said to be increased 40 times [48]. Because a morphologic spectrum of B-cell proliferation exists, we prefer the general term "lymphoproliferative diseases," which encompasses Epstein-Barr virus (EBV)-induced B-cell proliferations ranging from reactive, polyclonal hyperplasias to true monoclonal malignant lymphomas, as discussed below. The overall incidence of lymphoproliferative diseases now reported in renal, liver, heart, and heart-lung transplant recipients is 1% [40] to 2.5% [109], 2.3% [109], 5% [4] to 6.3% [109], and 33.3% [109], respectively. If only patients at risk (i.e., those alive with functioning grafts) were included, the incidence would no doubt be higher. Early concern that cyclosporine (CsA) therapy would lead to a higher incidence of lymphoproliferative diseases [10] has not materialized as experience with the drug has increased [82]. The degree of immunosuppression, rather than the particular type, is probably the most important predisposing factor.

In Penn's study of 316 patients with lymphoproliferative disorders (Table 3), extranodal involvement occurred in 76% of patients, compared with 24-48% of patients in the general population [89]. In 66% of these transplant patients, only a single organ was affected. The single organ most frequently involved was the brain (54%), although they were frequently multicentric. Hodgkin's disease occurred in only 11 patients (4%). The average

TABLE 3 Lymphomas in Organ Transplant Recipients

Type of tumor	No. of patients
Reticulum cell sarcomas[a]	182
Unclassified lymphomas	47
B-cell lymphomas	40
Lymphosarcomas	11[b]
Hodgkin's disease	11
Plasma cell lymphomas	7
B-cell hyperplasias (lymphomas?)	7
Lymphoreticular malignancies	4
T-cell lymphomas (one case of mycosis fungoides)	4
Burkitt's lymphoma	1
Histiocytic medullary reticulosis	1
True histiocytic lymphoma	1
Total	316

[a]Also classified as histiocytic lymphoma, microglioma, immunoblastic sarcoma, reticulosarcoma, and large cell lymphoma.
[b]One patient had a reticulum cell sarcoma, which underwent spontaneous regression. He developed a lymphocytic lymphoma 2 years later.
Source: Reproduced from I. Penn, Risk of cancer in the transplant patient. In *Principles in Organ Transplantation,* M. W. Flye, ed. W. B. Saunders, Philadelphia (in press, 1985). (By permission of publisher.)

age at the time of transplantation was 38 years (range, 5-70 years) [87], and the interval from transplant to diagnosis averaged 27 months (range, 2-146 months).

In the past 5 years we have attempted to systematically characterize the clinical, histologic, immunologic, cytogenetic, and virologic features of these lymphoproliferative diseases in order to delineate gaps in our knowledge and to predict the most appropriate therapy [26,35-43]. Our results will be summarized and compared with those of others. Of particular interest are the three largest well-studied series from Minnesota, Pittsburgh, and Stanford.

Clinical Syndromes

In the Minnesota series two main clinical groups have been identified (Table 4) [39,40, 43]. First, young patients (mean age, 21 years) present soon after transplantation (mean interval from transplantation to diagnosis, 7.8 months) or antirejection therapy (i.e., during periods of maximal immunosuppression) with an infectious mononucleosislike syndrome characterized by fever, pharyngitis, and lymphadenopathy. Second, older patients (mean age, 47 years) present at longer intervals after transplantation (mean interval, 5.3 years) with localized, extranodal tumor masses often with unusual clinical and radiologic manifestations [23,113].

Early reports from Penn's registry have emphasized a high (49%) incidence of CNS involvement (compared to less than 2% in the nontransplanted patients), including a high

TABLE 4 Summary of Patient Groups with Posttransplantation Lymphoproliferative Diseases

Group 1: Infectious mononucleosislike illness (42%)	Group 2: Localized solid tumor masses (58%)
Young patients	Older patients
Mean age, 21 years	Mean age, 47 years
Range, 11-46 years	Range, 22-68 years
Short interval from transplantation to diagnosis	Long interval from transplantation to diagnosis
Mean interval, 7.8 months	Mean interval, 5.3 years
Range, 1 week to 2.8 years	Range, 1.1-11 years
Symptoms of viral illness (fever, pharyngitis, lymphadenopathy)	Symptoms related to solid tumor masses (confined to CNS in 14%)
Widespread disease	More localized, primarily extranodal disease
Mortality rate (50%)	Mortality rate (75%)
Short clinical course when fatal	Longer clinical course when fatal
Mean survival, 2.3 months	Mean survival, 6.6 months
Range, 10 days to 8 months	Range, 2 weeks to 15 months
Responds to acyclovir	No response to acyclovir

proportion (82%) of disease limited to the CNS [83,97]. In our series, CNS involvement has occurred in 45% of patients and is usually indicative of widespread disease. Disease confined to the CNS occurred in only 14%. At Pittsburgh [109], 6 of 17 cases developed a syndrome of fever and of generalized lymphadenopathy, resembling infectious mononucleosis. Of the 17, however, 9 developed gastrointestinal lymphomas manifested by perforation, obstruction, or hemorrhage. A total of 11 patients developed solid tumors in a variety of extranodal sites. All 10 cardiac transplant patients reported from Stanford [4] had localized extranodal disease with the CNS the most common site (5 patients), followed by the lung, ATG injection site, and liver. This group noted a marked increased incidence of disease in patients treated with a combination of CsA, prednisone, and ATG (5 lymphomas in 39 recipients).

Histology

Morphologically, all these EBV-related lymphoid disorders have the features of polymorphic B-cell proliferation and produce extensive architectural obliteration of the organs involved [26]. However, some cases—classified as polymorphic diffuse B-cell hyperplasia (PDBH)—show marked plasmacytic differentiation, without atypia and necrosis, and others—classified as polymorphic B-cell lymphomas (PBL)—are characterized by nuclear atypia of the large cells and extensive necrosis. The lymphoproliferative diseases in cardiac allograft recipients have all been classified as diffuse large cell lymphomas [117]. No disorders resembling PDBH were apparently seen in either Stanford series. In the Pittsburgh series 2 patients had B-cell hyperplasia, 11 had large noncleaved cell lymphoma, and 3 had immunoblastic malignant lymphoma. Although these findings are consistent with our observations of a histologic spectrum including plasmacytoid and follicular center cell differentiation, a closer comparison between this and our series is not possible.

Immunologic Cell Typing

Using fluorescein-conjugated monospecific antibodies against each heavy and light Ig chains [26,36,39,40,43], we have shown that 8 of 11 lymphoid lesions studied were polyclonal B-cell proliferations. True monoclonal B-cell tumors (IgG-κ in all three cases) have also been documented. Furthermore, there is strong evidence that these B-cell monoclonal proliferations may progress from benign polyclonal B-cell hyperplasia to malignant lymphoma in a short period of time in association with the appearance of cytogenetic abnormalities [37,40]. In the Pittsburgh series, the lymphoproliferations were found to be polyclonal in six and monoclonal in three, and the clonality was indeterminate in six [109]. As was true in our series, all patients histologically interpreted as hyperplasia had polyclonal proliferations.

Cytogenetic Studies

Cytogenetic analysis has suggested that polyclonal B-cell proliferations may be precursors of monoclonal malignant lymphomas and may undergo malignant transformation identified by clonal cytogenetic abnormalities. We have been able to examine metaphase preparations from biopsy specimens in five patients [40]. In two patients with polyclonal PDBH, the karyotypes were normal diploid (46,XY) so that these tumors meet all the criteria for a benign, EBV-induced B-cell proliferation (hyperplasia, polyclonal, and diploid). In a second set of patients with polyclonal PBL, clonal cytogenetic abnormalities indicative of early malignant transformation were identified in a subpopulation of cells (trisomy-3 and trisomy-14, respectively). In one patient with a monoclonal (IgG-κ) PBL, a majority of cells contained a clonal cytogenetic translocation [t(2;19)(p23;p13)].

EBV Studies

The link between EBV and these lymphoproliferative diseases has been established further by means of serologic studies, ENBA staining of tumor tissue, and EBV DNA hybridization studies that demonstrate the presence of EBV-specific DNA sequences in biopsy specimens. In the Minnesota series, tumor-bearing patients with an infectious mononucleosislike illness may have serologic evidence of a primary (33%), reactivation (33%), or long-past EBV infection (33%) [40]. Of the three primary infections, two were heterophile positive. In older patients with tumor masses, no primary infections occurred, but serologic evidence of reactivation infection (63%) or long-past infection (37%) was found. Staining of tumor tissue for EBNA has been positive in several instances [13,39, 109], but false-negative results can occur for technical reasons, and EBV DNA hybridization techniques have provided a more sensitive method of detecting the EBV genome within tumor cells. Lymphoid lesions from 10 of 12 renal transplant recipients in the Minnesota series [39,40,95] and from four cardiac transplant recipients from Stanford [96] contained EBV-specific DNA sequences using EBV cRNA/DNA filter hybridization, vDNA/DNA reassociation kinetic analysis, or the Southern blot test. In the Pittsburgh series, 6 of 12 patients had EBNA-positive lymphoproliferations. Hybridization studies were not reported.

Therapy

Because most patients had EBV-carrying polyclonal B-cell proliferations and serologic evidence of a reactivated or primary EBV infection, we hypothesized that interruption of EBV replication with acyclovir (9-[(2-hydroxyethoxy)-methyl] guanine) may be effective therapy [37]. Acyclovir inhibits EBV DNA replication only in virus-producing cell lines by blocking the EBV-associated DNA polymerase but does not alter the synthesis of the latent EBV genome in nonproducer cell lines [37]. We have now treated seven patients with acyclovir and can predict, at least in part, the responsiveness to acyclovir based on the combined evaluation of clinical, histologic, immunologic, and cytogenetic characteristics [35,37,40]. Three groups of patients have been identified (Figure 3) [35,42].

Group 1 patients (three) have an EBV-induced IM-like illness characterized by a polyclonal PDBH, without cytogenetic abnormalities. All three had complete resolution of disease during acyclovir therapy [35]. This EBV-induced, benign (hyperplasia, polyclonal, diploid) B-cell proliferation is dependent on active viral replication (lytic cycle) which can be interrupted by blocking further viral synthesis using acyclovir. A reduction in immunosuppression may or may not be necessary depending on the severity of EBV infection and response to acyclovir.

Group 2 patients also have an IM-like illness, and cell marker studies demonstrate a polyclonal B-cell proliferation. Early malignant transformation, that is, progression from polyclonal to monoclonal, is suggested, however, by the findings of morphologic features of malignancy (polymorphic B-cell lymphoma) and clonal cytogenetic abnormalities in a small percentage of tumor cells. Because of the risk of progression from a polyclonal to a monoclonal B-cell proliferation, immunosuppression should be reduced or stopped in most of the kidney transplant patients with this lymphoproliferative disease

Group 1

Clinical	*Histology*
Infectious Mononucleosis-like Illness	Polymorphic Diffuse B-cell Hyperplasia
Immunologic Cell Typing	***Cytogenetics***
Polyclonal B-cell Proliferation	Normal Karyotype

Benign

Group 2

Clinical	*Histology*
Infectious Mononucleosis-like Illness	Polymorphic B-cell Lymphoma
Immunologic Cell Typing	***Cytogenetics***
Polyclonal B-cell Proliferation	Clonal Cytogenetic Abnormalities

Early Malignant Transformation

Group 3

Clinical	*Histology*
Localized Solid Tumor Masses	Polymorphic B-cell Lymphoma
Immunologic Cell Typing	***Cytogenetics***
Monoclonal B-cell Proliferation	Clonal Cytogenetic Abnormalities

Monoclonal Lymphoma

FIGURE 3 Summary of renal transplant recipients with EBV-related lymphoproliferative diseases. [Reproduced from D. W. Hanto, G. Frizzera, K. J. Gajl-Peczalska, and R. L. Simmons, Epstein-Barr virus, immunodeficiency, and B-cell lymphoproliferation. *Transplantation* 39:461-472, 1985. (By permission of the publisher.)]

and rejection allowed to proceed, should it occur. Serial biopsies should be performed as indicated to detect this transition.

Group 3 includes older patients who develop extranodal solid tumors that are morphologically malignant (PBL) and monoclonal and may contain clonal cytogenetic abnormalities. These lymphomas may begin as EBV-induced proliferations in association with cytogenetic transformation and are composed of latently infected (and therefore acyclovir-insensitive) B cells, as demonstrated in two patients. Standard chemotherapy or radiation therapy, combined with discontinuation of immunosuppressive drugs, should be used in these patients, whose mortality rates remain greater than 80%.

Other forms of treatment may be applicable in selected patients. Radiation therapy, combined with a reduction in immunosuppression, is still the treatment of choice in primary CNS lymphomas, although the recurrence rate is high and survival time is short [40]. They are histologically identical to the other EBV-related lymphomas and may be caused by EBV [47]. Therefore, the addition of acyclovir therapy might be helpful in these patients, although the clonality of the CNS lymphomas, an important determinant in acyclovir responsiveness in other patients, is not known.

GYNECOLOGIC CANCERS

McKann's 1969 report of a patient who developed squamous cell carcinoma of the cervix 2.5 years after renal transplantation [71] was the first of its kind. Subsequently other reports appeared of gynecologic cancers after transplantation [34,53,91,104,111]. They included cervical dysplasia, carcinoma in situ and invasive squamous cell carcinoma of the cervix, and metastatic malignant dysgerminoma of the ovary. In 1978, Penn reported 49 patients with gynecologic cancers—42 squamous cell carcinomas of the cervix, 3 adenocarcinomas of the uterus, and 4 ovarian carcinomas (not classified) [90]. Endometrial carcinoma was rare, either reflecting the younger age of transplant recipients or the different mechanisms responsible for development of disease.

Gynecologic cancers occur in 8.6% of patients who develop de novo neoplasms after transplantation and are the third most frequent type. However, cervical carcinoma alone occurred in 21% of women who developed cancer after transplantation. Of these 42 patients, 32 (76%) had carcinoma in situ, generally accepted as the precursor of invasive carcinoma, 6 (14%) had invasive carcinomas, and in 4 (10%) the depth of invasion was not reported. The risk of developing carcinoma of the cervix in situ has been calculated to be 14 times that of an age-matched control population [91]. The mean age at the time of diagnosis was 36 years (range, 22-50 years). The average interval between transplantation and diagnosis was 38 months (range, 6-97 months).

Conventional therapy for cervical carcinoma, including simple hysterectomy for minimally invasive disease and cone excision of the cervix or cryosurgery for carcinoma in situ, has been effective. As in the case of most skin cancers, a reduction in immunosuppression does not seem to be essential or even advisable. The morbidity and mortality are low. In one report only 2 of 18 patients with cervical carcinomas (16 carcinoma in situ and 2 invasive) treated in this fashion had progression of their disease [91]. One patient did well after a hysterectomy for recurrent cervical carcinoma after conization, but the other died of metastatic disease following a hysterectomy for invasive carcinoma and radiotherapy for a vaginal vault recurrence. All female transplant recipients who receive standard immunosuppressive therapy should have frequent, regular gynecologic examinations, including Pap smears.

The pathogenesis of cervical carcinomas in these patients is undoubtedly also multifactorial. There are many reports of cervical dysplasia and carcinoma developing in patients who receive therapy with busulfan, cyclophosphamide, azathioprine, prednisone, and methotrexate [91]. Although a clear cause and effect has not been established, the seroepidemiologic association between herpes simplex virus type 2 and cervical carcinoma in the general population [112] and the high frequency of herpesvirus infection in transplant patients are particularly interesting. Human papilloma virus (HPV) may also be important in the pathogenesis of these tumors [121].

TRANSPLANTATION OF KIDNEYS FROM DONORS WITH CANCER

Rarely, a malignant neoplasm is transplanted with the donor organ. Southam et al. reported the results of homotransplantation of human neoplastic cell lines into normal volunteers and terminal cancer patients [106], 8 years before the first report of a transplanted cancer [70,73]. An inflammatory response was evoked in the volunteers, and the transplanted tumor implants were rejected within 4 weeks. In the cancer patients, however, the inflammatory response was depressed, the tumor implants often grew for 1-3 weeks before regression occurred at 4-6 weeks, and the tumor implants of several patients continued to grow until excised several weeks later. In 1965, McPhaul and McIntosh described a recipient of a cadaver kidney from a patient who died of squamous cell carcinoma of the priform sinus [70,73]. The recipient died 8 months after transplantation of squamous cell carcinoma that had metastasized to the liver and transplanted kidney. The inadvertent transplantation of organs from donors with cancer has been reported many times since then [2,16,20,22,30,52,68,72,75,76,114,119,122].

Penn's series of 91 recipients of organs from donors with cancer (90 kidney and 1 heart) [89]. Donors with primary CNS cancers are excluded. Interestingly, one of the most common tumors in the donors were bronchogenic carcinomas, the most frequent metastatic tumor found in the kidney in the general population [80], and primary renal carcinomas. Transplanted cancers appeared in 37 recipients (41%). In 12 of 37 patients, the donor had a primary renal tumor either not detected at the time of transplant (7 patients) or biopsied at the time of donor nephrectomy (4 patients). In the other 25 patients with transplanted malignancies, the donor had disseminated bronchial carcinomas, breast carcinoma, or melanomas. Of the 37 patients, 10 had tumors confined to the allograft, 3 had invasion of surrounding structures, and in 24 there were distant metastases.

Malignant neoplasms were found in 6 of 13 kidneys transplanted from living donors [89], 4 of which involved cancers found during the donor nephrectomy. At the time, 2 of them were treated by wide excision; 1 patient underwent transplant nephrectomy after histologic confirmation 48 hr later, and the fourth patient had a partial nephrectomy 3 months posttransplant. None of these four patients have shown evidence of recurrent or metastatic disease. Two other cases of transplanted renal carcinomas have been reported in which one showed local spread and one developed distant metastases.

In summary, transplanted tumors appeared in 24 of 65 patients (37%) receiving kidneys from donors known to have cancer. As Penn has pointed out, the chance of transmission of cancer to the recipient is less for low-grade cancers that rarely metastasize and highest for bronchial and renal carcinomas. In 15 of 24 patients, widespread metastases occurred and resulted in death in a majority. Only three cases of "immunologic" rejection of the transmitted cancer after cessation of immunosuppressive medication have been reported. Prevention is critical.

To prevent transmission of malignant cells by the transplanted organ, the first priority is to not accept any donor with a known cancer, other than low-grade skin cancers or primary central nervous system neoplasms. Because occult primary tumors, especially of the bronchus, often appear to be a primary brain tumor, a firm tissue diagnosis should be obtained before transplantation from such a donor. If a suspicious lesion is found at the time of donor nephrectomy, a biopsy and frozen section diagnosis should be obtained. If the lesion is malignant, the organ probably should not be transplanted. If histologic evidence of cancer is not available or is later revised on permanent histologic section, a transplant nephrectomy (preferable) or wide excision of the lesion should be performed.

ACKNOWLEDGMENT

This study was supported by USPHS Grant AM 13083.

REFERENCES

1. Akhtar, M., Bunuan, B., Ali, M. A., and Godwin, J. T. Kaposi's sarcoma in renal transplant recipients—ultrastructural and immunoperoxidase study of four cases. *Cancer* 53:258-266, 1984.
2. Baird, R. N., White, H. J. O., and Tribe, C. R. Renal carcinoma in a cadaver kidney graft donor. *Br. Med. J.* 17:371, 1975.
3. Berger, H. M., Goldman, R., Gonick, H. C., and Waisman, J. Epidermoid carcinoma of the lip after renal transplantation. *Arch. Intern. Med.* 128:609-612, 1971.
4. Bieber, C. P., Heberling, R. L., Jamieson, S. W., et al. Lymphoma in cardiac transplant recipients associated with cyclosporin A, prednisone and anti-thymocyte globulin (ATG). In *Immune Deficiency and Cancer,* D. T. Purtilo, ed. Plenum, New York, 1984, pp. 309-320.
5. Birkeland, S. A. Malignant tumors in renal transplant patients—the Scandia transplant material. *Cancer* 51:1571-1575, 1983.
6. Blohmé, I., and Larko, O. Premalignant and malignant skin lesions in renal transplant patients. *Transplantation* 37:165-167, 1984.
7. Boyle, J., MacKie, R. M., Briggs, J. D., Junor, B. J. R., and Aitchison, T. C. Cancer, warts, and sunshine in renal transplant patients. *Lancet* 1:702-705, 1984.
8. Brady, R. S., Schottenfeld, D., and Reid, A. Multiple primary cancer risk after therapy for Hodgkin's disease. *Cancer* 40:1917-1926, 1977.
9. Broder, S., and Gallo, R. C. A pathogenic retovirus (HTLV-III) linked to AIDS. *N. Engl. J. Med.* 311:1292-1297, 1984.
10. Calne, R. Y., Rolles, K., White, D. J. G., et al. Cyclosporin A initially as the only immunosuppressant in 34 recipients of cadaveric organs: 32 kidneys, 2 pancreases, and 2 livers. *Lancet* 2:1033-1036, 1979.
11. Caron, G. A. Carcinoma at the site of herpes simplex infection. *JAMA* 243:2396, 1980.
12. Chaudhuri, P. K., Walker, M. J., and Das Gupta, T. K. Cutaneous malignant melanoma after immunosuppressive therapy. *Arch. Surg.* 115:322-323, 1980.
13. Crawford, D. H., Thomas, J. A., Janossy, G., et al. Epstein-Barr virus nuclear antigen positive lymphoma after cyclosporin A treatment in patient with renal allograft. *Lancet* 1:1355-1356, 1980.
14. Decker, J., and Goldstein, J. C. Current concepts in otolaryngology—risk factors in head and neck cancer. *N. Engl. J. Med.* 306:1151-1155, 1982.

15. DiGiovanna, J. J., and Safai, B. Kaposi's sarcoma–retrospective study of 90 cases with particular emphasis on the familial occurrence, ethnic background and prevalence of other diseases. *Am. J. Med.* 71:779-783, 1981.
16. Downes, M. E. Transplant of a kidney containing an occult metastasis. *Br. J. Radiol.* 53:908-909, 1980.
17. Drew, W. L., Conant, M. A., Miner, R. C., et al. Cytomegalovirus and Kaposi's sarcoma in young homosexual men. *Lancet* 2:125-127, 1982.
18. Durack, D. T. Opportunistic infections and Kaposi's sarcoma in homosexual men. *N. Engl. J. Med.* 305:1465-1467, 1981.
19. Eglin, R. P., Scully, C., Lehner, T., Ward-Booth, P., and McGregor, I. A. Detection of RNA complementary to herpes simplex virus in human oral squamous cell carcinoma. *Lancet* 2:766-768, 1983.
20. Fairman, R. M., Grossman, R. A., Barker, C. F., and Perloff, L. J. Inadvertent transplantation of a melanoma. *Transplantation* 30:328-330, 1980.
21. Filipovich, A. H., Zerbe, D., Spector, B. D., and Kersey, J. H. Lymphomas in persons with naturally occurring immunodeficiency disorders. In *Pathogenesis of Leukemias and Lymphomas: Environmental Influences,* I. T. Magrath, G. T. O'Conor, and B. Ramot, eds. Raven, New York, 1984, pp. 225-234.
22. Fox, M. Renal carcinoma in a living kidney graft donor. *Transplantation* 15:523-525, 1973.
23. Frick, M. P., Salomonowitz, E., Hanto, D. W., and Gedgaudas-McClees, K. CT of abdominal lymphoma after renal transplantation. *Am. J. Roentgenol.* 142:97-99, 1984.
24. Friedman-Kien, A. E., Laubenstein, L., Marmor, M., et al. Kaposi's sarcoma and pneumocystis pneumonia among homosexual men–New York City and California. *Morbid. Mortal. Weekly Rep.* 30:305-308, 1981.
25. Friedman-Kien, A. E., Laubenstein, L. J., Rubenstein, P., et al. Disseminated Kaposi's sarcoma in homosexual men. *Ann. Intern. Med.* 96:693-700, 1982.
26. Frizzera, G., Hanto, D. W., Gajl-Peczalska, K. J., et al. Polymorphic diffuse B-cell hyperplasias and lymphomas in renal transplant recipients. *Cancer Res.* 41:4262-6279, 1981.
27. Giraldo, G., Beth, E., and Haguenau, F. Herpes-type virus particles in tissue culture of Kaposi's sarcoma from different geographic regions. *JNCI* 49:1509-1526, 1972.
28. Giraldo, G., Beth, E., Henle, W., et al. Antibody patterns to herpesviruses in Kaposi's sarcoma. II. Serological association of American Kaposi's sarcoma with cytomegalovirus. *Int. J. Cancer* 22:126-131, 1978.
29. Gleichmann, E., Gleichman, H., Schwartz, R. S., Weinblatt, A., and Armstrong, M. Y. K. Immunologic induction of malignant lymphoma: Identification of donor and host tumors in the graft-versus-host model. *JNCI* 54:107-116, 1975.
30. Gokel, J. M., Rjosk, H. K., Meister, P., Stelter, W. J., and Witte, J. Metastatic choriocarcinoma transplanted with cadaver kidney. *Cancer* 39:1317-1321, 1977.
31. Graham, H. H., and Helwig, E. G. Cutaneous premalignant lesions. In *Advances in Biology of Skin: Carcinogenesis,* W. Montagna and R. L. Dobson, eds. Pergamon Press, New York, 1966, Vol. 7.
32. Granstein, R. D., and Sober, A. J. Current concepts in ultraviolet carcinogenesis (41406). *Proc. Soc. Exp. Biol. Med.* 170:115-125, 1982.
33. Greene, M. H., Young, T. I., and Clark, W. H., Jr. Malignant melanoma in renal-transplant recipients. *Lancet* 1:1196-1199, 1981.
34. Gupta, P. K., Pinn, V. M., and Taft, P. D. Cervical dysplasia associated with azathioprine (Imuran) therapy. *Acta Cytol.* (*Baltimore*) 13:373-376, 1969.
35. Hanto, D. W., Frizzera, G., Gajl-Peczalska, K. J., Balfour, H. H., Jr., Simmons, R. L., and Najarian, J. S. Acyclovir therapy of Epstein-Barr virus (EBV)-induced posttransplant lymphoproliferative diseases. *Transplant. Proc.* 17:89-92, 1985.

36. Hanto, D. W., Frizzera, G., Gajl-Peczalska, K. J., et al. The Epstein-Barr virus (EBV) in the pathogenesis of post-transplant lymphoma. *Transplant. Proc.* 13:756-760, 1981.
37. Hanto, D. W., Frizzera, G., Gajl-Peczalska, K. J., et al. Epstein-Barr virus induced B-cell lymphoma after renal transplantation. Acyclovir therapy and transition from a polyclonal to monoclonal B-cell proliferation. *N. Engl. J. Med.* 306:913-918, 1982.
38. Hanto, D. W., Frizzera, G., Gajl-Peczalska, K. J., et al. Epstein-Barr virus-induced B-cell lymphoma after renal transplantation. *N. Engl. J. Med.* 307:896-897, 1982.
39. Hanto, D. W., Frizzera, G., Purtilo, D. T., et al. A clinical spectrum of lymphoproliferative disorders in renal transplant recipients and evidence for the role of the Epstein-Barr virus. *Cancer Res.* 41:4253-4261, 1981.
40. Hanto, D. W., Gajl-Peczalska, K. J., Frizzera, G., et al. Epstein-Barr virus (EBV) induced polyclonal and monoclonal B-cell lymphoproliferative diseases occurring after renal transplantation. *Ann. Surg.* 198:356-369, 1983.
41. Hanto, D. W., and Simmons, R. L. Lymphoproliferative diseases in immunosuppressed patients. In *Progress in Transplantation,* P. J. Morris and N. L. Tilney, eds. Churchill-Livingstone, Edinburgh, 1984, pp. 186-208.
42. Hanto, D. W., Frizzera, G., Gajl-Peczalska, K. J., and Simmons, R. L. Epstein-Barr virus, immunodeficiency and B-cell lymphoproliferation. *Transplantation* 1985, in press.
43. Hanto, D. W., Sakamoto, K., Purtilo, D. T., et al. The Epstein-Barr virus in the pathogenesis of post-transplant lymphoproliferative disorders. Clinical pathologic, and virologic correlations. *Surgery* 90:204-213, 1981.
44. Hardie, I. R., Strong, R. W., Hartley, L. C. J., Woodruff, P. W. H., and Clunie, G. J. A. Skin cancer in Caucasian renal allograft recipients living in a subtropical climate. *Surgery* 87:177-183, 1980.
45. Hardy, M. A., Goldfarb, P., Levine, S., Dattner, A., Muggia, F. M., Levitt, S., and Weinstein, E. De novo Kaposi's sarcoma in renal transplantation. *Cancer* 38:144-148, 1976.
46. Harwood, A. R., Osoba, D., Hopstader, S. L., et al. Kaposi's sarcoma in recipients of renal transplant. *Am. J. Med.* 67:759-765, 1979.
47. Hochberg, F. H., Miller, G., Schooley, R. T., Hirsch, M. S., Florino, P., and Henle, W. Central-nervous-system lymphoma related to Epstein-Barr virus. *N. Engl. J. Med.* 309: 745-748, 1983.
48. Hoover, R., and Fraumeni, J. F., Jr. Risk of cancer in renal-transplant recipients. *Lancet* 2:55-57, 1973.
49. Hoxtell, E. O., Mandel, J. S., Murray, S. S., Schuman, L. M., and Goetz, R. W. Incidence of skin carcinoma after renal transplantation. *Arch. Dermatol.* 113:436-438, 1977.
50. Jablonska, S., Dabrowski, J., and Jakubowicz, K. Epidermodysplasia verruciformis as a model in studies on the role of papovaviruses in oncogenesis. *Cancer Res.* 32:583-589, 1972.
51. Jacobs, D., Brunner, F. P., Brynger, H., et al. Malignant diseases in patients treated by dialysis and transplantation in Europe. *Transplant. Proc.* 13:729-732, 1981.
52. Jeremy, D., Farnsworth, R. H., Robertson, M. R., Annetts, D. L., and Murnaghan, G. F. Transplantation of malignant melanoma with cadaver kidney. *Transplantation* 13:619-620, 1972.
53. Kay, S., Frable, W. J., and Hume, D. M. Cervical dysplasia and cancer developing in women on immunosuppression therapy for renal homotransplantation. *Cancer* 39: 1048-1052, 1970.
54. Kinlen, L. J., Sheil, A. G. R., and Peto, J. Collaborative United Kingdom-Australian study of cancer in patient treated with immunosuppressive drugs. *Br. Med. J.* 2:1461-1466, 1979.

55. Klein, G., and Klein, E. Immune surveillance against virus-induced tumors and non-rejectability of spontaneous tumors: Contrasting consequences of host versus tumor evolution. *Proc. Natl. Acad. Sci. USA* 74:2121-2125, 1977.
56. Koranda, F. C. Accelerated induction of skin cancers by ultraviolet radiation in hairless mice treated with immunosuppressive agents. *Surg. Forum* 26:145, 1975.
57. Koranda, F. C., Dehmel, E. M., Kahn, G., and Penn, I. Cutaneous complications in immunosuppressed renal homograft recipients. *JAMA* 229:419-424, 1974.
58. Krown, S. E., Real, F. X., Cunningham-Rundles, S., et al. Preliminary observations on the effect of recombinant leukocyte A interferon in homosexual men with Kaposi's sarcoma. *N. Engl. J. Med.* 308:1071-1076, 1983.
59. Little, P. J., Farthing, C. F., Khader, A. A., Bunuan, H., and Haleem, A. Kaposi's sarcoma in a patient after renal transplantation. *Postgrad. Med. J.* 59:325-326, 1983.
60. Lo, T. C. M., Salzman, F. A., Smedal, M. I., and Wright, K. A. Radiotherapy for Kaposi's sarcoma. *Cancer* 215:684-687, 1980.
61. Lund, H. Z. How often does squamous cell carcinoma of the skin metastasize? *Arch. Dermatol.* 92:635-637, 1965.
62. Lutzner, M. A., Orth, G., Dutronquay, V., Ducasse, M. F., Kreis, H., and Crosnier, J. Detection of human papillomavirus type 5 DNA in skin cancers of an immunosuppressed renal allograft recipient. *Lancet* 1:422-424, 1983.
63. Lutzner, M. A. Epidermodysplasia verruciformis: An autosomal recessive disease characterised by viral warts and skin cancer. *Bull. Cancer* 65:169-182, 1978.
64. Lutzner, M. A. Immunopathology of papillomavirus-induced warts and skin cancers in immunodepressed and immunosuppressed patients. *Semin. Immunopathol.* 5:53-62, 1982.
65. Maize, J. C. Skin cancer in immunosuppressed patients. *JAMA* 237:1857-1858, 1977.
66. Manny, N., Rosenman, E., and Benbassat, J. Hazard of immunosuppressive therapy. *Br. Med. J.* 2:291, 1972.
67. Marshall, V. Premalignant and malignant skin tumors in immunosuppressed patients. *Transplantation* 17:272-275, 1979.
68. Martin, D. C., Rubini, M., and Rosen, V. J. Cadaveric renal homotransplantation with inadvertent transplantation of carcinoma. *JAMA* 192:82-84, 1965.
69. Matas, A. J., Simmons, R. L., and Najarian, J. S. Chronic antigenic stimulation, herpesvirus infection, and cancer in transplant recipients. *Lancet* 1:1277-1279, 1975.
70. McIntosh, D. A., et al. Homotransplantation of a cadaver neoplasm and a renal homograft. *JAMA* 192:141-143, 1965.
71. McKhann, C. F. Primary malignancy in patients undergoing immunosuppression for renal transplantation. *Transplantation* 8:209-212, 1969.
72. MacLean, L. D., Dossetor, J. B., Gault, M. H., Oliver, J. A., Inglis, F. G., and MacKinnon, K. J. Renal homotransplantation using cadaver donors. *Arch. Surg.* 91:288-306, 1965.
73. McPhaul, J. J., and McIntosh, D. A. Tissue transplantation still vexes. *N. Engl. J. Med.* 272:105, 1965.
74. Miller, J. F. A. P., Grant, G. A., and Roe, F. J. C. Effect of thymectomy on the induction of skin tumors by 3,4-benzopyrene. *Nature* 199:920-922, 1963.
75. Mocelin, A. J., and Brandina, L. Inadvertent transplant of a malignancy. *Transplantation* 19:430, 1975.
76. Muiznieks, H. W., Berg, J. W., Laurence, W., Jr., and Randall, H. T. Suitability of donor kidneys from patients with cancer. *Surgery* 64:871-877, 1968.
77. Mullen, D. L., Silverberg, S. G., Penn, I., and Hammond, W. S. Squamous cell carcinoma of the skin and lip in renal homograft recipients. *Cancer* 37:729-734, 1976.
78. Munyon, W., et al. Transfer of thymidine kinase to thymidine kinaseless L cells by infection with ultraviolet-irradiated herpes simplex virus. *J. Virol.* 7:813-820, 1971.

79. O'Neill, F., and Miles, C. P. Chromosome changes in human cells induced by herpes simplex, types 1 and 2. *Nature* 223:851-852, 1969.
80. Olsson, C. A., Mozen, J. D., and LaFerte, R. O. Pulmonary cancer metastatic to the kidney—a common renal neoplasm. *J. Urol.* 105:492, 1971.
81. Ostrow, R. S., Bender, M., Niimura, M., Seki, T., Kawashima, M., Pass, F., and Faras, A. J. Human papillomavirus DNA in cutaneous primary and metastasized squamous cell carcinomas from patients with epidermodysplasia verruciformis. *Proc. Natl Acad. Sci. USA* 79:1634-1638, 1982.
82. Penn, I. Lymphomas complicating organ transplantation. *Transplant. Proc.* 15: 2790-2797, 1983.
83. Penn, I. The price of immunotherapy. *Curr. Prob. Surg.* 18:681-751, 1981.
84. Penn, I., Hammond, W., Brettschneider, L., and Starzl, T. Malignant lymphomas in transplantation patients. *Transplant. Proc.* 1:106-112, 1969.
85. Penn, I. Immunosuppression and skin cancer. *Clin. Plast. Surg.* 7:361-368, 1980.
86. Penn, I. Kaposi's sarcoma in organ transplant recipients. A report of 20 cases. *Transplantation* 27:8-11, 1979.
87. Penn, I. Lejkemias and lymphomas associated with the use of cytotoxic and immunosuppressive drugs. *Recent Results Cancer Res.* 69:7-13, 1979.
88. Penn, I. Malignancies associated with immunosuppressive or cytotoxic therapy. *Surgery* 83:492-502, 1978.
89. Penn, I. Risk of cancer in the transplant patient. In *Principles of Organ Transplantation,* M. W. Flye, ed. W. B. Saunders, Philadelphia, (in press, 1985).
90. Penn, I. Tumors arising in organ transplant recipients. *Adv. Cancer Res.* 28:31-61, 1978.
91. Porreco, R., Penn, I., Droegemueller, W., Greer, B., and Makowski, E. Gynecologic malignancies in immunosuppressed organ homograft recipients. *J. Am. Coll. Obstet. Gynecol.* 45:359-364, 1975.
92. Rapp, F., Editorial. *JNCI* 50:825, 1973.
93. Ruiter, M. On the histomorphology and origin of malignant cutaneous changes in epidermodysplasia verruciformis. *Acta Dermatovener. (Stockh.)* 53:290-298, 1973.
94. Ruiter, M., and Van Mullem, P. J. Further histological investigations on malignant degeneration of cutaneous lesions in epidermodysplasia verruciformis. *Acta Dermatovener. (Stockh.)* 50:205-211, 1970.
95. Saemundsen, A. K., Purtilo, D. T., Sakamoto, K., et al. Documentation of Epstein-Barr virus (EBV) infection in immunodeficient patients with life-threatening lymphoproliferative diseases by EBV cRNA/DNA and vDNA/DNA hybridization. *Cancer Res.* 41:4237-4242, 1981.
96. Saemundsen, A. K., Klein, G., Cleary, M., and Warnke, R. EBV-carrying lymphoma in cardiac transplant recipients. *Lancet* 2:158, 1982.
97. Schneck, S. A., and Penn, I. De novo brain tumors in renal transplant recipients. *Lancet* 1:983-986, 1971.
98. Scotto, J., Kopf, A., and Urbach, F. Non-melanoma skin cancer among Caucasians in four areas of the United States. *Cancer* 34:1333-1338, 1974.
99. Seligman, M., Chess, L., Fahey, J. L., et al. AIDS—an immunologic reevaluation. *N. Engl. J. Med.* 311:1286-1292, 1984.
100. Sheil, A. G. R., Mahony, J. F., Horvath, J. S., Johnson, J. R., Tiller, D. J., Stewart, J. H., and May, J. Cancer following successful cadaveric donor renal transplantation. *Transplant. Proc.* 8:733-735, 1981.
101. Sheil, A. G. R. Cancer in renal allograft recipients in Australia and New Zealand. *Transplant Proc.* 9:1133-1136, 1977.
102. Sheil, A. G. R., Mahoney, J. F., and Horvath, J. S. Cancer following renal transplantation. *Aust. N.Z. J. Surg.* 49:617, 1979.

103. Siegel, J. H., Janis, R., Alper, J. C., Schutte, H., Robbins, L., and Blaufox, M. D. Disseminated visceral Kaposi's sarcoma. *JAMA* 207:1493-1496, 1969.
104. Simmons, R. L., Kelly, W. D., Tallent, M. B., and Najarian, J. S. Cure of dysgerminoma with widespread metastases appearing after renal transplantation. *N. Engl. J. Med.* 283:190-191, 1970.
105. Silverberg, E. Cancer statistics, 1985. *CA* 35:19-35, 1985.
106. Southam, C. M., Moore, A. E., and Rhoads, C. P. Homotransplantation of human cell lines. *Science* 125:158-160, 1957.
107. Spector, B. D., Perry, G. S., III, and Kersey, J. H. Genetically determined immunodeficiency diseases (GDID) and malignancy: Report from the Immunodeficiency Cancer Registry. *Clin. Immunol. Immunopathol.* 11:12-29, 1978.
108. Spees, E. K., Jr., Kramer, K. K., Light, J. A., Oakes, D. D., and Zimmerman, L. E. Reactivation of malignant melanoma after renal transplantation. *Transplantation* 29:421-424, 1980.
109. Starzl, T. E., Nalesnik, M. A., Porter, K. A., et al. Reversibility of lymphomas and lymphoproliferative lesions developing under cyclosporin-steroid therapy. *Lancet* 1:583-587, 1984.
110. Stoll, H. L., Jr. Squamous cell carcinoma. In *Dermatology in General Medicine,* T. B. Fitzpatrick, ed. Mc-Graw-Hill, New York, 1979.
111. Tallent, M. B., Simmons, R. L., and Najarian, J. S. Primary carcinoma of the cervix appearing in immunosuppressed renal transplant recipient. *Am. J. Obstet. Gynecol.* 109:663-664, 1971.
112. Thomas, D. B., and Rawls, W. E. Relationship of herpes simplex virus type 2 antibodies and squamous dysplasia to cervical carcinoma in situ. *Cancer* 42:2716-2725, 1978.
113. Tubman, D. E., Frick, M. P., and Hanto, D. W. Lymphoma after organ transplantation: Radiologic manifestations in the central nervous system, thorax, and abdomen. *Radiology* 149:625-631, 1983.
114. Tunner, W. S., Goldsmith, E. I., and Witsell, J. C., II Human homotransplantation of normal and neoplastic tissue from the same organ. *J. Urol.* 105:18-20, 1971.
115. Wahren, B., Lampert, F., and Goetz, B. Herpes viruses and chromosomal alterations seen with light and whole-mount electron microscopy. *Exp. Cell Res.* 75:271-274, 1972.
116. Walder, B. K., Robertson, M. R., and Jeremy, D. Skin cancer and immunosuppression. *Lancet* 2:1282-1283, 1971.
117. Weintraub, J., and Warnke, R. A. Lymphoma in cardiac allograft recipients. *Transplantation* 33:347-351, 1982.
118. Westburg, S. P., and Stone, O. J. Multiple cutaneous squamous cell carcinomas during immunosuppressive therapy. *Arch. Dermatol.* 107:893-895, 1973.
119. Wilson, R. E., Hager, E. B., Hampers, C. L., Corson, J. M., Merrill, J. P., and Murray, J. E. Immunologic rejection of human cancer transplanted with a renal allograft. *N. Engl. J. Med.* 278:479-483, 1968.
120. Younis, F. M., Fernando, O. N., Sweny, P., Baillod, R., and Moorhead, J. Malignant melanoma in a patient with renal transplant. *Lancet* 2:1141, 1980.
121. Zachow, K. R., Ostrow, R. S., Bender, M., Watts, S., Okagaki, T., Pass, F., and Faras, A. J. Detection of human papillomavirus DNA in anogenital papillomavirus DNA in anogenital neoplasias. *Nature* 300:771-773, 1982.
122. Zukoski, C. F., Killen, D. A., Ginn, E., Matter, B., Lucas, D. O., and Seigler, H. F. Transplanted carcinoma in an immunosuppressed patient. *Transplantation* 9:71-74, 1970.

22

KIDNEY TRANSPLANT REJECTION

Overview and Update

James F. Burdick, G. Melville Williams, and Kim Solez
The Johns Hopkins University School of Medicine, Baltimore, Maryland

Transplantation is a rapidly changing field. To enable this to be in every sense a 1986 book, we have composed this update chapter while we were correcting the proofs for the other chapters. Much of the work discussed here is preliminary in the sense that it has appeared only in the form of an abstract or a meeting presentation, but we thought it would be useful to the reader to have an assessment of where things stood just at the point that this book was published.

It is clear from the preceding chapters that the process of rejection and/or acceptance of a grafted organ is even more complex than had been thought, involving many different types of cell interactions with the liberation of the innumerable factors which accelerate or decelerate the immune response to the allograft. This complexity is one of the factors which makes it difficult to interpret biopsy material taken at a single point in time.

The specific diagnosis of rejection remains an elusive goal, although in renal transplants the finding on biopsy of an intimal arteritis or of a tubulitis with Leu7 positive cells can be very helpful. The benign infiltrate that we have observed in biopsies of well-functioning transplanted kidneys (Chapter 10) also clouds the interpretation of biopsies of cardiac allografts if there is no myocytolysis. Physiological changes within the graft may be of great importance, and the advent of nuclear magnetic resonance as a tool to assess the biochemistry of various parts of the whole patient holds great promise. Early detection of rejection in both cardiac and renal allografts with nuclear magnetic resonance is beginning to be explored [11,39,40]. In renal allografts the loss of corticomedullary demarcation on magnetic resonance imaging, probably due to interstitial edema, is seen in acute rejection and not in cyclosporine nephrotoxicity [11,39]. This type of imaging has the added advantage that it can also detect perirenal fluid collection and aseptic necrosis of the femoral heads.

It appears that the FDA will soon license the first monoclonal antibody for clinical administration: OKT3. OKT3 has been employed successfully in a large series of patients to treat rejection unresponsive to conventional agents [15]. In our own practice, if evidence of rejection reversal fails to appear shortly after initiating OKT-3, acute rejection is very unlikely to be the cause of allograft dysfunction; generally, reversal is evident within 48 hours. We have found that OKT3 is of particular value in patients on cyclosporine in whom there is confusion about the degree to which renal dysfunction was due to cyclosporine toxicity and/or rejection [4,5]. Interesting bits of biology about the T3 molecule continue to accumulate, as exemplified by the report that, in addition to its ability to inhibit allogeneic cytotoxicity by activated T cells, it also activates T cells to cause nonspecific lysis of cells bearing irrelevant histocompatibility molecules [25,32]. The elucidation of the gene in the mouse that codes for one chain of the murine analogue of T3 [46] promises the means to create antibodies against the murine T3 equivalent in the near future, which will allow investigation of the several interesting biological questions that have arisen during clinical therapy with this antibody.

While the use of OKT3 represents a step forward in our specificity of treatment for rejection, it is likely that monoclonal antibodies to other important cell surface antigens will increase this specificity still further. An appealing alternative antigen against which one might create therapeutically useful monoclonal antibodies is the invariant segment of Ti, the T cell receptor. In some cases, antibodies against this invariant portion were not reactive against whole cells [12], indicating that it may be buried in the cell membrane. However, at least one antibody has been created which does react with the invariant portion of Ti on the cell surface [42] and this antibody would seem a logical candidate for further investigation of its potential as a specific immunosuppressive agent.

One of the best-characterized of the "adhesion molecules" (Chapters 11 and 15) on the surface of T cells is T8. It has been cloned and the protein sequence identified [28, 43]. This will allow the action of its component parts to be studied at a very basic level. It is a member of the immunoglobulin superfamily which is theoretically appealing with regard to its involvement with Class 1 antigens. A monoclonal antibody against human T8 has been discovered which appears to cross react with dog T8 [38] which should provide a useful reagent for study of the effect in vivo in this experimental animal. The interest in T8 is particularly relevant to transplantation in view of the fact that cultured cell lines from renal allograft biopsies are predominantly T8 positive [30]. An even more exciting approach to the fundamental mechanism of cell-mediated cytotoxicity is the actual characterization of the perforin molecule which inserts in the membrane of the target cell to create the pores that initiate cell lysis [29]. The pores formed are similar to those produced by complement [9]. It would seem that specific immunologic manipulation of this mechanism might be possible in the not too distant future.

Another cell surface antigen that might soon be exploited is the interleukin-2 receptor. The human IL2 has been cloned [20] and the gene encoding it has been localized on chromosome 10 [26]. Anti-IL2 receptor monoclonal antibody (interestingly, of the IgM class) has been shown to be a very effective immunosuppressive agent for primarily vascularized heart allograft in the mouse [22]. It initially seemed that interference with the interleukin-2 mechanism would be quite specific in its effect only on T-cell-mediated immunity. However, a developing controversy as to the degree of receptivity of B cells to interleukin-2 has given way to fairly clear evidence now that interleukin-2 receptors are very important in B-cell physiology, and indeed a large portion of B-cell growth factor activity from T lymphocytes may be actually ascribable to interleukin-2 [33].

The issue of differentiation of suppressor cells from cytotoxic cells remains difficult, but a slight further glimmer of hope is given by the antibody against 2H4 [27] which appears to provide this differentiation in humans. A further difficulty, particularly in the immunologic manipulation of cells on the basis of T-cell subsets, is the confirmation of our data [3] that co-expression of T4 and T8 clearly occurs at a low level in normal cells, and at a greatly increased level in activated T cells [2].

Cyclosporine has proved to be immensely important both clinically and experimentally. As recently pointed out by Cosimi [18], the early problems with primary nonfunction related to cyclosporine therapy have given rise to the fairly common approach of avoiding cyclosporine for the first five to ten days posttransplant, often with the use of ATGAM or Minnesota ALG during this time to provide a similar protection from early rejection [18,24,41]. In addition, our unit and others have developed a policy of switching the patients from cyclosporine to azathioprine several months posttransplant [35,44] which has provided some relief from the nephrotoxic effects and very little morbidity in terms of rejection episodes.

Although the renal failure observed in cyclosporine-treated cardiac allograft recipients appears to be progressive [34], recent data from the Canadian Multicenter Trial indicate that this is not the case in renal allograft recipients. Reduction in creatinine clearance after two, three, and four years of cyclosporine therapy is no greater than it is at one year [7]. The fact that the renal allograft is initially denervated may in some way protect it from progressive cyclosporine-induced renal failure. The lack of progression of cyclosporine-induced renal allograft dysfunction may indicate the absence of two factors believed to cause progression of renal failure in other settings—glomerular capillary hypertension [1] and extensive calcium phosphate deposition [45].

Along these lines, there is evidence that the structural basis of chronic cyclosporine nephrotoxicity is unique. Kidney weight is increased in patients with this disorder, not decreased as is the case in most types of chronic renal disease (Meyers, B., personal communication). It appears that cyclosporine is not concentrated in tubular cells as many other nephrotoxins are. Jackson and Humes found evidence for proliferation of an interstitial cell type, presumably fibroblasts, in rats treated with a high dose of cyclosporine (100 mg/kg subcutaneously/day) [21].

The fine needle aspiration technique described in Chapter 12 has begun to be applied in centers in the United States [16]. There remains a question as to whether a positive diagnosis of cyclosporine nephrotoxicity can be made by this method since it is clear that the polyclonal sheep anticyclosporine antibody used to demonstrate cyclosporine by immunofluorescence and immunoperoxidase in fine needle aspirate specimens also reacts with noncyclosporine materials [23], and the light microscopic changes brought about in the renal tubules by cyclosporine can be seen in settings other than cyclosporine nephrotoxicity [37].

There is mounting evidence that renal vasoconstriction rather than direct tubular toxicity is the primary mechanism in cyclosporine-induced renal dysfunction [10]. The rapid reversal of renal insufficiency commonly seen after therapy is stopped is more consistent with a vasoconstrictive rather than a tubular toxicity mechanism. Racusen et al. have shown that there is persisting vasoconstriction in a rat model of cyclosporine nephrotoxicity produced by intraperitoneal injection [37]. The ip route of administration of cyclosporine is associated with exceptionally high peak blood levels [47], which may account for the more severe renal failure observed in this model.

The vasoconstrictive component of experimental cyclosporine nephrotoxicity has prompted some investigators to try to alleviate nephrotoxicity experimentally using various vasoactive antihypertensive agents. Captopril has been shown not to be effective [14] but clonidine and calcium-channel blockers may lessen toxicity . Verapamil, one of the calcium-channel blockers, potentiates the immunosuppressive effect of cyclosporine [31] and prolongs the survival of rat cardiac allografts through an intrinsic immunosuppressive effect [13]. The apparent central role of calcium channels in T-cell activation via the T3/Ti complex or T11 [19,36,48] is intriguing in this regard.

It is possible that by the end of the 1980s cyclosporin A will be of only historical interest, having been replaced by its less nephrotoxic relative cyclosporin G. Preliminary studies indicate that cyclosporin G has immunosuppressive properties roughly comparable to cyclosporin A, while its nephrotoxicity is tenfold less than that observed with cyclosporin A [6,17].

Thus, in summary, there seem to be increasingly better paths through an increasingly more complicated forest. As we learn more about the complexities of the immune response, we become able to control or limit it more specifically and with greater safety. The problem in clinical transplantation is not that of controlling rejection, for this is virtually always possible given our current agents. The problem is to control rejection while sustaining the health of the patient. In this regard, cyclosporin A and OKT3 have obvious advantages over corticosteroids and azathioprine, and it is likely that even better agents for combating rejection lie just over the horizon.

REFERENCES

1. Anderson, S., Meyer, T. W., Rennke, H. G., and Brenner, B. M. Control of glomerular hypertension limits injury in rats with reduced renal mass. *J. Clin. Invest.* 76:612, 1985.
2. Blue, M-L., Daley, J. F., Levine, H., and Schlossman, S. F. Coexpression of T4 and T8 on peripheral blood T cells demonstrated by two-color fluorescence flow cytometry. *J. Immunol.* 134:2281, 1985.
3. Burdick, J. F., Beschorner, W. E., Smith, W. J., McGraw, D., Bender, W. L., Williams, G. M., and Solez, K. Characteristics of early routine renal allograft biopsies. *Transplantation* 38:679, 1984.
4. Burdick, J. F., Pennington, L. R., Smith, W., and Williams, G. M. Resetting the immunostat: OKT3 treatment for CYA confusion. *Transplant. Proc.* (in press, 1986).
5. Burdick, J. F., Pennington, L. R., Smith, W., Irwin, B., and Williams, G. M. Reversal of progressive renal allograft dysfunction with OKT3. (Submitted.)
6. Calne, R. Y., White, D. J. G., Thiru, S., Rollec, K., Drakopoulos, S., and Jamieson, N. V. Cyclosporin G: Immunosuppressive effect in dogs with renal allografts. *Lancet* 1:1342, 1985.
7. Canadian Multicentre Transplant Study Group. A randomized clinical trial of cyclosporine in cadaveric renal transplantation: Analysis at three years. *N. Engl. J. Med.* (in press, 1986).
8. Cosimi, A. B. Anti-lymphocyte globulin–A Final (?) Look. In *Progress in Transplantation,* Vol. 2, P. J. Morris and N. L. Tilyey, eds. Churchill Livingstone, Edinburgh, 1986, pp. 167-188.
9. Criado, M., Lindstrom, J. M., Anderson, C. G., and Dennert, G. Cytotoxic granules from killer cells: Specificity of granules and insertion of channels of defined size into target membranes. *J. Immunol.* 135:4245, 1985.
10. Curtis, J. J., Luke, R. G., Jones, P., Dubovsky, E. V., Whelchel, J. D., and Diethelm, A. G. Renal vasoconstriction in cyclosporine-treated (CY) transplant recipients (TXR) without other evidence of nephrotoxicity. *Kidney Int.* 29:428, 1986.
11. Dunbar, K., Salomon, D., Wingo, C., Peterson, J., Croker, B., Kaude, J., Thompson, R., and Tischer, C. Loss of corticomedullary demarcation on magnetic resonance

imaging: An index of biopsy-proven acute renal transplant dysfunction. *Kidney Int.* 29:429, 1986.
12. Fabbi, M. Production and characterization of antibody probes directed at constant regions of the a and b subunit of the human T cell receptor. *Eur. J. Immunol.* 15: 821, 1985.
13. Foegh, M. I., Khirabadi, B. S., and Ramwell, P. W. Prolongation of rat cardiac allograft survival by Ca^{++} blockers. *Transplantation* 40(2):211, 1985.
14. Gerkens, J. F. and Smith, A. J. Effect of captopril and theophylline treatment on cyclosporine-induced nephrotoxicity in rats. *Transplantation* 30:213, 1985.
15. Goldstein, G., Norman, D. J., Shield, C. F. III, Kreis, H., Burdick, J. F., Flye, M. W., Ponticelli, C., Starzl, T., and Monaco, A. OKT3 monoclonal antibody reversal of acute renal allograft rejection uncontrollable by conventional treatments. *N. Engl. J. Med.* (in press, 1986).
16. Helderman, J. A., Hernandez, J. A., Glennie, J. L., and Kokko, J. P. Confirmation of the utility of the fine needle aspiration biopsy of the transplanted kidney. *Kidney Int.* 29:430, 1986.
17. Hiestand, P. C., Gunn, H. C., Gale, J. M., Ryffel, B., and Borel, J. F. Comparison of the pharmacological profiles of cyclosporine, (Nva^2)-cyclosporine and (Val^2)dihydrocyclosporine. *Immunology* 55:249-255, 1985.
18. Hourmant, M., Soulillou, J. P., and Guenel, J. Comparison of three immunosuppressive regimens in kidney transplantation: A single-centre randomized study. *Proc. Eur. Dial. Transplant. Assoc. Ren. Assoc.* 21:982, 1985.
19. Imboden, J. B., and Stobo, J. D. Transmembrane signalling by the T cell antigen receptor. Perturbation of the T3-antigen receptor complex generates inositol phosphates and releases calcium ions from intracellular stores. *J. Exp. Med.* 161:446, 1985.
20. Ishida, N., Kanamori, H., Noma, T., Nikaido, T., Hisataka, S., Noboru, S., Shimizu, A., and Hanjo, T. Molecular cloning and structure of the human interleukin 2 receptor gene. *Nucl. Acids Res.* 13:7579, 1985.
21. Jackson, N. M., and Humes, H. D. Cyclosporine (CS) induces cell proliferation within the renal interstitium. *Kidney Int.* 29:303, 1986.
22. Kirkman, R. L., Barrett, L. V., Graulton, G. N., Kelly, V. E., Ythier, A., and Strom, T. B. Administration of an anti-interleukin-2 receptor monoclonal antibody prolongs cardiac allograft survival in mice. *J. Exp. Med.* 162:358, 1985.
23. Kolbeck, P. C., Wolfe, J. A., Burchette, J., and Sanfilippo, F. Differentiation of cyclosporine (CsA) nephrotoxicity from rejection by immunohistologic labeling of renal allograft biopsies. *Kidney Int.* 29:432, 1986.
24. Kupin, W. L., Venkatachalam, K. K., Oh, H. K., Dienst, S., and Levin, N. W. Sequential use of Minnesota antilymphoblast globulin and cyclosporine in cadaveric renal transplantation. *Transplantation* 40:601, 1985.
25. Leeuwenberg, J. F. M. Induction of nonspecific cytotoxicity by monoclonal anti-T3 antibodies. *J. Immunol.* 134:3770, 1985.
26. Leonard, W. J., Donlon, T. A., Lebo, R. V., and Greene, W. C. Localization of the gene encoding the human interleukin-2 receptor on chromosome 10. *Science* 228: 1547, 1985.
27. Letvin, N. L. Definition of the T-lymphocyte inducer of suppression in primates using a monoclonal antibody. *Cell. Immunol.* 94:360, 1985.
28. Littman, D. R., Thomas, Y., Maddon, P. J., Chess, L., and Axel, R. The isolation and sequence of the gene encoding T8: A molecule defining functional classes of T lymphocytes. *Cell* 40:237, 1985.
29. Masson, D. and Wschopp, J. Isolation of a lytic, pore-forming protein (perforin) from cytolytic T-lymphocytes. *J. Biol. Chem.* 260:9069, 1985.

30. Mayer, T. G. Characterization of in vivo-activated allospecific T lymphocytes propagated from human renal allograft biopsies undergoing rejection. *J. Immunol.* 134: 258, 1985.
31. McMillen, M. A., Tesi, R. J., Baumgarten, W. B., Jaffe, B. M., and Wait, R. B. Potentiation of cyclosporine by verapamil in vitro. *Transplantation* 40:444, 1985.
32. Mentzer, S. J., Barbosa, J. A., and Burakoff, S. J. T3 monoclonal antibody activation of nonspecific cytolysis: A mechanism of CTL inhibition. *J. Immunol.* 35:34, 1985.
33. Minger, M. C. Human interleukin-2 promotes proliferation of activated B cells via surface receptors similar to those of activated T cells. *Nature* 312:641, 1985.
34. Moran, M., Tomlanovich, S., and Myers, B. D. Cyclosporine-induced chronic nephropathy in human recipients of cardiac allografts. *Transplant. Proc.* 17 (Suppl. 1):185, 1985.
35. Morris, P. J., French, M. E., Dunnill, M. S., Hunnisett, A. G. W., Ting, A., Thompson, J. F., and Wood, R. F. M. A controlled trial of cyclosporine in renal transplantation with conversion to azathioprine and prednisolone after three months. *Transplantation* 36:273, 1983.
36. Oettgen, H. C., Terhorst, C., Cantley, L. C., and Rosoff, P. M. Stimulation of the T3-T cell receptor complex induces a membrane-potential-sensitive calcium influx. *Cell* 40:583, 1985.
37. Racusen, L. C., Kone, B. C., Whelton, A., and Solez, K. Renal blood flow, glomerular filtration rate, and renal morphology in cyclosporine-induced acute renal failure in Munich Wistar rats. *Am. J. Kidney Dis.* (in press, 1986).
38. Rieber, P. Monoclonal antibody to human cytotoxic-suppressor lymphocytes T cross reacts with canine lymphocytes and inhibits cell-mediated lympholysis of canine cells. *Exp. Hematol.* 13:641, 1985.
39. Ross, E. A., Barbaric, Z., Cohen, A., Salehmophaddam, S., and Danovitch, G. M. Magnetic resonance imaging (MRI) detection of renal allograft rejection. *Kidney Int.* 29:434, 1986.
40. Sasaguri, S. Early detection of cardiac allograft rejection with proton nuclear magnetic resonance. *Circulation* 72:231, 1985.
41. Sommer, B. G., and Ferguson, R. N. Three immediate post-renal transplant adjunct protocols combined with maintenance cyclosporine. *Transplant. Proc.* 17:1235, 1985.
42. Spits, H. Characteristics of a monoclonal antibody (WT-31) that recognizes a common epitope on the human T cell receptor for antigen. *J. Immunol.* 135:1922, 1985.
43. Sukhatme, V. P., Sizer, K. C., Vollmer, A. C., Hunkapiller, T., and Parnes, J. R. The T cell differentiation antigen Leu-2/T8 is homologous to immunoglobulin and T cell receptor variable regions. *Cell* 40:591, 1985.
44. Tegzess, A. M., Donker, A. J. M., Meijer, S., van Son, W. J., v/d Woule, F. J., Slooff, M. J. H., and v/d Slikke, L. B. The use of cyclosporine (C) only in cadaveric renal transplant recipients (CRTR): Conversion to prednisolone (P) and azathioprine (A) after 4 months. *Kidney Int.* 26:656, 1984.
45. Tomford, R. C., Karlinsky, M. L., Buddington, B., and Alfrey, A. C. Effect of thyroparathyroidectomy and parathyroidectomy on renal function and the nephrotic syndrome in rat nephrotic serum nephritis. *J. Clin. Invest.* 68:655-664, 1981.
46. van den Elsen, P. Isolation and characterization of a cDNA clone encoding the murine homologue of the human 20K T3/T-cell receptor glycoprotein. *Nature* 314:542, 1985.

47. Wassef, R., Cohen, Z., and Langer, B. Pharmacokinetic profiles of cyclosporine in rats. Influence of route of administration and dosage. *Transplantation* 40:489, 1985.
48. Weiss, M. J., Daley, J. F., Hodgdon, J. C., Reimberg, E. L. Calcium dependency of antigen-specific (T3-Ti) and alternative (T11) pathways of human T-cell activation. *Proc. Natl. Acad. Sci. U.S.-Biol. Sci.* 81:6836, 1984.

INDEX